Addison-Wesley's

LABORATORY AND DIAGNOSTIC TEST HANDBOOK

M. K. GAEDEKE, RN, MSN, CCRN, CS
Clinical Nurse Specialist, Nurse Practitioner
Children's Hospital of Buffalo
Buffalo, New York

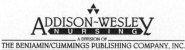

ADDISON-WESLEY
NURSING
A DIVISION OF
THE BENJAMIN/CUMMINGS PUBLISHING COMPANY, INC.

A Division of The Benjamin/Cummings Publishing Company, Inc.

Menlo Park, California • Reading, Massachusetts • New York • Don Mills, Ontario
Wokingham, UK • Amsterdam • Bonn • Paris • Milan • Madrid • Sydney
Singapore • Tokyo • Seoul • Taipei • Mexico City • San Juan • Puerto Rico

Executive Editor: Patricia L. Cleary
Acquisitions Editor: Erin Mulligan
Editorial Assistant: Suzanne Rotondo
Managing Editor: Wendy Earl
Production Supervisor: Sharon Montooth
Text and Page Designers: Belinda Fernandez and Brad Greene
Cover Designers: Belinda Fernandez and Yvo Riezebos
Copy Editor: Anita Wagner
Proofreader: Kristin Barendsen
Indexer: Katherine Pitcoff
Composition and Film Coordinator: Vivian McDougal
Compositor: Fog Press
Manufacturing Supervisor: Merry Free Osborne
Printer and Binder: Banta Company

Library of Congress Cataloging-in-Publication-Data
Gaedeke, M.K.
    Laboratory and diagnostic test handbook / M.K. Gaedeke.
        p.   cm.
    Includes bibliographical references and index.
    ISBN 0-8053-1359-1
    1. Diagnosis, Laboratory—Dictionaries. 2. Nursing—Dictionaries.
I. Title.
    [DNLM: 1. Diagnosis. Laboratory—nurses' instruction.
2. Diagnosis, Laboratory—handbooks. 3. Diagnostic Tests, Routine—nursing—handbooks.
QY 39 G127a   1995]
Rb37.A25G34   1995
616.07'56'03—dc20
DNLM/DLC
for Library of Congress   95-19476
                                                       CIP

ISBN 0-8053-1359-1
1 2 3 4 5 6 7 8 9 10-BAH-99 98 97 96 95

ADDISON-WESLEY
NURSING
THE BENJAMIN/CUMMINGS PUBLISHING COMPANY, INC.

A Division of Benjamin/Cummings Publishing Company, Inc.
2725 Sand Hill Road, Menlo Park, California, 94025

CONSULTANT

Carmel T. White, RN, MSN
Deaconess College of Nursing
St. Louis, MO

CONTRIBUTORS

Kathleen E. Andrews, RN, MN, CCRN
Missouri Western State College
St. Joseph, MO

Jeri L. Ashley, RN, MSN, OCN
Baptist Memorial Hospital—East
Memphis, TN

Suzanne Beyea, RN, CS, PhD
Saint Anselm College
Manchester, NH

Wendy Bodwell, RN, MSN, CNAA
Lifecare Center of Aurora
Aurora, CO

Susan Burchiel, RN, MSN, C
Cuesta College
San Luis Obispo, CA

Judith Gawlikowski, RN, MSN
Chester County Hospital
School of Nursing
West Chester, PA

Marcella J. Griggs, MS, RN, CS
Radford University School of Nursing
Radford, VA

Wendy Hollis, RN, MS
Los Angeles Harbor College
Wilmington, CA

Margaret Ludwikoski, RN, MSN, CCRN
St. Vincent Medical Center
School of Nursing
Toledo, OH

Elaine Marckx, RN, MSN
Chemeketa Community College
Salem, OR

Deborah Martin, RN, MSN
Baptist Memorial Hospital
School of Nursing
Memphis, TN

Becky Miner, RN, MSN, CS
St. Joseph's Hospital of Chewelah
Chewelah, WA

Rachel I. Rhude, RN, MSN, CCRN, CS
Franciscan Health System of
   Cincinnati, Inc.
Cincinnati, OH

Kathy Shuey, RN, MS, CS, OCN
Oncology Nurse Specialist
Presbyterian Healthcare Services
Albuquerque, NM

Kathy J. Shutler, RN, MSN
Belmont Technical College
St. Clairesville, OH

April Sieh, RN, MSN
Delta College
University Center, MI

Joyce Slusher, RN, BSN
Children's Hospital Medical Center
Cincinnati, OH

Elizabeth K. Wajdowicz, RN, PhD
St. Petersburg Junior College
St. Petersburg, FL

JoEllen Welborn, RN, MS
Palo Pinto General Hospital
Mineral Wells, TX

REVIEWERS

HOW TO USE THIS BOOK

Addison-Wesley's *Laboratory and Diagnostic Test Handbook* has been carefully conceived and developed to provide a comprehensive reference to more than 560 laboratory and diagnostic tests for nursing students and practicing nurses. A consistent two-column format, carefully reviewed by students and nurses, provides a quick and thorough reference with an emphasis on client teaching. All tests are listed in alphabetical order by their full name. The following features make this book unique and relevant to its users:

➤ The **Pediatric and Geriatric Tips for Performing Diagnostic and Lab Tests and Common Laboratory Values sections** provide specific information for the practitioner to keep in mind while administering laboratory tests to pediatric and elderly clients. The **pediatric** and **geriatric** sections each have a list of lab tips, along with a table containing variations in values for the most common laboratory tests.

➤ Category-specific lists of **universal precautions** explain how to handle body fluids and tissues.

➤ There is also a series of **collection techniques**, with step-by-step explanations of how to perform many commonly used procedures, such as venipuncture, radial arterial puncture, finger and heelstick method, 24-hour urine collection, clean-catch urine collection, routine urine specimen, sputum collection, and feces specimen.

➤ A list of the standard **collection tubes**, their colors, and their additives follows the explanation of techniques.

The following information is provided for each test:

Name of Test: The name of the test and a variety of alternate names, whenever relevant, are provided to assure that tests can be located promptly and easily. Tests are listed in the book alphabetically.

Pronunciation: A phonetic pronunciation guide follows the name of each test.

Normal Findings: Normal findings are listed for adults and, whenever possible, for infants, children, adolescents, pregnant women, and the elderly.

What This Test Will Tell You: This section begins with a simple, succinct statement of what the test is for, followed by an explanation of the test. The first sentence is crucial to the nurse who uses the book as a quick reference.

Action Alert! Critical findings or values, as well as appropriate responsive action, are clearly outlined whenever indicated.

Abnormal Findings: This section lists common abnormal findings related to the diagnostic or laboratory test.

Interfering Factors: Factors that can interfere with accurate test results are clearly outlined in this section.

Contraindications: This section identifies any clients who should not be undergoing the test, such as pregnant clients or those who are known to have allergic reactions.

Nursing Considerations

Prepare Your Client: This section will help the nurse/student prepare a client for a test. The first entry offers a clear explanation of the test in simple, non-medical terms, which the nurse can use with the client and/or family to help relieve anxiety and build trust.

Perform Procedure: This section will help the nurse/student perform the test. This is a critical part of its use as a reference, particularly for practicing nurses.

Care After Test: Specific care following the test is outlined here. Care related to the test itself (e.g., resuming fluid intake) is noted, as well as care related to the conditions for which the test is commonly ordered (e.g., assessing for signs of anemia or electrolyte imbalance.) The last entry in this section refers the user to appropriate related tests.

Educate Your Client and the Family: This is our most unique asset as to a laboratory and diagnostic reference. This book strongly emphasizes the role of the nurse in the life of the client and the client's family beyond the laboratory setting. This section provides information that encourages wellness education with a holistic approach, such as teaching about a low-salt diet, referring clients and families to appropriate resources, or stressing the importance of prenatal care.

Appendices: There are quick-reference tables for *common adult, pediatric, and geriatric laboratory values*. In addition, we have provided an extensive table of *therapeutic drug monitoring levels* for the reader's use. Finally, the tests are *cross-indexed by body system* and *alternate names* to increase accessibility. The index pages are a second color to allow easy access.

ACKNOWLEDGMENTS

To my boys, Jeff and Adam. You are my inspiration and my life. I love you both forever. To my best friend always, my teacher, my mentor, my life and my love, Jean-Michel. I've learned so much from you about matters of the heart. Frogs really do become princes . . .

Thank you to Addison-Wesley for inviting me to do this project. Patti Cleary's unwavering support and direction made this project a treasure to work on. Thanks to Alexa Stuart, who began the project and Suzanne Rotondo, who nursed it to the end. Without both of you being so dedicated to the quality and vision of this book we wouldn't have been able to achieve such great things. Many thanks to Carmel White for her tireless and invaluable reviewing of material. Finally, thank you Erin Mulligan, Acquisitions Editor, and production folks Sharon Montooth and Anita Wagner, for all of your hard work and vision.

CONTENTS

TIPS FOR PERFORMING DIAGNOSTIC AND LAB TESTS WITH PEDIATRIC CLIENTS

Age-associated differences have an impact on performing and interpreting diagnostic and laboratory procedures with infants and children. For instance, renal and pulmonary function are not fully developed in neonates. Also, many pediatric and neonatal health problems are related to congenital anomalies rather than acquired disease. The following are tips for performing test procedures with infants and children:

➤ Explain tests thoroughly to family members. Include such key information as any anticipated pain or discomfort, if parents can stay with or accompany the child, and how long they will be separated from their child, if at all.

➤ Whenever possible, allow parents or a significant other to stay with the child. The child is more likely to cooperate and the accuracy of tests will be enhanced.

➤ Include the child in the explanation of any tests whenever possible. Use age-appropriate language and simple explanations.

➤ Use play therapy whenever possible. This includes letting the child handle equipment and act out procedures on dolls.

➤ Do not perform any painful procedures in the child's room, especially their bed. Also do not perform any uncomfortable or painful procedures in the play room. Children need to feel their rooms and play areas are safe.

➤ Do not lie to children by telling them a procedure will not cause them pain or discomfort if it will.

➤ Fear can be as great a discomfort to a child as pain. Do not belittle their feelings by assuming that because a test isn't painful it shouldn't be upsetting to a child. Acknowledge and accept their feelings. Offer ways for the child to have control whenever possible.

➤ Be sure to provide extra safety measures. Infants and small children may roll off carts or sit up inappropriately and be at risk for injury.

➤ Sedation may be necessary in infants and small children, especially in imaging tests where movement will interfere with capturing clear pictures.

➤ Ensure maintenance of body temperature by providing warmth through clothing and/or blankets, since thermoregulation may be altered, especially in neonates.

➤ Prevent dehydration that may contribute to complications, especially when restricting food and fluids for testing.

COMMON PEDIATRIC LABORATORY VALUES

Laboratory Value	Conventional Units	SI units
Albumin	4.0–5.9 g/dL	40–59 g/L
Bilirubin		
Total	0.1–1.0 mg/dL	5.1–17.0 μmol/L
Direct (conjugated)	0.1–0.3 mg/dL	1.7–5.1 μmol/L
Indirect (unconjugated)	0.2–0.8 mg/dL	3.4–12.0 μmol/L
Blood urea nitrogen	5–18 mg/dL	1.8–6.4 mmol/L
Calcium		
Total	8.8–10.8 mg/dL	2.2–2.7 mmol/L
Ionized	4.8–5.9 mg/dL	1.12–1.37 mmol/L
Chloride	98–105 mEq/L	98–105 mmol/L
CO_2 content	20–28 mEq/L	20–28 mmol/L
Creatinine	0.3–0.7 mg/dL	26–61 μmol/L
Erythrocyte (RBC) count	4.6–5.5 million/mm^3(μL)	4.4–7.1×10^{12}/L
Glucose (fasting)		
<24 months of age	60–100 mg/dL	3.3–5.5 mmol/L
24 months to adolescence	70–105 mg/dL	3.8–5.8 mmol/L
Hematocrit	31%–43%	0.31–0.43
Hemoglobin	11–16 g/dL	6.8 9.9 mmol/L
Leukocyte (WBC) count	6,000–17,000/mm^3	6.0–17.0×10^9/L
Magnesium		
5 months–6 years	1.4–1.9 mEq/L	0.58–0.78 mmol/L
6–12 years	1.4–1.7 mEq/L	0.58–0.70 mmol/L
12–20 years	1.4–1.8 mEq/L	0.58–0.74 mmol/L
Partial thromboplastin time	60–70 seconds	
Phosphorus	4.5–5.5 mg/dL	1.45–1.78 mmol/L
Platelet count	150,000–450,000/mm^3	150–450×10^9/L
Potassium	3.4–4.7 mEq/L	3.4–4.7 mmol/L
Prothrombin time	11–14 seconds	85%–100%
Sodium	138–145 mEq/L	138–145 mmol/L

TIPS FOR PERFORMING DIAGNOSTIC AND LAB TESTS WITH GERIATRIC CLIENTS

Age-associated changes have an impact on performing and interpreting diagnostic and laboratory procedures with older adults, particularly for individuals over 75 years of age. Some laboratory parameters change with age. It is also important to pay attention to other confounding factors such as presentation of disease states, multiple chronic conditions, and polypharmacy, all of which may contribute to misinterpretation of diagnostic and laboratory data. The following are tips for performing test procedures on the older adult:

➤ Enhance communication by making sure eyeglasses, hearing aids, and dentures are in place and functioning.

➤ Allow more time for explanation by the clinician, response time from the client, and performance of the procedure. For confused clients, family involvement may be beneficial.

➤ Provide comfort by attending to positioning, support, and transfer of frail clients, especially those with decreased body mass and arthritic conditions.

➤ Ensure maintenance of body temperature by providing warmth through clothing and/or blankets, since thermoregulation may be altered.

➤ Prevent dehydration that may contribute to client confusion, especially when giving cleansing enemas or observing nothing-by-mouth.

➤ Use paper tape to avoid skin tears and blistering of fragile skin.

➤ Evaluate the medication regime to determine if the client will be adversely affected by withholding prescribed medications during the procedure.

➤ Give the laboratory a list of client medications since lab values may be altered by certain drugs.

➤ Assess the client for prolonged effects of any drug used for the procedure since decreased drug clearance is common in older adults.

➤ Don't misinterpret an abnormal laboratory value as a normal aging change. This can lead to misdiagnosis and failure to treat important conditions.

➤ Don't misinterpret an abnormal laboratory value as pathology when it is a normal aging change. This can lead to misdiagnosis and overtreatment of benign conditions.

➤ Laboratory tests that commonly are different with aging include a decrease in iron-binding capacity, a decrease in serum iron, a slight increase in potassium, a decrease in men's calcium level, an increase in oral glucose tolerance tests, an increase in postprandial blood sugars, an increase in erythrocyte sedimentation rate, a decrease in magnesium, a decrease in creatinine clearance, an increase in alkaline phosphatase, a decrease in albumin, an increase in low-density lipids (LDL), an increase in cholesterol, an increase in triglycerides, and a decrease in triiodothyronine.

COMMON GERIATRIC LABORATORY VALUES

Laboratory value	Conventional units	SI units
Albumin	3.2–5.0 g/dL	32–50 g/L
Bilirubin		
Total	0.1–1.0 mg/dL	5.1–17.0 µmol/L
Direct (conjugated)	0.1–0.3 mg/dL	1.7–5.1 µmol/L
Indirect (unconjugated)	0.2–0.8 mg/dL	3.4–12.0 µmol/L
Blood urea nitrogen	8–21 mg/dL	2.9–7.5 mmol/L
Calcium		
Total	8.5–10.5 mg/dL	1.98–2.44 mmol/L
Ionized	4.5–5.6 mg/dL	1.05–1.30 mmol/L
Chloride	95–110 mEq/L	95–110 mmol/L
CO_2 content	22–30 mEq/L	22–30 mmol/L
Creatinine	0.4–1.9 mg/dL	35–167 µmol/L
Erythrocyte (RBC) count		
Female	4.2–5.4 million/mm^3	4.2–5.4×10^{12}/L
Male	4.5–6.2 million/mm^3	4.5–6.2×10^{12}/L
Glucose (fasting)	52–135 mg/dL	2.9–7.4 mmol/L
Hematocrit		
Male	38%–54%	0.38–0.54
Female	35%–49%	0.35–0.49
Hemoglobin		
Male	10–17 g/dL	100–170 g/L
Female	11.5–15.5 g/dL	115–155 g/L
Leukocyte (WBC) count	3100–9000/mm^3	3.1–9.0×10^9/L
Magnesium	1.2–1.9 mEq/L	0.50–0.78 mmol/L
Partial thromboplastin time	60–70 seconds	
Phosphorus	2.7–4.5 mg/dL	0.87–1.45 mmol/L
Platelet count	130,000–450,000/mm^3	130–450×10^9/L
Potassium	3.5–5.1 mEq/L	3.5–5.1 mmol/L
Prothrombin time	11–14 seconds	85%–100%
Sodium	138–145 mEq/L	138–145 mmol/L

UNIVERSAL PRECAUTIONS

Universal precautions apply to blood and body fluids containing visible blood. They also apply to body tissues and to the following specific body fluids: vaginal secretions, seminal secretions, cerebrospinal fluid, synovial fluid, pleural fluid, peritoneal fluid, amniotic fluid, saliva in dental procedures, and body fluids in situations where it is difficult to differentiate among body fluids. Universal precautions *do not* apply to feces, urine, nasal secretions, sputum, saliva, sweat, tears or vomitus unless they contain visible blood.

Health care workers are at risk of exposure to blood-borne pathogens, i.e., hepatitis B virus (HBV), hepatitis C virus (HCV), and human immunodeficiency virus (HIV). Health care workers should consider *all* clients as potentially infected with blood-borne pathogens and must follow the infection control precautions for *all* clients.

The Centers for Disease Control recommend the following specific precautions to reduce the risk of exposure to potentially infective materials:

Handwashing
➤ Wash your hands thoroughly with warm water and soap (a) immediately, if contaminated with blood or other body fluids to which universal precautions apply, or potentially contaminated articles; (b) between clients; and (c) immediately after gloves are removed, even if the gloves appear to be intact. When hand-washing facilities are not available, use a waterless antiseptic hand cleaner in accordance with the manufacturer's directions.

➤ If you have a exudative lesion or weeping dermatitis, refrain from all direct client care and from handling client care equipment until the condition resolves.

Gloves
➤ Wear gloves when touching blood and body fluids containing blood, as well as when handling items or surfaces soiled with blood or body fluids as mentioned above.
➤ Wear gloves for all invasive procedures (i.e., any surgical entry into tissues, cavities, or organs or repair of major traumatic injuries).
➤ Change gloves after client contact.
➤ Wear gloves (a) if you have cuts, scratches, or other breaks in the skin; (b) in situations where hand contamination with blood may occur, e.g., with an uncooperative client; and (c) when you are performing venipuncture and other vascular procedures.

Other Protective Barriers
➤ Wear masks and protective eyewear (glasses, goggles) or face shields to protect the mucous membranes of your mouth, nose, and eyes during all *invasive* procedures and/or any procedure that is likely to generate droplets of blood or other body fluids to which universal precautions apply.
➤ Wear a disposable plastic apron or gown during procedures that are likely to generate splatters of blood or other body fluid (e.g., peritoneal fluid) and soil your clothing.

Sharps Disposal To prevent injuries, place used disposable needle-syringe units, scalpel blades, and other sharp items in puncture-resistant containers for disposal. Discard used needle-syringe units *uncapped* and *unbroken*. Place puncture-resistant containers as close as practicable to use areas.

Laundry Handle soiled linen as little as possible and with minimum agitation to prevent gross microbial contamination of the air and of persons handling the linen. Place linen soiled with blood or body fluids in leakage-resistant bags at the location where it is used.

Specimens Put all specimens of blood and listed body fluids in well-constructed containers with secure lids to prevent leakage during transport. When collecting specimens, take care to avoid contaminating the outside of the container.

Blood Spills Use a chemical germicide that is approved for use as a hospital disinfectant to decontaminate work surfaces after there is a spill of blood or other applicable body fluids. In the absence of a commercial germicide, a solution of sodium hypochlorite (household bleach) in a 1:100 dilution is effective.

Infective Wastes

➤ Follow agency policies for disposal of infective waste, both when disposing of, and when decontaminating, contaminated materials.

➤ Carefully pour bulk blood, suctioned fluids, and excretions containing blood and secretions, down drains that are connected to a sanitary sewer.

Sources U.S. Department of Health and Human Services, Public Health Service, Update: Universal precautions for prevention of transmission of human immunodeficiency virus, hepatitis B virus, and other blood-borne pathogens in health care settings, *Morbidity and Mortality Weekly Report*, June 24, 1988; 37:377–382, 387–388; *Morbidity and Mortality Weekly Report*, June 23, 1989, 39/No. S-6: 9–18.

VENIPUNCTURE PROCEDURE

Prepare Your Client

➤ Explain, in simple terms the client and family can understand, why the test is being performed. Do not use medical jargon or terminology unless the words and their meaning are explained fully.

➤ Explain that the test requires a small blood sample obtained by placing a needle into a vein (venipuncture).

➤ Instruct your client that they may feel some mild, brief discomfort or pain from the needle (venipuncture procedure). Assure the client that this discomfort will go away quickly after the needle is taken out.

➤ Ask client if they have ever fainted while having blood drawn or having a shot (injection). Take appropriate safety precautions with all clients by observing the environment and ensuring that if loss of consciousness occurs, injury is unlikely.

➤ Wash your hands prior to performance of venipuncture.

Perform Procedure

➤ Select a site for venipuncture, such as veins in the antecubital region. Apply a tourniquet or blood pressure cuff with sufficient pressure to obstruct venous return without occluding the arterial pulse.

➤ Wearing gloves, perform the venipuncture and collect a sample in the appropriate color collection tube.

➤ Release the tourniquet and apply pressure to the site as soon as the needle is withdrawn from the vein and skin. Pressure may be held for 2–3 minutes if needed for hemostasis at the site.

➤ Note interfering factors or medications on the laboratory requisition slip.

➤ Transport the sample to the laboratory immediately.

Care After Test

➤ Apply pressure to the site with a dry gauze and gloved hands for a minute for hemostasis.

➤ Inspect the site to be sure the bleeding has stopped and that no hematoma has developed.

➤ If a hematoma develops, reabsorption of the blood can be enhanced with applications of warm compresses, in 20-minute intervals, several times a day. Delay application of warm soaks until it is certain that the venipuncture site is stable and no longer bleeding.

➤ Apply an adhesive bandage.

➤ Instruct client and family that if bleeding begins again, they should press firmly with their fingers or hand over the area and notify the nurse right away.

➤ Support client in light of their fears and apprehensions about being tested and awaiting results. Obtain counseling or support services for client as indicated.

Interfering Factors

➤ Hemolysis of blood cells due to rough handling of the specimen will alter many test results.

➤ Collection of a sample above an existing IV fluid line may produce a diluted sample.

➤ If the tourniquet is left in place for longer than 1–2 minutes, hemoconcentration may occur within that extremity and affect the sample values.

➤ Failure to place the sample in a collection tube with the proper anticoagulant, or failure to mix the sample sufficiently with the anticoagulant in some collection tubes, may affect the values.

Potential Complications

➤ Infection, bleeding, or hematoma formation may occur at the venipuncture site.

Prepare Your Client

➤ Explain that the test is being performed to see how much oxygen and carbon dioxide are in the blood. Tell your client that this helps evaluate how well the lungs and heart are working. Use simple terms that the client and family can understand. Do not use medical jargon or terminology unless the words and their meaning are explained fully.

➤ Explain that the test requires a small blood sample obtained by placing a needle into an artery (arterial puncture) or painlessly by drawing blood from an already indwelling arterial catheter.

➤ Instruct your client and family that there may be a feeling of brief discomfort or pain from the needle (arterial puncture procedure). Assure the client that this discomfort will go away soon after the needle is taken out.

➤ Wash your hands.

Perform Procedure

➤ Arterial puncture for blood gas analysis is appropriate only for single or very infrequent sampling. If cardiorespiratory compromise is significant, an indwelling arterial catheter should be placed for frequent arterial blood sampling.

➤ Identify the radial artery for arterial puncture.

➤ Perform the Allen test to assure adequate ulnar (collateral) arterial blood flow to the hand:

—Elevate the hand and arm above the heart.

—Instruct the client to open and close the hand, or do this for them.

—With the hand and arm still elevated, compress both the radial and ulnar arteries of the client's hand simultaneously for approximately 5 seconds. The hand should blanch during this time.

—Lower the hand and arm to the level of the heart while still holding both arteries. Release pressure from *only* the ulnar artery.

—Make sure that color returns to the hand within 5 seconds with the radial artery still compressed.

—Normal return of color is described as a *negative* or *normal* finding. A positive test is a sluggish or absent return to normal coloring.

➤ A small amount of local anesthetic may be administered over the arterial puncture site electively.

➤ Prepare a syringe and needle by flushing them with a small amount of sodium heparin (1000 U/mL) or obtain a prepackaged unit specifically designed for arterial blood gas collection.

➤ Wearing gloves, perform the arterial puncture by inserting the needle at a 45-degree angle through the skin over the palpable pulse.

➤ Collect 0.2–0.5 mL of arterial blood as required by your laboratory.

➤ Ensure that all air is removed from the syringe and the sample is transported to the laboratory on ice.

➤ Gently rotate the syringe to ensure the blood sample is well mixed with the anticoagulant to prevent clotting of the specimen.

➤ Mark the client's temperature and FiO_2 (fraction of inspired oxygen) of any oxygen therapy clearly on the laboratory slip.

Care After Test

➤ Apply pressure to the arterial site with a dry gauze and gloved hands for at least 5 minutes to ensure hemostasis.

➤ Inspect the site to be sure the bleeding has stopped and that no hematoma has developed.

➤ If a hematoma develops, reabsorption of the blood can be enhanced with applications of warm compresses, in 20-minute intervals, several times a day. Delay application of warm soaks until it is certain that the venipuncture site is stable and no longer bleeding.

➤ Apply an adhesive bandage.

➤ Instruct client and family that if bleeding should begin again, they should press firmly with their fingers or hand over the area and notify the nurse right away.

➤ Assess for complications such as arterial spasm or inadequate arterial blood flow as evidenced by a cold, mottled hand. Paresthesia and numbness may also be present.

➤ Support client and family in light of their fears and apprehensions about being tested and awaiting results. Obtain counseling or support services for your client as indicated.

Interfering Factors

➤ Failure to use an anticoagulant or adequately mix the blood with the anticoagulant will result in clotting of the blood sample and inability to analyze the specimen.

➤ Failure to remove any air from the sample prior to analysis will result in inaccuracies in P_{O_2} and P_{CO_2} results.

➤ Failure to transport the sample on ice will result in inaccurate findings.

Potential Complications

➤ Infection, bleeding, or hematoma formation may occur at the arterial puncture site.

➤ Impairment of peripheral arterial circulation to the hand may result in ischemia or necrosis.

Prepare Your Client

➤ Explain why the test is being performed; use simple terms without medical jargon so the client and family can understand.

➤ Explain that the test requires a small blood sample obtained by poking the end of a finger or the heel of a foot with a sharp object only deeply enough to get a small blood sample.

➤ Instruct your client and family that mild, transient discomfort from the stick may be felt. Assure the client that this pain or discomfort will go away after completion of the blood collection procedure.

➤ Wash your hands prior to performance of the finger or heel stick.

Perform Procedure

➤ Select a lateral aspect of one of the fingers and cleanse prior to the finger stick procedure (avoid the central tip area of the fingers as the nerve supply is more dense in this area). Alternately, the heel is used in infants with the lower back portion of the heel as the puncture site.

➤ Wearing gloves and using a lancet or autolet device, make a small puncture in the skin at the collection site. Avoid using excessive pressure to express blood for collection. Firm or rough pressure on the fingers during collection of blood may cause hemolysis of the sample.

➤ Collect the sample in a heparinized capillary tube (red-banded tube) and seal one or both ends after collection.

➤ Note interfering factors or medications on the laboratory requisition slip.

➤ Transport the sample to the lab immediately. The sample will require processing in a centrifuge before analysis.

Care After Test

➤ Apply pressure to the site with a dry gauze and gloved hands for a minute for hemostasis.

➤ Inspect the site to be sure the bleeding has stopped.

➤ Apply an adhesive bandage.

➤ Instruct client and family that if bleeding begins again, they should press firmly with their fingers or hand over the area until the bleeding stops.

➤ Support client in light of their fears and apprehensions about being tested and awaiting results. Obtain counseling or support services as indicated.

Interfering Factors

➤ If the finger or heel is squeezed too roughly to try to get a blood sample, hemoconcentration or hemolysis may occur in the blood sample and affect the results.

➤ Failure to place the sample in a capillary tube and send it to the laboratory immediately to be processed may affect the values.

Potential Complications

➤ Infection, bleeding, or hematoma formation may occur at the puncture site.

Prepare Your Client

➤ Explain, in simple terms the client and family can understand, why the test is being performed. Do not use medical jargon or terminology unless the words and their meaning are explained fully.

➤ Explain that the test requires collection of *all* urine during a 24-hour period by collecting it in a sterile container.

➤ Check to see if the client is receiving any medications that may alter the test results. If so, discuss with the primary health care provider whether these should be discontinued 2 weeks prior to the test.

➤ Provide the client or family with appropriate instructions to collect the specimen.

Perform Procedure

➤ Wear gloves if there is a possibility that your hands will touch the client's urine.

➤ Make sure the collection container is the one required by your institution and has preservative in it. The urine generally needs to be refrigerated or kept on ice during the 24-hour collection period.

➤ Have the client urinate and discard this urine. Note this time as the start of the 24-hour collection time.

➤ Put a notice of the collection time at the bedside and also post it in the bathroom.

➤ Collect *all* the urine for 24 hours.

➤ Tell the client to void 24 hours after the test began. Put this urine into the collection container and take it to the laboratory.

➤ Compare output records with the amount of urine in the collection container. If they are not equal, the test is likely to be invalid.

➤ Indicate on the lab slip any medications that may alter results.

Care After Test

➤ Ensure that the specimen is free of fecal and menstrual discharge contamination and toilet tissue.

➤ Assess color, odor, and character of the urine.

➤ Ensure that the specimen labels and the laboratory requisition have the correct information on them and are attached securely to the specimen containers.

➤ Take the specimen immediately to the laboratory, or refrigerate it.

➤ Note medications the client is receiving that may discolor urine or affect the test results.

➤ Support client in light of their fears and apprehensions about being tested and awaiting results. Obtain counseling or support services for your client as indicated.

Interfering Factors

➤ Fecal contamination
➤ Menstrual discharge contamination
➤ Toilet tissue contamination
➤ Failure to collect all urine during the collection period

Potential Complications

None

Adapted from Kozier, B., Erb, G., Blais, K., Johnson, J. Y., Temple, J. S. (1993). *Techniques in Clinical Nursing*. Redwood City, CA: Addison-Wesley Nursing.

Prepare Your Client

➤ Explain, in simple terms the client and family can understand, why the test is being performed. Do not use medical jargon or terminology unless the words and their meaning are explained fully.

➤ Explain that the test requires a sample of urine obtained by collecting it in a sterile container.

➤ Provide the client or parent with appropriate instructions to collect the specimen.

Perform Procedure

➤ Use aseptic technique.

➤ Wear gloves if there is a possibility that your hands will touch the client's urine.

➤ Ensure that the specimen is free of fecal and menstrual discharge contamination and toilet tissue.

➤ Instruct the client or parent on how to clean the genitals and perineum before the collection or clean the client's vulvar area or tip of the penis with an antiseptic before the collection.

➤ Collect the urine midstream.

Care After Test

➤ Assess color, odor, and character of the urine.

➤ Ensure that the specimen labels and the laboratory requisition have the correct information on them and are attached securely to the specimen containers.

➤ Take the specimen immediately to the laboratory, or refrigerate it.

➤ Note medications the client is receiving that may discolor urine or affect the test results.

➤ Support client in light of their fears and apprehensions about being tested and awaiting results. Obtain counseling or support services for your client as indicated.

Interfering Factors

➤ Fecal contamination
➤ Menstrual discharge contamination
➤ Toilet tissue contamination
➤ Failure to use aseptic technique

Potential Complications

None

Adapted from Kozier, B., Erb, G., Blais, K., Johnson, J. Y., Temple, J. S. (1993). *Techniques in Clinical Nursing*. Redwood City, CA: Addison-Wesley Nursing.

ROUTINE URINE SPECIMEN COLLECTION FOR ADULT OR CHILD

Prepare Your Client

➤ Explain, in simple terms the client and family can understand, why the test is being performed. Do not use medical jargon or terminology unless the words and their meaning are explained fully.

➤ Provide the client or parent with appropriate instructions to collect the specimen.

Perform Procedure

➤ Use clean technique.

➤ Wear gloves if there is a possibility that your hands will touch the client's urine.

➤ Ensure that the specimen is free of fecal or menstrual discharge contamination and toilet tissue.

➤ Direct the client to void approximately 120 mL of urine in a collection cup. Assist as necessary.

Care After Test

➤ Assess color, odor, and character of the urine.

➤ Ensure that the specimen labels and the laboratory requisition have the cor-rect information on them and are attached securely to the specimen containers.

➤ Note medications the client is receiving that may discolor urine or affect the test results.

➤ Take the specimen immediately to the laboratory, or refrigerate it.

➤ Support client in light of their fears and apprehensions about being tested and awaiting results. Obtain counseling or support services for your client as indicated.

Interfering Factors

➤ Fecal contamination

➤ Toilet tissue contamination

➤ Menstrual discharge contamination

➤ Failure to use aseptic technique

Potential Complications

None

Adapted from Kozier, B., Erb, G., Blais, K., Johnson, J. Y., Temple, J. S. (1993). *Techniques in Clinical Nursing*. Redwood City, CA: Addison-Wesley Nursing.

Prepare Your Client

➤ Explain, in simple terms the client and family can understand, why the test is being performed. Do not use medical jargon or terminology unless the words and their meaning are explained fully.

➤ Explain that the test requires a sample of sputum obtained by collecting it in a sterile container.

➤ Instruct the client not to touch the inside of the sputum container and to expectorate directly into the container.

Perform Procedure

➤ Use aseptic technique.

➤ Wear gloves if there is a possibility that your hands will touch the client's sputum.

➤ Instruct the client to obtain 1–2 teaspoons (5–10 mL).

➤ Direct the client to take a deep breath before coughing up secretions so they will have enough air to force secretions out of the lungs and into the pharynx.

➤ Cover the container immediately after specimen is collected to avoid contamination.

Care After Test

➤ Assess color, odor, consistency, and character of the sputum.

➤ Ensure that the specimen labels and the laboratory requisition have the correct information on them and are attached securely to the specimen containers.

➤ Take the specimen immediately to the laboratory, or refrigerate it.

➤ Note antibiotics the client is receiving that may affect the test results.

➤ Provide oral care.

Interfering Factors

➤ Contamination by saliva and oral flora

➤ Failure to use aseptic technique

Adapted from Kozier, B., Erb, G., Blais, K., Johnson, J. Y., Temple, J. S. (1993). *Techniques in Clinical Nursing*. Redwood City, CA: Addison-Wesley Nursing.

FECES SPECIMEN COLLECTION

Prepare Your Client

➤ Explain, in simple terms the client and family can understand, why the test is being performed. Do not use medical jargon or terminology unless the words and their meaning are explained fully.

➤ Explain that the test requires a sample of stool or bowel movement obtained by collecting it in a container. Verify that the client understands these words and the intended method of collection.

➤ Check with the primary care provider about whether the client needs to be placed on a diet free of red meat and whether to discontinue oral iron preparations before an occult blood test.

➤ Instruct the client or parent to collect the specimen directly into a specimen cup or a collection container while on the toilet. Tell them not to contaminate with urine, menses, water, or toilet paper.

Perform Procedure

➤ Wear gloves if there is a possibility that your hands will touch the client's feces.

➤ Use clean technique.

➤ Prevent contamination of the specimen by urine or menstrual discharge.

➤ Ensure that the appropriate amount of stool is collected for ordered tests.

Care After Test

➤ Ensure that the specimen labels and the laboratory requisition have the correct information on them and are attached securely to the specimen containers.

➤ Take the specimen *immediately* to the laboratory. Do *not* refrigerate.

➤ Note medications the client is receiving that may interfere with testing for culture and sensitivity.

➤ Support client in light of their fears and apprehensions about being tested and awaiting results. Obtain counseling or support services for your client as indicated.

Interfering Factors

➤ Urine contamination
➤ Menstrual discharge contamination
➤ Toilet tissue contamination
➤ Failure to use aseptic technique

Potential Complications

None

Adapted from Kozier, B., Erb, G., Blais, K., Johnson, J. Y., Temple, J. S. (1993). *Techniques in Clinical Nursing*. Redwood City, CA: Addison-Wesley Nursing.

GUIDE TO THE MOST COMMON BLOOD COLLECTION TUBES

Color	Additive	Purpose
Red top	None	To allow blood sample to clot, allowing serum to be separated and and the test to be performed on the serum only.
Purple or lavender top	EDTA	To prevent blood from clotting, which allows testing of blood sample as a whole. This is particularly important when red and white blood cells need to be tested.
Green top	Heparin	To prevent the blood sample from clotting when the plasma needs to be tested.
Blue top	Sodium citrate and citric acid	To prevent the blood sample from clotting when the plasma needs to be tested.
Gray top	Glycolytic inhibitor, such as sodium fluoride	To prevent glycolysis and to help keep glucose in its in vivo state.

Acetylcholine Receptor Antibody

ah **set** il **koe** leen • ree **sep** tur • an ti **bod** ee
(AChR antibodies)

Normal Findings
ADULT AND CHILD
(Results are reported as percent loss of AChR)
Loss of less than 20% of AChR (SI units: Loss of ≤0.03 nmol/L)
NEWBORN
AChR antibodies can be detected in most neonates born to mothers with myasthenia gravis. The antibodies are passed from maternal to fetal circulation, but only about 12% of these newborns will actually develop symptoms of myasthenia gravis.

What This Test Will Tell You
This blood test diagnoses myasthenia gravis and monitors the client's response to therapy.

Acetylcholine (a parasympathetic neurotransmitter) and intact acetylcholine receptor sites at the myoneural junction are necessary for impulse transmission to the muscle for voluntary movement. Myasthenia gravis occurs when autoantibodies form that block and bind acetylcholine receptor sites. Acetylcholine receptor–blocking antibodies are present in 90% of patients with symptoms. Titers decrease significantly when a client goes into remission.

The antibody binding test is positive for myasthenia gravis in most clients with severe or acute disease and in 80% of clients with mild disease, 50% of clients with ocular myasthenia, and 25% of clients in remission. A sustained decrease of 50% or greater in titer levels is associated with clinical improvement. The blocking assay is usually performed when the binding test is negative and symptoms continue to suggest myasthenia gravis. Testing for both blocking and binding AChR antibodies increases the accuracy of this test.

Abnormal Findings
▲ INCREASED LEVELS (in this case more than 20% loss of AChR) may indicate myasthenia gravis.

ACTION ALERT!
Rising antibody titers correlate with a worsening clinical condition in untreated or undertreated myasthenia gravis. As this disease progresses, it can deteriorate into a myasthenic crisis and acute respiratory failure.

Interfering Factors
➤ False positive results occur in clients with amyotrophic lateral sclerosis treated with cobra venom.
➤ False positive results occur in clients with rheumatoid arthritis treated with penicillamine.
➤ Failure to maintain the sample at room temperature or not processing the sample quickly will alter results.
➤ Muscle-relaxing and immunosuppressive medications can alter results.

NURSING CONSIDERATIONS
Prepare Your Client
➤ Explain that this test will measure levels of antibodies in blood cells. These antibodies can damage the connection between nerves and muscles, causing weakness and fatigue. Where indicated, explain also that this test will be used to measure the client's response to therapy.

Perform Procedure

> Collect 7–10 mL of venous blood in a red-top tube.

Care After Test

> If the test is positive for myasthenia gravis, assess client's depth and rate of respirations. Carefully note any symptoms of respiratory distress signaling a myasthenic crisis.

> If test is positive, assess the client's ability to swallow and chew safely. Myasthenia gravis causes weakness in those muscles innervated by the cranial nerves and can lead to choking hazards.

> If test is positive, space activity with rest; client will quickly fatigue.

> Protect client from extremes of temperature and other stressors, which can exacerbate symptoms.

> Initiate safety precautions to protect client from falls and other accidents secondary to muscle weakness.

> Evaluate the results of other tests such as the tensilon test, anti-DNA antibodies, antiparietal cell antibodies, anti-smooth-muscle antibodies, and rheumatoid factor.

Educate Your Client and the Family

> Emphasize the importance of eating slowly and choosing soft, easily chewed foods to prevent choking problems.

> Encourage client to pace activities and to set priorities to avoid undue fatigue.

> Teach client to plan rest periods. Clients with myasthenia become progressively fatigued during a day.

> Teach the symptoms of an exacerbation or crisis such as breathlessness, inability to hold up the head, and difficulty swallowing secretions.

> Encourage client to wear medical alert identification.

Acid-Fast Bacilli
ass id fast • bah sil ie
(AFB)

Normal Findings
Negative for AFB

What This Test Will Tell You
This test of various body fluids identifies tubercle bacilli (*Mycobacterium tuberculosis*) in order to diagnose and monitor the treatment of tuberculosis. Findings of acid-fast bacilli (AFB) on microscopic examination indicate possible tuberculosis and allow for timely initiation of antituberculosis therapy. However, a definitive diagnosis of tuberculosis may take several weeks. Smears and cultures, primarily of sputum but also of other body specimens such as urine, skin biopsies, cerebrospinal fluid, gastric washings, and blood, are stained to detect acid-fast bacilli.

Abnormal Findings
Positive AFB results may indicate tuberculosis, infection with other strains of the *Mycobacterium* genus, or infection with *Nocardia* or *Actinomyces* species.

■■■■ ACTION ALERT!

If tuberculosis is strongly suspected, initiation of therapy may be instituted prior to confirmation by AFB test, but after specimens are collected.

Interfering Factors

➤ Improper specimen collection
➤ Delay in sending specimen to the laboratory

Contraindications

➤ Gastric aspirate for sampling may be contraindicated in clients with esophageal or gastric disease such as varices, strictures, and active ulcers.

Potential Complications

➤ Sputum collected by tracheal suctioning may produce transient hypoxia and require administration of supplemental oxygen.
➤ Gastric aspiration for collection may cause esophageal or gastric trauma resulting in hemorrhage and perforation.

NURSING CONSIDERATIONS

Prepare Your Client

➤ Explain that this test is to detect possible infection with tuberculosis.
➤ Inform the client that it may take several weeks before results of the tests are available.
➤ Inform the client that it may be necessary to obtain several specimens over several days.
➤ Check to see if client is receiving broad-spectrum antibiotics at the time of the collection because these may destroy the mycobacteria in the urine.

Perform Procedure

The procedure varies with the type of specimen collected.

SPUTUM

➤ Obtain the specimen from the lungs: saliva and nasal drainage are not sputum.
➤ Collect an early morning specimen, after secretions have collected overnight.
➤ Determine and explain the procedure by which the specimen will be collected (coughing or tracheal suctioning).
➤ If the client is unable to produce sputum, contact respiratory therapy for postural drainage and chest percussion to stimulate production of acceptable sputum.
➤ Increase fluid intake the night before or have the client breathe humidified air to help liquify secretions and aid in coughing up sputum.
➤ The material from the first deep productive cough of the morning should be expelled and collected without contaminating the inside of the sterile container or lid by touching it with the mouth or hands.
➤ Producing sputum may be especially difficult for women who are unaccustomed to spitting.

GASTRIC ASPIRATES

➤ Clients unable to produce sputum usually swallow sputum during the night, and it pools in the stomach. Gastric contents can then be collected for culture first thing in the morning by a gastric tube passed through the nose or mouth.
➤ Explain to the client the procedure for inserting a gastric tube.
➤ Instruct the client to fast for at least 8 hours prior to the test.
➤ After the gastric tube has been passed into the stomach, withdraw gastric contents into a sterile syringe and immediately place into a sterile container, avoiding contamination.

➤ Transport the specimen to the laboratory immediately to prevent destruction of the tubercle bacilli by gastric acids.

BLOOD

➤ Explain the venipuncture process clearly to the client.

➤ Tell the client that there is no need to restrict foods, fluids, or medications for this test.

URINE

➤ Inform the client that the first morning midstream specimen is most useful.

➤ Explain the procedure for collecting a midstream urine sample.

OTHER BODY FLUIDS AND TISSUES

➤ Explain to the client that when noninvasive techniques have not provided a diagnosis, the physician may need to perform invasive procedures to obtain a specimen, such as bronchoscopy, lumbar puncture, or biopsies.

➤ Assist the physician performing the procedure to obtain the specimen according to established protocols.

➤ Collect the specimen, label the container, and send to the laboratory immediately.

Care After Test

➤ Assess for symptoms of tuberculosis such as malaise, fever, night sweats, and weight loss.

➤ Institute AFB or respiratory isolation pending diagnostic results if tuberculosis is suspected.

➤ Observe for symptoms of hypoxia and administer oxygen after collection of sputum specimens if indicated.

➤ Observe for bleeding and/or possible hemorrhage after gastric washing.

➤ Review results of related tests such as the white blood count, skin tests, and chest x-ray.

Educate Your Client and the Family

➤ Instruct client to turn their head away from others and cover their mouth and nose when coughing or sneezing. Tell them to dispose of tissues in an appropriate receptacle.

➤ Explain respiratory or AFB precautions to hospitalized clients if indicated.

➤ Inform client and family that several weeks may be needed for conclusive results.

➤ Explain that respiratory isolation is not necessary in the home setting because family members have already been exposed.

➤ Teach client about drug therapy when instituted.

➤ Instruct client on the importance of compliance with therapy and follow-up sputum cultures.

➤ Listen to client's and family's concerns and offer a positive outlook for the client if they comply with the drug regimen.

Acid Phosphatase, Serum
ass id • fos fah tase • see rum

Normal Findings
ADULT AND ELDERLY
0.11–0.60 U/L (Roy, Brower, Hayden; at 37°C) (SI units: 0–0.60 U/L)
CHILD
8.6–12.6 U/mL (at 30°C)
NEWBORN
10.4–16.4 U/mL (at 30°C)

What This Test Will Tell You
This blood test diagnoses, stages, and monitors the efficacy of treatment of prostatic cancer. Acid phosphatase is one of a group of enzymes located primarily in the prostate gland and in prostate secretions. Smaller amounts are found in the bone marrow, spleen, liver, kidneys, and blood components such as erythrocytes and platelets. Elevated levels are seen in clients with prostatic cancer that has metastasized beyond the capsule to other parts of the body, especially the bone.

Abnormal Findings
▲ INCREASED LEVELS may reveal prostatic cancer, bone fracture, cancer metastasis to the bone, multiple myeloma, Paget's disease, sickle cell crisis, Gaucher's disease, renal impairment, cancer of the breast, obstructive jaundice, Laënnec's cirrhosis, leukemia (myelogenous), osteogenesis imperfecta, thrombocytosis, thromboembolism, idiopathic thrombocytopenic purpura (with bone marrow megakaryocytes), partial translocation trisomy 21, or hyperparathyroidism.

Interfering Factors
➤ Rectal examination, prostatic massage, urinary catheterization, or instrumentation of the prostate within 2 days prior to the test may cause falsely high acid phosphatase levels in males due to prostatic stimulation.
➤ Drugs including androgens (in females), clofibrate (Atromid-S.), and antilipidemic agents may cause elevated levels.
➤ Specimens received more than 15 minutes after collection or hemolyzed specimens invalidate results.
➤ The test is more accurate for diagnosis in advanced prostatic cancer than in early prostatic cancer.

NURSING CONSIDERATIONS
Prepare Your Client
➤ Explain that this test is important to help determine whether there is a problem in the prostate gland and if other parts of the body have been affected.
➤ Explain that you will need to draw blood from the vein for the test.
➤ Do not restrict food, fluids, activities, or medications before the test.

Perform Procedure
➤ Collect 5 mL of venous blood in a red-top tube.
➤ Label the sample and note any interfering factors (i.e., prostatic exam or instrumentation, or medications).
➤ Request that the test be performed without delay, or freeze the specimen.
➤ Do not leave specimen at room temperature for 1 hour or longer

because the enzyme is heat- and pH-sensitive and its activity will decrease.

Care After Test
➤ Assess for signs and symptoms of urinary outflow obstruction at the bladder neck and prostatic urethra, which are bladder distention, urinary frequency, nocturia, urgency, hesitancy, diminished force of the urinary stream, overflow incontinence, and postvoid dribbling.
➤ Observe client for symptoms of bone metastasis, which are pain in low back, pelvis, and upper thighs. Offer a variety of pain relief measures.
➤ Review other diagnostic studies and findings such as digital rectal exam, prostate-specific antigen, closed or open fine needle biopsy, transrectal ultrasonography, pelvic computed tomography, magnetic resonance imaging, and lymphangiography.

Educate Your Client and the Family
➤ Explain the need for adequate fluid intake, exercise, and rest.
➤ Describe the benefits of a variety of pain relief measures such as heat, massage, and combinations of medications.
➤ Provide a written list of signs and symptoms of renal insufficiency and instruct the client to notify the primary health care provider or nurse if these occur.

Acoustic Stimulation
a koos tik • stim yu lay shun
(Fetal Acoustic Stimulation Test, FAST, Vibroacoustic Stimulation Test, VST)

Normal Findings
Reactive
Fetal heart rate acceleration of at least 15 beats per minute for at least 120 seconds or two accelerations of at least 15 beats per minute for at least 15 seconds within 5 minutes of stimulus.

What This Test Will Tell You
This fetal stimulation test evaluates fetal well-being in conjunction with nonstress testing by attempting to induce accelerations of the fetal heart rate (FHR). The test is used for fetuses who do not show normal reactivity. Acoustic stimulation is noninvasive and produces a buzzing sound and a low-frequency vibration. It is unknown if the fetus moves in response to the sound or to the vibration. Fetal movement produces increases in the FHR.

Acoustic stimulation is also used during labor if a fetus has decreased variability (fluctuation) in the FHR or is in a sleep cycle and to evaluate fetal activity for mothers who have decreased perception of fetal movement.

Abnormal Findings
Nonreaction or other reactions may indicate fetal distress, anesthesia, anencephaly, fetal tachycardia, anomalies, fetal arrhythmias, or fetal complete heart block.

ACTION ALERT!

A negative response or lack of movement may indicate a serious health threat to the fetus that requires emergency delivery and immediate resuscitation of the infant.

Interfering Factors

➤ Maternal administration of narcotics, sedatives, tranquilizers, antihypertensive agents, barbiturates, magnesium sulfate, methadone, and alcohol may decrease the fetal response to acoustic stimulation.

➤ A preterm fetus may not respond to acoustic stimulation as a term fetus would. The ability to perceive sound increases with gestation.

NURSING CONSIDERATIONS

Prepare Your Client

➤ Explain to the client that the test is performed to wake up the baby and to make the baby move.

➤ Assess the client for the need for the acoustic stimulus: nonreactivity of the FHR during a nonstress test, decreased variability in the FHR in labor, and women who have decreased feeling of fetal movement.

➤ Show the acoustic stimulator (or an artificial larynx can be used) to the client and demonstrate the use on the client's hand if possible.

➤ Tell the client that the test may need to be repeated.

Perform Procedure

➤ Place the client in a semi-Fowler's position.

➤ Connect the acoustic stimulator to the fetal monitor if it is being used for nonstress testing, or for a client in labor. If connection is not possible, press the mark button on the fetal monitor to mark the time of the acoustic stimulus.

➤ Use after 5-minute wait when used with nonstress testing.

➤ Apply the acoustic stimulator for 1–3 seconds on the woman's abdomen.

➤ Repeat the acoustic stimulation in 10 minutes if no response occurs to the first stimulation.

➤ Instruct the client to tell the nurse when the fetus moves.

➤ Notify the primary health care provider if the client in labor or nonstress testing does not have a fetal response to acoustic stimulation.

Care After Test

➤ Assess the response of the fetus to the acoustic stimulation, including increases in the FHR; what the rate increased to and for how long; changes in variability of the FHR; and how many times the acoustic stimulation was performed and the response to each.

➤ Evaluate other related tests such as nonstress test, biophysical profile, daily fetal movement count, and amniocentesis.

Educate Your Client and the Family

➤ Explain to the client that further testing will be done if the fetus does not respond to acoustic stimulation.

➤ Tell client to notify their primary health care provider if they have less than three movements in 1 hour. A nonstress test or biophysical profile may be ordered.

Acquired Immune Deficiency Syndrome Serology

ah kwie erd • im yoon • dee fish en see • sin drome

(AIDS Screen, AIDS Serology, HIV Antibody Test, HIV Test, Enzyme-Linked Immunosorbent Assay for HIV, ELISA for HIV, Western Blot Test for HIV, Indirect Fluorescent Antibody [IFA] for HIV)

Normal Findings

ADULT

ELISA seronegative

Western Blot seronegative

(Serum tests negative for human immunodeficiency virus [HIV] antibody)

NEWBORN

Seronegative

Infants born to mothers who have HIV may become infected during gestation, delivery, or breastfeeding.

What This Test Will Tell You

This blood test detects the presence of antibodies to the human immunodeficiency virus (HIV) in the blood.

To ensure absolute accuracy, serum from individuals and serum samples for blood donation are first screened by the ELISA (enzyme-linked immunosorbent assay) and, if positive, the ELISA is repeated. A positive sample is retested by a Western Blot or Indirect Fluorescent Antibody (IFA). If both tests are positive, the client is informed. If the ELISA alone is positive but follow-up tests are negative, the client should be retested in 3–6 months. In some states, positive testing must be reported to state or county health departments.

Once HIV infection has been confirmed, CD4 (helper T cell) counts are routinely measured to monitor the progression of HIV and to assess the effectiveness of therapy. Epstein-Barr virus, cytomegalovirus, and hepatitis B titers are obtained to assist in diagnosis and treatment.

Abnormal Findings

▲INCREASED LEVELS (seropositive) may indicate HIV exposure, HIV infection, AIDS, or AIDS-related complex.

After exposure and subsequent infection by HIV, the immune system does not mount an immediate response. It takes 6 weeks to 12 months or longer before antibodies to HIV can be detected. An infected, asymptomatic individual who tests sero-negative (negative for HIV antibody) may transmit the virus before antibodies appear.

Interfering Factors

➤ Antibodies for HIV do not appear in the early stages of the disease. It may take 6–12 weeks or longer for antibodies to appear and result in a positive titer.

➤ Clients with clinical symptoms of the advanced stages of AIDS may no longer have detectable antibodies due to severe immunological depression.

➤ Not all strains of HIV are as easily detected by present methods.

➤ Previous pregnancy or blood transfusion may cause an individual to be previously sensitized to the media used for testing. This can result in a false positive result because the serum sample reacts to the culture media rather than the virus itself.

NURSING CONSIDERATIONS

Prepare Your Client

➤ Obtain informed consent, or verify that it has been obtained. The client must give permission and understand the implications of HIV testing including possible effect on insurability. Some states require anonymity in testing and results are reported only by identification numbers. Check with your own institution's and state's policies regarding anonymity.

➤ Reassure the client that absolute confidentiality of test results will be observed. Test results should not be given by telephone.

➤ If you are working with blood donors, be sure potential donors understand their blood will be tested for HIV.

➤ Offer counseling before testing and when the results are given to the client. Counseling regarding HIV transmission, accuracy of the test, and behavioral changes is essential.

➤ Explain that this test detects exposure to and infection by HIV, not active AIDS. They may have no symptoms of illness despite infection with the virus.

➤ Be sure to inform the client when results will be available, because the waiting period is likely to be stressful.

Perform Procedure

➤ Using universal precautions, collect 5–10 mL of venous blood in a red-top tube.

➤ Apply pressure to site, and check for continued bleeding or hematoma

formation. Apply a pressure dressing. Clients with HIV may be thrombocytopenic.

Care After Test

➤ Evaluate client for symptoms of AIDS such as fever, night sweats, weight loss, anorexia, swollen lymph nodes (lymphadenopathy), history of respiratory infections, or change in mentation.

➤ Protect client from falls or other accidents if level of consciousness is impaired.

➤ Inspect the oral mucosa carefully, checking for candida, herpes, or other painful lesions that will make eating difficult.

➤ Perform frequent, gentle oral care using a non-alcohol-based solution.

➤ Offer frequent small meals and snacks to help achieve or maintain ideal weight.

➤ Evaluate client for activity intolerance or shortness of breath, which is an initial symptom of pneumocystis carinii.

➤ Offer support to client, family, and significant others.

➤ Refer client to an AIDS program if one is available in the area. Counseling and support by experienced health care professionals is critical in living with HIV infection and AIDS.

➤ Review related tests such as complete blood count with differential, lymphocyte marker assay, and body fluid cultures.

Educate Your Client and the Family

➤ Teach client and family that HIV is not transmitted by casual contact such as kissing or touching, but it is found in secretions and blood. Tell them not to share razors or toothbrushes.

➤ Discuss behavioral changes with client. The disease may be transmitted by sharing needles or having unprotected sex. Encourage client to wear a condom during intercourse. An inexpensive female condom is now available. Inform client that condoms do experience failure.

➤ Explain to client that repeated exposure to HIV or other viruses, such as cytomegalovirus, hepatitis, or herpes, taxes the immune system and can hasten the clinical onset of AIDS. Avoiding those practices that expose the client to viruses and other illnesses may help them stay healthier longer.

➤ Review the signs and symptoms of AIDS with your client, and encourage them to seek medical care when symptoms such as shortness of breath begin.

➤ Recommend that the client use soft toothbrushes, and gentle mouth rinses to maintain integrity of the oral mucosa.

➤ Stress the importance of maintaining normal weight, and consult with a registered dietician to design a well-balanced, high-calorie diet, especially if the client develops diarrhea, constipation, or severe weight loss.

Adrenal Angiography

ah dree nal • an jee og rah fee
(Adrenal Angiogram)

Normal Findings
Normal adrenal vasculature

What This Test Will Tell You
This radiographic test is used primarily to visualize the adrenal arteries and diagnose tumors and other pathology of the adrenal glands. It will determine glandular blood flow, the presence or absence of tumors, and the size of the adrenal gland.

Abnormal Findings
Abnormalities may indicate adrenal carcinoma, adrenal adenoma, pheochromocytoma, adrenal hyperplasia, or adrenal hypoplasia.

ACTION ALERT!

➤ If pheochromocytoma is suspected, alpha- and beta-adrenergic blockers are usually administered several days before the test to prevent severe or even fatal hypertension from occurring.

➤ Assess client carefully for allergic reaction to contrast material including dyspnea, itching, urticaria, flushing, hypotension, and shock. Life-threatening anaphylactic reactions can occur and need to be recognized and treated immediately.

Interfering Factors
➤ Movement during the test

Contraindications
➤ Allergy to iodinated dye or shellfish
➤ Bleeding disorders
➤ Anticoagulation
➤ Pregnancy
➤ Atherosclerosis

Potential Complications
➤ Allergic reaction, anaphylaxis
➤ Hemorrhage from arterial access site
➤ Embolism or infarction due to

dislodging of atherosclerotic plaque
➤ Exacerbation of hypertension in client with a pheochromocytoma (epinephrine-secreting tumor)
➤ Adrenal hemorrhage or necrosis from pressure of dye injection

NURSING CONSIDERATIONS
Prepare Your Client
➤ Explain to the client that this test is to look for problems in a gland that sits on the kidneys and produces important hormones.
➤ Tell your client or family that once needles are inserted, the procedure itself is painless, but some pressure may be felt while lines are passed and there may be warmth from the dye.
➤ Ensure that an informed consent is obtained, because of the possible complications associated with this procedure.
➤ Restrict food or fluids for 8–12 hours before the test.
➤ Assess for history of dye or shellfish allergies and anticoagulant use (including aspirin).
➤ Evaluate prothrombin and partial thromboplastin times.
➤ Mark radial, dorsalis pedis, and femoral pulses with a pen prior to the procedure. This will assist with the pulse monitoring after the procedure. Note quality of pulses prior to the procedure on the care plan.
➤ Have the client void prior to the procedure.
➤ Give sedation if ordered.
➤ Obtain baseline vital signs before the procedure.
➤ Inform client that the test usually takes about an hour.

Perform Procedure
Nurses do not perform this procedure but should understand the process to prepare the client and assist the physician.

Place client on a special x-ray table and instruct them to lie very still while pictures are being taken and the needle for the catheter (long thin tube) is inserted. Assist in administering a local anesthetic to numb the area where the catheter will be inserted. Warn the client this may produce a brief burning sensation before the area becomes numb. A catheter is threaded through a needle placed in the leg vessel. The catheter is advanced under fluoroscopy into the inferior adrenal artery. Films are taken. The catheter is removed and a pressure dressing is applied.

Care After Test
➤ Monitor vital signs closely until stable, usually every 15 minutes for the first hour, every 30 minutes for the next hour, and then every 4 hours for 24 hours. Monitor the arterial puncture site or dressing for hemorrhage/hematoma formation with each vital sign assessment.
➤ Assess peripheral pulses for preprocedure quality.
➤ Look for signs and symptoms of emboli dislodgement or clot formation (loss of peripheral pulse, pain, temperature changes in the extremity, numbness, tingling).
➤ Compare color and temperature of procedural leg with that of the other leg.
➤ Assess for signs/symptoms of allergic dye reaction such as itching, rash, and difficulty breathing. Delayed reactions usually occur 2–6 hours after the test.
➤ Instruct client to keep the affected leg straight and to rest in bed for 6–12 hours to minimize bleeding and bruising.

➤ Encourage drinking fluids to replace fluid volume lost from the diuretic effect of the contrast medium.

➤ Apply ice and pressure to the puncture site to minimize bleeding, hematoma formation, and swelling.

➤ Evaluate other related tests such as computed tomography, adrenocorticotropic (ACTH) hormone levels, ACTH stimulation test, and urine vanillylmandelic acid levels.

Educate Your Client and the Family

➤ Instruct the client and family to monitor for bleeding or bruising at the puncture site because bleeding may occur several days later.

➤ Advise client to keep the area clean and dry, and to contact their primary health care provider if signs of infection such as redness, tenderness, swelling, or drainage occur.

Adrenal Venograph
ad **ree** nal • **vee** noe graf
(Adrenal Venography, Adrenal Venogram)

Normal Findings
Patent and normal adrenal vasculature bilaterally
Normal size, absence of tumors, cysts, or congenital anomalies of both adrenals
Hormone assay within normal limits for adrenal veins

What This Test Will Tell You
This x-ray with contrast is used to visualize the adrenal veins to detect if the gland has the proper blood flow, assess the presence or absence of tumors, and determine the size of the adrenal gland. It can also be used to sample the blood returning from each adrenal gland, giving an indication of the amount of cortisol and epinephrine produced. If the serum level is elevated unilaterally, one of the glands is overproducing the hormones. If the serum level is subnormal, one or both of the glands are not producing adequate amounts of the hormone.

Abnormal Findings
Abnormalities may indicate unilateral or bilateral adrenal hyperplasia, unilateral or bilateral pheochromocytoma, or extra-adrenal pheochromocytoma.

ACTION ALERT!
➤ Assess clients carefully for allergic reaction to contrast material including dyspnea, itching, urticaria, flushing, hypotension, and shock. Life-threatening anaphylactic reactions can occur and need to be recognized and treated immediately.

➤ Administer beta- and alpha-adrenergic blocking agents as ordered to clients with suspected pheochromocytoma to prevent severe or fatal hypertensive crisis related to catecholamine release.

Interfering Factors
➤ Movement may interfere with imaging.

Contraindications
➤ Allergies to iodinated dye or shellfish, unless modifications in the test-

ing procedure are made

➤ Bleeding disorders, anticoagulation therapy

Potential Complications

➤ Allergic reaction to contrast material

➤ Hemorrhage from puncture site

➤ Dislodgement of atherosclerotic plaque causing emboli formation

➤ Exacerbation of hypertension in clients with a pheochromocytoma (epinephrine-secreting tumor)

➤ Adrenal hemorrhage or necrosis from pressure of dye injection that may lead to Addison's disease

➤ Bacteremia, sepsis

➤ Thrombophlebitis

NURSING CONSIDERATIONS

Prepare Your Client

➤ Explain that this test is performed to look at two important glands in the body, the adrenal glands, which produce hormones.

➤ Assess for history of dye or shellfish allergies.

➤ Ensure that an informed consent is obtained, because of the possible complications associated with this procedure.

➤ Assess for anticoagulant use (including aspirin).

➤ Assess for prothrombin and partial thromboplastin times.

➤ Restrict food and fluids for 8 hours prior to the test.

➤ Tell clients that a local anesthetic will be used to numb the injection site (usually the femoral vein). Warn them there will be a brief burning sensation as the anesthetic is injected into the skin.

➤ Obtain baseline vital signs and have the client void prior to the procedure.

➤ If client has suspected pheochromocytoma, administer beta-adrenergic medications to prevent catecholamine-induced hypertension as ordered.

➤ Administer sedation if ordered.

Perform Procedure

Nurses do not perform this procedure but should understand the process to prepare the client and assist the physician. The usual procedure time is 1–2 hours. The client is assisted to a supine position on the x-ray table. The groin is cleansed and draped with sterile towels. A small catheter is passed from the femoral vein to the adrenal veins, dye is injected, and x-rays are obtained of the areas. Blood is obtained and sent to the laboratory. Following the test, the catheter is removed and a sterile pressure dressing is applied.

Care After Test

➤ Monitor vital signs closely until stable; usually every 15 minutes for the first hour, every 30 minutes for the next hour, and then every 4 hours for 24 hours. Check puncture site/dressing for hemorrhage/hematoma formation with each vital sign assessment. Apply ice as a comfort measure or to reduce hematoma formation and bleeding as indicated.

➤ For client with suspected pheochromocytoma, assess for tachycardia, hypertension, diaphoresis, tremor, pallor, flushing, anxiety, and hyperglycemia, which may signal a crisis.

➤ Check for signs/symptoms of emboli dislodgement including loss of peripheral pulse, pain, temperature changes in the extremity, numbness, and tingling, which would signify vascular occlusion. Compare the leg used for the procedure to the other leg.

➤ Check for signs/symptoms of allergic dye reaction, which may occur as late as 2–5 hours following administration.

➤ Encourage drinking fluids to replace fluids lost during diuresis that may occur from the contrast material.

➤ Review related tests such as adrenal angiography and serum and urine catecholamines.

Educate Your Client and the Family

➤ Teach the client with pheochromocytoma to avoid stress and physical exertion, which can precipitate a hypertensive crisis.

➤ Inform family that evaluation of other family members should be undertaken if client is diagnosed with pheochromocytoma.

➤ Teach client and family not to discontinue or alter medications ordered by the primary health care provider without consultation.

Adrenocorticotropic Hormone

ah **dree** noe **kor** ti koe **troe** pik • **hor** mone
(ACTH, Corticotropin)

Normal Findings

ADULT, ADOLESCENT, CHILD, ELDERLY

8 A.M. fasting: 15–100 pg/mL (SI units: 10–80 ng/L)

4 P.M. nonfasting: 10–50 pg/mL (SI units: 10–50 ng/L)

These values vary greatly depending upon the laboratory and methods used. Times for collection should be verified with laboratory, but circadian rhythms require approximately these morning and afternoon times.

PREGNANT OR MENSTRUATING CLIENT

Levels may vary from expected norms during pregnancy or menstruation.

NEWBORN

10–185 pg/mL

What This Test Will Tell You

This test measures the production of adrenocorticotropic hormone (ACTH) by the anterior pituitary in order to diagnose primary and secondary adrenal gland dysfunction. ACTH stimulates the adrenal cortex to make mineralocorticoids, glucocorticoids, and adrenogenitalcorticoids. Because of the complex feedback system of hormones, elevations or decreased levels of ACTH may alter other gland functions.

ACTH levels vary with the client's daily circadian cycle. Levels obtained upon awakening will be $1/2$ to $2/3$ higher than those obtained 10–12 hours later.

Abnormal Findings

▲INCREASED LEVELS may indicate primary adrenal insufficiency (Addison's disease), ectopic ACTH syndrome, oat-cell carcinoma, physical or mental stress, obesity, or congenital adrenal hyperplasia.

▼DECREASED LEVELS may indicate

pituitary insufficiency, Cushing's syndrome, adrenal adenoma or carcinoma, or steroid or oral contraceptive administration.

Interfering Factors
➤ Glucocorticoids, estrogen, and oral contraceptives can decrease levels.
➤ Stress (mental and physical) and obesity can elevate levels.
➤ Physical activity may increase levels.
➤ Blood glucose levels may interfere with accurate results.
➤ Radioactive scans within 1 week of this test may interfere with accurate results.

NURSING CONSIDERATIONS

Prepare Your Client
➤ Explain that this test is to see how well the pituitary gland, which produces hormones, is working.
➤ Consider diurnal variations by asking your client if they work night shifts or are awake much of the night. If so, consider a later testing time.
➤ Instruct the client not to eat or drink after midnight on the night before levels are drawn.
➤ Note any use of steroids on the lab slip because these medications can increase ACTH levels.
➤ Encourage client to relax, and reduce environmental stress because stress levels increase ACTH. Report high stress levels to the primary

health care provider because they will invalidate the test.

Perform Procedure
➤ Collect 20 mL of venous blood in a *chilled* green-top tube, or in a *chilled* plastic collection tube.
➤ Transport the sample to the laboratory immediately on ice.

Care After Test
➤ Ensure that the client receives food and any medications that were withheld for this test.
➤ Evaluate related tests such as cortisol level and ACTH stimulation test.

Educate Your Client and the Family
➤ Discuss the correlation between high stress levels and production of ACTH and cortisol. Suggest methods the client may use to decrease stress level.
➤ Assess the need for supplemental glucocorticoids if ACTH levels are decreased. Explain the drug therapy of glucocorticoids. Instruct the client not to abruptly stop medications.
➤ Teach client and family the need to wear medical alert identification and to inform primary health care providers and surgeons of the need for glucocorticoids for surgery or stressful procedures.
➤ Coordinate the client's activity schedule of physical therapy, rest periods, and visitation to decrease the physical stress level.

Adrenocorticotropic Hormone Stimulation

ah **dree** noe **kor** ti koe **troe** pik • hor mone • **stim** yu lay shun
(ACTH Stimulation, Cosyntropin Test)

Normal Findings

ALL AGES

Rapid test: >7 µg/dL above baseline
24-hour test: >40 µg/dL above baseline
3-day test: >40 µg/dL above baseline

What This Test Will Tell You

This test diagnoses disorders in the adrenal glands, anterior pituitary gland, or both in order to differentiate between primary and secondary adrenal insufficiency. The test measures the relationship between ACTH and the production of cortisol by the adrenal cortex. Normally, an increase in ACTH produces an increase in cortisol. For this test, synthetic ACTH is given to the client and after a set amount of time, a serum cortisol is drawn.

ACTH released by the anterior pituitary stimulates the adrenal cortex to secrete cortisol. When optimal cortisol levels are reached, there is a negative feedback effect, inhibiting ACTH and thus inhibiting further cortisol production.

If the client shows a marked increase in cortisol following the ACTH administration, adrenal hyperplasia is suspected, as in Cushing's syndrome. An ACTH-producing tumor will not demonstrate an increase in cortisol following ACTH administration because its stimulus to produce cortisol does not occur from ACTH, but rather within the tumor itself.

If there is not an increase in cortisol production following the administration of ACTH, adrenal or ante-rior pituitary insufficiency is suspected.

Abnormal Findings

▲ INCREASED LEVELS may indicate pituitary insufficiency and adrenal cortical hyperplasia/Cushing's disease.

▼ DECREASED LEVELS may indicate primary adrenal insufficiency and Addison's disease.

Interfering Factors

➤ Long-term glucocorticoid therapy, which suppresses ACTH release
➤ Estrogens
➤ Oral contraceptives

NURSING CONSIDERATIONS

Prepare Your Client

➤ Explain that the test measures how well the body produces a hormone, cortisol.
➤ Restrict food and fluids for 8 hours prior to the test.
➤ Assess for glucocorticoid use.

Perform Procedure

RAPID

➤ Draw a baseline serum cortisol level. Place 4 cc venous blood in red-top tube.
➤ Inject the synthetic cosyntropin intramuscularly.
➤ Obtain serum cortisol level in 30 minutes and 60 minutes.

24-HOUR TEST

➤ Obtain a baseline serum cortisol level. Place 4 cc venous blood in red-top tube.
➤ Start an IV of synthetic cosyntropin in normal saline solution.

➤ Administer 2 units/hour for 24 hours.

➤ Obtain serum cortisol level 24 hours after the start of the IV cosyntropin infusion. Make sure to draw this sample in the arm that did not have the IV cosyntropin solution.

3-DAY

➤ Obtain a baseline serum cortisol level. Place 4 cc venous blood in red-top tube.

➤ Start an IV of synthetic cosyntropin in normal saline solution.

➤ Administer 3–4 units/hour for 8 hours. This will be done daily for 2–3 days.

➤ Obtain serum cortisol level 72 hours from the start of the initial IV cosyntropin infusion. Make sure to draw the sample in the arm that did not have the IV cosyntropin solution.

Care After Test

➤ Evaluate for alteration in glucose metabolism by monitoring blood glucose levels.

➤ Evaluate related tests such as ACTH level.

Educate Your Client and the Family

➤ Instruct client on the importance of not stopping glucocorticoid treatment suddenly or without medical supervision.

➤ Teach client with adrenal abnormalities to wear medical alert identification.

➤ Provide emotional support for altered self-concept.

A

Alanine Aminotransferase, Serum

al ah neen • am in oe • trans fur ase • see rum
(ALT, SGPT, Serum Glutamic-Pyruvic Transaminase)

Normal Findings

ADULT
Male: 10–32 U/L
Female: 9–24 U/L
Pregnant: Values unchanged

NEWBORN
Normal values for infants may be twice as high as those for adults.

CHILD, ADOLESCENT
5–35 U/L

ELDERLY
Values may be slightly higher than adult levels.

What This Test Will Tell You

This blood test measures liver function and diagnoses liver disease. Ala-nine aminotransferase is an enzyme found in the cytoplasm of hepatic cells and to a lesser degree in kidney, heart, and skeletal muscle tissues. It is often used in conjunction with a related test, aspartate aminotransferase (AST, or serum glutamic oxatoacetic transaminase, SGOT). These two tests are sometimes referred to as liver enzyme tests and are typically part of a liver function panel, which also includes direct and indirect bilirubin and alkaline phosphatase levels.

Abnormal Findings

▲INCREASED LEVELS (*Very high*

levels—*up to 50 times normal*) may indicate acute viral hepatitis, acute hepatotoxic hepatitis or liver necrosis (related to drug or chemical toxicity).

Moderately increased to high levels may indicate infectious mononucleosis, chronic hepatitis, cholestasis, cholecystitis, chronic congestive heart failure leading to hepatomegaly, or prodromal or improving hepatitis.

Slightly to moderately increased levels may indicate cirrhosis, myocardial infarction, congestive heart failure, or resolving or prodromal hepatitis.

▼ DECREASED LEVELS may indicate resolution of pathology.

ACTION ALERT!

Values greater than 2000 U/L may indicate severe liver necrosis. Jaundice may not be present initially. Impaired clotting is a complication of liver dysfunction and can lead to bleeding and hemorrhage.

Interfering Factors

➤ Many drugs may falsely elevate ALT levels, including antibiotics such as carbenicillin, clindamycin, erythromycin, gentamicin, cephalosporins, tetracycline and ampicillin; narcotic agents such as meperidine, morphine, and codeine; antihypertensives such as methyldopa guanethidine and propranolol; and other drugs such as digitalis, salicylates, heparin, acetaminophen, isoniazid (INH), methotrexate, and chlorpromazine.

➤ Ingestion of lead or exposure to tetrachloride injures hepatic cells and causes high elevations of ALT.

➤ Hemolysis of the blood sample may interfere with the results.

➤ Exercise may decrease levels.

NURSING CONSIDERATIONS

Prepare Your Client

➤ Explain that this test is used to help determine how well the liver is working.

Perform Procedure

➤ Collect 5–7 mL of venous blood in a red-top tube.

➤ Handle tube gently to prevent hemolysis of specimen, which could interfere with results.

➤ Closely observe the venipuncture site for hematoma formation or excessive bleeding due to coagulopathies from hepatic dysfunction. Apply a pressure dressing.

Care After Test

➤ Assess client for unusual bruising or prolonged bleeding from venipuncture site. Delayed clotting is a complication of severely impaired liver function.

➤ Assess skin, sclera of eyes for jaundice and note findings.

➤ Consult with a registered dietician to design a high-calorie, well-balanced diet. People with advanced liver disease have poor absorption of nutrients due to decreased bile flow into the intestines. As appropriate, reduce sodium or protein in the diet if edema and ascites, or increased ammonia levels are present.

➤ Evaluate other liver function tests such as aspartate aminotransferase (AST), direct and indirect bilirubin levels, alkaline phosphatase, serum ammonia, and prothrombin time.

Educate Your Client and the Family

➤ Instruct client and family to report any jaundice—yellow discoloration of the skin or the whites of eyes.

> Instruct client and family on a high-calorie, well-balanced diet as appropriate. If sodium or protein restrictions are indicated, help client and family make dietary selections with these limitations.
> Clients with impaired liver function have prolonged bleeding times. Instruct client and family on safety measures such as electric razors, non-skid shoes, and soft toothbrushes.
> Instruct client and family to report prolonged or unusual bleeding or bruising. Also report very dark colored or tarry stools or esophageal varices, as they are complications of liver disease.

A

Aldolase, Serum

al doe lase • see rum
(ALD, ALS)

Normal Findings
ADULT AND ELDERLY
3.0–8.2 U/dL (SI units: 22–59 mU at 37°C)
Levels are slightly higher in men than women because of greater muscle mass.
NEWBORN
Normal results are 2–4 times the adult level.
CHILD
Normal results are approximately twice adult levels.

What This Test Will Tell You
This blood test is used in conjunction with assays of other enzymes to diagnose hepatic and muscular diseases and to differentiate muscular from neurological pathology in muscular weakness. Aldolase is an enzyme present in skeletal, cardiac, and hepatic tissue that is important in the breakdown of glucose. It is most commonly used to diagnose and monitor the progression of skeletal muscle diseases such as muscular dystrophy and dermatomyositis. Note: if the muscle pathology is related to neurologic disease, serum aldolase levels are normal.

Abnormal Findings
▲INCREASED LEVELS may indicate acute hepatitis (viral or toxic), Duchenne's muscular dystrophy, trauma involving muscles, myocardial infarction, trichinosis, hemolytic anemia, gangrene, melanoma, leukemia, or cancer involving lung, breast, liver, gastrointestinal tract, or genitourinary system.
▼DECREASED LEVELS may indicate late muscular dystrophy, hereditary fructose intolerance, or resolution of pathology.

Interfering Factors
> Thiabendazole, intramuscular injections, hemolysis, and exposure to chlorinated insecticides may increase levels.
> Phenothiazines may cause decreased values.

NURSING CONSIDERATIONS

Prepare Your Client

➤ Explain that this test is to help diagnose acute liver or skeletal muscle disease.

➤ Review the client's environmental and work history for exposure to interfering agents.

Perform Procedure

➤ Collect 2–5 mL of venous blood in a red-top tube.

➤ Carefully inspect the venipuncture site for hematoma formation or prolonged bleeding if liver disease is suspected, and apply a pressure dressing.

Care After Test

➤ If test is used to evaluate acute liver disease, evaluate client for other signs of liver disease such as jaundice, unusual bruising, prolonged bleeding, or ascites.

➤ If test is used to help diagnose or monitor the progression of skeletal muscle disease, evaluate client for muscle weakness, ataxia, and problems with coordination.

➤ Assess for occult gastrointestinal bleeding with routine stool guaiac testing. Esophageal varices and mucosal bleeding are complications of liver disease.

➤ Provide a safe environment that protects the client from injury if muscle weakness or bleeding tendencies are suspected.

➤ Consult with a registered dietician to design a high-calorie, well-balanced diet. Clients with advanced liver disease have poor absorption of nutrients due to decreased bile flow into the intestines. As appropriate, reduce sodium or protein in the diet if edema and ascites, or increased ammonia levels are present.

➤ Review related tests such as serum aminotransferase (AST), alanine aminotransferase (ALT), lactic dehydrogenase (LDH), direct and indirect bilirubin, alkaline phosphatase, prothrombin time, ammonia levels, and creatine phosphokinase (CK or CPK).

Educate Your Client and the Family

➤ Instruct client with liver disease to report any jaundice, excessive bruising, or fullness in abdomen to physician.

➤ Instruct client with suspected muscle disease and their family on proper rest, restricting strenuous activity, and monitoring for difficulty ambulating.

➤ Teach client with liver disease and their family about a high-calorie, well-balanced diet. If sodium or protein restrictions are indicated, help client and family make dietary selections with these limitations.

➤ Clients with impaired liver function have prolonged bleeding times. Instruct client and family on safety measures such as electric razors, non-skid shoes, and soft toothbrushes.

Aldosterone, Serum and Urine

al dos tur one • see rum • and • yur in
(Aldosterone Assay)

Normal Findings

ADULT, ADOLESCENT:
STANDING
Male: 6–22 ng/dL (SI units: 0.17–0.61 nmol/L)
Female: 5–30 ng/dL (SI units: 0.14–0.8 nmol/L)
PREGNANT
Values are 2–4 times higher in pregnancy.
NEONATE
5–60 ng/dL (SI units: 0.14–1.7 nmol/L)
INFANT
1 week–1 year old: 1–160 ng/dL (SI units: .03–4.6 nmol/L)
CHILD
1–3 years old: 5–60 ng/dL (SI units: 0.14–1.7 nmol/L)
3–5 years old: 5–80 ng/dL (SI units: 0.14–2.3 nmol/L)
5–7 years old: 5–50 ng/dL (SI units: 0.14–1.5 nmol/L)
7–11 years old: 5–70 ng/dL (SI units: 0.14–2.0 nmol/L)
ADOLESCENT
11–15 years old: 5–50 ng/dL (SI units: 0.14–1.5 nmol/L)
SUPINE
3–10 ng/dL (SI units: 0.08–0.3 nmol/L)
URINE
2–16 µg/24 hours (SI units: 5.5–45 nmol/24 hours)

What This Test Will Tell You

This blood or urine test measures adrenal cortex function and disorders associated with the adrenal glands. The adrenal cortex secretes numerous hormones, including aldosterone, a mineralocorticoid that regulates retention of sodium and chloride and elimination of potassium and hydrogen. This process has a direct effect upon blood pressure and fluid volume. This test can detect primary or secondary aldosteronism. The most common cause of primary aldosteronism is tumors of the adrenal cortex.

Abnormal Findings

▲INCREASED LEVELS may indicate primary aldosteronism, hyponatremia, hyperkalemia, stressful conditions (mental, physical), obesity, sodium-restricted diet, prolonged physical upright position, Cushing's syndrome, pregnancy, or diuretic or steroid therapy.

▼DECREASED LEVELS may indicate Addison's disease, adrenal destruction, prolonged recumbent position, high sodium diet, hypokalemia, pregnancy, toxemia, or diabetes mellitus.

Interfering Factors

➤ Dietary intake of licorice for 2 weeks prior to the test because it exerts an aldosterone-like effect on the body.

➤ Stress and increased exercise can increase aldosterone levels.

➤ Medications that can increase aldosterone levels include diuretics, diazoxide, estrogen, hydralazine, and nitroprusside.

➤ Medications that can decrease aldosterone levels include fludrocortisone, propranolol, oral contraceptives, and intravenous glucose.

➤Hypokalemia causes decreased

levels.

➤ High or low salt diet.

➤ Supine (lower levels) or standing position (higher levels).

NURSING CONSIDERATIONS

Prepare Your Client

➤ Explain to client that these tests help identify problems with a particular hormone, aldosterone, that helps regulate water balance and blood pressure.

➤ Instruct client that the diet for 2 weeks prior to the test should include at least 3 g of sodium each day. Tell them also not to eat licorice.

➤ Check to see if they are receiving any medications that may alter the test results. If so, consult the primary health care provider to decide whether these should be discontinued 2 weeks prior to the test.

Perform Procedure

SERUM LEVEL

➤ Obtain 5–10 mL venous blood and place in red-top tube.

➤ Draw the sample while the client is in the supine position *before* first rising for the day.

➤ If serum level in standing position is required, draw that *after* the supine level is drawn. Obtain 5–10 mL venous blood and place in red-top tube.

➤ Indicate client position during each blood draw on the lab slip.

➤ Indicate any medications that may alter result on the lab slip.

➤ Send sample on ice to the lab immediately.

URINE

➤ Make sure the collection container is the one required by your institution and has preservative in it. The urine generally needs to be refrigerated during the 24-hour collection period. Carefully follow procedure for 24-hour urine collection.

Care After Test

➤ Monitor blood pressure for hypertension when increased levels are suspected or confirmed.

➤ Monitor for fluid retention with increased levels. Assess blood pressure, lung sounds for crackles, and peripheral edema.

➤ Evaluate skin care precautions carefully in edematous patients.

➤ Evaluate related tests such as serum cortisol and plasma renin.

Educate Your Client and the Family

➤ Explain to both client and family that increased stress increases aldosterone levels.

➤ Teach client who is receiving glucocorticoid treatment not to stop taking it abruptly or without medical supervision. Tell client to inform any other health care providers about steroid therapy (especially prior to surgical or invasive procedures).

➤ Instruct client to wear medical alert identification.

Alkaline Phosphatase, Serum

al kah line • fos fah tase • see rum

(ALP)

Normal Findings

Note: Values vary depending on method used.

ADULT (AGE 20–60)

30–120 U/L

ELDERLY

Slightly higher than adult values.

INFANT

85–230 U/L

CHILD

Values remain high until epiphyses close.

Females, ages 2–10: 100–350 U/L

Females, ages 10–13: 110–400 U/L

Males, ages 2–10: 100–350 U/L

Males, ages 13–15: 125–500 U/L

ISOENZYMES

Liver isoenzyme: 20–130 U/L

Bone isoenzyme: 20–120 U/L

Intestinal isoenzyme: 0–18 U/L

Placental isoenzyme: 50% of total in third trimester (appears from first trimester to 1 month postpartum)

What This Test Will Tell You

This blood test determines the presence of liver and bone disorders. Alkaline phosphatase (ALP) is an enzyme that is normally found in the liver, biliary tract, and bone. Smaller amounts are found in the placenta. ALP levels rise during periods of bone growth (osteoblastic activity), liver disease, and bile obstruction. Isoenzymes of ALP are used to distinguish between liver, bone, and placental disease by separating them with heat fractionalization.

Abnormal Findings

▲INCREASED LEVELS may indicate cirrhosis, rheumatoid arthritis, normal bones of growing children, healing fractures, metastatic bone tumor, intrahepatic or extrahepatic biliary obstruction, primary or metastatic liver tumor, Paget's disease, normal pregnancy or early postpartum, or intestinal ischemia or infarction.

▼DECREASED LEVELS may indicate abnormal bone formation in prepubescent children, scurvy, cretinism, pernicious anemia, hypophosphatemia, celiac disease, pernicious anemia, hypophosphatemia, celiac desease, secondary growth retardation, or hypothyroidism.

Interfering Factors

➤ Hemolyzed specimens should be rejected because results will be inaccurate.

➤ Many medications can cause high readings. These drugs include vitamin D, barbiturates, chlorpropamide, allopurinol, many antibiotics, azathioprine, colchicine, fluorides, indomethacin, isoniazid (INH), methotrexate, methyldopa, nicotinic acid, oral contraceptives, phenothiazine, probenecid, and tetracyclines.

➤ Failure to fast for 10–12 hours prior to collection or specimens left at room temperature can produce falsely elevated results.

> Albumin made from placental tissue can cause elevated ALP.

> Drugs that may cause decreased levels include fluorides, nitrofurantoin, oxylates, and zinc salts.

NURSING CONSIDERATIONS

Prepare Your Client

> Explain that this test is important to help understand how well the liver and bones are working.

> Explain that you will need to draw blood from the vein for the test.

> Tell the client that they will need to fast for 12 hours prior to the test and suggest that the blood be drawn before breakfast. Overnight fasting may be required for isoenzymes.

> Confer with the primary health care provider about which medications the client is taking that will need to be restricted for this test.

Perform Procedure

> Collect 3–10 mL venous blood in a red-top tube.

> Label the sample and note any interfering factors or medications.

> Send to the lab immediately for testing or for spinning and refrigeration.

Care After Test

> Assess fluid and nutritional status for impaired liver function manifested by ascites, spider angiomas, bleeding, decreased albumin level, and decreased muscle mass.

> Evaluate for increased fluid volume manifested by ascites, lower leg edema, and hepatomegaly.

> Watch for bleeding due to hypoprothrombinemia.

> Initiate safety precautions such as night lights and frequent bed checks for client with liver disease because hepatic encephalopathy may impair cognitive functioning.

> Assess client suspected of having bone tumors, metastasis to the bone, or other bone disease for evidence of bone pain, pathological fractures, swelling, and deformities.

> Evaluate other liver and biliary function studies such as biliary excretion, direct and indirect bilirubin, total serum protein, aspartate transaminase (SGOT), alanine transaminase (SGPT), lactic dehydrogenase (LDH), and serum cholesterol.

> Evaluate other indicators of bone function such as serum calcium, phosphorus, complete blood count, and sedimentation rate.

Educate Your Client and the Family

> Explain that eating high-fat food or taking any of several drugs prior to the test can cause falsely high readings.

> Teach the client and family the value of a nutritious diet. Educate them about foods that provide essential proteins and vitamins to avoid or minimize complications of bleeding or encephalopathy.

> Instruct the client and family on safety measures at home to reduce injuries and bleeding if advanced liver or bone disease are present.

Alpha₁-antitrypsin, Serum

al fa an ti trip sin • see rum

(A1AT, AAT, ATT)

Normal Findings

Note: Normal values vary widely. Check with your own laboratory for normal values.

ADULT, CHILD, ADOLESCENT, AND ELDERLY

85–400 mg/dL or ≥250 mg/dL

PREGNANT

Levels may increase by 100% in late pregnancy.

NEWBORN

145–270 mg/dL

What This Test Will Tell You

This blood test screens for high risk of emphysema and liver disease associated with a congenital absence of the alpha₁-antitrypsin (AAT) protein. Other uses for this test include nonspecific detection of inflammatory, infectious, and necrotic processes because AAT levels are often increased with inflammatory conditions.

AAT is a protein produced by the liver. Inherited deficiencies of this protein are associated with early onset of lung and liver disorders in which functional tissue is destroyed and replaced with excessive connective tissue.

Abnormal Findings

▲INCREASED LEVELS may indicate inflammatory disorders, pulmonary infections, cancer, thyroid infections, use of oral contraceptives, pregnancy, stress, strenuous exercise, hyaline membrane disease, rheumatoid arthritis, or bacterial infections.

▼DECREASED LEVELS may indicate early onset of emphysema, cirrhosis, hepatic damage, pulmonary disease, nephrotic syndrome, or malnutrition.

A

Interfering Factors

➤ Serum levels may increase by 100% in pregnancy.

➤ Strenuous exercise, stress, and oral contraceptives may falsely elevate values.

➤ Failure to follow prescribed dietary restrictions prior to the test may alter results, particularly if the client has elevated levels of cholesterol or triglycerides.

NURSING CONSIDERATIONS

Prepare Your Client

➤ Explain that the test is to determine whether there is a protein deficiency that can cause a lung or liver disease.

➤ Instruct the client to fast from food for 8 hours before the test if required by your laboratory. Water is not restricted.

➤ If indicated, advise the client not to take oral contraceptives for 24 hours prior to the test.

Perform Procedure

➤ Perform a venipuncture to collect 5–10 mL of blood in a red-top tube.

➤ Label the tube and send to the laboratory immediately.

Care After Test

➤ If test results show the client is at risk for developing emphysema, begin client education. Include such factors as avoidance of smoking, avoidance of air pollution, avoidance of infection, and education about the disease process of emphysema.

➤ Evaluate related tests such as chest x-ray, pulmonary function, and liver enzymes.

Educate Your Client and the Family

➤ Encourage the client with an AAT deficiency to stop smoking and avoid areas having high air pollution, because AAT deficiencies are associated with emphysema.

➤ Instruct client to use preventive methods to protect their lungs, such as avoiding persons with upper respiratory infections, seeking medical care when they have a respiratory infection, etc.

➤ Suggest that client with AAT deficiency seek genetic counseling because this is an inherited disorder.

Alpha-fetoprotein
al fa fee toe proe teen

Normal Findings

ADULT
<15 ng/mL
PREGNANT
38–45 ng/mL at 16–18 weeks' gestation
CHILD UNDER 1 YEAR
<30 ng/mL; recedes rapidly to adult values.

What This Test Will Tell You

This blood test is used during pregnancy to screen for fetal anomalies, particularly open fetal neural tube defects (e.g., myelomeningocele or spina bifida, and anencephaly). Additionally, this test is used to screen nonpregnant clients for various types of cancer, hepatic disease, and inflammatory bowel diseases, and to monitor the effects of cancer treatment. Alpha-fetoprotein (AFP) is a glycoprotein initially produced by the fetal yolk sac and later by the parenchymal cells of the liver. It is transmitted to maternal blood through the placenta. Maternal serum alpha-fetoprotein (MSAFP)

peaks at 16–18 weeks' gestation, rendering this the optimal time for testing. Fetal serum AFP begins to decline at 34 weeks' gestation and recedes to adult levels after the first year of life. In the event of an elevated MSAFP, an amniocentesis and/or ultrasonography may be recommended for definitive diagnosis. For nonpregnant clients, an elevated serum AFP will be followed by further testing before making a conclusive diagnosis.

Abnormal Findings

▲ INCREASED LEVELS *for pregnant client* may reveal open neural tube defects, multiple pregnancy, omphalocele, esophageal or duodenal atresia, congenital nephrosis, Meckel's syndrome, hydrocephalus, tetralogy of Fallot, Turner's syndrome, intrauterine fetal death, or impending spontaneous abortion.

▲ INCREASED LEVELS *for nonpregnant client* may reveal hepatocellular carcinoma; ovarian or testicular germ-cell tumors; renal tumors; carcinoma of the pancreas, stomach, colon, or lung; Hodgkin's disease; lymphoma; cirrhosis; hepatitis; or inflammatory bowel disease.

▼ DECREASED LEVELS *for pregnant client* may reveal trisomy 13, 18, or 21.

Interfering Factors

➤ Inaccurate dating of pregnancy for estimation of fetal age will affect interpretation of test results.

➤ Multiple pregnancy or fetal death will elevate MSAFP levels and require differentiation from fetal malformations.

➤ Results will need to be adjusted for African-Americans, who have a 10% higher MSAFP, and for diabetics and heavier females, who have a lower MSAFP.

➤ Minimal contamination of amniotic fluid or maternal serum with fetal serum will result in very high values.

➤ Recent radioisotope administration can affect results.

➤ Gentle handling of blood sample is required to prevent hemolysis.

NURSING CONSIDERATIONS

Prepare Your Client

➤ Tell the pregnant client that this test is to help see if her baby is developing normally and if she is having more than one baby.

➤ Explain to pregnant client that if the MSAFP test results are too high or too low, the test will be repeated. If the results are still not normal, other tests may be recommended to find out why the results are not in the normal range.

➤ Explain to nonpregnant client that

this test is to see if there is an indication to check for some types of cancer, liver diseases, and intestinal (bowel or gut) diseases.

➤ Inform client that if the results are high additional testing may be recommended to find the cause.

➤ Explain to client being treated for hepatocellular carcinoma that a drop in AFP levels indicates that the cancer is responding to treatment (the client is getting better).

Perform Procedure

➤ Collect 7–10 mL of venous blood in a 10–15 mL red-top tube.

➤ Label sample and indicate gestational age for pregnant client.

Care After Test

➤ Assess client and family for anxiety related to outcome of test. Offer information and referral as indicated.

➤ Evaluate related tests, such as amniocentesis for pregnant client or other cancer-related studies for nonpregnant client.

Educate Your Client and the Family

➤ Explain to the pregnant client that test results do not prove that the baby is normal or abnormal; if the results are high or low, then further testing may be recommended to find out why the results are different than expected.

➤ Explain to the nonpregnant client that a high test result does not mean that they have cancer or any particular disease. Other tests will be done to find out why the results are different than expected.

➤ Provide an opportunity for client to ask questions.

Amebiasis Antibody

am eh bie a sis • an ti bod ee

(*Entamoeba histolytica* Antibody)

Normal Findings

➤ Normal value: negative.

➤ Titer < 1:32 usually indicates a negative result.

➤ Titer of 1:32–1:64 is inconclusive and needs to be repeated.

➤ Titer of 1:128 or greater indicates active or recent *Entamoeba histolytica* infection.

➤ Titer of 1:256–1:2,048 indicates current infection.

What This Test Will Tell You

This blood test measures and detects antibodies to *Entamoeba histolytica*, the parasite that causes amebic dysentery. Infection by *Entamoeba histolytica* ranges from an asymptomatic carrier state to severe diarrhea and extraintestinal involvement. Antibodies may persist months to years after complete cure.

Serologic testing is important because barium, antibiotics, antiprotozoal agents, and soap or oil enemas make detection of the parasite in the stool impossible. It is recommended for diagnostic workup of clients with inflammatory bowel disease. Those clients with amebic liver infection and/or colonic invasion will test positive for the antibody while the asymptomatic cyst passers will not.

Abnormal Findings

▲ INCREASED LEVELS (positive titers) may indicate amebic liver abscess, intestinal infection, or amebic dysentery/diarrhea.

▼ DECREASED LEVELS (negative titers) may indicate normal, healthy individuals and asymptomatic cyst passers.

ACTION ALERT!

Clients with positive amebiasis antibody and diarrhea are infectious.

NURSING CONSIDERATIONS

Prepare Your Client

➤ Explain that this blood test will look for a parasite infection that can cause dysentery.

Perform Procedure

➤ Collect 5 mL of venous blood in a red-top tube.

Care After Test

➤ Assess your client for dehydration and electrolyte depletion if client has diarrhea.

➤ Treat dehydration with fluid and electrolyte replacement.

➤ Assess your client for fever, abdominal tenderness, and hepatomegaly.

Educate Your Client and the Family

➤ Teach your client that the infection is transmitted by drinking contaminated water or eating contaminated food. It can also be spread by oral or anal sex.

➤ Stress the importance of handwashing.

➤ Explain that it is possible to carry the cysts in the bowel and pass them along to others but never develop the diarrhea or other major symptoms (cyst passer).

> Teach client to scald fresh fruits and vegetables if contamination is suspected. The cysts are very difficult to kill and can survive outside the body. They are even resistant to chlorine.

> If the client has diarrhea, recommend a diet free from milk and lactose as well as high in potassium. Stress the importance of fluid replacement.

Ammonia, Plasma
ah **moe** nya • **plaz** mah

A

Normal Findings
ADULT, PREGNANT, ADOLESCENT, ELDERLY
15–50 µg/dL (SI units: 11–36 µmol/L)
NEWBORN
64–150 µg/dL (SI units: 47–110 µmol/L)
CHILD
40–80 µg/dL (SI units: 29–58 µmol/L)

What This Test Will Tell You
This blood test evaluates hepatic function and estimates the amount of hepatic dysfunction in liver disease. Ammonia is a by-product of protein metabolism and an important part of acid-base balance. Intestinal bacteria break down protein taken in, producing ammonia as a waste product. The body uses the nitrogen product of this metabolic process, and the liver has to convert ammonia to urea, which can then be excreted by the kidneys. Often in severe hepatic failure the liver is unable to carry out this conversion, causing blood levels of ammonia to become elevated.

Abnormal Findings
▲ INCREASED LEVELS may indicate hepatic damage, Reye's Syndrome, congestive heart failure, renal failure, emphysema, erythroblastosis fetalis, pericarditis, bronchitis, cor pulmonale, or leukemia.
▼ DECREASED LEVELS may indicate hypertension.

ACTION ALERT!
Elevated levels, beyond 100–150 µg/dL, are associated with mental status changes. Monitor client for confusion and take safety precautions as indicated.

Interfering Factors
> Hemolysis of blood sample may increase results.
> High-protein diet may increase levels, while a low-protein diet may lower results.
> Exercise may temporarily increase levels.
> Medications and therapy that may increase results include some antibiotics, diphenhydramine, thiazide, ammonium salts, furosemide, and total parenteral nutrition.
> Medications that may decrease results include lactulose, neomycin, kanamycin, potassium salts, and tetracycline.

NURSING CONSIDERATIONS
Prepare Your Client
> Explain that this test measures how well the liver is working.

> Some laboratories may require a fasting sample because protein intake may affect results. If this is required by your laboratory, instruct client about the required fasting time.

Perform Procedure
> Collect 3–10 mL of venous blood in a green-top tube.
> Gently invert the tube several times, place the sample on ice, and send to the lab immediately. Note any antibiotic therapy on the laboratory slip.

Care After Test
> Assess client for unusual bruising or prolonged bleeding from venipuncture site. Delayed clotting is a complication of severely impaired liver function.
> Assess skin, sclera of eyes for jaundice and note findings.
> Consult with a registered dietician to design a high-calorie, well-balanced diet. Clients with advanced liver disease have poor absorption of nutrients due to decreased bile flow into the intestines. As appropriate, reduce sodium or protein in the diet if edema and ascites, or increased ammonia levels are present.
> Administer lactulose as ordered to increase frequency of bowel movements and therefore intestinal excretion of ammonia.
> Administer neomycin or kanamycin as ordered to decrease the amount of intestinal bacteria and ammonia levels.

> Note mental status and document. Increasing plasma levels can be a sign of approaching hepatic coma.
> Evaluate other liver function tests such as aspartate aminotransferase (AST), direct and indirect bilirubin levels, alkaline phosphatase, serum ammonia, and prothrombin time.

Educate Your Client and the Family
> Instruct the client or family to report any jaundice, the yellow discoloration of skin or whites of eyes.
> As appropriate, instruct client and family on a high-calorie, well-balanced diet. If sodium restrictions or protein restrictions are indicated, assist client and family in choosing dietary selections with these limitations.
> Clients with impaired liver function have prolonged bleeding times. Instruct the client and family on safety measures such as electric razors, non-skid shoes, and soft toothbrushes.
> Instruct the client or family to report prolonged or unusual bleeding or bruising. Also tell them to report very dark colored or tarry stools, as esophageal varices are a complication of liver disease.
> If ammonia levels are high, mental alertness may be decreased. Have the family notify staff of any changes in mental status. They know the client better than anyone and may pick up on changes sooner than the medical personnel could.

Amniocentesis
am nee oe sen tee sis

Normal Findings
PREGNANT CLIENT
Normal amniotic fluid is clear, but may contain some white flecks of vernix caseosa if the fetus is near term. (See *Amniotic Fluid Analysis* for further detail.)

What This Test Will Tell You
This test analyzes amniotic fluid to evaluate fetal maturity, fetal health, fetal gender with concern for sex-linked disorders, and fetal abnormalities including chromosomal, metabolic, hemolytic, and neural tube defects. Amniocentesis may also be done to accomplish amniography and fetography. The skilled practitioner who performs the amniocentesis may conduct a gross analysis for clarity of the amniotic fluid. The test is conducted at different points during pregnancy, depending upon the diagnostic purpose, but cannot be conducted until the amniotic fluid volume reaches 150 mL, usually about the 16th week of pregnancy. At that time, tests may be conducted for women and/or couples who have genetic, teratogenic, and age-related factors that create concern for fetal well-being. Tests later in pregnancy may be conducted to evaluate fetal maturity when fetal/maternal/placental factors and timing of delivery may be critical to the health of the newborn.

Abnormal Findings
➤ *Gross analysis of amniotic fluid* may indicate maternal/fetal/placenta/umbilical cord bleeding or meconium-stained amniotic fluid

from fetal distress or breech presentation.

➤ *Analysis for fetal condition* may reveal fetal distress, immature fetal lungs/immature fetus, autosome or sex chromosome abnormalities, open neural tube defects, inborn errors of metabolism, erythroblastosis fetalis, fetal hypoxia, sickle-cell anemia, thalassemia, fetal sepsis, or fetal or umbilical cord bleeding.

➤ *Analysis for maternal condition* may reveal maternal bleeding, abruptio placenta, chorioamnionitis, Rh isoimmunization, or infection.

ACTION ALERT!
➤ Amniotic fluid with a port wine appearance contains blood and suggests maternal, fetal, umbilical cord, or placental needle trauma during the procedure. The fluid is analyzed to determine whether the bleeding is maternal or fetal in origin. Immediate assessment and intervention needs to occur.
➤ Meconium-stained amniotic fluid may indicate fetal distress.

Interfering Factors
➤ Morbid obesity may inhibit transabdominal uterine access due to the depth of subcutaneous tissue.
➤ An anteriorly placed placenta may inhibit transabdominal uterine access.
➤ Oligohydramnios will increase the difficulty of obtaining amniotic fluid.
➤ Blood and meconium in the amniotic fluid will adversely affect the fluid analysis.
➤ Disorders including some cancers and liver diseases can increase alpha-fetoprotein levels.

➤ Disposable plastic syringes may alter amniotic fluid cells.

➤ Room must be darkened to withdraw amniotic fluid being analyzed for bilirubin; fluid is placed immediately in an amber or aluminum foil–wrapped tube and covered to protect it from light and prevent a breakdown in the bilirubin.

Contraindications

➤ Anteriorly placed placenta that prohibits access without placental disruption
➤ Abruptio placenta
➤ History of premature labor
➤ Incompetent cervix

Potential Complications

➤ Trauma to the fetus, umbilical cord, or placenta
➤ Maternal bleeding
➤ Abruptio placenta
➤ Rh sensitization from fetal bleeding into maternal circulation
➤ Leak of amniotic fluid
➤ Infection
➤ Spontaneous abortion
➤ Premature labor
➤ Amniotic fluid embolism
➤ Puncture of bladder or intestines

NURSING CONSIDERATIONS

Prepare Your Client

➤ Explain that this test is to get information about the baby including age and sex as well as any possible problems or abnormalities.

➤ Ensure that an informed consent is obtained, because of the possible complications associated with this procedure.

➤ Tell the client that there are no restrictions on food or fluid prior to the test.

➤ Ask the client if she is allergic to iodine, because a povidone-iodine (Betadine) skin prep may be done prior to the test.

➤ Ensure the client has voided before the procedure if she is 20 or more weeks' pregnant so that the bladder will not be inadvertently punctured. If the client is less than 20 weeks' pregnant, the bladder should not be emptied because it helps to support the uterus in an accessible position.

➤ Take baseline vital signs and fetal heart rate before the procedure.

Perform Procedure

Nurses do not usually perform this procedure, but need to understand it so that it can be explained to client. Explain that ultrasound will be used to locate the placenta and determine the position of the baby so that neither will be damaged during the procedure. Position the client on her back with her hands behind her head or across her chest to avoid touching the sterile field. The procedure takes about 20–30 minutes. Darken the room during the procedure. Shave and cleanse the client's abdomen with a disinfecting solution at the site selected for needle entry. A local anesthetic may be given at the entry site. (Note: Some practitioners do not use local anesthetics as they find equal discomfort with the anesthetic and amniocentesis needle sticks.) Tell the client that she may experience some mild cramping when the needle is inserted into the uterus, and a pulling or suction sensation when the amniotic fluid is removed.

A needle long enough to reach the uterus (spinal needle) that is encased in a special cover known as a stylet is inserted; the stylet facilitates passage of the needle. The stylet is removed and a syringe is attached to the needle. 5–10 mL of amniotic fluid are drawn up into the syringe and the needle is removed. Place the fluid in a light-resistant container. Cleanse the abdomen to remove disinfecting solution and apply a sterile bandage to the needle insertion site.

Care After Test

➤ Assess and record client vital signs and fetal heart rate; report deviations from normal to primary health care provider.

➤ Assess the client for rupture of membranes and uterine contractions by looking for a leak or gush of fluid from the vagina and rhythmical tightening of the uterine muscles resulting in effacement (taking up) and dilatation (opening) of the cervix.

➤ Instruct the client to rest on her left side to prevent and/or correct supine hypotensive syndrome. This position decreases pressure on the vena cava by the gravid uterus, thus increasing venous return and cardiac output.

➤ Assess fetal heart rate and evaluate for changes from baseline or normal heart rate.

➤ Assess the puncture site for drainage.

➤ Determine whether the Rh-negative client has had her prenatal injection of Rh_o immune globulin; if not, the primary maternity care provider may prescribe it at this time to prevent Rh sensitization.

➤ Explain that it takes approximately 2 weeks to get the test results.

➤ Explain that negative results do not ensure a normal baby, but mean that the baby does not appear to have any of the conditions that can be detected by this test.

➤ Explain that the test may be repeated, particularly if monitoring fetal maturity is a critical concern.

➤ Review related tests such as alpha-fetoprotein and fetal ultrasonography.

Educate Your Client and the Family

➤ Instruct the client to notify her primary maternity care provider if she has abdominal pain or cramping, her water breaks, she has bleeding from the vagina, the baby moves less or not at all, or she has chills and a fever.

➤ If a fetal disorder is diagnosed, ensure that the family receives written information in addition to counseling about the diagnosed condition.

Amnioscopy
am nee oss koe pee
(Embryoscopy)

Normal Findings
PREGNANT CLIENT
Clear amniotic fluid, approximately 1000 mL

What This Test Will Tell You
This endoscopic test assesses fetal well-being, especially after the 37th week of gestation, by directly visual-

izing the fetus through an optical device inserted into the vagina and through the cervical opening. In the event of fetal hypoxic insult, intestinal activity of the fetus is stimulated and meconium is expelled. The characteristic color for recently expelled meconium is green or yellow-brown. Oligohydramnios and depressed response of the fetus to the stimulus of a bright light may also indicate fetoplacental insufficiency.

Abnormal Findings

Amnioscopy may reveal fetal abnormalities including breech presentation, post-term fetus, or fetal distress manifested by meconium staining, fetoplacental insufficiency, cord compression, or insertion of umbilical vessels between amnion and chorion.

ACTION ALERT!

Meconium-stained amniotic fluid may indicate fetal distress. Immediate assessment of the fetus is indicated.

Interfering Factors

➤ Spasm of levator muscles
➤ Tight cervical os

Contraindications

➤ Premature rupture of membranes
➤ Active vaginal or cervical infections such as gonorrhea or chlamydia
➤ Placenta previa
➤ Unstable fetal lie

Potential Complications

➤ Rupture of membranes
➤ Stimulation of the onset of labor
➤ Interference with a low-lying placenta
➤ Infection

NURSING CONSIDERATIONS

Prepare Your Client

➤ Explain that this test is to make sure the fluid the baby is in is clear and that the baby is receiving enough oxygen.
➤ Make sure that an informed consent form is signed by the client prior to the procedure.
➤ Tell the client that the procedure will take about 10–15 minutes.
➤ Explain that the client will be lying on her back with her legs supported in stirrups.
➤ Tell the client that she may be uncomfortable during cervical dilatation and may experience vaginal discomfort and menstrual-like cramps after the procedure.
➤ Ask the client if she is allergic to iodine, because a povidone-iodine (Betadine) vaginal prep may be done.
➤ Have the client void before the procedure.
➤ Assess and record the client's vital signs and the fetal heart rate before the procedure.

Perform Procedure

Nurses do not perform this procedure but should understand the process to prepare the client and assist the primary maternity care provider. The primary maternity care provider performs a vaginal examination and cervical assessment. The cervix is dilated or expanded to about 2 fingertips in diameter (2 cm). An amnioscope is inserted into the dilated cervical canal using sterile procedure. A light source is connected to the instrument and visualization of the amniotic fluid is done through the amnioscope.

Care After Test

➤ Assess and record client's vital signs and fetal heart rate; report deviations from normal to primary maternity care provider.

➤ Assess the client for rupture of membranes and uterine contractions by looking for a leak or gush of fluid from the vagina and rhythmical tightening of the uterine muscles resulting in effacement (taking up) and dilatation (opening) of the cervix.

➤ Instruct the client to rest on her left side after the procedure to prevent and/or correct supine hypotensive syndrome. This position decreases pressure on the vena cava by the gravid uterus, thus increasing venous return and cardiac output.

➤ Review related tests such as nonstress test, daily fetal movement count, and obstetric ultrasound.

Educate Your Client and the Family

➤ Instruct the client to notify her primary maternity care provider if she has cramping, her water breaks, she has bleeding from the vagina, the baby moves less or not at all, or she has a fever.

➤ Teach client to perform a daily fetal movement count.

Amniotic Fluid Analysis

am nee ot ik • floo id • ah nal ah sis

Normal Findings

PREGNANT CLIENT

➤ Acetylcholinesterase: Absent.

➤ Alpha-fetoprotein: Level decreases with gestational age.

➤ Bacteria: Absent.

➤ Bilirubin: Optical density (OD) of pigments at 450 nm is 0.015 or less at 36–38 weeks' gestation. This is not a highly reliable measure of fetal maturity.

➤ Biochemical analysis of enzymes: Negative.

➤ Chromosome: Normal karyotype.

➤ Color: Clear; white flecks of vernix caseosa will be found in fluid if the fetus is near term.

➤ Creatinine: ≥2 mg/dL of amniotic fluid indicates mature fetal renal functioning (36+ weeks). <2 mg/dL of amniotic fluid suggests an immature fetus.

➤ DNA analysis: Normal.

➤ Fat cells: 10% or greater at 36–38 weeks' gestation.

➤ Foam stability index (FSI): >0.48 indicates fetal lung maturity.

➤ Lecithin/sphingomyelin (L/S) ratio: 2:1 (3:1 in diabetic mothers) indicates fetal lung maturity; considered the most accurate indicator of fetal lung maturity.

➤ Meconium: Absent.

➤ Phosphatidylglycerol: Present.

What This Test Will Tell You

This fluid analysis evaluates fetal maturity, fetal health, fetal gender with concern for sex-linked disorders, and fetal abnormalities including chromosomal, metabolic, hemolytic, and neural tube defects. The specimen is obtained by performing an amniocentesis. The test is conducted at different points during pregnancy, depending upon the diagnostic purpose, but cannot be conducted until the amniotic fluid volume reaches 150 mL, usually about the 16th week of pregnancy. At that time, tests may be conducted for women and/or couples who have genetic, teratogenic, and age-related factors that create concern for fetal well-being. Tests later in pregnancy may be conducted to evaluate fetal maturity when fetal/maternal/placental factors and timing of delivery may be critical to the health of the newborn.

Abnormal Findings

➤ Acetylcholinesterase: Increased in the presence of open fetal neural tube defects.

➤ Alpha-fetoprotein: Peaks at 13–14 weeks' gestation with a median range of 14–20 mg/L. Median range at 16–18 weeks is 5–15 mg/L.

➤ Bacteria: Presence may indicate fetal infection and/or chorioamnionitis.

➤ Bilirubin: High levels indicate hemolytic disease of the fetus in Rh isoimmunized mother.

➤ Biochemical analysis of enzymes: Abnormal findings indicate inborn errors of metabolism as well as other genetic disorders.

➤ Chromosome: Abnormal karyotype indicates autosomal or sex chromosome anomalies.

➤ Color: Red indicates bleeding from maternal, placental, fetal, or umbilical cord trauma; important to identify source. A yellow discoloration may occur with increased bilirubin and a yellow-brown color may be associated with fetal death.

➤ Creatinine: <2 mg/dL of amniotic fluid suggests an immature fetus.

➤ DNA analysis: Abnormal findings can reveal sickle-cell anemia and thalassemia.

➤ Fat cells: <10% indicates gestational age <35–36 weeks.

➤ Foam stability index (FSI): <0.48 suggests immature fetal lungs.

➤ Lecithin/sphingomyelin (L/S) ratio: <2:1 (<3:1 in diabetic mothers) indicates immature fetal lungs; also, 2:1 ratio may not indicate fetal lung maturity in the event of erythroblastosis fetalis or fetal sepsis.

➤ Meconium: Presence may indicate fetal hypoxic insult or post-term fetus; may be associated with breech presentation.

➤ Phosphatidylglycerol: Absent with fetal lung immaturity.

ACTION ALERT!

➤ Amniotic fluid with a port wine appearance contains blood and suggests maternal, fetal, umbilical cord, or placental needle trauma during the procedure. The fluid is analyzed to determine whether the bleeding is maternal or fetal in origin. Immediate assessment and intervention needs to occur.

➤ Meconium-stained amniotic fluid may indicate fetal distress.

Interfering Factors

➤ Oligohydramnios may cause inaccurate test results.

➤ Blood and meconium in the amniotic fluid will adversely affect the fluid analysis.

➤ Disorders including some cancers and liver diseases can increase alpha-fetoprotein levels.

➤ Disposable plastic syringes may alter amniotic fluid cells.

➤ Room must be darkened to withdraw amniotic fluid being analyzed for bilirubin; fluid is placed immediately in an amber or aluminum foil–wrapped tube and covered to protect it from light and prevent a breakdown in the bilirubin.

Contraindications
See *Amniocentesis.*

Potential Complications
See *Amniocentesis.*

NURSING CONSIDERATIONS
See *Amniocentesis.*

A

Amylase, Serum
am il ase • see rum
(Blood Amylase)

Normal Findings
ADULT, ADOLESCENT, AND CHILD
50–190 IU/L
80–150 Somogyi units/dL
(SI units: 25–125 U/L)
PREGNANT
Values may show slight increases during pregnancy.
NEWBORN
<80 Somogyi units/dL
ELDERLY
Levels may be slightly increased in elderly clients.

What This Test Will Tell You
This blood test differentiates between pancreatitis, trauma to the pancreas, and other abdominal symptoms. Amylase is an enzyme produced in both the salivary glands and pancreas, and secreted into the gastrointestinal (GI) tract. Most commonly, obstruction of the pancreatic duct (from inflammation, pancreatic tumor, or a gallstone) or trauma to the pancreas leads to an outpouring of amylase into the peritoneum and lymph system. The amylase is then absorbed into the bloodstream by blood vessels in the peritoneum, leading to elevations in blood levels of amylase.

Abnormal Findings
▼ DECREASED LEVELS *of serum amylase* may indicate chronic pancreatitis, cirrhosis, pancreatic cancer, toxemia of pregnancy, or hepatitis.
▲ INCREASED LEVELS *of serum amylase* may indicate acute pancreatitis, perforated peptic ulcer, perforated bowel, obstruction of the common bile duct, obstruction of the pancreatic duct, trauma to the pancreas, parotitis (mumps), pulmonary infarction, chronic pancreatitis with exacerbation, acute cholecystitis, ectopic pregnancy, or diabetic ketoacidosis.

ACTION ALERT!
Levels increased threefold may indicate severe disease. Permanent loss of pancreatic functions or death may result from pancreatic dysfunction or secondary complications such as adult respiratory distress syndrome.
Do not use morphine for pain management in clients with known or suspected pancreatitis. It may produce spasms of the pancreatic duct and worsen the symptoms of pancreatitis.

Interfering Factors

➤ Medications and substances that may elevate serum amylase levels include narcotics, aminosalicylic acid, indomethacin, pentazocine, rifampin, salicylates, asparaginase, sulfasalazine, bethanechol, corticosteroids, dexamethasone, ethyl alcohol, glucocorticoids, azathioprine, loop diuretics, methyldopa, oral contraceptives, iodine-containing contrast media, and diatrizoate.

➤ Medications that may reduce serum levels of amylase include oxalates, glucose, and citrates.

➤ Intravenous dextrose may lower serum amylase, resulting in a deceptively lower value.

➤ Hemolysis of the blood sample due to rough handling during collection or transport of the specimen may alter test results.

➤ Spasm of the sphincter of Oddi may produce elevations of serum amylase without an existing injury or disease of the pancreas.

➤ Contamination of the blood sample with saliva by coughing or sneezing near an open sample container may introduce added amylase to the sample.

➤ Individuals with an acute episode of mumps will have elevated amylase due to the involvement of the parotid glands, which produce amylase.

➤ Clients who have recently had pancreatic surgery or have confirmed perforated ulcer, perforated intestine, or abdominal abscess will display increased levels of serum amylase.

➤ Clients with chronic pancreatic disorders may have lower levels because the diseased pancreas loses its ability to produce as much amylase.

NURSING CONSIDERATIONS

Prepare Your Client

➤ Explain that this test helps to determine whether an important gland of the body called the pancreas is healthy or damaged.

➤ Instruct client to avoid ingestion of alcohol for 24 hours prior to testing.

➤ If narcotic analgesics must be used, selection of a medication *other than* morphine will be preferable. Morphine is more likely than other narcotics to cause spasm of the sphincter of Oddi.

Perform Procedure

➤ Collect 5–7 mL of venous blood in a red-top tube.

Care After Test

➤ Evaluate for signs and symptoms of pancreatitis including abdominal and back pain, nausea, vomiting, fever, and abdominal tenderness. In severe cases, look for respiratory distress, shock, electrolyte imbalances, and mental status changes.

➤ Maintain careful and accurate intake and output records of fluid balance.

➤ Assess for disturbances in glucose metabolism by assessing for hypoglycemia and hyperglycemia.

➤ If changes in mentation occur, institute safety precautions to avoid injury.

➤ If electrolyte imbalances are suspected or known, monitor the electrocardiogram continuously.

➤ Assess for occult blood in the stool.

➤ If a perforated peptic or duodenal ulcer is suspected, assess your client for fresh gastric bleeding using a nasogastric tube and saline lavage. If positive, continued iced saline lavage and IV access is advisable.

➤ Review related tests such as urine amylase, serum albumin, serum glucose, hemoglobin, arterial blood gases, hematocrit, red blood cell count, blood urea nitrogen, serum and urine creatinine, white blood cell count and differential, haptoglobin, and liver enzyme studies.

Educate Your Client and the Family

➤ Inform client and family that fat, caffeine-containing drinks, and alcohol will worsen symptoms because they increase the activity of the pancreas.

➤ Stress the importance of long-term follow-up with the primary health care provider to monitor recovery and any future problems with the pancreas.

➤ If the client is presenting with acute abdominal symptoms, explain that test samples must be obtained *before* therapeutic intervention. Some interventions may influence amylase levels or affect other testing used in differential diagnosis.

Amylase, Urine
am il ase • yur in

Normal Findings

ALL AGES

10–80 amylase units/hour, or 0–17 U/hour) (Mayo Clinic)

3–35 IU/hour

6–30 Wohlgemuth units/mL

Up to 6000 Somogyi units/24 hours, 60 275 Somogyi units/hour

(SI units: 6.5–48.1 U/hour)

PREGNANT

Elevations during pregnancy may indicate an ectopic pregnancy.

What This Test Will Tell You

This timed urine test is performed in clients with suspected pancreatitis or gastrointestinal disorders. In the presence of normal renal function, urine and serum amylase levels rise in the presence of acute pancreatitis and similar conditions. However, urine amylase levels remain elevated for 5–7 days after serum amylase has returned to normal. Urine amylase levels rise when excess amylase is absorbed into the circulating bloodstream and cleared by the kidneys.

An amylase to creatinine clearance ratio of 5% or more is diagnostic criteria for pancreatitis. Elevations of urine amylase may be 40 times normal levels during acute episodes of pancreatitis.

Abnormal Findings

▼ DECREASED LEVELS *of urine amylase* may indicate chronic pancreatitis, cirrhosis, hepatitis, alcoholism, cachexia, liver cancer, or hepatic abscess.

▲ INCREASED LEVELS *of urine amylase* may indicate acute pancreatitis, obstruction of the pancreatic duct, pancreatic cancer, parotitis (mumps), trauma to the pancreas or spleen, diabetic ketoacidosis, perforated peptic or duodenal ulcer, cholecystitis, cholelithiasis, intestinal obstruction, renal failure, ectopic pregnancy, necrotic bowel, or pulmonary infarction.

Do not use morphine for pain management in client with known or suspected pancreatitis. It may produce spasms of the pancreatic duct and worsen the symptoms of pancreatitis.

Interfering Factors

➤ Medications that increase urine amylase levels include aspirin, thiazide diuretics, narcotic analgesics, indomethacin, bethanechol, and pentazocine, and alcohol ingested within 24 hours of testing.

➤ Fluoride may lower urine amylase levels.

➤ Contamination with blood, feces, toilet paper, or bacteria may interfere with accuracy of results.

➤ Failure to keep the urine collection refrigerated or on ice during collection and when transported to the lab may alter the test results.

➤ Contamination of the specimen with saliva (which contains amylase) by coughing, sneezing or talking over the uncovered specimen may contaminate the specimen.

➤ Failure to collect all of the urine produced during the collection period may affect the test results.

Contraindications

➤ Menstruation; may need to reschedule for after the completion of menstrual cycle

➤ Disorder producing blood in the urine

NURSING CONSIDERATIONS

Prepare Your Client

➤ Explain that this test helps to evaluate how well a gland in the body called the pancreas is working.

➤ Explain the process of a 24-hour collection of urine to the client and family.

➤ Instruct the client to drink generous amounts of fluids, unless otherwise indicated.

➤ Explain to your client that the urine specimen must be kept free of contaminants of blood, feces, bacteria, saliva, and toilet paper. Describe how to collect the specimen without contaminating it.

Perform Procedure

➤ Closely follow the procedure for collection of a 24-hour urine sample.

➤ Place the urine in a clean container which does *not* contain a preservative.

➤ Maintain this container under refrigerated conditions or on ice throughout the collection period.

Care After Test

➤ Evaluate for signs and symptoms of pancreatitis including abdominal and back pain, nausea, vomiting, fever, and abdominal tenderness. In severe cases, look for respiratory distress, shock, electrolyte imbalances, and mental status changes.

➤ Maintain careful and accurate intake and output records of fluid balance.

➤ Assess for disturbances in glucose metabolism by assessing for hypoglycemia and hyperglycemia.

➤ If changes in mentation occur, institute safety precautions to avoid injury.

➤ If electrolyte imbalances are suspected or known, monitor the electrocardiogram continuously.

➤ Assess for occult blood in the stool.

➤ If a perforated peptic or duodenal ulcer is suspected, assess client for fresh gastric bleeding using a naso-gastric tube and saline lavage. If positive, continued iced saline lavage and IV access is advisable.

➤ Review related tests such as serum amylase, serum albumin, serum glucose, hemoglobin, arterial blood gases, hematocrit, red blood cell count, blood urea nitrogen, serum and urine creatinine, white blood cell count and differential, haptoglobin, and liver enzyme studies.

Educate Your Client and the Family

➤ Inform client and family that fat, caffeine-containing drinks, and alcohol will worsen symptoms because they increase the activity of the pancreas.

➤ Stress the importance of long-term follow-up with the primary health care provider to monitor recovery and any future problems with the pancreas.

Androstenedione
an droe steen dee one

Normal Findings
ADULT
Premenopausal Female: 60–300 ng/dL
Postmenopausal Female: 30–800 ng/dL
Male: 90–170 ng/dL
NEWBORN
20–290 ng/dL
CHILD
8–50 ng/dL
ADOLESCENT
8–240 ng/dL

What This Test Will Tell You
This blood test facilitates diagnosis, evaluation, and management of androgen dysfunction, including ovarian, testicular, menstrual, and menopausal disorders as well as premature development of secondary sexual characteristics. Androstenedione is one of the major types of androgens normally secreted by men and women. It is produced by adrenal glands and the stromal cells of the ovaries and then converted to

estrone by adipose tissue and blood.

Abnormal Findings
▲ INCREASED LEVELS may indicate Cushing's syndrome, polycystic ovary syndrome; congenital adrenal hyperplasia; female pseudohermaphroditism; a gonadal, adrenocortical, or ectopic tumor producing adreno-corticotropic hormone (ACTH); hirsutism; Stein-Leventhal Syndrome; osteoporosis in females; or gynecomastia in males.

▼ DECREASED LEVELS may indicate sickle-cell anemia, adrenal failure, or ovarian failure.

Interfering Factors
➤ Intake of steroid or pituitary hormones.

➤ Serum samples must be refrigerated and processed within 1 hour of collection for accurate analysis. Frozen serum may be sent to specially equipped laboratories for analysis.

➤ Gentle handling of blood sample is required to prevent hemolysis.

> Timing of the menstrual cycle.

NURSING CONSIDERATIONS
Prepare Your Client
> Explain that this test helps evaluate the amount of a hormone being produced by the body. The test may be used in the diagnostic or treatment phases.
> Consult with the primary health care provider about withholding hormone therapy before the test.

Perform Procedure
> Collect 8–10 mL of venous blood in a 10-mL red-top tube; blood amount must be adequate to collect 2 mL of serum. Collect sample in the morning to account for temporal changes in levels.
> Label sample including age and gender of client and, if pertinent to client, phase of menstrual cycle, and the name of each prescribed steroid or pituitary hormone and last date taken.
> Collect sample 1 week before or after menstruation.

Care After Test
> Instruct the client to resume taking prescribed hormones unless otherwise directed by the primary health care provider.
> Refer as indicated for counseling for body image disturbances.
> Review related tests such as serum estrogen and progesterone levels.

Educate Your Client and the Family
> Explain that this test is one of several that will help to find out how much of this hormone the body is making.
> Explain that it may be necessary to repeat the test.
> Explain that other tests will also be used to help determine the best course of treatment.

Angiotensin-Converting Enzyme, Serum
an jee oe ten sin • con vurt ing • en zime • see rum
(ACE, SACE)

Normal Findings
ADULT, PREGNANT, AND ELDERLY
18–67 U/L
NEWBORN, CHILD, AND ADOLESCENT
ACE levels are higher in people under age 20 than in adults.

What This Test Will Tell You
This blood test is used primarily in clients with sarcoidosis to evaluate the severity of the disease and the response to therapy. Angiotensin-converting enzyme (ACE) is found mainly in lung epithelial cells and in smaller amounts in blood vessels and renal tissue. It converts angiotensin I to angiotensin II, a vasopressor that stimulates the adrenal cortex to produce aldosterone and is important in regulating arterial blood pressure. Elevated ACE levels are found in a high percentage of clients with sarcoidosis. However, about 5% of the normal adult population have ele-

vated levels. If sarcoidosis is suspected, a tissue biopsy is performed to confirm the diagnosis.

Abnormal Findings

▲ INCREASED LEVELS may indicate sarcoidosis, Gaucher's disease, diabetes mellitus, leprosy, cirrhosis, tuberculosis, chronic renal disease, hyperthyroidism, silicosis, Hodgkin's disease, myeloma, scleroderma, active histoplasmosis, amyloidosis, pulmonary embolism, idiopathic pulmonary fibrosis, or hyperthyroidism.

▼ DECREASED LEVELS may indicate steroid therapy, adult respiratory distress syndrome, or hypothyroidism.

Interfering Factors

➤ Steroid therapy can cause decreased ACE levels.
➤ Hemolysis of the blood sample will result in inaccurate ACE levels.
➤ Failure to properly store or promptly transport the specimen will result in lower ACE levels.

Contraindications

➤ The test should not be performed on persons under age 20 because they normally have very high levels of ACE.

NURSING CONSIDERATIONS

Prepare Your Client

➤ Explain, as appropriate, that the test is to evaluate sarcoidosis or is one of several tests to diagnose their condition.
➤ Explain that you will need to draw blood from the vein for the test.

Describe the venipuncture process clearly.

Perform Procedure

➤ Perform a venipuncture to collect 5–7 ml of blood in a red-top tube. Some laboratories may require a green-top tube.
➤ Apply pressure to the venipuncture site.
➤ Write the client's age on the laboratory slip.
➤ Note on the laboratory slip if the client is taking steroids.

Care After Test

➤ Assess client with elevated ACE levels for symptoms of pulmonary sarcoidosis such as shortness of breath, cough, fatigue, weight loss, and fever.
➤ Evaluate related tests such as chest x-ray, pulmonary function, or tissue biopsies.

Educate Your Client and the Family

➤ Inform client that about 5% of healthy people have elevated ACE levels.
➤ If a diagnosis of sarcoidosis is made, describe the disease process and explain that treatment with steroids often results in dramatic improvement in symptoms.
➤ Teach client and family to observe for adverse responses to steroid therapy, if appropriate.
➤ Teach client and family how to take blood pressure, if indicated.
➤ Teach client to pace activities, conserve energy, and improve nutritional intake.

Anion Gap

an ie on • gap

(Anion Gap, Blood, R Factor)

Normal Findings

All ages: 8–18 mEq/L (SI units: 8–18 mmol/L)

A normal anion gap in the presence of acidosis may indicate renal tubular acidosis, diarrhea, parenteral hyperalimentation, administration of sodium chloride, fistulas of the gastrointestinal tract, sickle-cell nephropathy, or hydronephrosis.

What This Test Will Tell You

This blood test helps in the diagnosis and treatment of different types of acidosis by measuring the difference between serum cations (positively charged particles) and anions (negatively charged particles). When a metabolic acidosis is caused by an increased production of usually *unmeasured* ions from acids such as ketone bodies, lactic acid, phosphates, and sulfates, the gap is increased. However, the gap remains unchanged in metabolic acidosis caused by a loss of bicarbonate ions or an increase in chloride ions because compensatory mechanisms balance with an increase or decrease in the measured anions Cl^- and HCO_3^-.

The anion gap is calculated from the following formula:

$$\text{Anion gap} = (Na^+ + K^+) - (Cl^- + HCO_3^-)$$

Abnormal Findings

▲ INCREASED LEVELS (>18 mEq/L) may indicate lactic acidosis, ketoacidosis, alcohol intoxication, renal failure, severe dehydration, severe salicylate intoxication, starvation and fasting, antifreeze ingestion, or paint thinner ingestion.

▼ DECREASED LEVELS (<8 mEq/L) may indicate high values of electrolytes including sodium, calcium, and magnesium; nephrosis; or multiple myeloma.

ACTION ALERT!

Levels greater than 18 mEq/L may indicate life-threatening metabolic acidosis from a lack of oxygen or normal metabolism in the tissues. Be especially diligent for cardiac dysrhythmias and respiratory distress that can occur in acidosis and lead to cardiopulmonary arrest.

Interfering Factors

➤ Hemolysis of blood sample increases potassium and bicarbonate levels.

➤ Lithium, vasopressin, chlorpropamide, high doses of penicillin, diuretics, carbenicillin, salicylates, paraldehyde, methanol ingestion, dieting, and starvation may elevate levels.

➤ Licorice, adrenocorticotropic hormone, cortisone, phenylbutazone, and diuretics may decrease levels.

➤ Falsely low results occur from iodine absorption if wounds are packed with povidone-iodine.

➤ A normal anion gap may exist with acidosis in the presence of diarrhea, hyperalimentation, renal tubular acidosis, and ureterostomies.

➤ A normal anion gap exists with metabolic acidosis when bicarbonate is lost in the body fluids and chloride is retained. These conditions include pancreatic fistulas, renal tubular acidosis, and renal loop hypofunctioning.

NURSING CONSIDERATIONS

Prepare Your Client
➤ Explain that this test tells how well the body is taking care of important chemicals and acids.

Perform Procedure
➤ Collect 7–10 mL of venous blood in a red-top tube.
or
➤ Calculate the anion gap from recently compiled electrolyte values of sodium, potassium, chloride, and bicarbonate. Use the formula from the section What This Test Will Tell You.

Care After Test
➤ Assess for signs and symptoms of metabolic acidosis if anion gap is greater than 18 mEq/L. Look for rapid, vigorous breathing (Kussmaul's respirations); increased pulse rate; and flushed skin.

➤ Assess for signs and symptoms of metabolic alkalosis if anion gap is less than 8 mEq/L. Look for shallow, slow breathing; disorientation; lethargy; and possible convulsions.
➤ Initiate safety precautions for client with metabolic alkalosis (anion gap less than 8 mEq/L) because cognitive functioning may be impaired.
➤ Obtain order for cardiac arrhythmia monitoring if hyperkalemia (potassium level greater than 5.5 mEq/L) is present.
➤ Review related tests including sodium, potassium, chloride, and bicarbonate levels and arterial blood gases.

Educate Your Client and the Family
➤ If metabolic alkalosis is present, explain the importance of safety precautions to the client and family.
➤ If hyperkalemia is present, explain that cardiac monitoring is required for possible heart rhythm problems.

Antegrade Pyelography
an teh grayd • pie eh log grah fee
(Pyelography, Antegrade)

Normal Findings
ADULTS
Following injection of contrast medium, the upper collecting system of the urinary tract should fill uniformly and appear normal in size and course. The normal bladder and bilateral ureters should be outlined clearly to determine their shape, size, and location.

PREGNANT
Slight-to-moderate hydroureter and hydronephrosis; right kidney larger than left kidney.
INFANT
Urinary bladder is an abdominal organ in infants because of the small conical pelvis.
CHILD
Bladder size differs widely among

individual children and is generally greater in girls than in boys.

Defects in the ureters are related to the vesicoureteral junction and the possible reflux of urine into the ureter or subsequent renal pelvis. Bladder capacity is reduced. Bladder muscles weaken, causing incomplete emptying. Bladder outlet changes may cause obstruction in the male (benign prostatic hypertrophy) or incontinence in the female. Progressive loss of the whole nephrons and renal mass (mainly cortex) occurs in the kidney, resulting in smaller size.

What This Test Will Tell You

This radiographic procedure examines the upper collecting system when there is a urinary tract obstruction and (1) retrograde ureteropyelography is contraindicated, and/or (2) poor renal function prohibits adequate visualization through an intravenous pyelogram. The test can determine the shape, size, and location of the bladder and bilateral ureters, and it can assess the filling of the upper collecting system of the urinary tract. It can also measure renal pressure. Urine collected during the test can be evaluated for culture, cytologic studies, and renal functional reserve. This procedure may also be used for therapeutic procedures to treat urinary tract anomalies, including the placement of a nephrostomy tube or a ureteral stent (catheter) to allow the kidney to drain.

Abnormal Findings

Abnormalities may indicate ureteral strictures, ureteral stones, ureteral obstructive tumors, intrarenal reflux, hydronephrosis, antegrade pyelo-nephrosis, or urinary tract dilation.

█████ ACTION ALERT!

Any intrarenal pressure value that exceeds 20 cm H$_2$O indicates obstruction that, if left untreated, can lead to chronic end stage renal disease. Monitor for signs of kidney damage from back pressure (costovertebral angle [CVA], tenderness, hypertension and dysuria).

Interfering Factors

➤ Movement of the person during the procedure may cause inadvertent puncture of other area structures.
➤ Visualization of the kidney can be impaired if feces or gas is present in the bowel, or if barium procedures have recently been performed.

Potential Complications

Hemorrhage
Extravasation of urine
Infection/sepsis
Allergic reactions/anaphylaxis
Hematoma
Pneumothorax
Nephrostomy tube obstruction

Contraindications

➤ Pregnancy, unless test is absolutely necessary. Because of the fetal radiation hazard it is best postponed until 6 weeks postpartum.
➤ Allergy to the contrast medium, unless test is modified.
➤ Clotting disorder. Be aware of baseline prothrombin time (PT) and partial thromboplastin time (PTT).

NURSING CONSIDERATIONS

Prepare Your Client

➤ Explain that this test is to examine the shape, size, and location of the bladder and ureters (long, thin tubes that carry urine from the kidneys to the bladder) and kidneys and to

make sure they are working properly.
➤ Make sure an informed consent is obtained, because of the possible complications associated with this procedure.
➤ Assess the chart for history of allergic reaction to iodine, shellfish, or radiographic dye.
➤ Instruct client to remain as motionless as possible during the procedure.
➤ Record baseline vital signs.
➤ Restrict food and fluids for 4 hours before the procedure.
➤ Administer sedatives or tranquilizers as ordered before the client goes to the radiology department.
➤ Do not remove glasses, dentures, or hearing aids unless dictated by your institution's policy. The client may need these to communicate and cooperate during the procedure.
➤ Assess the client's history and recent coagulation studies for indications of bleeding disorders.

Perform Procedure

Nurses do not perform this procedure, but should understand the process to prepare the client. Assist the client into a face-down position on the table. Specific positioning will depend on the x-ray or ultrasound identification of kidney position. The site over the renal pelvis is cleansed and local anesthetic is injected. Warn the client this may cause a brief stinging sensation.

Under fluoroscopy a 1.5-inch, 14-gauge needle with stylet is inserted percutaneously into selected site. A manometer is used if intrarenal pressure monitoring is required. Obtain urine specimen and send it to the laboratory. Contrast medium is injected equal to amount of urine

removed. Fluoroscopic x-rays are taken of urinary structures. Apply percutaneous nephrostomy tube if drainage is needed.

Care After Test

➤ Monitor vital signs closely until stable; usually every 15 minutes for the first hour, every 30 minutes for the next hour, and then every 4 hours for 24 hours.
➤ Assess dressing for bleeding, hematoma, or urine leakage at the puncture site at each check of vital signs. Report urine leakage to the primary health care provider.
➤ Monitor fluid intake and urine output for at least 24 hours. Notify the health care provider if client is unable to void for 8 hours. Observe urine for hematuria. Report hematuria that persists after third voiding.
➤ Observe for and report signs of sepsis or leaking of contrast medium (chills, fever, rapid pulse or respirations, hypotension).
➤ Check patency and drainage of nephrostomy tube if present.
➤ Notify the primary health care provider immediately if abdominal or flank pain are present, or if a pneumothorax is suspected due to respiratory difficulty that indicates adjacent organ puncture.
➤ Administer analgesics and antibiotics as prescribed.
➤ Encourage fluids, if not contraindicated, due to diuretic effect of contrast material.
➤ Enforce bed rest for 8–12 hours after the procedure to reduce risk of bleeding.
➤ Evaluate related tests such as renal ultrasound, blood urea nitrogen, and serum creatinine.

Educate Your Client and the Family

➤ Encourage the client to drink fluids, if permitted, to rid the body of contrast material faster.

➤ If renal calculi are present, teach the client dietary modifications that may help reduce stone formation, including getting enough fluids, and acidification or alkalinization of urine as indicated.

Antidiuretic Hormone

an ti die yu reh tic • hor mone
(ADH, Vasopressin)

Normal Findings

1–5 pg/mL (SI units: <1.5 ng/L)

What This Test Will Tell You

This blood test measures the level of antidiuretic hormone (ADH), particularly in the diagnosis of syndrome of inappropriate antidiuretic hormone or diabetes insipidus. Antidiuretic hormone is made in the hypothalamus, but stored and released by the posterior pituitary. Its principle function is to control fluid balance by regulating the renal excretion of water in response to serum osmolality. If serum osmolality increases, signaling dehydration, then ADH is released to decrease renal excretion of water. Conversely, if serum osmolality is decreased, signaling fluid overload, then ADH secretion is decreased to increase fluid excretion.

In addition to serum osmolality, other conditions can cause ADH release, including abnormalities in the pituitary or hypothalamus, neurological trauma, neoplasms, pulmonary disease, and renal disease.

Abnormal Findings

▲ INCREASED LEVELS may indicate syndrome of inappropriate ADH (SIADH), hypovolemia, dehydration, severe trauma, postoperative condition, central nervous system tumors, pneumonia, or pulmonary tuberculosis.

▼ DECREASED LEVELS may indicate diabetes insipidus, overhydration, hypervolemia, surgical trauma to pituitary, or renal disease.

Interfering Factors

➤ Medications that may elevate ADH levels include acetaminophen, nicotine, carbamazepine, estrogen, tricyclic antidepressants, oral hypoglycemic agents, and thiazide diuretics.

➤ Positive pressure ventilation, pain, and stress may increase levels of ADH.

➤ Medications which may decrease ADH levels include morphine agonists, alcohol, beta-adrenergics, and phenytoin.

➤ Alcohol may decrease ADH levels.

➤ Radioactive scan within 1 week of

blood sampling will interfere with results.

➤ Glass tubes or syringes for sampling may affect results.

NURSING CONSIDERATIONS
Prepare Your Client
➤ Explain that this test is to measure ADH, which regulates water balance in the body.
➤ Restrict food for 12 hours prior to blood sampling.
➤ Ask the client to refrain from engaging in significant physical activity for 10–12 hours before the sampling.
➤ Instruct the client to lie down for 30 minutes prior to sampling.

Perform Procedure
➤ Collect 7 mL of venous blood in a *plastic* red-top tube.

Care After Test
➤ Monitor intake and output closely.
➤ Observe for signs and symptoms of fluid imbalance. For overhydration, note pitting edema, dyspnea, weight gain, tachycardia, and hypertension. For dehydration, note poor skin turgor, postural hypotension, increased body temperature, and thirst.
➤ Review related tests such as serum electrolytes and serum osmolality.

Educate Your Client and the Family
➤ If stress or excessive alcohol consumption appear to be factors in elevated ADH levels, instruct client on stress-reducing exercises and refer for counseling as indicated.

Anti-Insulin Antibody
an tee **in** suh lin • an ti **bod** ee
(Anti–Beta Cell Antibody, Anti–Insulin Receptor Antibody)

Normal Findings
No antibodies present
<3% binding of labeled beef and/or pork insulin by client's own serum

What This Test Will Tell You
This blood test determines insulin resistance and can determine the most appropriate therapeutic agent for a diabetic client. Diabetics may form antibodies to the insulin they are given thereby requiring larger doses of insulin to control glucose levels. They may also form antibodies to the insulin-producing beta cells of the pancreas, or to insulin receptors.

Abnormal Findings
Abnormal results may reveal insulin resistance or insulin allergies.

Interfering Factors
➤ Radioactive scanning within 7 days prior to the test

NURSING CONSIDERATIONS
Prepare Your Client
➤ Explain that this test will help determine if antibodies are being formed by the body to keep the insulin from working well.

Perform Procedure

➤ Collect 7 mL of venous blood in a red-top tube.

Care After Test

➤ Assess glucose control of the client closely. Monitor for increasing insulin needs without a known reason such as an increase in activity or change in diet.

➤ Evaluate any signs and symptoms of diabetic ketoacidosis including deep, rapid respirations, change in level of consciousness, thirst, polyuria, and hunger.

➤ Consult with a registered dietician for client demonstrating abnormal glucose levels related to diabetes mellitus.

➤ Review related tests such as serum glucagon, random glucose level, and urine glucose level.

Educate Your Client and the Family

➤ Teach family and client to monitor the amount of insulin required to maintain a normal glucose level, and to notify the primary health care provider of any upward trends in amount of insulin required.

➤ If test is positive, instruct client to use only human insulin and assist in the switch from the beef or pork insulin to the human insulin.

➤ Reinforce previous teaching on insulin injection and rotation of sites to maximize absorption.

Antimitochondrial Antibody

an ti mie toe kon dree al • an ti bod ee
(AMA)

Normal Findings

Negative
Titer levels < 1:5

What This Test Will Tell You

This blood test helps diagnose primary biliary cirrhosis (PBC) by measuring the presence of antimitochondrial antibody. PBC is characterized by a necrotizing and inflammatory process that destroys the bile duct cells and damages liver cells, leading to hepatic failure. Other forms of biliary cirrhosis are caused by obstruction of the bile ducts, primarily by stones. The causes of PBC are unknown, but are thought to be autoimmune or endocrine in nature.

Abnormal Findings

▲INCREASED LEVELS may indicate primary biliary cirrhosis, secondary biliary cirrhosis, chronic active hepatitis, hepatic impairment related to hepatotoxic agents, cryptogenic cirrhosis, myasthenia gravis, systemic lupus erythematosus, rheumatoid arthritis, pernicious anemia, thyroid disease, or Addison's disease. High titers of 1:40–1:80 indicate primary biliary cirrhosis (PBC).

Interfering Factors

➤ Failure of laboratory methods to clearly differentiate antimitochondrial antibodies from other antibodies can result in false positive reports.

NURSING CONSIDERATIONS

Prepare Your Client

➤ Explain that this test is used to help determine the cause of liver problems.

Perform Procedure

➤ Collect 7 mL of venous blood in a red-top tube.

➤ Observe the venipuncture site closely for hematoma formation or bleeding. Coagulopathies are common in liver disease. Apply a pressure dressing to the venipuncture site.

Care After Test

➤ Assess client for unusual bruising or prolonged bleeding. Delayed clotting is a complication of severely impaired liver function.

➤ Assess skin, sclera of eyes for jaundice and note findings.

➤ Consult with a registered dietician to design a high-calorie, well-balanced diet. Clients with advanced liver disease have poor absorption of nutrients due to decreased bile flow into the intestines. As appropriate, reduce sodium or protein in the diet if edema and ascites, or increased ammonia levels are present.

➤ Consult with the primary health care provider to review drug dosages of any prescribed medications which are metabolized by the liver.

➤ Evaluate client for increased fluid volume such as ascites, edema, dyspnea.

➤ Measure abdominal girths daily if ascites is present.

➤ Consult with the primary health care provider regarding the need for vitamin supplementation of fat-soluble vitamins: vitamins K, D, A.

➤ Consult with the primary health-care provider about the benefit in prescribing antihistamines such as diphenhydramine to relieve itching or topical lotions that contain menthol.

➤ Evaluate other tests such as aspartate aminotransferase (AST), alanine aminotransferase (ALT), direct and indirect bilirubin levels, alkaline phosphatase, serum ammonia, prothrombin time, cholangiography, and liver biopsy.

Educate Your Client and the Family

➤ Teach your client that liver disease can have many causes and that PBC is not caused by alcohol.

➤ For client with severely impaired liver function, instruct client and family to report unusual or increased bruising and tarry stools. Instruct them to use electric razors and to use non-skid shoes to avoid falls and injuries.

Antinuclear Antibody

an ti noo klee ur • an ti bod ee

(ANA, Smith Antigen, Sm Antigen, Ribonucleoprotein, RNP)

Normal Findings

Negative at a titer of 1:32 or less.

What This Test Will Tell You

This blood test helps diagnose a variety of autoimmune diseases, especially lupus erythematosus, by detecting and measuring antinuclear antibodies. Antinuclear antibody testing (ANA) is most helpful in screening and diagnosing systemic lupus erythematosus (SLE), a variable, unpredictable disease with multisystem involvement.

ANA titers are strongly positive in 95%–99% of clients with SLE, making it highly sensitive. However, it has a low specificity resulting in many false positive results. Because a negative ANA titer rules out SLE in most cases, this test is often drawn to diagnose or rule out SLE when a client presents with joint pain, lethargy, or other diffuse symptoms.

Indirect immunofluorescence is a method of detecting ANA patterns of antibody activity characteristic of various disorders. SLE has a typical homogenous pattern of staining. A speckled pattern reveals antibodies to nonnuclear components, called extractable nuclear antigen antibodies, the Smith antigen (Sm) and the ribonucleoprotein (RNP). The Sm antigen is highly specific for SLE. Elevated levels of RNP antigen are indicative of mixed connective disease.

Abnormal Findings

▲INCREASED LEVELS may indicate systemic lupus erythematosus, scleroderma, rheumatoid arthritis, Sjögren's disease, dermatomyositis, polyarteritis, infectious mononucleosis, viral disease, leukemia, myasthenia gravis, or chronic hepatitis.

Interfering Factors

➤ False positives may occur.
➤ Medications that may result in false positive results include procainamide, hydralazine, isoniazid, salicylates, acetazolamide, chlorothiazide, penicillin, phenytoin, and many antibiotics.
➤ 1%–5% of normal population may test positive.
➤ Increased age is associated with false positive results.
➤ Steroid therapy may result in false negatives.

NURSING CONSIDERATIONS

Prepare Your Client

➤ Explain that this test will help determine if your client has a disease where the body attacks its own tissues, called autoimmune disease.

Perform Procedure

➤ Collect 7–10 mL of venous blood in a red-top tube.

Care After Test

➤ Monitor blood pressure, intake and output of fluids, daily weight, blood urea nitrogen, and serum and urine creatinine to detect signs of renal impairment.
➤ Document fever, decreased range of motion, joint pain, and activity intolerance.
➤ Space activity to allow for periods of rest.

> Ensure a physical therapy evaluation is made for client with impaired mobility.

> Assess client for signs of gastrointestinal bleeding. Therapy for SLE and other autoimmune diseases often includes steroids, which can cause impairments in intestinal mucosa.

> Refer client for home health care evaluation if activities of daily living are impaired.

> Review related tests including complement levels, sedimentation rate, white blood cell count with differential, lupus erythematosus test (LE prep), and Hep-2 antigen test.

Educate Your Client and the Family

> Give hope to the client and family.

Let them know spontaneous remissions often occur for indefinite periods of time.

> If steroid therapy is initiated, teach client to take steroids with food or milk. Review symptoms of gastrointestinal bleeding.

> Remind client to schedule an eye examination at least once a year. Blindness is a complication of SLE.

> Tell client that fatigue, emotional stress, infection, and surgery can cause the disease to flare up.

> Teach client to avoid prolonged exposure to the sun, which worsens photophobia and the facial rash.

> Encourage client to join a support group and an exercise program to help alleviate the arthritis. The Arthritis Foundation is a good resource.

Antiparietal Cell Antibody

an ti pah rie eh tahl • sel • an ti bod ee
(APCA)

Normal Findings

No antiparietal cell antibodies are found in the serum.

What This Test Will Tell You

This blood test helps diagnose an autoimmune cause of pernicious anemia (PA) by detecting the presence of antiparietal cell antibodies (APCA). Parietal cells lining the gastric mucosa secrete the intrinsic factor necessary for vitamin B_{12} (extrinsic factor) absorption. Vitamin B_{12} is crucial in the formation of normal red blood cells (RBCs) and for neurological function.

Testing for antiparietal cell antibodies alone often results in false positive findings. For this reason, APCA testing is done in conjunction with other tests for a definitive diagnosis. APCA titers are negative in other types of anemias.

Abnormal Findings

▲INCREASED LEVELS may indicate pernicious anemia, chronic or atrophic gastritis, gastric ulcer, thyroid disease, diabetes mellitus, or iron deficiency anemia.

ACTION ALERT!

Untreated pernicious anemia can cause irreversible neurological impairment and death.

Interfering Factors

➤ 10%–15% of normal population will have positive antibody titers, but anti-intrinsic-factor antibody is usually absent in these individuals.

➤ 2% of normal children will have false positive results.

➤ Gastric atrophy, diabetes mellitus, thyroid disorders, and iron deficiency may also cause the formation of APCAs.

➤ Hemolyzed blood or elevated serum lipid levels may interfere with results.

NURSING CONSIDERATIONS

Prepare Your Client

➤ Explain that this test will help diagnose the cause for abnormal red blood cells. The test will help determine if the body is creating and destroying its own abnormal red blood cells.

Perform Procedure

➤ Collect 7–10 mL of venous blood in a red-top tube.

➤ Handle the specimen carefully to avoid hemolysis.

Care After Test

➤ If pernicious anemia is diagnosed, plan scheduled injections of vitamin B_{12} for the patient. Vitamin B_{12} therapy is essential. Without it, PA is fatal within 1–3 years.

➤ Protect client from injury and burns. Heat and pain sensation are diminished because of peripheral neuropathy. Nerve damage may be permanent.

➤ Evaluate neurological status. PA can cause ataxia, numbness, and poor fine motor coordination.

➤ Assess client for tachycardia, chest pain, and palpitations related to anemia.

➤ Evaluate tissue oxygenation status. Pallor, weakness, shortness of breath may be common findings indicating the need for oxygen therapy or transfusion even in the presence of a normal arterial oxygenation level.

➤ Review related tests such as the red blood cell count, hemoglobin, hematocrit, red blood cell indices, anti-intrinsic-factor antibody, Schilling test, and gastric acid stimulation results.

Educate Your Client and the Family

➤ Teach client and family how to administer intramuscular injections of vitamin B_{12}. Stress the importance of regular injections and the consequence of noncompliance.

➤ Inform family of the need to evaluate relatives for PA. Early therapy with vitamin B_{12} can prevent permanent nerve damage.

➤ Teach client to be very careful in extremes of temperature, especially guarding against thermal injury and frostbite.

➤ Encourage client to wear shoes and to inspect the feet for cuts and abrasions often. Because sensation may be decreased, foot injuries may go unnoticed.

➤ Tell client to obtain regular health assessments and follow-up. Clients with PA are prone to develop gastric carcinoma. Teach them to seek medical attention immediately for any gastrointestinal symptoms.

➤ Encourage client to plan rest periods and to space activity. Client will have more energy when the hemoglobin builds up.

Anti-Smooth-Muscle Antibody

an tee • smooth • muss sul • an ti bod ee
(ASMA)

Normal Findings

Normal titer of anti-smooth-muscle antibodies is less than 1:20.

What This Test Will Tell You

This blood test detects the presence of smooth-muscle antibodies, which are found in autoimmune diseases of the liver and bile duct. Positive ASMA titers are found in 2/3 of the clients with chronic active hepatitis, and in some clients with primary biliary cirrhosis. ASMAs are helpful in the differential diagnosis of these autoimmune diseases because they generally do not appear in the other forms of hepatitis and liver disease.

Abnormal Findings

▲ INCREASED LEVELS may indicate chronic active hepatitis, primary biliary cirrhosis, acute viral hepatitis, hepatic cancer, intrinsic asthma (20%), infectious mononucleosis, or myasthenia gravis.

NURSING CONSIDERATIONS

Prepare Your Client

➤ Explain that this test will help diagnose specific problems in the liver and gallbladder caused by the body's own defense mechanisms.

Perform Procedure

➤ Collect 7–10 mL of venous blood in a red-top tube.
➤ Observe the venipuncture site closely for hematoma formation or bleeding. Coagulopathies are common in liver disease. Apply a pressure dressing to the venipuncture site.

Care After Test

➤ Assess fluid and nutritional status for evidence of liver dysfunction.
➤ Check daily weights, abdominal girth measurements, and intake and output records for signs of volume overload related to edema or ascites.
➤ Evaluate client for symptoms of liver damage such as increased bleeding tendencies, jaundice, and ascites.
➤ Consult with the primary health care provider about drug dosages of all ordered medications which are metabolized or excreted by the liver.
➤ Consult with a registered dietician to design a high-calorie, well-balanced diet. Clients with advanced liver disease have poor absorption of nutrients due to decreased bile flow into the intestines. As appropriate, reduce sodium or protein in the diet if edema and ascites, or increased ammonia levels are present.
➤ Review related tests such as pro thrombin time, alanine aminotransferase, aspartate aminotransferase, alkaline phosphatase, antinuclear antibodies, serum ammonia, antimitochondrial antibodies, and liver biopsy.

Educate Your Client and the Family

➤ Reassure your client that chronic active hepatitis (autoimmune hepatitis) is not due to drugs or alcohol. It is not contagious.
➤ Instruct client and family on a high-calorie, well-balanced diet as appropriate. If sodium or protein restrictions are indicated, help client

and family make dietary selections with these limitations.

➤ Clients with chronic active hepatitis may be treated in the long term with corticosteroids, especially if symptoms are severe. Teach your client about the side effects of long-term steroid use, such as weight gain, irritable stomach, moon-face, and mood swings.

➤ Reassure client that steroids are very helpful in reducing symptoms.

Antispermatozoal Antibody

an tee spur mat ah zoe al • an ti bod ee
(Sperm Antibody Agglutination, Sperm Antibody Assay, Sperm Immobilization Antigen-Antibody Reaction, Antisperm Antibodies, Infertility Screen)

Normal Findings
Negative

What This Test Will Tell You
This blood and fluid test detects immunologic infertility, and is one of multiple diagnostic evaluations completed as part of a fertility profile for couples. The test detects the presence of sperm antibodies, and determines the sperm antibody binding site. Both the male and female are checked for antispermatozoal antibodies. Agglutination of sperm when incubated in the female partner's blood serum or cervical mucus indicates formation of antibodies to partner's sperm. Agglutination or immobilization of sperm also occurs when antibodies are produced by the male against his own sperm.

Abnormal Findings
Positive results may reveal infertility and autoimmunity to sperm.

Interfering Factors
➤ Use of condoms for specimen collection; they contain spermicidal agents.

➤ Delayed delivery of semen to the laboratory for testing; testing must occur within 2 hours after collection.

➤ Refrigeration of semen.

➤ Improper timing of collection of cervical mucus. Collection of the sample should be as close as possible to time of ovulation.

NURSING CONSIDERATIONS
Prepare Your Client
➤ Explain that this test will check whether either of the partners is "allergic" to the sperm and has formed antibodies (cells to destroy sperm) against it.

➤ Instruct clients that ejaculation should be avoided for at least 3 days prior to collecting semen.

➤ Discuss the methods of obtaining semen with the clients. Recognize that this may be embarrassing for them, making it difficult for them to respond and ask questions.

➤ If the semen is collected at home, it should be transported to the laboratory for testing within 2 hours of collection.

➤ Explain that semen obtained by masturbation or coitus interruptus should be collected in a clean glass receptacle with an adequate opening in which to direct the tip of the erect ("hard") penis and with adequate capacity for the ejaculate (2–5 mL, or $^1/_2$ to 1 teaspoon). Semen obtained through intercourse (or sex) should be collected in a sheath (or special condom or rubber) without a spermicide or lubricant; the sheath with ejaculate should be placed in a clean glass receptacle.

➤ Instruct client that semen specimen must not be chilled; container can be held during transport to keep close to body temperature.

➤ Instruct the clients in methods to determine when ovulation occurs (e.g., basal body temperature and spinnbarkheit test), as this is the optimal time for specimen collection.

➤ Explain that blood will be drawn from the vein from both the male and female partners. Explain the venipuncture process clearly.

➤ Tell the female client that there are no fluid or food restrictions prior to the test; advise the male client to avoid alcohol consumption for at least 24 hours before collecting semen for sperm analysis.

Perform Procedure

➤ Give the male client an appropriate receptacle and have him collect his semen as directed. Submit the sample to the laboratory with his name, date, time of collection, and date of last previous ejaculation.

➤ Female client will have cervical mucus collected by the primary care provider at an office visit.

➤ Collect 7–10 mL of venous blood from both male and female partners in 10–15 mL red-top tubes.

➤ Label samples carefully.

Care After Test

➤ Explain that this test is one of several that will be done to diagnose, evaluate, and determine the optimal course of action for impaired fertility.

➤ Evaluate related tests such as semen analysis, cervical mucus test, and progesterone assay.

Educate Your Client and the Family

➤ Instruct the couple that the primary care provider will meet with them when all test results have been received to review the findings and make recommendations for further testing or for the best plan of action to follow.

➤ Teach clients about influences on fertility including basal body temperature, stress, and environmental factors.

➤ If applicable, inform clients about infertility support groups.

A

Anti-Streptolysin O Titer

an ti strep tuh lie sin • oe • tie ter
(Anti-Streptolysin Antibody Test, ASO, Streptococcal Antibody Test,
Streptozyme, Antideoxyribonuclease Antibody, Anti-DNase B, ADB,
Streptodornase)

Normal Findings

Normal values vary with age and geographic location. School-age children will have higher normal titers than adults or preschoolers. See the chart below.

What This Test Will Tell You

This blood test detects antibodies to beta-hemolytic streptococcus group A. An elevation in the ASO and anti-DNase indicates that a recent streptococcus infection has occurred, which if untreated can lead to rheumatic fever or glomerulonephritis.

Antibodies to strep appear 1 week to 1 month after the initial strep infection, usually before systemic symptoms appear. Antibody titers may fall as systemic symptoms arise or remain elevated through the course of the disease. Anti-DNase titers tend to stay elevated longer than ASO, making it more valuable in detecting late manifestations of rheumatic fever. Serial titers are more useful than isolated readings.

ASO titers alone detect 80%–85% of streptococcal infections; together with anti-DNase, accuracy increases to 95%. Unfortunately, approximately 15%–20% of clients with poststreptococcal syndrome do not have elevated ASO titers, which makes diagnosis more difficult.

Abnormal Findings

▲INCREASED LEVELS may indicate streptococcal pharyngitis, rheumatic fever, rheumatic heart disease, glomerulonephritis, scarlet fever, or bacterial endocarditis. Titers above 250 Todd units suggest dormant rheumatic fever, while titers from 500–5,000 Todd units suggest acute glomerulonephritis or rheumatic heart disease. Serial titers for 4–8 weeks or more provide the best information regarding the acute and resolving stages of poststreptococcal disease.

ACTION ALERT!

Clients with untreated streptococcal pharyngitis (beta-hemolytic strep group A) may develop rheumatic fever or glomerulonephritis.

Interfering Factors

➤ Antibiotic therapy lowers titers.
➤ Adrenocorticosteroid therapy will lower titers.
➤ Positive titers are found in healthy individuals.

	ASO	Anti-DNase*
Adult:	<85–120 Todd units/mL	<340 units
Preschool:	<85–120 Todd units/mL	<170 units
School-age:	<170 Todd units/mL	<480 units

*Values are often reported using different scales and values according to the laboratory method used. Carefully check your own laboratory for appropriate values.

➤ False positives occur with tuberculosis and liver disease.

NURSING CONSIDERATIONS

Prepare Your Client

➤ Explain that this test will see if they have recently had a strep throat infection, which may be causing the symptoms.

➤ Evaluate client's recent history of pharyngitis and any antibiotic therapy. When determining a history of antibiotic therapy, be sure to evaluate compliance with duration of therapy.

Perform Procedure

➤ Collect 10 mL of venous blood in a red-top tube.

➤ Notify lab if the client has been treated with antibiotics. Note on the lab slip the name, dose, and duration of therapy.

Care After Test

➤ Assess client for fever (usually low-grade), malaise, and abdominal pain characteristic of rheumatic fever. Administer antipyretics and non-steroidal anti-inflammatory drugs (NSAIDS) for comfort.

➤ Assess client for signs of cardiac compromise including tachycardia, dyspnea, fatigue, and moist rales.

➤ Auscultate the heart sounds, listening for new murmurs which may be from valve damage secondary to rheumatic heart disease.

➤ Assess the client for weight gain and edema. Check the urine for protein and blood, which are symptoms of glomerulonephritis.

➤ Place client on strict intake and output measurements. Restrict fluids and salt if edema and fluid retention occur.

➤ Assess skin for subcutaneous nodules and rashes characteristic of rheumatic fever.

➤ Maintain client on bed rest until signs of cardiac symptoms and inflammation subside. Activity can resume when anti-inflammatory medications are discontinued.

➤ Position client comfortably to alleviate joint pain. Consider warm, moist soaks to ease painful, inflamed joints.

➤ Review related tests such as the complete blood count and differential, creatinine clearance, serum creatinine, blood urea nitrogen, blood cultures, and echocardiogram.

Educate Your Client and the Family

➤ Teach your client and family the signs and symptoms of strep throat, fever, sore throat, and malaise. DO NOT let a strep throat go untreated.

➤ Emphasize the fact that untreated strep infections can lead to heart damage. Rheumatic heart disease is more likely to occur in people with previous histories of rheumatic fever.

➤ Teach client to take antibiotics as ordered. DO NOT stop taking them until the prescription is finished.

➤ If client does have rheumatic fever, explain that prophylactic antibiotics will be required before dental work, invasive instrumentation for diagnostic testing, and surgery.

Antithrombin III
an tee throm bin • three
(AT-III)

Normal Findings
Normal findings may vary with method; check with the laboratory used.

ADULT, CHILD, ADOLESCENT, AND ELDERLY
Plasma: >50% of control value
Serum: 15%–35% lower than plasma value
Immunologic: 65%–120% of normal
Functional: 77%–122% of normal

PREGNANT
May be increased depending upon the stage of pregnancy.

NEWBORN AND INFANT
Functional method used from birth to 5 months:
Premature: 26%–61%
Full-term: 44%–76%

What This Test Will Tell You
This blood test diagnoses disseminated intravascular coagulation and other hypercoagulation disorders. Antithrombin III (AT-III) is a naturally occurring IgG immunoglobulin, synthesized by the liver, that inhibits coagulation. Thrombin and other clotting factors are inactivated by AT-III, creating an equilibrium between clotting and nonclotting factors. If AT-III levels are increased, clotting decreases; if decreased, clotting increases.

Abnormal Findings
▲INCREASED LEVELS may reveal deficiency of Factors V and VII, hepatitis, menstruation, vitamin K deficiency, renal transplantation, or hemophilia A or B.
▼DECREASED LEVELS may be found with arteriosclerosis, burns, cardiovascular disease, cerebrovascular accident, cirrhosis, congenital antithrombin III deficiency, deep vein thrombosis, diabetes mellitus (type II), disseminated intravascular coagulation (DIC), malignancy, malnutrition, nephrotic syndrome, recent surgery, postpartum, pulmonary embolism, septicemia, or thromboembolism.

▮ ACTION ALERT!
Levels under 50% indicate a significant risk for thrombosis. Be prepared to begin heparin therapy.

Interfering Factors
➤ Medications that increase the value include anabolic steroids, androgens, bishydroxycoumarin, progesterone-containing oral contraceptives, progesterone, and warfarin sodium.
➤ Medications that decrease levels include fibrinolytics, heparin calcium, heparin sodium, L-asparaginase, and estrogen-containing oral contraceptives.
➤ Hemolyzed or lipemic specimens will alter results.
➤ Renal transplantation may result in elevated levels.

NURSING CONSIDERATIONS
Prepare Your Client
➤ Explain that this test measures one part of the process of blood clotting.
➤ Restrict food and fluids other than water for 10–12 hours prior to the test.

Perform Procedure

➤ Collect 5 mL of venous blood in a red-top tube or in a blue-top tube containing sodium citrate.

Care After Test

➤ Assess for signs and symptoms of blood clot formation including swelling of extremities, positive Homan's sign, and deep calf pain.

➤ Assess for signs of pulmonary embolism including chest pain, dyspnea, apprehension, cough, and crackles.

➤ Review related tests such as pro-thrombin time, partial thromboplastin time, bleeding time, and activated clotting time.

Educate Your Client and the Family

➤ Teach client and family the signs and symptoms of clotting including pain, swelling, change in normal color, and changes in sensation.

➤ Instruct client to alert health care providers to an AT-III deficiency because surgery and other procedures causing inactivity will put the client at risk for clot formation.

A

Antithyroglobulin Antibody
an ti thie roe glob yoo lin • an ti bod ee
(Thyroid Autoantibody, Thyroid Antithyroglobulin Antibody, Thyroglobulin Antibody)

Normal Findings
ADULT
Titer of less than 1:100

What This Test Will Tell You

This blood test monitors for thyroid disease caused by autoimmune diseases, particularly Hashimoto's disease. In these diseases, the thyroid is inflamed and releases thyroglobulin from the thyroid gland. Antithyroglobulin antibodies combine with thyroglobulin and increase the inflammatory process in the thyroid gland. These autoantibodies attack and injure the thyroid tissue.

Abnormal Findings

▲ INCREASED LEVELS may indicate Hashimoto's thyroiditis, rheumatic diseases, lupus erythematosus, thyroid cancer, thyrotoxicosis, myxe-dema, pernicious anemia, hypothyroidism, hemolytic anemia, or Sjögren's syndrome.

Interfering Factors

➤ Low titers of antibodies may be normally present in healthy people, especially geriatric women, without thyroid disease.

NURSING CONSIDERATIONS

Prepare Your Client

➤ Explain that this test is done to detect a problem with the thyroid gland.

➤ Do not restrict food or fluids for this test.

Perform Procedure

➤ Collect 5 cc of venous blood in a red-top tube.

Care After Test

➤ Assess client for signs and symptoms of hypothyroidism including complaints of being cold, weight gain, dry skin, thinning hair, hypotension, cold extremities, fatigue, stonelike facial expression, constipation, dysrhythmias, slowed mental function, and clumsiness.

➤ Provide safety precautions for client with impaired cognitive or motor function.

➤ Review diet and promote exercise for complaints of fatigue and constipation.

➤ Initiate continuous cardiac monitoring for clients with dysrhythmias.

➤ Review related tests such as antithyroid microsomal antibody test, serum thyroxine levels, T_3 levels, thyroid-stimulating hormone levels, and electrocardiogram.

Educate Your Client and the Family

➤ Teach client and family that Hashimoto's thyroiditis is an autoimmune disease, usually treated with steroids. Explain that an autoimmune disease occurs when the body doesn't properly recognize its own tissues and tries to destroy them.

➤ Inform client of the importance of eating properly, getting plenty of rest, and taking the medication as prescribed.

➤ Tell client that the steroids prescribed can cause side effects such as fluid retention, mood swings, nausea, stomach ulcers, and even weak bones. If any of these symptoms occur, instruct client to inform the primary health care provider.

➤ Tell client to take the steroid medication with milk, food, or an antacid to minimize stomach upset.

Antithyroid Microsomal Antibody

an ti thie roid • mie cro soe mul • an ti bod ee
(Thyroid Autoantibody, Thyroid Antimicrosomal Antibody, Antimicrosomal Antibody, Microsomal Antibody)

Normal Findings

ADULT
Titer of less than 1:100
Positive findings may be present in 5%–10% of the normal population.

What This Test Will Tell You

This blood test monitors for a particular thyroid disease, Hashimoto's thyroiditis. In this disease, the thyroid is inflamed and releases microsomes from the thyroid follicle. These microsomes act as foreign antigens, causing the body to produce microsomal antibodies to fight the antigen. These microsomal antibodies in turn also attack and injure the thyroid tissue.

Abnormal Findings

▲ INCREASED LEVELS may indicate Hashimoto's thyroiditis, rheumatic disease, lupus erythematosus, thyroid cancer, myxedema, Sjögren's syndrome, thyroiditis, goiter, autoimmune hemolytic anemia.

Interfering Factors

➤ Low titers of antibodies may be normally present in 5%–10% of healthy people without thyroid disease.

NURSING CONSIDERATIONS

Prepare Your Client

➤ Explain that this test is done to detect a problem with the thyroid gland.

➤ Do not restrict food or fluids for this test.

Perform Procedure

➤ Collect 5 cc of venous blood in a red-top tube.

Care After Test

➤ Assess client for signs and symptoms of hypothyroidism including complaints of being cold, weight gain, dry skin, thinning hair, hypotension, cold extremities, fatigue, stonelike facial expression, constipation, dysrhythmias, slowed mental function, and clumsiness.

➤ Provide safety precautions for client with impaired cognitive or motor function.

➤ Review diet and promote exercise for complaints of fatigue and constipation.

➤ Initiate continuous cardiac monitoring for client with dysrhythmias.

➤ Review related tests such as antithyroglobulin antibody test, serum thyroxine levels, T_3 levels, thyroid-stimulating hormone levels, and electrocardiogram.

Educate Your Client and the Family

➤ Teach client and family that Hashimoto's thyroiditis is an autoimmune disease, usually treated with steroids. Explain that an autoimmune disease occurs when the body doesn't properly recognize its own tissues and tries to destroy them.

➤ Inform client of the importance of eating properly, getting plenty of rest, and taking the medication as prescribed.

➤ Inform client that the steroids prescribed can cause side effects such as fluid retention, mood swings, nausea, stomach ulcers, and even weak bones. If any of these symptoms occur, instruct client to inform the primary health care provider.

➤ Instruct client to take the steroid medication with milk, food, or an antacid to minimize stomach upset.

Arterial Blood Gases

ar teer ee ahl · blud · gas es
(ABGs, Blood Gases)

Normal Findings

ADULT AND ADOLESCENT

➤ pH: 7.35–7.45
➤ pCO_2: 35–45 mm Hg
➤ pO_2: 80–105 mm Hg
➤ HCO_3^-: 22–26 mEq/L
➤ O_2 saturation: 95%–100%
➤ Base excess: −2 to +2

PREGNANT

➤ pH: 7.35–7.45
➤ pCO_2: Values may be as low as 30 by the end of the second trimester because of hyperventilation.
➤ HCO_3^-: Values may be as low as 20 by the end of the second trimester. The bicarbonate level falls to balance

the drop in the pCO_2 and maintain a normal pH.

➤ pO_2: 85–100 mm Hg
➤ O_2 saturation: 95%–100%
➤ Base excess: May be decreased if the bicarbonate level is decreased.

NEWBORN

➤ pH: 7.30–7.40. Decreased values reflect the low bicarbonate levels normally present in newborns.
➤ pCO_2: 26–41mm Hg.
➤ HCO_3^-: 16–24 mEq/L. Premature infants may have even lower reference values.
➤ pO_2: 60–70 mm Hg. Decreased values persist until the lungs are fully developed.
➤ O_2 saturation: 40%–90%. Decreased values persist until the lungs are fully developed.
➤ Base excess: May be decreased if bicarbonate level is decreased.

CHILD (2 MONTHS TO 2 YEARS)

➤ pH: 7.34–7.46
➤ pCO_2: 26–41 mm Hg
➤ Other values are similar to adult values.

ELDERLY

➤ pO_2 and O_2 saturation values decrease in the elderly as functional lung capacity decreases. The pO_2 decreases 3–5 mm Hg for each decade of life after age 30. After age 70, a pO_2 of approximately 85 mm Hg should be considered a maximum value.

HIGH ALTITUDE

In high altitudes, such as Denver, values for pO_2, O_2 saturation, and pCO_2 are lower because the atmospheric pressure is lower.

What This Test Will Tell You

Blood gases are used to determine the acid-base balance and/or the respiratory or metabolic status of the client.

pH: The pH is the measurement of the free hydrogen ion (H^+) concentration in the blood. The body maintains a normal range by regulating the ratio of acid to base via the blood buffering system, the lungs, and the kidneys. A pH of less than 7.35 indicates acidemia; a pH of greater than 7.45 indicates alkalemia. Significant deviations in pH can be life threatening.

pCO_2: The pCO_2 represents the partial pressure carbon dioxide exerts in the arterial blood. Because pCO_2 is primarily controlled by the lungs, it is referred to as the respiratory component of blood gas measurements. When there is excess CO_2 in the blood, as occurs with hypoventilation, CO_2 combines with water to form carbonic acid (H_2CO_3), causing an acidotic state referred to as respiratory acidosis. When hyperventilation occurs, the CO_2 in the blood decreases and results in respiratory alkalosis.

HCO_3^- and base excess: HCO_3^-, or bicarbonate, is an alkaline substance that functions as an important buffer in the bloodstream. Because HCO_3^- levels are regulated by the kidneys and become elevated or decreased by metabolic derangements, HCO_3^- is referred to as the metabolic component of blood gas measurements. When the bicarbonate level decreases, as occurs with diabetic acidosis, renal failure, or cardiac arrest, metabolic acidosis occurs. When the bicarbonate level increases, as with excess loss of acids through the kidneys or gastrointestinal tract, metabolic alkalosis occurs.

Most laboratories also measure base excess. A value of < –2, referred to as base deficit, indicates metabolic acidosis. A value of > +2, referred to as base excess, indicates metabolic alkalosis.

pO_2: pO_2 represents the partial pressure of oxygen in the blood; its measurement identifies how well the lungs are oxygenating the blood. pO_2 is the amount of oxygen dissolved in the plasma that is available to bind with hemoglobin. A decrease in pO_2 is referred to as hypoxia. An increase in pO_2 above normal levels occurs only as a result of administration of high doses of oxygen.

O_2 saturation: Oxygen saturation (O_2% Sat) is the amount of oxygen actually bound to the hemoglobin and available for transport throughout the body. Hemoglobin should be completely (100%) saturated with oxygen. When 95%–100% of the hemoglobin carries oxygen, the tissues are being adequately oxygenated. When O_2 saturation levels fall below 75%, the tissues are unable to extract enough oxygen to carry out their vital functions. O_2 saturation is affected by the pO_2, body temperature, pH, and the chemical and physical structure of the hemoglobin itself. The combination of O_2 saturation, pO_2, and hemoglobin levels reflect tissue oxygenation. Oxygen saturation can also be measured continuously by pulse oximetry.

Abnormal Findings

➤ *Respiratory acidosis* (pH is decreased, pCO_2 is increased, HCO_3^- is normal) may indicate respiratory depression due to a cause such as sedation, narcotic overdose, or central nervous system depression; pulmonary disease such as chronic obstructive lung disease, pneumonia, atelectasis, or pneumothorax; or pri-

mary respiratory failure.
➤ *Respiratory alkalosis* (pH is increased, pCO_2 is decreased, HCO_3^- is normal) may indicate hyperventilation due to a cause such as pain, anxiety, or overventilation via a mechanical ventilator; or compensation for severe metabolic acidosis.
➤ *Metabolic acidosis* (pH is decreased, pCO_2 is normal, HCO_3^- is decreased) may indicate diabetes mellitus, shock, renal failure, diarrhea, respiratory failure, hepatic disease, Addison's disease, or sepsis.
➤ *Metabolic alkalosis* (pH is increased, pCO_2 is normal, HCO_3^- is increased) may indicate prolonged vomiting, nasogastric suctioning, diuretic therapy without potassium replacement, sodium bicarbonate ingestion, or compensation for chronic respiratory acidosis.

ACTION ALERT!

Critical values
➤ pH: <7.2 or >7.6
➤ pCO_2: <20 or >70 mm Hg
➤ HCO_3^-: <10 or >40 mEq/L
➤ pO_2: <40 mm Hg
➤ O_2 saturation: <75%
Abnormal arterial blood gas (ABG) values indicate problems with pulmonary ventilation, oxygenation, or metabolism that may require prompt intervention. Assess the client's mental status and vital signs, and notify the primary health care provider immediately if any values in the critical range are obtained because they could lead to respiratory or cardiac arrest.

Interfering Factors

➤ Hyperthermia may falsely elevate pO_2 and pCO_2; hypothermia may lower these values.
➤ Allowing the sample to sit at room temperature for longer than 2 minutes may result in a decreased pH and pO_2.

➤ Tracheobronchial suctioning within 20 to 30 minutes prior to obtaining the sample may cause a decrease in the pO_2 and O_2 saturation levels.

➤ Excess heparin in the syringe may result in a decreased pH, pCO_2, and pO_2.

➤ Hemolysis of the blood sample causes inaccurate results.

➤ Failure to expel air bubbles from the syringe causes falsely elevated pO_2 or falsely decreased pCO_2.

Contraindications

➤ Clients with significantly prolonged bleeding times should have arterial punctures performed only if absolutely necessary. It may be necessary to apply pressure to the puncture site for 10–15 minutes or longer.

➤ Radial or ulnar artery puncture should not be performed when arterial circulation to the hand is compromised.

Potential Complications

➤ Thrombosis of the artery may follow arterial puncture.

➤ Bleeding from the puncture site may occur if adequate pressure is not applied after the arterial puncture.

NURSING CONSIDERATIONS

Prepare Your Client

➤ Explain that this test is important to determine how well the lungs are functioning and the acid-base status of the blood.

➤ Inform the client that the blood must be drawn from an artery and thoroughly describe this procedure.

➤ Tell the client there is no need to restrict food or fluids.

➤ Note the settings for oxygen therapy or mechanical ventilator. Verify that no changes have been made in settings for 30 minutes prior to the test.

➤ Verify that the client has not been suctioned for 20 minutes prior to the test.

➤ Ensure that the client has rested for 30 minutes prior to the test.

➤ Perform the Allen test to assess collateral circulation before performing the arterial puncture on the radial artery. Occlude both the ulnar and radial arteries in the wrist with two fingers for 10 seconds until the hand blanches, then release the finger over the ulnar artery and look for pink coloring coming back into the hand distal to the wrist. If coloring returns, the ulnar artery will provide adequate circulation and blood gases can be drawn from the radial artery. If the pink color does not return on either hand, select another artery for puncture.

➤ Describe any anticipated discomforts (arterial punctures cause brief, sharp pain).

Perform Procedure

Arterial Puncture

➤ Obtain a blood gas collection kit or heparinize a 3-mL syringe with 1 mL of heparin and expel all but 0.2 mL of heparin. Attach a 20-gauge needle to the syringe.

➤ Palpate the artery to be used. The radial artery is usually preferred, but the brachial or femoral artery may be used if institutional policies permit.

➤ Cleanse the puncture site with an antiseptic agent and allow to dry.

➤ Puncture the artery and draw 3–5 mL of blood. Withdraw the needle and apply pressure to the arterial site for at least 5 minutes.

➤ Expel any air from the syringe, cap the syringe, and gently mix the specimen. Place the syringe in ice to inhibit metabolic activity.

➤ Indicate on the ABG requisition slip the time the sample was drawn, the client's temperature, and whether the client was breathing room air or supplemental oxygen or is on mechanical ventilation.

➤ Transport the sample to the laboratory immediately.

INDWELLING ARTERIAL LINE

If the client has an indwelling arterial line, the sample may be drawn from this line, avoiding the necessity of an arterial puncture.

➤ Obtain a 5-mL syringe and a 3-mL syringe, preheparinized or heparinized as described above.

➤ Attach the 5-mL syringe to an in-line stopcock on the arterial line, withdraw 5 mL of blood from the line, and discard. Then immediately attach the 3 mL heparinized syringe, withdraw 3 mL of blood, expel any excess air, cap the syringe, and place it in ice.

➤ Label the syringe as described above and transport to the laboratory immediately.

➤ Flush the stopcock, cap the port, and then flush the arterial line back to the client.

Care After Test

➤ Apply direct digital pressure to the arterial puncture site for at least 5 minutes, then apply a pressure bandage.

➤ Observe the puncture site for bleeding or hematoma formation.

➤ Check for the presence of pulses or for signs of nerve or circulatory impairment distal to the puncture site. Report to the primary health care provider immediately if the hand becomes cold, pale, or pulseless or if the client complains of paresthesia.

➤ Assess the client closely for signs of inadequate ventilation or acid-base imbalance, especially with a history of fluid loss. Observe vital signs and mental status closely if indicated.

➤ Institute continuous cardiac monitoring if results are significantly abnormal.

➤ Evaluate results of related tests such as hemoglobin, electrolytes, pulmonary function, and chest x-ray.

Educate Your Client and the Family

➤ Inform the client that although results will be available quickly, several samples may need to be obtained to determine response to therapy.

➤ If respiratory acidosis is present, encourage deep breathing and perform chest physiotherapy if indicated. Administer only low-flow oxygen when emphysema is present.

➤ If respiratory alkalosis is present, assess for tachypnea and encourage slow, regular breathing. Relieve pain and anxiety if indicated.

➤ If metabolic acidosis is present, assess for the cause of this disorder and institute appropriate intervention. Instruct the client on appropriate treatment for diabetes, renal failure, or other metabolic diseases present.

➤ If metabolic alkalosis is present, assess for drug ingestion or other causes of this disorder. Instruct the client not to ingest large quantities of antacids containing bicarbonate, which could result in alkalosis.

➤ If hypoxia is present, administer oxygen therapy and assist ventilation if necessary. Encourage the client to breathe deeply.

A

Arteriography of the Arms and Legs

ar tee ree og rah fee

(Angiography, Angiogram, Peripheral Arteriography, Femoral Angiography)

Normal Findings

All ages: Normal vascular anatomic structure, normal and patent arteries

What This Test Will Tell You

This radiographic test diagnoses arterial occlusive disease as well as anatomic abnormalities of arteries in the legs and the arms. The test can help diagnose peripheral vascular disease, aneurysms, congenital and acquired anomalies, injuries, emboli, and other pathology. An arterial catheter is inserted into the femoral or brachial artery under fluoroscopy. Contrast material is injected and motion films are taken to record the flow of contrast (dye) through the arterial tree. The structure of the arterial system can be visualized and occlusive areas identified.

This test may also be used as a therapeutic procedure to treat emboli and occlusions. Balloon angioplasty may be done during the procedure to dilate occluded arteries. Special catheters may also be inserted to attempt to remove clots found in the arterial system.

Abnormal Findings

Abnormalities may indicate peripheral vascular disease, atherosclerotic occlusive disease, arterial occlusion from thrombus formation or embolus, arterial aneurysms, arterial trauma, tumors, congenital arterial malformations, popliteal artery entrapment syndrome, or Buerger's disease.

ACTION ALERT!

Assess client carefully for allergic reaction to contrast material including dyspnea, itching, urticaria, flushing, hypotension, and shock. Life-threatening anaphylactic reactions can occur and need to be recognized and treated immediately.

Contraindications

➤ Allergy to contrast material without modifications
➤ Renal insufficiency or renal failure, because contrast material is excreted through the kidneys and is nephrotoxic
➤ Pregnancy, due to radiation exposure of the fetus
➤ Dehydration

Potential Complications

➤ Allergic reactions including anaphylaxis
➤ Hemorrhage
➤ Vasospasm
➤ Thrombus or embolus resulting in arterial occlusion in the extremity
➤ Embolus of blood clot or atherosclerotic plaque to other body areas
➤ Infection

NURSING CONSIDERATIONS

Prepare Your Client

➤ Explain that this test is used to diagnose and sometimes treat problems in the blood vessels and circulation.
➤ Ensure that an informed consent is obtained, because of the possible complications associated with this procedure.

➤ Ensure the client has no allergy to contrast material or iodine.

➤ Explain to the client or family that a local anesthetic is used to numb the area where the catheter will be inserted. This may produce a brief burning sensation before the area becomes numb.

➤ Explain that the catheter (long thin tube) is threaded through a needle placed in a thigh or arm artery (femoral or brachial artery). The catheters are threaded through the artery to the part of the body the physician needs to see. Assure the client that threading the catheters is not painful.

➤ Tell your client or family that once needles are inserted, the procedure itself is painless, but some pressure may be felt while lines are passed and there may be warmth from the contrast medium.

➤ Record baseline vital signs.

➤ Locate peripheral pulses and mark with a pen to assist in monitoring them after the procedure.

➤ Restrict food and fluids for 4–6 hours prior to the test.

➤ Administer sedatives or tranquilizers as ordered.

➤ Assure that adults and older children have voided before the procedure.

➤ Do not remove glasses, dentures, or hearing aids unless dictated by your hospital policy. The client may need these in order to communicate and cooperate during the procedure.

Perform Procedure

Nurses do not perform this procedure but should understand the process to prepare the client and assist the physician.

The site for arterial entry is anesthetized with a local anesthetic such as mepivacaine or lidocaine. Percutaneous puncture or a cutdown is performed to gain arterial access. Fluoroscopy is used to confirm placement of a guide wire introduced through the arterial catheter and to visualize the catheter throughout the procedure. Films are taken during injection of radiopaque contrast material to visualize the arterial vasculature.

Carefully assess the client for signs and symptoms of allergic reaction to contrast material. Apply pressure to the arterial puncture site after the catheter is removed until bleeding stops. Apply a pressure dressing to the site.

Care After Test

➤ Monitor vital signs closely until stable; usually every 15 minutes for the first hour, every 30 minutes for the next hour, and then every 4 hours for 24 hours.

➤ Maintain pressure on the arterial puncture site with either a sandbag or pressure dressing.

➤ Maintain bed rest with the extremity extended for 6–12 hours following the procedure to minimize complications of bleeding, hematoma formation, headaches, nausea, and vomiting.

➤ Assess the arterial puncture site(s) carefully for bleeding and hematoma.

➤ Assess circulation with each vital sign assessment of the affected extremity. Assess presence and strength of pulses, capillary refill, color, temperature, and sensation. Report immediately any abnormal findings.

➤ Assess for signs of a cerebral vascular accident resulting from a catheter-induced emboli including change in level of consciousness, dif-

A

ficulty with speech, and hemiparesis.

➤ Observe for signs of allergic reaction to the contrast material, including urticaria, pruritus, conjunctivitis, dyspnea, and apprehension.

➤ Encourage drinking fluids, because the contrast material has a diuretic effect. Delayed reactions usually occur within 2–6 hours of the test.

➤ If arterial circulation is compromised, adjust exercise and physical demands to meet limitations and prevent claudication.

➤ Evaluate related tests such as Doppler studies.

Educate Your Client and the Family

➤ Teach client and family a heart-healthy diet, including no added salt, if there is evidence of atherosclerosis.

➤ Teach client with compromised arterial circulation how to pace activities to prevent claudication. Also instruct client not to wear restrictive clothing that could further impair circulation to the extremity.

Arthrocentesis
ar throe sen tee sis
(Synovial Fluid Analysis, Joint Aspiration)

Normal Findings
All ages: Gross analysis finds a clear, pale yellow, viscous liquid with a pH of 7.2–7.4 and a good mucin clot. Most joints contain 3 mL or less. The knee contains 3–3.5 mL.
RBC—less than 2,000/mm
WBC—less than 200/mm
Neutrophils—less than 25%
Culture—negative
Glucose—nearly equal to serum (fasting)
Crystals—none
Uric acid—approximately equal to the serum
Rheumatoid factor—none
Lupus erythematosus cells—none

What This Test Will Tell You
This fluid analysis test is performed primarily to determine the cause and type of joint disorder and effusion. This procedure is also performed therapeutically to drain fluid from a joint or administer local pharmaco-

logical therapy. A differential diagnosis of arthritis is possible with this procedure; it is especially useful in identifying septic or crystal-induced arthritis. Fluid may also be drained to relieve the distention and pain resulting from the accumulation of fluid (effusion) in the joint. Local drug therapy, such as corticosteroids or gold, may also be administered using this procedure.

Abnormal Findings
▲INCREASED OR ABNORMAL LEVELS may indicate *noninflammatory abnormalities* such as degenerative joint disease (osteoarthritis), traumatic arthritis, osteochondritis dissecans, or subsiding or early inflammation; or *inflammatory abnormalities* such as rheumatoid arthritis, gout, pseudogout, ankylosing spondylitis, systemic lupus erythematosus, or rheumatic fever; or *septic abnormalities* such as septic arthritis

or tuberculous arthritis; or *hemorrhagic abnormalities* such as hemophilia, trauma, synovioma, hemangioma (benign neoplasm).

Interfering Factors
➤ Failure to mix the specimen with an anticoagulant, or delay in sending the specimen to the lab immediately, may result in inaccurate findings.
➤ Contamination of specimen may cause erroneous results.
➤ Exposing the specimen to an acid diluent will alter the white cell count and cause the mucin to precipitate.
➤ An elevated blood glucose level, such as with uncontrolled diabetes mellitus, or failure to adhere to dietary restrictions prior to testing, may affect the glucose level of the specimen.
➤ The microscopic examination may not reflect an infection or inflammatory process in its early stages.

Contraindication
➤ Skin or wound infections near joint, due to the risk of sepsis

Potential Complications
➤ Inflammation at needle insertion site
➤ Sepsis of joint, which may lead to osteomyelitis

NURSING CONSIDERATIONS
Prepare Your Client
➤ Explain as appropriate to the client that this procedure is to help find the reason for pain and swelling, or to help relieve discomfort by draining extra fluid and administering medication.
➤ Explain that the procedure is usually done by first giving a shot to numb the area, and this will cause a burning or stinging sensation before the area is numbed. The procedure takes approximately 10 minutes. A sedative may be needed for young children.
➤ Warn client that there may be some transient discomfort when the needle enters through the synovial membrane into the joint capsule.
➤ Restrict food or fluids, other than clear nonsweetened liquids, for 6–12 hours prior to the test if glucose determinations are planned.
➤ Ask the client if they currently take aspirin or anticoagulants. Consult with the primary health care provider about withholding these medications and ordering clotting studies.
➤ Ask the client and check the chart for a history of sensitivity to antiseptics such as betadine and local anesthetics such as lidocaine, carbocaine, and procainamide.
➤ Ensure that an informed consent is obtained, because of the possible complications associated with this procedure.

Perform Procedure
➤ Apply an elastic bandage around the joint to be aspirated in order to compress fluid into the sac, if ordered by the primary health care provider.
➤ Clean the site with an antiseptic.
➤ Administer a local anesthetic and insert a sterile aspiration needle into the joint space using strict aseptic technique.
➤ 10–15 mL of fluid is withdrawn.
➤ If injecting a corticosteroid or other medication, detach the first syringe and replace with the syringe containing medication while leaving the needle in place.
➤ Withdraw the needle and apply pressure with a sterile dressing for 2–3 minutes to prevent bleeding.

A

> Apply a dry sterile dressing.
> Prepare specimens for ordered microscopic exams using sterile technique. Add anticoagulants as specified by tests ordered. Gently invert several times to mix. For cultures, crystal examination, and cytologic studies, add heparin. For glucose measurements of fluid, add the preservative potassium oxalate. Do not add an anticoagulant for other studies, such as general appearance and mucin examination. Most tests require 2–5 mL of fluid, but refer to specific laboratory for exact amounts of fluid and type and amount of anticoagulant.
> Perform a venipuncture using a red-top tube for blood glucose if synovial fluid glucose is to be measured.
> Send all specimens to the lab immediately. Label specimens clearly as "Synovial Fluid" and "Do not use acid diluents."

Care After Test

> Apply ice packs (with cover) for 24–36 hours to decrease pain and swelling.
> Maintain good body alignment of affected joint. Use pillows or other aids as necessary.
> Apply an elastic bandage for joint stability if a large amount of fluid was removed.
> Use caution when handling soiled dressings, especially if septic arthritis is suspected.
> Observe the puncture site for erythema, tenderness, warmth, or exudate.
> Evaluate related tests such as arthrogram, arthroscopy, rheumatoid factors, serum calcium and phosphorus factors, coagulation studies, erythrocyte sedimentation rate (ESR), and antibody studies.

Educate Your Client and the Family

> Instruct client to resume activities when they feel ready, but to use frequent rest periods and support.
> Explain that the pain will increase after local anesthetic wears off, but should diminish in 2–3 days.
> Explain that client should expect some transient pain, swelling, and stiffness in the joint with increased use. Instruct client to report an increase in these feelings to the primary health care provider.
> Teach client about the symptoms of a joint infection—redness, tenderness, and fever—and to report them to the primary health care provider.

Arthrogram
ar throe gram
(Arthrography)

Normal Findings

Knee: Normal meniscus. Wedge-shaped shadow pointed toward the interior of the joint. Intact cartilage, ligaments, and tendons.
Shoulder: Intact subscapular bursa and joint capsule, bicipital tendon sheath.

What This Test Will Tell You

This radiographic test with contrast dye evaluates joint damage, usually in the knee or shoulder. It is usually indicated when a person is complaining of persistent pain in the knee or shoulder. This test is also commonly performed prior to arthroscopy or surgery. Because surgery cannot be performed immediately following the arthrogram due to the contrast medium, the physician may prefer to perform the arthroscopy rather than the arthrogram for direct visualization of the joint and for performing minor surgical repairs.

Arthrography provides visualization of soft tissues of encapsulated joints not seen on standard x-rays. These tissues include the meniscus, cartilage, ligaments, joint capsule, rotator cuff, and subacromial bursa. Although the knee is most common, other joints that can also be inspected include the shoulder, temporomandibular, elbow, wrist, and hip. The examination is made after air, contrast medium, or both are injected into the joint capsule.

Abnormal Findings

Abnormal knee results may indicate tears and lacerations of medial meniscus, tears and lacerations of joint ligaments and tendons, osteochondritis dissecans, osteochondral fractures, dislocation of bone or cartilage structures, joint capsule abnormalities, synovial abnormalities, arthritis, congenital abnormalities, or chondromalacia.

Abnormal shoulder results may indicate tears of the rotator cuff, tears of tendons, damage from recurrent joint dislocations, adhesive capsulitis, or bicipital tenosynovitis.

Interfering Factors

➤ Client's inability to perform the required maneuvers for visualization and spread of contrast medium (running in place or moving joint through full range of motion).
➤ Incomplete aspiration of joint fluid prior to instilling contrast medium dilutes the medium, diminishing the quality of the film.
➤ Improper injection technique puts contrast medium in the wrong position, causing inability to visualize.

Contraindications

➤ Acute arthritic attack; risks are infection and aggravation of inflammation.
➤ Infections of the joint or skin; risk is bone sepsis.
➤ Pregnancy; risk is radiation exposure to the fetus.
➤ Allergy to contrast material or iodine unless modifications in testing are made.
➤ Arthroscopy may be the test of choice for minor surgical repairs.

Potential Complications

➤ Infection at puncture site or in joint capsule
➤ Allergic or anaphylactic reaction to contrast medium
➤ Hemorrhage
➤ Thrombophlebitis

NURSING CONSIDERATIONS

Prepare Your Client

➤ Explain that this test is used to look at the soft tissue structures of the joint capsule, which are not seen on a regular x-ray.
➤ Explain that the client will remain alert and be given local anesthetics. The procedure takes approximately 30 minutes. Sedatives may be used for small children.
➤ Tell client that the procedure is performed in the radiology department in order for the examiner to

track the contrast medium on a special x-ray machine called a fluoroscope.

➤ Explain that discomfort may be experienced when the needle enters into the joint space and when manipulation of the joint is needed to spread the dye.

➤ Assess the client for a history of sensitivities or allergies to iodine, seafood, or to contrast medium used for other tests such as an IVP.

➤ Ensure that an informed consent is obtained, because of the possible complications associated with this procedure.

➤ Ask the client to bring someone to drive them home after the test is performed on an outpatient basis, because joint rest is required afterward.

Perform Procedure

➤ Nurses do not perform this procedure, but should understand the process to prepare the client. First, the area is cleansed using aseptic technique. Local anesthetic is administered to the puncture site. A needle is inserted into the joint space and synovial fluid is aspirated. A sample of synovial fluid is sent to the laboratory for synovial fluid analysis. (See *Arthrocentesis*.) Air and/or contrast medium is injected into the joint space. The joint is manipulated in order to distribute the contrast medium. This may be done with range-of-motion activities or running in place. Fluoroscopic x-rays are taken. A sterile dressing is applied.

Care After Test

➤ Apply elastic bandage for 12–24 hours.

➤ Apply ice bags, with cover, for first 12–24 hours to reduce swelling and possible bleeding.

➤ Apply warm soaks after the first 12–24 hours to relax tense muscles, decrease pain, and facilitate absorption of contrast medium.

➤ Assess puncture site for redness, bleeding, exudate, or swelling.

➤ Assess extremity below (distal to) the examined joint for pulses, capillary refill, temperature, color, and sensation.

➤ Administer mild analgesics as needed.

➤ Maintain joint rest for 12 hours.

➤ Observe for signs of allergic reaction to the contrast medium, which include urticaria, pruritus, conjunctivitis, dyspnea, and apprehension.

➤ Encourage client to drink fluids to facilitate renal excretion of the contrast medium and because the medium is a diuretic.

➤ Evaluate related tests such as the synovial fluid analysis and arthroscopy (done at least 24 hours later).

Educate Your Client and the Family

➤ Teach client that a slight grating in the joint is normal for up to 48 hours due to the removal of the synovial fluid, the joint's lubricant. Grating observed after this time should be reported to the primary health care provider.

➤ Teach application of elastic bandage if ordered.

➤ Instruct client not to use the joint for the first 24 hours. This includes driving, cooking, and other daily activities.

➤ Instruct the client not to perform strenuous activities such as jogging, weight lifting or exercise programs until after consulting with the primary health care provider.

> Teach client strengthening exercises, depending on results of tests and consultation with primary health care provider.

> Teach client about low-impact activities, depending on findings and consultation with physician.

Arthroscopy
ar thrah scoe pee

Normal Findings

ADULT AND ELDERLY

The normal synovial or diarthrodial joint is surrounded by muscles, ligaments, tendons, and cartilage. It is lined by a synovial membrane, which contains a viscous lubricating fluid. The synovial membrane is smooth with a fine vascular network. Cartilage is smooth and white. The ligaments and tendons are intact, silvery in color, and are cable-like. The articular cartilage and joint surfaces are smooth and white.

INFANT AND CHILD

The thick outer edges of the menisci (curved cartilage) of the knee are attached to the joint capsule, while the inner edges are unattached and lie snugly against the rounded surfaces of the bones.

ADOLESCENT

The expected findings are the same as for the adult. Changes from degenerative disease often begin in adolescence.

What This Test Will Tell You

This test uses a fiber-optic endoscope to visualize selected joints for injuries or abnormalities, monitor degenerative processes, and evaluate the effects of medical and surgical therapy. It is also used to perform minor surgical repairs. Biopsies and synovial fluid analysis are frequently done in conjunction with this test. The minor surgical repairs attempted through the use of an arthroscope provide a safer alternative to open surgery of a joint. The procedure is usually performed after a thorough history, x-rays, and arthrography. If surgery is anticipated, this visualization of the joint may be preferred to an arthrogram, whose contrast medium will delay arthroscopy and surgery.

Abnormal Findings

Abnormal results may indicate meniscal abnormalities (injury, tears), patellar abnormalities (dislocation, fracture, subluxation, chondromalacia), synovial abnormalities (synovitis, rheumatoid arthritis, degenerative arthritis, gout, pseudogout, osteochondromatosis), extrasynovial abnormalities (torn ligaments, Baker's cysts, ganglion cyst), or condylar abnormalities (osteochondritis dissecans, degenerative articular cartilage, bone fragments from fractures).

Interfering Factors

> Contrast medium used in arthrogram requires that arthroscopy be scheduled 24–48 hours later to allow the dye to be excreted.

Contraindications

> Wound or skin infections; risk is infecting the joint

➤ Bleeding disorders or anticoagulant therapy unless extreme caution is used and the benefits clearly outweigh the risks

➤ Severe fibrous ankylosis or joint flexion of less than 50 degrees, because joint cannot be positioned properly for fluid aspiration

Potential Complications

➤ Infection leading to osteomyelitis

➤ Untoward reactions to general or local anesthetics (includes topical anesthetics and narcotics)

➤ Injury or perforation to area

➤ Thrombophlebitis

➤ Hemorrhage, especially when biopsy is performed

➤ Infrapatellar anesthesia

➤ Synovial rupture

NURSING CONSIDERATIONS

Prepare Your Client

➤ Explain that this examination allows the physician to look inside the joint to find the injury or problem.

➤ Explain that minor surgical repairs may be done with the use of microscopic surgical instruments without the risks of an open surgery of the joint. This type of surgery is frequently referred to as "Band-Aid" surgery.

➤ Explain that the procedure usually takes approximately 15–30 minutes, and is performed by an orthopedic surgeon in the operating room.

➤ Inform client that the procedure is usually done using only numbing medicine in the area unless a surgical procedure is anticipated.

➤ Explain to the client receiving a local anesthetic that there will be transient discomfort from the injection, from the needle entering the joint cavity, and from the pressure of the tourniquet.

➤ Teach crutch walking prior to procedure to allow for practice before pain and swelling occur.

➤ Restrict food and fluids for at least 8 hours prior to the procedure.

➤ Assess the health history for a history of allergies to topical, local, or general anesthetics.

➤ Ensure that an informed consent is obtained, because of the possible complications associated with this procedure.

➤ Administer an IV antibiotic, if ordered, to prevent infection of the bone following manipulation.

➤ If hospital policy dictates, remove the hair from the area involved with a razor or depilatory cream. This may be done in the hospital room, preoperative waiting area, or in the operating room.

➤ Assess joint area for rashes or signs of infection.

➤ Evaluate the results of any coagulation studies performed.

Perform Procedure

Nurses do not perform this procedure but should understand the process to prepare the client. Position client on their back on the operating room table. Scrub area according to surgical procedure. Local anesthetic is administered. A spinal or general anesthetic may be administered by an anesthesiologist if surgical repair is indicated. Blood is drained from the leg (or joint) by applying a tourniquet and/or elastic wrap from toes to lower thigh. Elevate the leg. The foot of the table is lowered to put knee at a 45-degree angle.

A cannula is inserted into the joint capsule through a 3–5 mm incision. The obturator penetrating the synovial sac may cause some pain. The arthroscope is inserted in and out through the obturator to visualize various spaces. Usually one incision allows for viewing of entire joint. A camera may be attached to the arthroscope to photograph specific spaces. A normal saline and epinephrine solution is instilled for better viewing and to distend the joint capsule while minimizing bleeding. A synovial biopsy or reparative surgery is performed.

The arthroscope is removed and the joint irrigated with saline prior to removing cannula. Massage and apply pressure to the joint to remove saline solution. 1–2 stitches are made or steri-strips are applied before covering with an adhesive and compression dressings. A long leg cast is applied if extensive surgery is performed.

Care After Test
➤ Monitor for fever, bleeding, swelling, redness, heat, or tenderness at incision site.
➤ Monitor for deep pain and administer analgesics as indicated.
➤ Assess extremity for sensation, color, temperature, and capillary refill.
➤ Perform postoperative assessment

if client had a general anesthetic. This includes vital signs and level of consciousness until alert and stable.
➤ Apply covered ice bags to reduce swelling.
➤ Maintain adhesive dressing for 24 hours, then apply a small adhesive bandage.
➤ Administer intravenous antibiotics when ordered to prevent osteomyelitis.
➤ Resume client's preoperative diet.
➤ Evaluate related tests such as arthrogram, x-rays, and coagulation studies.

Educate Your Client and the Family
➤ Teach client that the joint may be used for mild to moderate activities, such as crutch walking, but excessive use should be avoided for 2–3 days and until after consultation with the primary health care provider.
➤ Instruct client to walk only with crutches for 2 days or until they can walk without a limp.
➤ Teach client leg strengthening exercises if ordered. A common exercise for the knee is straight-leg raises every hour with the gradual addition of weight. Within 7 days the client should raise 5–7 pounds.

Arylsulfatase A, Urine
air il sul fah tase • A • yur in
(ARS-A)

Normal Findings
ADULT, ELDERLY, ADOLESCENT
Male: 1.4–19.3 U/L
Female: 1.4–11 U/L
CHILD
1 U/L

What This Test Will Tell You
This urine test diagnoses a variety of cancers and other disorders. Arylsulfatase A (ARS-A) is an enzyme present throughout the body, except in fully developed erythrocytes. The

ARS-A enzyme is important in the detoxification of material to ester sulfates. Excessive levels interfere with this process, causing metabolic abnormalities.

Abnormal Findings

▲INCREASED LEVELS may indicate cancer of the bladder, colon, or rectum; genetic lyposomal disorders; or myeloid (granulocytic) leukemia.

▼DECREASED LEVELS may indicate metachromatic leukodystrophy.

Interfering Factors

➤ Specimen contaminated with toilet tissue, stool, mucus, or menses.
➤ Improper storage of specimen.
➤ Surgery performed within 1 week of testing will result in elevated levels.
➤ Failure to collect all urine during 24-hour testing period.

NURSING CONSIDERATIONS

Prepare Your Client

➤ Explain that this test measures a substance (enzyme) that is normally present throughout the body but can be increased or decreased in certain conditions.
➤ Explain that the test requires that all urine be collected during the 24 hours of the test.
➤ Instruct the client to make sure that urine is not contaminated with toilet tissue, stool, mucus, or menses.

Perform Procedure

➤ Obtain a 24-hour urine collection in a container with preservative.
➤ Keep the specimen on ice or in refrigerator during the test.

Care After Test

➤ Assess for signs and symptoms of metastatic cancer including bone pain, fatigue, and recurring symptoms of the tumor.

➤ Refer client and family to a cancer support group.
➤ Assess for the client's ability to cope with changes in body image such as weight loss or gain, loss of hair, changes in body functions, decreased sexual function, and role changes. Refer to social services to assist with the financial and economic impact of cancer.
➤ Consult with a registered dietician for client with anorexia, weight loss, or special dietary needs.
➤ Assess for signs and symptoms of infection such as chills, fever, and drop in the absolute neutrophil count. Institute precautions to protect the client such as no fresh fruits or vegetables. Remove fresh flowers and plants, enforce good handwashing, and have client avoid persons with upper respiratory tract infections.
➤ Review related tests such as complete blood count with differential, carcinoma antigen 19-9, carcinoembryonic antigen level, urinalysis, fecal occult blood, computed tomography scan, alkaline phosphatase, acid phosphatase, and metachromatic granules in urine.

Educate Your Client and the Family

➤ As appropriate, instruct client and family on a high-calorie, well-balanced diet.
➤ Assess for alterations in patterns of bowel or bladder elimination. Promote more normal patterns by encouraging adequate fluid intake and a well-balanced diet unless contraindicated.
➤ If a lipid storage decrease is suspected, assess family history and refer concerned client of childbearing age to a genetic counselor.

Ascorbic Acid, Urine and Plasma

ah skor bik • ass id • yur in • and • plaz mah
(Vitamin C)

Normal Findings

ALL AGES
Plasma: 0.2–2.0 mg/dL (SI units: 10–120 µmol/L)
Urine: 30 mg/24 hours (SI units: 180 µmol/24 hours)
PREGNANT
Values may be lower during pregnancy and in the immediate postpartum period.

What This Test Will Tell You

These blood and urine tests diagnose metabolic and nutritional abnormalities related to ascorbic acid intake or utilization. Ascorbic acid, also known as vitamin C, is necessary for capillary synthesis, capillary formation, and resistance to infection. It is necessary for adequate iron absorption, and it plays a critical role in wound healing.

Abnormal Findings

▼DECREASED LEVELS may indicate anorexia, malnutrition, smoking, pregnancy or postpartum period, fever, infection, burns, cancer, malabsorption syndromes, tissue healing, scurvy, or cancer.
▲INCREASED LEVELS may indicate massive ascorbic acid therapy or excessive dietary intake.

Interfering Factors

➤ Aspirin, estrogens, oral contraceptives, aminopyrine, barbiturates, paraldehyde, nitrosamines, and heavy metals can lower the serum ascorbic acid level.
➤ Vitamin C levels are lower in smokers than nonsmokers, and may be depleted following prolonged stress.
➤ Ascorbic acid can interfere with tests that detect glucose in the urine.
➤ Excessive oral intake of vitamin C within 24 hours of testing will cause elevated test results.

NURSING CONSIDERATIONS

Prepare Your Client

➤ Explain that this test is used to determine the amount of vitamin C in the blood, so that problems with getting enough or with the body being able to use it can be found.
➤ Check with your laboratory regarding the need to restrict food and fluids for 8 hours prior to the test.
➤ For the urine test, explain the 24-hour urine collection process to the client or family.

Perform Procedure

➤ For the plasma test, collect 10 mL of venous blood in a green-top tube.
➤ For the urine test, collect a 24-hour urine specimen, refrigerating it or keeping it on ice during the collection period.

Care After Test

➤ Assess health history for infection, fever, anemia, ascorbic acid replacement therapy, tissue trauma, and malignancies that may affect levels.
➤ Evaluate for signs and symptoms of scurvy, a rare but severe disorder resulting from prolonged ascorbic acid deficiency. Symptoms include petechiae, ecchymoses, gum changes,

hyperkeratosis, arthralgia, dyspnea, edema, weakness, lethargy, and aching legs.

➤ Consult with a registered dietician to assist the family and client in meeting special dietary needs.

➤ If the client has anorexia or malnutrition related to an eating disorder, advise that counseling and/or family therapy can help treat eating disorder symptoms and prevent relapses.

➤ Evaluate other laboratory tests that help determine nutritional status, such as the serum albumin and the complete blood count.

Educate Your Client and the Family

➤ Teach client and family dietary sources of ascorbic acid, especially fresh fruits and vegetables.

➤ If the client is a smoker, stress the importance of smoking cessation, and refer to a smoking cessation support group.

Aspartate Aminotransferase, Serum

ass par tate • am in oe trans fur ase • see rum
(AST, Serum Aspartate Transaminase, Formerly Called Serum Glutamic-Oxaloacetic Transaminase or SGOT)

Normal Findings

ADULT
5–40 IU/L (SI units: 8–20 U/L)
Values may be slightly lower in females.
Exercise may increase values.

PREGNANT
Labor and delivery cause slight increases in levels.

NEWBORN
25–75 U/L
Normal values may be 2–4 times higher than adult levels.

INFANT
15–60 U/L

CHILD AND ADOLESCENT
Similar to adult levels.

ELDERLY
Values are slightly higher than adult's.

What This Test Will Tell You

This blood test helps determine the extent of damage to the liver, heart or musculoskeletal system. This test is often performed in conjunction with the alanine aminotransferase (ALT) test. Both AST and ALT are enzymes found mainly in liver, heart, and skeletal muscle tissue; only small amounts are found in kidney tissue. Serum levels of these enzymes rise proportionately to the amount of tissue damage present when intracellular enzymes are released from injured cells.

Values differ in different pathophysiologic conditions. In alcoholic hepatitis, the AST level is usually greater than the ALT level. In viral and chronic hepatitis, the ALT level is greater than the AST level. Values of AST may be as high as 20 times that of normal in fulminant forms of hepatitis. In myocardial infarction, the AST level begins to rise 6–10 hours after the infarction occurs and levels peak 12–48 hours following infarction. Levels do not return to normal until 72–96 hours following the infarction.

Abnormal Findings

▲ INCREASED LEVELS (*Very high levels—10–20 times normal*) may indicate acute viral hepatitis, mononucleosis, alcoholic cirrhosis, extensive musculoskeletal trauma, extensive burns, or hepatotoxicity from medications.

Moderately increased to high levels (5–10 times normal) may indicate chronic hepatitis, muscular dystrophy, dermatomyositis, or resolving or prodromal stages of viral hepatitis, mononucleosis, or alcoholic cirrhosis.

Slightly to moderately increased levels (2–5 times normal) may indicate hemolytic anemia, acute pancreatitis, pulmonary emboli, or metastatic hepatic tumors.

▼ DECREASED LEVELS may indicate pregnancy, diabetic ketoacidosis, or beriberi.

Interfering Factors

➤ Many drugs may increase results either by causing cholestasis or by hepatotoxic effects. These include antibiotics such as ampicillin, clindamycin, and erythromycin; vitamins including folic acid, pyridoxine, and vitamin A; narcotics; salicylates; digitalis; cortisone; indomethacin; isoniazid (INH); and oral contraceptives.

➤ Intensive exercise or musculoskeletal trauma, including intramuscular injections may increase levels.

➤ Hemolysis of specimen may cause elevated levels.

➤ Failure to draw samples during rising or peak periods may result in normal serum results despite organ injury.

NURSING CONSIDERATIONS

Prepare Your Client

➤ Explain that this test is important to help understand either how well the liver is functioning or to help diagnose a heart attack. If appropriate, explain that this test also helps evaluate how well either the liver or the heart is healing after liver disease or a heart attack has been diagnosed.

➤ Do not administer intramuscular injections prior to drawing the blood sample for AST to be sure results are not altered by muscular trauma.

Perform Procedure

➤ Collect 7–10 cc of venous blood in a red-top tube.

➤ If serial samples are being obtained to measure fluctuation of enzyme levels, carefully note the time and sample number. Note on the lab slip the time of the onset of chest pain where indicated.

➤ Unless otherwise ordered or indicated, draw serial samples at the same time each day.

➤ Handle the sample gently to avoid hemolysis.

Care After Test

➤ Assess client for unusual bruising or prolonged bleeding from venipuncture site. Delayed clotting is a complication of severely impaired liver function.

➤ Assess skin and sclera of eyes for jaundice and note findings. Protect the skin from damage due to pressure or friction.

➤ Assess for occult gastrointestinal bleeding with routine stool guaiac testing. Esophageal varices and mucosal bleeding are complications of liver disease.

> If myocardial infarction is suspected, assess for pertinent signs/symptoms such as chest or arm pain, nausea, or diaphoresis.

> Consult with a registered dietician to design a high-calorie, well-balanced diet for patients with liver disease. As appropriate, reduce sodium or protein in the diet if edema or increased ammonia levels are present.

> Consult with a registered dietician to design a low-fat, low-sodium diet for clients with heart disease.

> Review related tests such as serum alanine aminotransferase (ALT), direct and indirect bilirubin levels, alkaline phosphatase, and prothrombin time.

Educate Your Client and the Family

> Instruct the client and family to report any jaundice—yellow discoloration of skin or whites of the eyes.

> For client with severely impaired liver function, instruct client and family to report unusual or increased bruising and tarry stools. Instruct them to use electric razors and non-skid shoes to avoid falls and injuries.

> For client with suspected heart attack (myocardial infarction), tell client and family to report any chest or arm pain, indigestion, nausea, or profuse sweating to staff immediately.

> Instruct client and family on a high-calorie, well-balanced diet as appropriate. If sodium or protein restrictions are indicated, help client and family make dietary selections with these limitations.

> Assist client with heart disease to achieve a low-sodium, low-fat diet.

Aspergillus Antibody, Serum
ass per gill uss • an ti bod ee • see rum

Normal Findings
Negative, no aspergillus antibodies found

What This Test Will Tell You
This blood test detects the presence of circulating antibodies to the fungal organism *Aspergillus*. *Aspergillus* is commonly found in our environment but becomes a pathogen when inhaled by an immunocompromised host. Systemic infection by *Aspergillus* is most likely to occur in clients with low white blood cell counts and those taking large doses of steroids, immunosuppressant agents, or cyto-toxic drugs. *Aspergillus* can also invade and form a fungus ball (aspergilloma) in lungs previously damaged by tuberculosis, bronchiectasis, or cancer, or it may infect the eye, ear, or heart valves after surgical replacement.

Antibodies to *Aspergillus* are not always detectable when the client has a systemic infection, but a positive titer is helpful in diagnosis. *Aspergillus* antibodies are more likely to be present if the client has a pulmonary fungus ball or the allergic manifestation called allergic bronchopulmonary disease. Because antibody titers are not always present and cultures and sputum smears are not always positive, *Aspergillus* is difficult to diagnose. Clinicians should rely on symptoms, history, cultures, x-rays, and antibody titers.

Abnormal Findings

▲ INCREASED LEVELS may indicate fungus ball in the lungs, allergic bronchopulmonary disease, *Aspergillus* infection of the heart valves, or systemic infection.

Interfering Factors

➤ Antibody testing is often negative in immunocompromised clients.

NURSING CONSIDERATIONS

Prepare Your Client

➤ Tell your client that this test will look for evidence that a mold or fungus is causing problems.

Perform Procedure

➤ Perform a venipuncture, drawing at least 7 mL of venous blood in a red-top tube.

Care After Test

➤ Monitor your client's temperature. Fever in spite of antibiotics is characteristic of fungal infections.
➤ Check the color of the sputum. *Aspergillus* has a golden brown color.
➤ Assess the respiratory system for dyspnea, uncontrolled coughing, hemoptysis, and hypoxia, which indicate pulmonary involvement.
➤ If your client has a low white blood cell count and is neutropenic, institute neutropenic precautions. Calculate the absolute neutrophil count to ascertain if the client is truly neu-

tropenic. Use the following formula: % neutrophils of total white blood cell count × (bands + segs) = absolute count

If the absolute count is < 1000, then there is a moderate chance of severe bacterial infection. If the absolute count is < 500, there is a strong possibility of severe bacterial infection.

➤ Institute precautions for client with neutropenia, including impeccable handwashing, no rectal temperatures or suppositories, no intramuscular injections, no fresh fruit or flowers in the room, and no visitors or caregivers with upper respiratory tract infections.
➤ Client with severe fungal infections is likely to be treated with amphotericin, which requires premedication with diphenhydramine, steroids, and acetaminophen.
➤ Review related tests such as the white blood cell count and differential, sputum cultures, and chest x-ray.

Educate Your Client and the Family

➤ Explain that *Aspergillus* is not contagious; it cannot be transmitted from person to person.
➤ Teach your client and family that all visitors and staff who come in contact with a neutropenic person must wash their hands before contact.
➤ Ask family and significant others not to visit if they have a cold or other infection.
➤ Inform your client that the unpleasant side effects of amphotericin will be lessened by premedication.

Atrial Natriuretic Factor

ay tree al • nay tree yu ret ik • fak tor

(Natriuretic Hormone, Atrial Natriuretic Hormone, Atrionatriuretic Peptides)

Normal Findings
All ages: 20–77 pg/mL

What This Test Will Tell You
This blood test helps in the diagnosis of congestive heart failure (CHF) and circulatory volume overload. The test measures the blood levels of atrial natriuretic factor (ANF), a hormone produced by the heart in response to stretching from increased blood volume. ANF has several important actions in the body that all work to decrease blood pressure and circulating volume. ANF's actions to reduce total blood volume mean less stretch occurs within the heart and ANF levels should be reduced.

Abnormal Findings
▲INCREASED LEVELS may indicate congestive heart failure or myocardial dysfunction.

▼DECREASED LEVELS may indicate dehydration, hypovolemia, hemorrhage, or distributive shock.

Interfering Factors
➤ Cardiac medications
➤ Antihypertensive and other vasoactive medications
➤ Diuretics
➤ Steroids
➤ Oral contraceptives
➤ Antibiotics
➤ Non-steroidal anti-inflammatory medications

NURSING CONSIDERATIONS
Prepare Your Client
➤ Explain that this test helps determine how well the heart is able to pump and circulate all of the blood volume.

➤ Discuss with the primary health care provider the need to withhold cardiac and vasoactive medications for 24 hours preceding the test. Normally these medications are not given during this time.

➤ Instruct the client not to eat for 12–14 hours before the test. Water is allowed.

➤ Advise the client not to greatly change salt intake in the days preceding the sampling.

Perform Procedure
➤ Collect 7 mL of venous blood in a *chilled* lavender-top tube.

Care After Test
➤ Evaluate the client's diet for the average daily sodium intake.

➤ Evaluate the client's history for coronary and vascular disease. Especially note nocturnal dyspnea and dependent edema.

➤ Review related tests such as serum sodium and serum osmolarity.

Educate Your Client and the Family
➤ Explain that this test is important in determining how well the heart is able to pump blood throughout the body.

➤ Teach the client with elevated ANF levels that sodium restriction is important to prevent the heart from being overloaded by too much fluid and blood to pump.

➤ Emphasize foods that are part of a heart-healthy diet, rather than dwelling on foods that are not healthy.

➤ Stress the importance of regularly scheduled exercise.

➤ Instruct the client to notify the primary health care provider if increased swelling in the ankles, feet, back, or surrounding the eyes should be noticed. Difficulty breathing, including at night, or using more pillows to sleep at night should also be reported.

A

Bacterial Meningitis Antigen
bak teer ee ahl • men in jie tis • an ti jen

Normal Findings
Normally, results are negative for bacterial antigens.

What This Test Will Tell You
This test detects the presence of bacteria antigen in cerebral spinal fluid (CSF), which confirms a diagnosis of meningitis. This test is used only as an adjunct to CSF Gram stain and culture.

Bacteria can be found in CSF by Gram stain 80% of the time when a client has bacterial meningitis. Antigen testing is a quick and accurate way to detect bacteria when Gram stain is negative, before cultures come back, or when it is crucial to identify a specific organism. A negative test for bacterial antigen, however, is not conclusive.

Two methods to detect bacterial antigens are in common use: latex agglutination (LA) and countercurrent immunoelectrophoresis (CIE). Both detect antigens to *H. influenzae*, *N. meningitidis*, meningococcal groups A, B, C, and *S. pneumoniae*, all of which are common causes of meningitis. The LA method is faster and more accurate. Antigens may also be found in blood and urine, but CSF testing yields the most reliable results.

Abnormal Findings
▲ INCREASED LEVELS (or a positive result) may indicate bacterial meningitis.

███████ ACTION ALERT!
The presence of bacterial antigen in cerebral spinal fluid confirms a diagnosis of bacterial meningitis. Antibiotic therapy should be started immediately.

Interfering Factors
➤ *E. coli* and *N. meningitidis* antigen may cause false positive reaction with group B meningococcal reagent.
➤ Previous antibiotic therapy may interfere with accurate test results.

NURSING CONSIDERATIONS
Prepare Your Client
➤ Explain that this test is to help diagnose an infection in the brain.
➤ See *Lumbar Puncture* for information on how to prepare client for CSF test.

Perform Procedure
➤ See *Lumbar Puncture* for information on CSF procedure.
➤ Collect at least 1 mL of CSF in a sterile container using aseptic technique.
➤ If urine is being tested, collect 10 mL of urine by clean catch in a sterile container.

Care After Test
➤ See *Lumbar Puncture.*
➤ Make sure client is in a quiet, darkened room. Clients with meningitis are often photophobic and suffer from meningeal irritation.
➤ Perform frequent neurological checks to detect changes in level of consciousness and other focal neurological changes.
➤ If client has meningococcal meningitis, they must be placed on respiratory isolation.
➤ Observe client carefully for onset of seizures. Institute seizure precautions.
➤ Begin appropiate antibiotics as soon as cultures are drawn.
➤ Administer antipyretics for fever

and pain management. Narcotics are not indicated.

➤ Review related tests such as CSF culture and sensitivity, CSF analysis, and CSF pressure.

Educate Your Client and the Family

➤ If client has meningococcal meningitis, then all recent contacts must begin prophylactic antibiotic therapy.

➤ Discuss recent health history with client and family. Inquire if there is a recent history of upper respiratory infection, ear infection, or exposure to others with recent illnesses.

➤ Reassure them that recovery is usually complete if appropiate therapy is instituted.

Barium Enema
ba ree um • en e mah
(Barium Enema, Air Contrast Study, BE, Lower Gastrointestinal Series, Lower GI Series)

Normal Findings

Absence of ulcerations, polyps, mass lesions, strictures/stenoses, diverticula, and acute inflammatory structural changes
Normal filling, emptying, and colonic wall movement

What This Test Will Tell You

This x-ray with contrast test is used primarily to diagnose diseases of the colon and large intestine such as colorectal cancer, inflammatory disease, polyps, diverticula, and structural changes in the lower gastrointestinal (GI) tract. The colon of the normal client allows unobstructed fecal passage through peristalsis. Peristaltic movements can be viewed during fluoroscopic visualization of the barium enema.

Abnormal Findings

Abnormalities may indicate precancerous and cancerous polyps, colon cancer, lower GI tract ulceration/bleeding, inflammatory bowel disease, ulcerative colitis, diverticulitis, Crohn's disease, appendicitis, external compression of bowel from tumors or abscesses, fistulas, diverticulosis, or intussusception.

ACTION ALERT!

Rare but life-threatening complications of this procedure include intestinal perforation and anaphylaxis. Assess for signs of intestinal perforation, which include severe pain, fever, rigid abdomen, and shock symptoms.

Interfering Factors

➤ Stool in the intestinal tract.
➤ Inability to retain the barium in the lower intestine.
➤ Inability to remain on the fluoroscopy table until all areas of the large intestine have been visualized may decrease the information available.
➤ Barium used in an upper GI study done in the previous 2–4 days may impair visualization.
➤ Hospitalized elderly clients with dementia, acute febrile illness,

cachexia, fecal incontinence, or diarrhea may be less likely to tolerate the preparations necessary to adequately interpret the barium enema.

Contraindications

➤ Fulminant ulcerative colitis
➤ Toxic megacolon
➤ Intestinal obstruction
➤ Unstable cardiovascular status
➤ Inability to cooperate
➤ Suspected perforation, since colonic wall distention with barium during the procedure can worsen hemorrhage and colonic inflammation, and increase the risk of perforation and bacteremia

Potential Complications

➤ Rectal or vaginal perforation induced by the balloon enema tip
➤ Bowel perforation
➤ Mild allergic reactions with pruritus, urticaria, and edema
➤ Vasovagal reactions
➤ Anaphylaxis
➤ Fecal impaction with barium

NURSING CONSIDERATIONS

Prepare Your Client

➤ Tell the client that this test is used to visualize the lower GI tract, in order to see if any abnormalities exist. Let them know it will take about 45–60 minutes.
➤ If they are needed, roentgenographic (x-ray) and diagnostic studies of the colon such as ultrasound and colonoscopy should be done prior to barium studies, since barium may obscure other films.
➤ Explain that the procedure is done with the client awake. Intravenous sedation may be given to promote comfort and relaxation, but it is not usually required.

➤ Inform the client that although the procedure is uncomfortable, it should not be painful. Tell the client that they may feel abdominal cramping, but that they should notify the nurse if they feel severe abdominal pain.
➤ Tell the client they may be asked to change positions on the fluoroscopy table in order to ensure that barium solution covers the entire bowel wall and that the barium-filled colon is adequately visualized.
➤ Ensure that an informed consent is obtained, because of the possible complications associated with this procedure.
➤ Note the presence of allergies, asthma, or atopic disease on the medical record before a barium enema is performed, since there is a small potential for allergens associated with balloon-equipped enema tips to be absorbed through the rectal mucosa and result in an anaphylactic reaction.
➤ Ensure the adequacy of the bowel preparation. In adults, this is usually a cathartic and enema preparation or a balanced electrolyte lavage solution. A liquid diet for 24–48 hours before the procedure is necessary.
➤ Check for individualized bowel preparations for clients with intestinal ostomies.
➤ Administer the appropriate bowel preparation for pediatric clients. The solution is usually magnesium citrate, 30 mL per year of age to a maximum of 300 mL, given the day before the procedure, along with saline enemas the night before and the morning of the procedure. A liquid diet for 48 hours before the procedure is recommended.
➤ Have the client urinate before the procedure.

Perform Procedure

Nurses do not perform this procedure, but should understand the process to prepare the client and to assist the gastroenterologist in obtaining the best results from the procedure. After the bowel is cleansed to prepare the colon for the procedure, barium sulfate (a chalky, radiopaque, water-soluble, inert substance) is administered rectally to provide a contrast medium, and radiographic pictures of the bowel are taken under fluoroscopy. Fluoroscopy allows visualization of bowel filling and colonic movements. Spot films may be taken at intervals. A single-contrast barium enema uses only barium as a contrast agent, whereas a double-contrast barium enema uses a combination of barium and air as contrast agents.

Encourage the client to retain the enema, despite abdominal cramping or urge to defecate. Position the client as needed to promote barium-filling of the colon and to adequately visualize the bowel: prone, prone 45 degrees, Trendelenburg, supine, and left lateral decubitus are positions that may be used. Apply pressure to areas of the client's abdomen as needed, to assist with adequate barium filling and visualization of the colon. Assess the client's vital signs, oxygenation status, level of abdominal distention, level of consciousness, vagal response, and pain tolerance during the procedure.

Care After Test

➤ Monitor vital signs every 15–30 minutes until the client is stable.

➤ Observe for signs of complications, such as bleeding, vomiting, change in vital signs, severe abdominal pain and/or distention, and abdominal rigidity.

➤ Administer cleansing enema or laxative as ordered, to help evacuate barium from the GI tract.

➤ Increase oral fluids to help the evacuation of the barium.

➤ Evaluate related tests such as colonoscopy, fecal occult blood, hemoglobin, and carcinoembryonic antigen.

Educate Your Client and the Family

➤ Inform the client that following a double-contrast procedure some abdominal discomfort may be felt, due to the air forced into the bowel lumen during the procedure. Getting up and walking around can help get rid of the air and minimize the discomfort.

➤ Advise the client that increasing fluid intake after the procedure can help clear barium from the system.

➤ Teach client to expect stools to be chalky and light-colored for 24–72 hours after the barium.

➤ Instruct the client to call the primary care provider if barium is not passed after 2–3 days; cathartics or enemas may be prescribed to avoid constipation or obstruction.

➤ Teach client and family an anti-cancer diet, including the need for adequate fluid and fiber intake.

Barium Swallow

ba ree um • swal oe

(Upper Gastrointestinal Test, Upper GI Test, Upper GI Series, Esophageal Radiography)

Normal Findings

Absence of ulcerations, polyps, mass lesions, strictures/stenoses, foreign bodies, varices, diverticula, motility disorders, and hiatal hernia

What This Test Will Tell You

This radiographic test visualizes the esophagus, stomach, duodenum, and jejunum and diagnoses diseases such as peptic ulcer disease, cancer, inflammatory disease, polyps, and diverticula. Fluoroscopic examination uses barium sulfate to visualize the structures of the upper gastrointestinal system. In some agencies, a barium swallow is used to visualize and diagnose problems in the esophagus only. In other agencies, this test is used to visualize the entire upper gastrointestinal tract.

Abnormal Findings

Gastrointestinal abnormalities may indicate obstructions, ulcerations, strictures, foreign bodies, lower esophageal rings, esophageal motility disorders, esophagitis, diverticula, varices, polyps, tumors, hiatus hernia, chalasia, achalasia, or compression of the esophagus.

ACTION ALERT!

If barium studies are performed as the initial diagnostic tool for clients with peptic ulcer disease, and gastrointestinal (GI) bleeding ensues or worsens, barium will obscure and delay tests that can verify bleeding sites, such as endoscopy and angiography. Performing an upper GI series before angiography and endoscopy must be carefully considered in the presence of actual or potential bleeding.

Interfering Factors

➤ Roentgenographic (x-ray) and diagnostic studies of the GI tract including abdominal scans, ultrasounds, and endoscopy should be done prior to barium studies, since barium may limit the information obtained from these tests.

➤ Food in the upper gastrointestinal tract, especially the esophagus, will impair visualization.

➤ Barium studies may not be accurate in identifying shallow superficial ulcers, due to failure of the barium to properly fill the ulcer crater.

Contraindications

➤ Intestinal obstruction, since esophageal wall distention with barium during the procedure can worsen esophageal inflammation and increase the risk of perforation and bacteremia. Diatrizoate (Gastrografin) rather than barium is the preferred contrast medium for clients with suspected perforations.

➤ Unstable cardiovascular status.

Potential Complications

➤ Mild allergic reactions with pruritus, urticaria, and edema

➤ Vasovagal reactions

➤ Fecal impaction with barium

NURSING CONSIDERATIONS

Prepare Your Client

➤ Explain that this test is used to look at the stomach, swallowing tube, and other parts of the upper intestinal tract to see if any problems exist. The test usually takes less than 30 minutes.

➤ Ensure that an informed consent is obtained, because of the possible complications associated with this procedure.

➤ Make sure food, fluids, and oral medications are withheld after midnight prior to the procedure.

➤ Explain that the procedure is done with the client awake. Intravenous sedation may be given to promote comfort and relaxation, but it is not usually required.

➤ Tell the client that although the procedure may be uncomfortable, it should not be painful.

➤ Instruct the client that changing positions on the fluoroscopy table may be needed to ensure that barium solution covers the entire esophagus and that the barium-filled lumen can be adequately visualized.

➤ Ensure adequacy of esophageal preparation. In adults, this means that the client swallows a barium mixture while in the supine position. Dysphagic clients should swallow a barium tablet or a food/marshmallow bolus in addition to liquid barium, to aid in better visualization of esophageal strictures.

Perform Procedure

Nurses do not perform this procedure, but should understand the process to prepare the client and to assist the gastroenterologist in obtaining the best results from the procedure.

Barium sulfate (a chalky, radiopaque, water-soluble, inert substance) is swallowed while in a supine position to provide a contrast medium. Radiographic pictures of the esophagus, stomach, duodenum, and jejunum are taken under fluoroscopy. Position the patient as needed to promote barium-filling of the esophagus and other organs and to promote adequate visualization; supine and Trendelenburg are positions that may be used.

Assess the client's vital signs, oxygenation status, level of abdominal distention, level of consciousness, vagal response, and pain tolerance during the procedure.

Care After Test

➤ Monitor vital signs closely until stable; usually every 25 minutes for the first hour, every 30 minutes for the next hour, and then every 4 hours for 24 hours.

➤ Observe for signs of complications, such as bleeding, vomiting, change in vital signs, severe abdominal pain and/or distention, and abdominal rigidity.

➤ Administer cleansing enema or laxative as ordered, to help evacuate barium from the GI tract.

➤ Evaluate related tests such as gastrointestinal endoscopies, esophageal function studies, chest x-rays, and scans that visualize the gastrointestinal tract.

Educate Your Client and the Family

➤ Advise the client that increasing fluid intake after the procedure can help clear barium from the system.

➤ Teach client to expect stools to be chalky and light-colored for 24–72 hours after the barium.

➤ Tell the client to call their primary health care provider if the barium is not passed after 2–3 days; cathartics or enemas may be prescribed to avoid constipation or obstruction.

➤ Teach client and family an anti-cancer diet, including the need for adequate fluid and fiber intake.

Barr Body Analysis
bar • bod ee • ah nal ah sis
(Sex Chromatin Mass, Sex Chromatin Body, Sex Chromatin Test, Chromatin-Positive Body, Buccal Smear)

Normal Findings
FEMALES
Chromatin positive (one Barr body in the cell nucleus). 25%–50% of the cells tested will be chromatin positive.
MALES
Chromatin negative (no Barr bodies).

What This Test Will Tell You
This microscopic examination screens for sex chromosome abnormalities and helps determine the gender of a newborn with ambiguous genitalia. During embryonic implantation, one of the two normal X chromosomes in a female becomes inactivated, forming a chromatin mass or Barr body. In a normal female (XX), only one X chromosome in a cell will be active. The most common sex chromosome abnormality in females is Turner's syndrome, in which there are either no chromatin bodies or less than 20% Barr chromatin bodies (XO).

A normal male (XY) will have no Barr chromatin bodies, as he has only one X chromosome. In males, the most common abnormality is Klinefelter's syndrome, in which Barr chromatin bodies are present (XXY).

The Barr body analysis is used for screening only. A full karyotype (chromosome analysis) is needed if abnormalities are detected, or may be used instead of the Barr analysis. Chromosome analysis is a simple, more accurate test.

Abnormal Findings
▲ INCREASED LEVELS may indicate Klinefelter's syndrome in males.
▼ DECREASED LEVELS may indicate Turner's syndrome in females.

Interfering Factors
➤ Poor sampling technique resulting in inadequate numbers of buccal cells.
➤ Inadequate fixation of cells on the microscopic slide results in cell deterioration.
➤ Adrenocorticosteroid or estrogen therapy.
➤ Age of client less than 7 days.

NURSING CONSIDERATIONS
Prepare Your Client
➤ Explain to the client or parents that this test is to determine the cause of abnormal sexual development.
➤ Explain that although other body cells can be used, the specimen is usually taken from the inside of the cheek (buccal mucosa) because it is easy to obtain cells from that site.

➤ Assure client or family that there will be little to no discomfort during the procedure, although light pressure will be used to obtain the specimen.
➤ Do not restrict food or fluid prior to the test.

Perform Procedure
➤ Have client rinse mouth well before procedure if they are old enough to do so.
➤ Scrape buccal mucosa with a wooden or metal spatula twice; discard the first specimen and spread the second specimen over a glass slide. Buccal mucosa must be scraped firmly to collect an adequate number of cells and to avoid collection of saliva without cells.
➤ Spray the slide with a cell fixative.
➤ Label specimen with client's name, gender, age, date specimen was obtained, and the specimen site.
➤ Send the specimen to the laboratory.

Care After Test
➤ Observe client for discomfort in area from which the specimen was collected.

➤ Explain to client or family that it may take up to 4 weeks to obtain test results.
➤ Answer client and family's questions and make referrals as indicated.
➤ Review related tests such as chromosome analysis.

Educate Your Client and the Family
➤ Explain that this test is for screening; in the event of abnormal findings, additional tests may be done to confirm the diagnosis.
➤ Be supportive of client and family, recognizing anxiety that may be associated with a diagnosis of sex chromosome abnormalities.
➤ If testing is to determine the child's gender, explain that a medical team will work together to identify the sex of the child. Explain the importance of doing this at an early age to avoid gender identification and developmental problems.

B

Bence-Jones Protein
benss joenz • proe teen
(Urine Immunoelectrophoresis)

Normal Findings
All ages: Absence of Bence-Jones protein in urine

What This Test Will Tell You
This urine test diagnoses multiple myeloma and Waldenström's macroglobulinemia. Bence-Jones protein is a specific, low-molecular-weight protein made by cancerous plasma

cells in the bone marrow. It is rapidly cleared by the kidneys and then excreted in the urine. When the renal tubular load is exceeded by the increased amounts of protein, tubular cells may become damaged and renal failure can result.

These proteins are found in only 50–80% of clients with multiple myeloma, but they are found in almost all clients with Waldenström's macroglobulinemia.

Abnormal Findings

▲ INCREASED LEVELS may indicate multiple myeloma, Waldenström's macroglobulinemia, tumor metastases to the bone, amyloidosis, macroglobulinemia, or chronic lymphocytic leukemia.

Interfering Factors

➤ Connective tissue disease.
➤ Renal insufficiency.
➤ Contamination with menstrual blood may yield false positive results.
➤ Prostatic secretion or semen may yield false positive results.
➤ Failure to keep specimen refrigerated may result in false positive findings.
➤ Contamination with stool or toilet paper.
➤ Very dilute urine may result in false negative findings.

NURSING CONSIDERATIONS

Prepare Your Client

➤ Explain that this test is important to help diagnose some types of cancer, especially multiple myeloma.
➤ Instruct client to provide an early morning urine sample.
➤ Tell the client not to contaminate specimen with stool, menses, or toilet paper.

Perform Procedure

➤ Instruct the client to collect an early morning specimen of at least 50 cc (about 2 ounces) of urine in sterile container.
➤ Refrigerate specimen; heat coagulates the protein and can cause decomposition, which results in false positive findings.

Care After Test

➤ Assess for signs and symptoms of metastatic cancer including bone pain, fatigue, and recurring symptoms of the tumor.
➤ Assess the client for signs and symptoms of hypercalcemia, renal failure, or neurological deficits such as weakness. Take special safety precautions if motor weakness or neurological deficits are noted.
➤ Assess carefully for chronic and acute pain. Obtain pain management consultation if indicated.
➤ Assess for signs and symptoms of infection such as chills, fever, and drop in the absolute neutrophil count. Institute precautions to protect the client such as no fresh fruits or vegetables. Remove fresh flowers and plants, and enforce good handwashing.
➤ Refer client and family to a cancer support group.
➤ Assess the client for signs and symptoms such as bleeding from injection sites, petechia, or ecchymosis, occult blood, and decreasing platelet count related to increased risk for bleeding.
➤ Clients with impaired bone marrow function may have prolonged bleeding times. Institute safety measures such as electric razors, nonskid shoes, no intramuscular injections, no rectal temperatures, and soft toothbrushes.
➤ Encourage verbalization of fears related to cancer, prognosis, treatment, and death.
➤ Inform client that result should be available in 1–3 days.
➤ Review related diagnostic tests such as bone marrow, total serum protein, red blood cell count, platelet count, white blood cell count with differential, and serum protein

electrophoresis.

Educate Your Client and the Family

➤ Provide answers to questions and emotional support for possible diagnosis of multiple myeloma.

➤ Clients with cancer often have prolonged bleeding times. Instruct client and family on safety measures such as electric razors, non-skid shoes, and soft toothbrushes.

B

Bilirubin, Serum

bil i roo bin • see rum
(Direct Bilirubin Level, Indirect Bilirubin Level, Conjugated Bilirubin Level, Unconjugated Bilirubin Level, Total Bilirubin Level)

Normal Findings

ADULT, CHILD, ADOLESCENT, ELDERLY

Total: 0.1–1.0 mg/dL (SI units: 5.1–17.0 µmol/L)
Direct (conjugated): 0.1–0.3 mg/dL (SI units: 1.7–5.1 µmol/L)
Indirect (unconjugated): 0.2–0.8 mg/dL (SI units: 3.4–12.0 µmol/L)
Unconjugated bilirubin is normally 70%–85% of total bilirubin.

NEWBORN

Total: 1–12 mg/dL (SI units: 17.1–20.5 µmol/L)

What This Test Will Tell You

This blood test evaluates liver and erythropoietic function, and helps differentiate types of jaundice. This test measures the blood levels of bilirubin, the orange-yellow pigment in bile. Bilirubin is produced mainly from hemoglobin catabolism; the hemoglobin is released from old erythrocytes destroyed in the reticuloendothelial cells of the liver, spleen, and bone marrow. Bilirubin is changed chemically (conjugated) in the normal liver and then excreted in bile.

Measuring unconjugated and conjugated bilirubin helps differentiate the cause of jaundice in a client. Elevated conjugated (direct) bilirubin is usually related to obstructed flow of the processed bilirubin via the bile into the intestine, causing bilirubin to back up and enter the bloodstream. This blockage may be either extrahepatic from strictures, stones, or tumors, or intrahepatic from biliary atresia or strictures. Unconjugated (indirect) levels may be elevated by hepatocellular injury such as hepatitis or advanced cirrhosis where the liver can no longer conjugate the bilirubin. Unconjugated levels may also be elevated due to the excessive destruction of red blood cells, in hemolytic anemia. If hepatic damage progresses, both direct and indirect levels may be elevated. In cases of severe chronic hepatic disease, the indirect bilirubin level may actually return to a nearly normal level but the direct bilirubin level remains elevated. Jaundice usually is clinically observable at serum levels greater than 2.5 mg/dL.

Abnormal Findings

▲ INCREASED LEVELS *of indirect or unconjugated bilirubin* may indicate hemolytic diseases, physiological jaundice (neonate), erythroblastosis fetalis, hemolytic jaundice, Gilbert's syndrome, Crigler-Najjar syndrome, large amount of internal bleeding, transfusion reaction, or sickle-cell anemia.

▲ INCREASED LEVELS *of direct (conjugated) bilirubin* are usually due to obstruction in the biliary tree, and may indicate intrahepatic biliary obstruction such as viral hepatitis, drug-induced cholestasis, cirrhosis, or extrahepatic biliary obstruction such as gallstones, hepatic or pancreatic carcinoma, bile duct disease, or biliary atresia.

▲ INCREASED LEVELS *of combined indirect and direct bilirubin* may indicate hepatocellular disease, hepatitis, Dubin-Johnson syndrome, or cirrhosis.

 ACTION ALERT!

A total bilirubin level greater than 15 mg/dL in a neonate requires phototherapy; a value greater than 20 mg/dL (>340 μmol/L) will be treated with an exchange transfusion. If untreated, neonates with elevated bilirubin levels can develop kernicterus, leading to permanent neurologic impairment.

Interfering Factors

➤ Exposure of the sample to sunlight or ultraviolet light may decrease levels.

➤ Hemolysis.

➤ Lipemia.

➤ Hepatotoxic drugs such as phenothiazines, monoamine oxidase (MAO) inhibitors, methotrexate, allopurinol, anabolic steroids, antibiotics, acetaminophen, ascorbic acid, chlorpropamide, codeine, dextran, morphine, many diuretics, codeine, cholinergics, meperidine, theophylline, quinidine, salicylates, and estro-

gens may increase levels.

➤ Use of drugs causing hemolysis such as chloramphenicol, sulfonamide, indomethacin, and arsenic-containing agents may also cause increased levels.

➤ Medications that may decrease serum bilirubin levels include caffeine, penicillin, and barbiturates.

NURSING CONSIDERATIONS

Prepare Your Client

➤ Explain to your client and family that this test helps see how well the liver is working.

➤ Although fasting is not required, it is preferred that clients do not have anything by mouth except water for 4–8 hours prior to the test. Check with your own laboratory for guidelines. This is not usually necessary for infants.

Perform Procedure

➤ Perform a venipuncture to collect a 5–7 mL sample of venous blood in a red-top tube. For a neonate, perform a heelstick and fill the microcapillary tube to designated level.

➤ Apply pressure or pressure dressing to venipuncture site. Clients with impaired liver function have a tendency for prolonged bleeding.

➤ Handle specimen gently to prevent hemolysis.

➤ Send specimen to lab immediately, protecting sample from direct sunlight or ultraviolet light.

Care After Test

➤ Assess client for presence of jaundice, noting color of skin, sclera, and mucous membranes.

➤ Take special precautions to prevent skin breakdown due to pressure or abrasion. Jaundice increases complications associated with skin integrity.

➤ Assess client for unusual bruising or prolonged bleeding from venipuncture sites. Prolonged bleeding is a complication of severely impaired liver function.

➤ Protect from potential injury which could result in internal or external bleeding.

➤ Assess client for presence of gastrointestinal bleeding by testing all stools routinely for occult blood. Esophageal varices and mucosal bleeding are common complications of liver disease.

➤ In a neonate, bilirubin levels greater than 15 mg/dL require treatment with phototherapy. Explain this procedure and rationale to parents clearly.

➤ Consult with a registered dietician to design a well-balanced, high-calorie diet with appropriate amounts of sodium and protein.

➤ Review related tests such as prothrombin time and liver function studies.

Educate Your Client and the Family

➤ Instruct client with liver disease to report any jaundice, excessive or easy bruising, or fullness of the abdomen (ascites) to the primary health care provider.

➤ Instruct client to report any bloody vomit and/or tarry stools to staff. Esophageal varices are a complication of severe liver disease.

➤ For client with chronic liver disease, educate client and family on the importance of complying with prescriptions and avoiding over-the-counter medications unless approved by the primary health care provider, because many medications are detoxified by the liver.

➤ Instruct family on a well-balanced, high-calorie diet. Clients with advanced liver disease absorb nutrients poorly due to decreased bile flow into the intestines. Clients with ascites or peripheral edema should have a low-sodium diet. Client with elevated ammonia levels should limit protein intake.

B

Bilirubin, Urine
bil i roo bin • yur in

Normal Findings
Bilirubin is normally absent in urine.

What This Test Will Tell You
This urine test evaluates liver and erythropoietic function, and helps differentiate types of jaundice. This test measures the urine levels of bilirubin, the orange-yellow pigment in bile. Bilirubin is produced mainly from hemoglobin released from old erythrocytes destroyed in the reticuloendothelial cells of the liver, spleen, and bone marrow. Bilirubin is changed chemically (conjugated) in the normal liver and then excreted in bile. Measuring unconjugated and conjugated bilirubin helps differentiate the cause of jaundice. Elevated conjugated (direct) bilirubin usually occurs when flow of the processed bilirubin is obstructed, and therefore enters the bloodstream. This blockage may be either extrahepatic from

strictures, stones, or tumors, or intra-hepatic from biliary atresia or strictures. Unconjugated (indirect) levels are elevated in primary liver dysfunction, when the liver can no longer process the bilirubin. Unconjugated levels may also be elevated when excessive destruction of red blood cells occurs, as in hemolytic anemia. If hepatic damage progresses, both direct and indirect levels may be elevated. In cases of severe chronic hepatic disease the indirect bilirubin level may actually return to a nearly normal level but the direct bilirubin level remains elevated. Jaundice usually is clinically observable at serum levels greater than 2.5 mg/dL.

Unconjugated bilirubin is not water soluble, so it is not excreted in urine. However, conjugated bilirubin is water soluble, and is excreted in urine when serum levels are elevated. This test is used less often now that serum determination of bilirubin is easily performed.

Abnormal Findings

▲ INCREASED LEVELS may indicate conjugated hyperbilirubinemia, calculi or tumor of common bile duct, viral or toxic hepatitis, cirrhosis, drug-induced cholestasis, primary biliary cirrhosis, tumor, or Dubin-Johnson syndrome.

▼ NEGATIVE RESULTS in the presence of hyperbilirubinemia may indicate hemolytic anemia, erythroblastosis fetalis, Gilbert's syndrome, or Crigler-Najjar Syndrome.

Interfering Factors

➤ Exposure of specimen to light and/or room temperature may alter results.
➤ Large amounts of ascorbic acid or nitrites as well as indomethacin may decrease or cause false negative results with some testing methods.
➤ Medications that may increase urine bilirubin levels include phenothiazines, phenazopyridine, allopurinol, antibiotics, barbiturates, diuretics, estrogen, and oral contraceptives.

NURSING CONSIDERATIONS

Prepare Your Client

➤ Explain that this test is used to help diagnose the reason for the client's yellow coloring (jaundice) and to evaluate if the liver and red blood cells are working normally.
➤ Explain that you will need a fresh urine specimen for this test. Provide the client with the proper container and privacy to obtain the specimen.
➤ Check with the primary health care provider about restricting prescribed medications that may affect test results.

Perform Procedure

➤ Send the sample immediately to the laboratory. Protect sample from light.
➤ For bedside testing, refer to manufacturer's guidelines on packaging. For all methods, use a freshly voided specimen within 30 minutes of voiding and protect from light.

Care After Test

➤ Assess client for presence of jaundice, noting color of skin, sclera, and mucous membranes.
➤ Assess client for other signs and symptoms of liver disease such as fatigue, lethargy, malaise, anorexia, abdominal discomfort, abdominal distention, pruritus, and edema.
➤ Take special precautions to prevent skin breakdown due to pressure or abrasion. Jaundice increases complications associated with skin integrity.

➤ Assess client for unusual bruising or prolonged bleeding from venipuncture sites. Prolonged bleeding is a complication of severely impaired liver function.

➤ Protect client from potential injury which could result in internal or external bleeding.

➤ Assess client for gastrointestinal bleeding by testing all stools routinely for occult blood. Esophageal varices and mucosal bleeding are common complications of liver disease.

➤ Consult with a registered dietician to design a high-calorie, well-balanced diet. Clients with advanced liver disease absorb nutrients poorly due to decreased bile flow into the intestines. As appropriate, reduce sodium or protein in the diet if edema and ascites, or increased ammonia levels are present.

➤ Evaluate related tests such as aspartate aminotransferase (AST), direct and indirect bilirubin levels, alkaline phosphatase, serum ammonia, prothrombin time, red blood cell count, red blood cell indices, hematocrit, and hemoglobin.

Educate Your Client and the Family

➤ Instruct client with liver disease to report any jaundice, excessive or easy bruising, or fullness of the abdomen (ascites) to the primary health care provider.

➤ Tell client to report any bloody vomit and/or tarry stools to staff.

➤ For client with chronic liver disease, educate client and family on the importance of complying with prescriptions. Tell then to avoid over-the-counter medications unless approved by the primary health care provider, because many medications are detoxified by the liver.

➤ Instruct the family on a well-balanced, high-calorie diet. Clients with advanced liver disease absorb nutrients poorly due to decreased bile flow into the intestines. Client with ascites or peripheral edema should have a low-sodium diet. Client with elevated ammonia levels should limit protein intake.

B

Bleeding Time
(Ivy Method, Duke Method, Mielke or Template Method)

Normal Findings

ADULT, ADOLESCENT, ELDERLY, PREGNANT
Template method: 2.0–8.5 minutes
Ivy method: 1–10 minutes
Duke method: 1–3 minutes
NEWBORN
Ivy method: 1–5 minutes
CHILD
Ivy method: 1–6 minutes

What This Test Will Tell You

This blood test diagnoses bleeding problems related to abnormalities with platelet function and vascular responses to injury. The test measures the length of time bleeding continues after a standardized incision is made in the skin. Normal bleeding time is dependent upon normal quantities and function of platelets. The elasticity of blood vessel walls is also an influencing factor in bleeding time, as the vessel wall's ability to constrict is one of the clotting mechanisms. This test is performed either as a preoperative screening to evaluate the stability of the client's hemostatic mechanisms, or to detect the presence of a variety of coagulation disorders.

The template method, also called the Mielke bleeding time, is the most commonly performed method and considered the most accurate. The Duke and Ivy methods were earlier-developed methods of assessing bleeding time.

Abnormal Findings

▲ INCREASED BLEEDING TIME may indicate thrombocytopenia, platelet dysfunction syndromes, disseminated intravascular coagulation (DIC), prolonged anticoagulant therapy, severe liver disease (as in advanced cirrhosis), acute leukemia, Hodgkin's disease, bone marrow failure, von Willebrand's disease, deficiency of clotting factors (I, II, V, VII, VIII, IX, or XI), hemolytic disease of the newborn, Cushing's disease, aplastic anemia, or pernicious anemia.

▼ DECREASED BLEEDING TIME may indicate severe polycythemia.

ACTION ALERT!
>12 minutes, adults, Ivy and template methods
>5 minutes, adults, Duke method
>6 minutes, infants and children, Ivy method
These prolonged bleeding times may point to a potentially dangerous bleeding disorder. Protect client from injury and observe closely for signs of hemorrhage including tachycardia, pallor, hypotension, and anxiety.

Interfering Factors

➤ Heparin, warfarin, streptokinase, salicylates, dextran, indomethacin, and non-steroidal anti-inflammatory drugs administered before the test will prolong bleeding time. As little as 10 grains of acetylsalicylic acid (ASA) up to 5 days before the test will prolong bleeding time.

➤ Sulfonamide, thiazide, antineoplastic drugs, some narcotics, and mithramycin may prolong bleeding time.

➤ Corticosteroid will increase platelet counts and decrease bleeding times.

➤ Heavy alcohol consumption may increase bleeding time, especially with alcohol abuse.

➤ Deviation from standard depth and width of the incision alters bleeding time results.

➤ Touching the incision during the test disturbs fibrin particles and increases bleeding time.

Contraindications

➤ Clients with a platelet count less than 75,000/mm^3

➤ Clients with a history of keloid formation

➤ Clients who are unable to cooperate with testing

➤ Clients with cellulitis in the arms or with inflammatory conditions of the skin in the area to be tested

Potential Complications

➤ Infection at the test site
➤ Excessive bleeding at the test site
➤ Keloid scar formation

NURSING CONSIDERATIONS

Prepare Your Client

➤ Explain to your client that this test measures the time required to form a clot and stop bleeding.

➤ Tell your client that the test requires about 20 minutes or less to perform.

➤ Explain that the test will leave two small, hairline scars that will be minimally visible when healed.

Perform Procedure

➤ Position the client sitting or lying with one arm extended and supported. The ventral surface of the forearm is usually selected.

➤ Situate a blood pressure cuff on the client's arm and inflate to 40 mm Hg. The cuff must remain inflated for 30–60 seconds before beginning the test.

➤ Select an area on the forearm that is free of superficial veins and cleanse the test area with an antiseptic.

➤ Apply the template device to the test site (for standardized and modified template methods).

➤ Make an incision 1 mm deep and 9 mm long (standard template method) or activate the spring-loaded blades (modified template method) to make two incisions, 1 mm deep and 5 mm long. Some institutions use one incision only. For the Ivy method, clean the earlobe with antiseptic and make a puncture in the earlobe 2–4 mm deep with a lancet. Note the time that bleeding begins by activating a stopwatch.

➤ Blot the drops of blood from the incision or puncture sites with filter paper every 30 seconds. Take care not to touch the wound. The filter paper is brought close to the incision without touching the edge of the wound and disturbing the platelet plug. Stop the timer when blood no longer stains the filter paper.

➤ If two incisions are used, average the bleeding time of the two incisions

or the puncture marks and record the average as a bleeding time. If one incision is used, record the actual bleeding time as observed.

Care After Test

➤ Apply pressure to the site if bleeding time has been greater than 12 minutes.

➤ Maintain close approximation of the wound edges with an adhesive bandage or a bandage dressing.

➤ Inspect the test site each shift for signs of infection, bleeding, or hematoma.

➤ Review related tests such as prothrombin time, activated partial thromboplastin time, platelet count, platelet aggregation, hemoglobin, hematocrit, and complete blood cell count.

Educate Your Client and the Family

➤ If a bleeding tendency is identified, instruct the client and family to protect the client from trauma. Injuries may result in uncontrolled bleeding, which is difficult to manage.

➤ Instruct the client to use an electric razor rather than a safety razor and to use a soft-bristle toothbrush for oral care. Electric razors or depilatory creams may be used by women.

➤ Instruct the client and family in diet, activity, and/or medication regimens to prevent constipation. Hard stools may be traumatic to anal and rectal mucosa.

➤ Teach the client and family how to apply pressure to a bleeding wound, should an injury occur. Discuss possible responses to injuries should an emergency arise. Posting phone numbers in an accessible location near the telephone at home will help the client or family should the primary health care provider or emergency medical system need to be alerted.

➤ Instruct the client to carry or wear medical alert identification indicating a bleeding disorder.

➤ Instruct the client with prolonged bleeding time to avoid taking over-the-counter medications that pro-long bleeding time, such as aspirin or products containing aspirin. Client should be instructed to avoid large quantities of alcohol and its regular use. A written list of products to avoid will provide the client or family with a reference when shopping or selecting home remedies for minor ailments.

Blood Culture and Sensitivity
blud • kul chur • and • sen sih tiv ih tee

Normal Findings
All ages: Negative, or no growth. Blood is normally sterile and exhibits no organism growth.

What This Test Will Tell You
This blood test diagnoses bacteremia or septicemia and identifies the type of pathogenic microorganisms present in the blood and the most effective antibiotics. Pathogens in blood may be reported initially as gram-negative or gram-positive (Gram stain technique), as rods or cocci bacteria, or as fungi. Given sufficient time to grow, the organism is identified by name on the report. A culture report that identifies pathogens often requires a minimum of 24 hours (67% of pathogens are identified in 24 hours) to 72 hours (90% of pathogens are identified by 72 hours). Some pathogens, such as some fungi and mycobacteria, may take weeks to incubate and provide identifiable growth on culture.

After identification, the organism is tested with a variety of medicated discs impregnated with different antimicrobial agents. Sensitivity reports may take an additional 24 hours or more, after the organism has been identified. The sensitivity report will state that the pathogen is either resistant to, moderately sensitive to, or very sensitive to (most effective) selected antimicrobial medications.

Abnormal Findings
Abnormalities may include transient bacteremia or septicemia from common pathogens such as *Pseudomonas aeruginosa, Escherichia coli, Klebsiella pneumoniae, Staphylococcus aureus, Streptococcus pneumoniae, Neisseria meningitidis, Hemophilus influenzae,* and species of the Enterobacteriaceae family and the *Brucella, Serratia,* and *Candida* genera.

ACTION ALERT!

The mortality rate in an overwhelming septicemia may be as high as 20% in debilitated or immunocompromised clients. Therapeutic intervention may be required before positive identification of bacteria or the most effective antibiotic therapy can be identified. Broad-spectrum antibiotic therapy needs to be initiated to treat the suspected infection.

Interfering Factors

➤ Contamination of the specimen with bacteria from the client's skin, errors in the phlebotomist's sampling technique, and exposure of the culture media to organisms in the air or environment may introduce organisms into the culture media that do not reflect the client's clinical circumstances.

➤ Antimicrobial therapy prior to collection of the blood sample may result in negative results, even in the presence of bacteremia, or in delayed growth.

➤ Use of an inappropriate culture media or container may interfere with aerobic growth.

➤ Removal of culture media bottle caps at the bedside may prevent anaerobic growth and could become a source of culture media contamination.

➤ Inadequate growth time, temperature, or culture conditions may fail to produce enough organism growth for identification.

NURSING CONSIDERATIONS

Prepare Your Client

➤ Explain to your client or the family that the test is to determine whether a bacteria has entered the blood, and to find out what bacteria it might be.

➤ Explain to the client or family that if an organism is identified in the blood, the lab will test for what medications the organism is sensitive to and find the most effective treatment.

➤ Inform the client or family that the culture process will require a minimum of 24 hours and may take several days or even several weeks. Discuss the need for the lengthy sensitivity portion of the testing to determine the most effective medication regimen.

Perform Procedure

➤ Check with specific laboratory policies before doing this test. Some facilities require specimens to be collected from two different venipuncture sites.

➤ Cleanse the rubber tops of the culture media bottles with povidone-iodine and allow to air dry.

➤ Cleanse the skin at the venipuncture site with 70% alcohol and allow to air dry.

➤ Collect 10–15 mL of venous blood into a syringe. Remove the needle used for venipuncture and replace with a second sterile needle.

➤ Inoculate the anaerobic bottle first, and the aerobic bottle second, if both anaerobic and aerobic cultures are being obtained.

➤ Mix the inoculated culture media gently.

➤ Transport the labeled culture samples to the lab promptly.

Care After Test

➤ Observe for signs and symptoms of infection including high or persistent fever, hypotension, poor peripheral perfusion, metabolic acidosis, and markedly elevated white blood cell count.

➤ If antibiotic therapy has been delayed pending completion of the culturing process, begin the ordered antibiotic therapy.

➤ Review related tests such as culture and sensitivity of other body fluids, and white blood cell count with differential.

➤ Explain to your client or family that treatment for the suspected organism may begin before there is a final report because of the time required to grow cultures. The culture report then serves to confirm or alter the original diagnosis.

➤ Explain to your client or family the treatment plan for the suspected infection and any expected results.

Blood Glucose, Random

blud • gloo cose • ran dum

(Serum Glucose, Blood Glucose, Random Glucose, Blood Sugar)

Normal Findings

ADULT

70–110 mg/dL (SI units: 3.9–6.1 mmol/L)

PREGNANT

80–150 mg/dL (SI units: 4.4–8.3 mmol/L)

PREMATURE INFANT

20–60 mg/dL (SI units: 1.1–3.3 mmol/L)

NEWBORN

30–70 mg/dL (SI units: 1.7–3.9 mmol/L)

Fetal cord blood in newborn: 45–96 mg/dL (SI units: 2.5–5.3 mmol/L)

CHILD, ADOLESCENT

<24 months of age: 60–100 mg/dL (SI units: 3.3–5.5 mmol/L)

24 months through adolescence: 70–105 mg/dL (SI units: 3.9–5.8 mmol/L)

ELDERLY

80–140 mg/dL (SI units: 4.4–7.7 mmol/L)

What This Test Will Tell You

This blood test detects alterations in glucose metabolism, and is most often used as a random screen for glucose level or when a client is unconscious for unknown reasons. It may also help diagnose diabetes mellitus or evaluate the control of this disease. Two hormones are needed for glucose metabolism: insulin and glucagon. Insulin allows glucose into the cells, thereby lowering blood glucose. Glucagon encourages the breakdown of glycogen in the liver, causing the blood glucose to increase. Blood glucose fluctuates depending upon the person's activity level and the length of time from the last meal. A fasting blood glucose is used as a baseline measurement, as it is not influenced by dietary intake as a variable factor.

Abnormal Findings

▲ INCREASED LEVELS may indicate diabetes mellitus, stress, Cushing's disease, steroid use, or pheochromocytoma.

▼ DECREASED LEVELS may indicate cachexia, hypothyroidism, insulin overdose, increased exercise, or liver disease.

■ ACTION ALERT!

➤ Adult male: <50 or >400 mg/dL
➤ Adult female: <40 or >400 mg/dL
➤ Infant: <40 mg/dL
➤ Newborn: <30 or >300 mg/dL

Any of these obtained values in the indicated population signifies either severe hypoglycemia or hyperglycemia necessitating immediate intervention. Prolonged hypoglycemia, especially in the neonate, can result in permanent and irreversible brain damage.

Interfering Factors
➤ Factors that may increase levels include steroids, anesthesia, stress, infection, caffeine, nicotine, beta blockers, diuretics, estrogen, and phenytoin.
➤ Factors that may decrease levels include alcohol, anabolic steroids, insulin, and oral antidiabetic agents.

NURSING CONSIDERATIONS
Prepare Your Client
➤ Explain that this test is to measure the amount of sugar in the bloodstream and is often used to look for any sign of sugar diabetes (diabetes mellitus).
➤ Do not give insulin, oral antidiabetic agents or food until after the blood is drawn.
➤ There is no period of fasting for this random analysis of blood glucose.

Perform Procedure
➤ Perform a venipuncture and collect 5 cc of blood into a red-top or green-top tube.
➤ Client or staff may instead use a bedside glucometer after obtaining a sample from a fingerstick. Follow the manufacturer's directions for usage.

Care After Test
➤ Administer any medications withheld for this test.
➤ Resume client's normal diet immediately to prevent hypoglycemia.
➤ Assess for symptoms such as nausea, light-headedness, hunger, and tremors, which may signify hypoglycemia.
➤ If the blood glucose is extremely low, i.e. <50, hold the insulin and consult the primary health care provider. Administer a source of carbohydrates by offering crackers, orange juice, or other high-carbohydrate foods to client who has no alteration in level of consciousness.
➤ Evaluate related tests such as fasting blood sugar, glucose tolerance test, 2-hour postprandial glucose level, and urine glucose and ketones.

Educate Your Client and the Family
➤ Inform client and family that continued elevated blood glucose levels may indicate sugar diabetes (diabetes mellitus).
➤ Begin or reinforce diabetic teaching as indicated.
➤ Encourage client to self-monitor blood glucose. Many insurance companies will provide the monitors and test strips.
➤ Encourage client and family to join diabetes support groups.

Blood Smear

blud • smeer

(Peripheral Blood Smear, Red Blood Cell Morphology, RBC Smear, WBC Smear, Heinz Bodies, Howell-Jolly Bodies, Spicule Cell)

Normal Findings

ALL AGES

Normal number, size, shape, and color of red blood cells (RBCs)

Normal number of white blood cells (WBCs)

Normal WBC differential count (see *White Blood Cell with Differential Count*)

Normal number of platelets

What This Test Will Tell You

This microscopic examination of a blood smear provides descriptive information about the red and white blood cells and platelets, and helps to diagnose anemias. Usually incorporated into the complete blood count (CBC), the blood smear examines the appearance of red cells for variations in size, shape, color, or intracellular appearance. Additionally, the white blood cells are examined for total quantity, degree of maturity, and the variation of cell types (see *White Blood Cell with Differential Count*). The report generally focuses on abnormal cell types for RBCs and the differential count of white cell variations.

Abnormal Findings

WHITE BLOOD CELLS

➤ *Elevated WBC count (leukocytosis)* may indicate infection, leukemia, trauma, pertussis, sepsis, stress, inflammation, hemorrhage, tissue trauma or injury, malignancy, toxins, uremia, eclampsia, thyroid storm, pain, cold, heat, cigarette smoking, anesthesia response, or tissue necrosis.

➤ *Elevated neutrophil count (neutrophilia)* may indicate stress, myelocytic leukemia, trauma, Cushing's syndrome, inflammation, rheumatic fever, sepsis, malignancy, pernicious anemia, chronic morphine addiction, hemolytic transfusion reaction, thyroiditis, rheumatoid arthritis, hemorrhage, diabetic ketoacidosis, eclampsia, gout, or acute infection.

➤ *Elevated lymphocyte count (lymphocytosis)* may indicate chronic bacteria infection, viral infection, upper respiratory tract infections, atypical pneumonia, tuberculosis, brucellosis, syphilis, pertussis, toxoplasmosis, Graves' disease, lymphocytic leukemia, lymphoma, multiple myeloma, radiation, hepatitis, or mononucleosis.

➤ *Elevated monocyte count (monocytosis)* may indicate chronic inflammatory disorders, bacterial endocarditis, viral infections, tuberculosis, chronic ulcerative colitis, mononucleosis, myelogenous leukemia, polycythemia vera, multiple myeloma, Hodgkin's disease, or parasitic infections.

➤ *Elevated eosinophil count (eosinophilia)* may indicate parasitic infections, Addison's disease, tumors, allergic reactions, chronic skin infections, ulcerative colitis, Crohn's disease, leukemia, eczema, or autoimmune diseases.

➤ *Elevated basophil count (basophilia)* may indicate leukemia, polycythemia vera, hemolytic anemia, radiation therapy, viral infections, recovery from bone marrow suppression, tuberculosis, iron deficiency, or myelofibrosis.

➤ *Decreased WBC count (leukopenia)* may indicate bone marrow failure, leukemia, myeloma, aplastic anemia, Schwachman-Diamond syndrome, drug toxicity, dietary deficiency, ingestion of heavy metals, radiation, or autoimmune disease.

➤ *Decreased neutrophil count (neutropenia)* may indicate aplastic anemia, viral infections, hepatitis, influenza, measles, radiation therapy, dietary deficiency, bacterial infection, Addison's disease, overwhelming infection, or chemotherapy.

➤ *Decreased lymphocyte count (lymphopenia)* may indicate leukemia, sepsis, Hodgkin's disease, burn or traumatic injuries, uremia, lupus erythematosus, late stages of HIV infection, immunosuppression, drug therapy (corticosteroids, antineoplastics), aplastic anemia, tuberculosis, or radiation therapy.

➤ *Decreased monocyte count (monocytopenia)* may result from prednisone therapy, rheumatoid arthritis, HIV infection, or hairy cell leukemia.

➤ *Decreased eosinophil count (eosinopenia)* may indicate increased adrenosteroid production, mononucleosis, congestive heart failure, or Cushing's syndrome.

➤ *Decreased basophil count (basopenia)* may indicate acute allergic reactions, myocardial infarction, peptic ulcer, steroid therapy, stress reactions, or hyperthyroidism.

RED BLOOD CELLS

➤ *Microcytes (small RBCs)* may indicate iron deficiency anemia, thalassemia, or hereditary spherocytosis.

➤ *Macrocytes (large RBCs)* may indicate vitamin B_{12} or folic acid deficiency, postsplenectomy, liver disorder, or reticulocytosis secondary to

increased erythropoiesis.

➤ *Spherocytes (small, round RBCs)* may indicate hereditary spherocytosis or acquired immunohemolytic anemia.

➤ *Elliptocytes (crescent, sickle-shaped)* may indicate sickle-cell anemia or hereditary elliptocytosis.

➤ *Leptocytes (thin, low-hemoglobin RBCs)* may indicate thalassemia or hemoglobinopathies.

➤ *Spicule cells (small, needle-shaped RBCs)* may indicate uremia, bleeding ulcer, or liver disease.

➤ *Hyperchromasia (highly colored RBCs)* may indicate dehydration.

➤ *Hypochromasia (pale RBCs)* may indicate thalassemia, iron deficiency anemia, or cardiac disease.

➤ *Nucleated RBCs* may indicate physiologic response to anemias, transfusion reaction, other RBC deficiency, congestive heart failure, hypoxemia, leukemia, or myeloma, or be normal in infants.

➤ *Basophilic stippling* may indicate lead poisoning or reticulocytosis.

➤ *Howell-Jolly bodies* may indicate hemolytic anemia or megaloblastic anemia, or be seen following splenectomy.

➤ *Heinz bodies* may indicate hemolytic anemia, drug-induced RBC damage, coagulopathies, or hemoglobinopathies.

ACTION ALERT!

➤ A white blood cell, neutrophil, or lymphocyte count of less than 500/mm³ demonstrates that the client is at extreme risk for infection. Institute protective isolation measures immediately.

➤ If results indicate anemia from blood loss, red blood cell destruction, or abnormalities in the formation of red blood cells, client must be assessed for clinical evidence of anemia, bleeding disorders, or adverse response to medication therapies. Be especially alert for hypoxemia symptoms including angina, myocardial ischemia, and activity intolerance.

Interfering Factors

➤ In hemolytic anemias, red cell appearance may be affected by stress, strenuous exercise, exposure to temperature extremes, dehydration, fever, or acute illness.

➤ Early morning generally is associated with lower WBC and late afternoon with higher WBC.

➤ Pregnancy, labor, stress, exercise, and digestion may produce elevations in the white cell count.

➤ Neutrophils decrease with debilitation and overwhelming infection.

➤ Medications that may increase the white cell count include corticosteroids, aspirin, allopurinol, chloroform, epinephrine (adrenaline), heparin, quinine, and triamterene.

➤ Medications that may decrease the white cell count include barbiturates, antineoplastics, antibiotics, diuretics, sulfonamides, anticonvulsants, antithyroid medications, non-steroidal anti-inflammatory drugs, and arsenic derivatives.

➤ Splenectomy may produce a mild elevation of white cell counts; in some anemias, splenectomy reduces damage to red cells.

➤ Medications that may produce false positive results for Heinz bodies include antimalarial medications, nitrofurantoin, phenacetin, procarbazine, sulfonamides, and furazolidone.

➤ Children have greater elevations of neutrophils in response to infection.

➤ Elderly clients may not have a neutrophilic response to infection.

NURSING CONSIDERATIONS

Prepare Your Client

➤ Explain that this test looks at the blood and its cells to discover any problems there may be in the number, size, shape, and content of the cells.

Perform Procedure

➤ Collect 7 mL of venous blood in a lavender-top tube. Additionally, collect a drop of blood onto a slide for microscopic examination (slide can be obtained by venipuncture, heel stick or finger stick).

Care After Test

➤ Encourage rest periods for client experiencing fatigue related to anemia.

➤ Evaluate client's ability to perform activities of daily living.

➤ Refer to community health care services as needed if client is unable to perform basic daily needs.

➤ Client with leukocytopenia, lymphocytopenia, or neutropenia needs to be protected from infection. Stress importance of handwashing to family and all caregivers. Avoid exposure to anyone with recent or current illness.

➤ Review related tests such as hemoglobin, hematocrit, complete blood cell count, reticulocyte count, red blood cell indices, globin chain analysis, white blood cell count, hemoglobin electrophoresis, serum bilirubin, urine bilirubin, and Schilling test.

Educate Your Client and the Family

➤ Teach client to continue light physical activity if experiencing fatigue, but to rest when needed and not to plan too strenuous or prolonged activities.

➤ Inform client with anemia that maintaining regular patterns of sleep, rest, and activity is important to prevent fatigue.

➤ Stress the importance of a well-balanced diet to provide optimal energy stores.

➤ If a deformity of the red cells, such as sickle cell, is identified, teach your client/family about behaviors or circumstances that could exacerbate symptoms (sickling crisis): stress, cold exposure, fever, dehydration, strenuous exercise.

➤ If your client is identified as having a genetically transmitted disorder of the blood cells (sickle-cell ane-

mia), offer genetic counseling to your client and/or family.

➤ If an alteration in white blood cells is identified that indicates a viral or bacterial infection, instruct your client/family in the responses to infection that may help facilitate recovery or promote comfort. These responses may include use of antipyretic medications, fluid intake, rest, reduction of visitors to limit transmission of disease, administration of antibiotics or other medications as prescribed.

➤ If white blood cell counts are low, teach the client and family about preventing infection, avoiding crowds and small children, and not eating fresh fruits due to danger of pseudomonas and fungi.

Blood Typing
blud • tie ping

Normal Findings

A, Rh-positive   O, Rh-positive
A, Rh-negative   O, Rh-negative

B, Rh-positive   AB, Rh-positive
B, Rh-negative   AB, Rh-negative

What This Test Will Tell You

This blood test is performed to match donor blood with the recipient who requires a blood transfusion. Blood typing identifies the inherited antigens that comprise one of four possible blood types: A, B, AB, and O. Blood typing also determines the Rhesus or Rh factor, another inherited trait. These two antigens, in a variety of combinations, compose the eight basic blood types.

The ABO typing process identifies the presence or absence of A or B antigens on the surface of red blood cells.

Rh typing is a test for the presence or absence of the Rh_o (D) antigen on the surface of the red blood cells.

Abnormal Findings

There are no high or low levels of any test parameters. Blood type is limited to A, B, AB, or O. Rh is limited to negative or positive.

ACTION ALERT!

Failure to administer donor blood of the same type (and usually Rh factor) will result in a potentially fatal hemolytic transfusion reaction. Blood is rarely given without a cross-match, and then only in extreme emergencies using blood of the same type or type O. Less severe transfusion reactions (antigen-antibody response) may also result in chills, fever, low back pain, chest pain, hypotension, nausea, bleeding disorders (may precipitate disseminated intravascular coagulation), pruritus, and urticaria.

In case of a reaction during administration of donor blood, stop the blood transfusion immediately. DO NOT remove the IV access. Infuse normal saline through the IV site. Send the unused portion of donor blood to the laboratory for repeat cross-matching. Notify the primary health care pracitioner and the blood bank in the laboratory. Monitor the client's vital signs every 15 minutes until stable. For some reactions, a urine sample will be sent to the lab (for analysis of hemoglobinuria) and a blood sample drawn for another cross-match. Prepare to administer intravenously an antihistamine, such as diphenhydramine, or acetaminophen for treatment of fever.

Interfering Factors

➤ Recent administration of dextran or intravenous contrast media causes cellular aggregation similar to the agglutination seen in the ABO and Rh typing processes, obscuring results.

➤ Transfusion of blood within the preceding 3 months may have stimulated the production of antibodies to that donor blood, making cross-matching more difficult.

➤ Hemolysis of red cells due to rough handling during or after collection may interfere with the reliability of test results.

➤ Testing for the D^u antigen may be obscured by administration of methyldopa, cephalosporins, or levodopa, resulting in false positive results.

Contraindications

➤ Cultural, religious, or moral beliefs of the client may be opposed

to transfusion of donor blood products, presenting a potential contraindication from the client's point of view.

NURSING CONSIDERATIONS

Prepare Your Client

➤ Explain that the test will determine the client's blood type and Rh so that blood or blood products can be administered safely, should it be necessary. Blood typing is common prior to major surgery, during pregnancy, and prior to collection of donor blood.

➤ Explain to the client who is a potential recipient of donor blood that the typing process is conducted under careful protocols to ensure the safety of the donor blood. Many institutions require a written consent by the client or responsible party prior to administration of donor blood products.

➤ Explain to the pregnant client that Rh blood typing is necessary to see if she is Rh-negative exposed to antigens during a pregnancy with an Rh-positive fetus. If so, she must be treated with Rh_o (D) immune globulin (RhoGAM) within 72 hours of the completion of an Rh-positive pregnancy.

Perform Procedure

➤ Collect 5–15 mL of venous blood in a red-top tube. If cross-matching of client blood with multiple units of donor blood is anticipated, two tubes of blood may be required.

➤ Transport the sample to the lab immediately, handling it gently.

Care After Test

➤ If blood transfusion is planned, assess client for signs and symptoms of bleeding or anemia including pallor, dyspnea, chest pain, and fatigue.

➤ Encourage rest periods for client experiencing fatigue related to anemia.

➤ Evaluate client's ability to perform activities of daily living.

➤ Refer to community health care services as needed if client is unable to perform basic daily needs.

➤ Obtain a dietary consult to assist the client and family in choosing a well-balanced diet, including foods high in iron and vitamin B_{12}.

➤ Encourage the client to carry identification that states the ABO and Rh blood group identified during the typing process.

➤ Administer Rh_o (D) immune globulin to Rh-negative female with an Rh-positive baby within 72 hours of the completion or termination of the pregnancy.

➤ Review related tests such as hemoglobin, hematocrit, reticulocyte count, red blood cell indices, hemoglobin electrophoresis, ferritin level, total iron-binding capacity (TIBC), bone marrow and liver biopsies, and iron absorption and excretion studies.

Educate Your Client and the Family

➤ Explain to your client the reason why blood typing has been ordered.

Such reasons may include preparation for surgery, cross-matching, tissue typing, and donating blood, and during pregnancy to see if the fetus is at risk for fetal hemolytic Rh incompatibilities.

➤ Explain to your client that ABO blood type and Rh factor are inherited characteristics, and do not change. Once they are accurately identified, the client can carry identification stating their blood type and Rh to speed up treatment in case of an emergency transfusion.

➤ Examine with your client any religious, cultural, moral, or ethical objections to receiving blood products. Provide access to a spiritual adviser or counselor should the client wish to explore these conflicts.

➤ Assure your client that the typing and cross-matching process does not expose the client to any blood-borne pathogens.

➤ Explain that although the typing process to determine the client's ABO and Rh blood group will need to be done only once, blood samples will have to be drawn for subsequent cross-matching. For each unit of donor blood, cross-matching requires sufficient blood from the client to monitor for an interaction.

Bone Biopsy
bone • bie op see

Normal Findings

ADULT, PREGNANT, ADOLESCENT, AND ELDERLY

Bone tissue consisting of fibers of collagen, osteocytes, and osteoblasts. Two histologic types of tissue include (1) compact, dense, concentric layers of mineral deposits, and (2) widely spaced (cancellous) layers of mineral deposits with osteocytes and red and yellow marrow between them. No abnormal cells or tissues.

NEWBORN

The cancellous bone tissue consists of red marrow only.

CHILD

The amount of yellow marrow (fat cells) depends upon the age of the client. Red marrow cells are replaced with adipose (fat) cells with maturity. The yellow marrow can revert to red marrow if needed.

What This Test Will Tell You

Microscopic examination of bone is usually performed to diagnose a lesion found by radiologic (x-ray) examination. This test may also differentiate benign and malignant tumors and identify the primary site of a cancer that has metastasized to the bone.

The test is frequently performed as an open biopsy immediately prior to surgical intervention for bone disease, after the incision has been made. A needle biopsy may also be performed using a special serrated biopsy needle.

Abnormal Findings

➤ Benign conditions may indicate bone cyst, infection, fibroma, osteoid osteoma, osteoblastoma, or osteochondroma.
➤ Malignant conditions may indicate metastasis of cancer from breast, lung, prostate, kidney, or thyroid; multiple myeloma; osteosarcoma; or Ewing's sarcoma.

Interfering Factors

➤ Failure to use proper fixative or to send specimen to the laboratory immediately

Contraindications

➤ Coagulopathies

Potential Complications

➤ Bone fracture
➤ Damage to surrounding soft tissue
➤ Infection (osteomyelitis)
➤ Hemorrhage

NURSING CONSIDERATIONS

Prepare Your Client

➤ Explain that this procedure will provide a sample of bone needed to discover any problems that may exist in the bone.
➤ Evaluate health history and coagulation studies closely for any signs of coagulopathies.
➤ Inform the client whether the biopsy will be by needle aspiration in the room or by open biopsy in the operating room.
➤ Ensure that an informed consent is obtained, because of the possible complications associated with this procedure.
➤ Restrict food and fluids for at least 8 hours prior to the procedure if an open biopsy is performed. Do not restrict foods and fluids if the client is having a needle biopsy.
➤ Take and record vital signs for a baseline assessment.
➤ Administer intravenous (IV) antibiotics if ordered to prevent postoperative infection (osteomyelitis).
➤ Assess for a history of sensitivity to local anesthetics such as mepivacaine, lidocaine, or novocaine.
➤ Explain that a transient discomfort or pain is experienced during the needle biopsy when the numbing medication is injected into the tissue and when the covering to the bone (periosteum) is entered.
➤ Teach relaxation and distraction methods of pain management for use

when the bone is entered, because the local anesthetic does not relieve this pain.

➤ Administer pain medication prior to the procedure.

➤ Explain to the client having an open biopsy that they will be asleep during the procedure.

➤ Inform the client that discomfort will be experienced for several days after the anesthetic has worn off.

Perform Procedure

OPEN BIOPSY

Nurses do not usually perform this procedure but should understand the process to prepare the client and assist the physician. Position the client for access to biopsy site. Prepare the area by cleaning with a topical antiseptic and draping. Surgical protocols for orthopedic preparation are followed. A biopsy sample is removed through surgical excision. Send the specimen to the laboratory in a formalin solution. The incision is closed as indicated for the extent of surgical intervention. Clean the site and apply a sterile dressing.

NEEDLE BIOPSY

Nurses do not usually perform this procedure but should understand the process to prepare the client and assist the physician. Position the client for access to biopsy site. Prepare area by cleaning with a topical antiseptic and draping. A local anesthetic is injected into subcutaneous tissues to the periosteum. A small incision is made at the biopsy site. A biopsy needle with trocar is inserted, twisting it into the bone. A bone tissue plug is extracted and placed in a marked formalin-prepared specimen container. The incision is closed with sutures or steri-strips. Apply a sterile dressing.

Care After Test

➤ Monitor vital signs closely until stable; usually every 15 minutes for the first hour, every 30 minutes for the next hour, and then every 4 hours for 24 hours.

➤ Administer analgesics as indicated.

➤ Apply ice bags to decrease pain and swelling.

➤ Assess dressing for drainage.

➤ Assess for signs of bone infection: fever, headache, or redness, warmth, tenderness, drainage, abscess, or necrosis at the site.

➤ Evaluate related tests such as x-rays, bone scans, and tumor markers.

Educate Your Client and the Family

➤ Teach the client the signs and symptoms of infection.

➤ Teach the client precautions to prevent pathological fractures if indicated by results. This includes body mechanics and prevention of falls.

➤ Teach methods of pain management when cancer is diagnosed. This should include effective use of medications, as well as relaxation, distraction, and positioning techniques.

B

Bone Marrow Biopsy

bone • mare oe • bie op see

(Bone Marrow Aspiration, Bone Marrow Examination)

Normal Findings

ADULT

Active erythroid, myeloid, and megakaryocyte cells. Myeloid cell (white blood cell) to erythrocyte cell (red blood cell) ratio (M:E) is 3:1. Refer to chart on page 115. The bone marrow is made of both red marrow and yellow marrow.

NEWBORN

Bone marrow is red. The composition is primarily erythrocytic and granulocytic cells (precursors to red blood cells and white blood cells).

CHILD

The activity and composition of cells varies with age. As many red blood cell precursors are replaced by fat cells, a yellow marrow is produced. The yellow cells can return to red if needed.

ELDERLY

Expected values are the same as for the adult except there is frequently a decreased number of leukocyte precursors (myelocytes). Concentrations and ratios remain the same.

What This Test Will Tell You

Microscopic analysis of bone marrow is performed to further investigate abnormal types of cells found on a peripheral blood smear or to evaluate response to medical treatment. The studies will indicate the presence or absence of types of cells and provide a ratio of cells that is characteristic of certain disease states, including anemias, toxic states producing bone marrow destruction, tumors, leukemia, platelet disorders, and agranulocytosis (decreased produc-

tion of certain types of red blood cells).

The bone marrow biopsy is used in conjunction with other findings to determine and diagnose conditions leading to abnormal blood cell formation. Specific evaluation of results usually requires a hematologist.

Abnormal Findings

▲ INCREASED LEVELS *of RBC precursors (erythrocytes)* may indicate physiologic compensation for hemorrhagic, hemolytic anemias, or polycythemia vera.

▼ DECREASED LEVELS *of RBC precursors* may indicate erythroid hypoplasia caused by radiation, chemotherapy treatment, or consumption of agents toxic to bone marrow, or marrow replacement with fibrotic tissue or tumor.

▲ INCREASED LEVELS *of platelet precursors (megakaryocytes)* may indicate chronic myeloid leukemia, hemorrhage, infection, thrombocytopenia, thrombocytopenic purpura, compensation for hypersplenism, polycythemia vera, or megakaryocytic myelosis.

▼ DECREASED LEVELS *of platelet precursors* may indicate chemotherapy, tumor of fibrotic marrow, aplastic anemia, polycythemia vera, megakaryocytic myelosis, myelofibrosis, idiopathic thrombocytopenia, cirrhosis, irradiation, or pernicious anemia.

▲ INCREASED LEVELS *of leukocyte precursors (myelocytes)* (increased myelocyte to erythrocyte ratio [M:E ratio]) may indicate compensation

Cell type	Newborn(%)	Children(%)	Adult(%)
Undifferentiated	0–1.0	0–1.0	0–1.0
Reticulocytes	0.4–2.5	0.4–2.5	0.4–2.5
Promyelocytes	0.76	1.4	1.0–8.0
Myelocytes	2.5	18.4	4.2–19
neutrophilic	5.0–19	5.0–19	5.0–19
eosinophilic	0.5–3.0	0.5–3.0	0.5–3.0
basophilic	0.0–0.5	0.0–0.5	0.0–0.5
Myeloblasts	0.3–6.0	0.3–6.0	0.3–6.0
Lymphocytes	49.0	16.0	3.0–20.7
Monocytes	0.1–4.3	0.1–4.3	0.1–4.3
Bands (stabs)	14.1	0	13.0–34.0
Plasma Cells	0.02	0.4	0.1–3.9
Megakaryocytes	0.05	0.1	0.0–3.0
Pronormoblasts	0.1	0.5	0.2–4.2
Normoblasts			
basophilic	0.34	1.7	0.25–4.8
polychromatophilic	6.9	18.2	3.5–29.0
orthochromic	0.54	2.7	1.0–25.0
Granulocytes (segmented)			
neutrophilic	11.6–30.0	11.6–30.0	11.6–30.0
eosinophilic	0.5–4.0	0.5–4.0	0.5–4.0
basophilic	0.0–3.7	0.0–3.7	0.0–3.7
Neutrophils	32.4	57.1	34–82.7
Myeloid/Erythroid ratio	4.4:1	2.9:1	2.3–3.5:1

for infection or leukemia.

▼ DECREASED LEVELS of leukocyte precursors may indicate metastatic neoplasia or agranulocytosis.

▲ INCREASED LEVELS of lymphocytes may indicate mononucleosis, lymphocytic leukemia, lymphoma, aplastic anemia, macroglobulinemia, or myelofibrosis.

▲ INCREASED LEVELS of plasma cells may indicate infection, chronic inflammatory disorders, hypersensitivity states, multiple myeloma, Hodgkin's disease, rheumatic fever, cancer, agranulocytosis, amyloidosis, aplastic anemia, collagen disease, carcinomatosis, cirrhosis, infection, irradiation, macroglobulinemia, rheumatoid arthritis, syphilis, or ulcerative colitis.

▲ INCREASED LEVELS of normoblasts may indicate polycythemia vera.

▼ DECREASED LEVELS of normoblasts may indicate folic acid and vitamin B_{12} deficiency or anemia.

▲ INCREASED LEVELS of neutrophils may indicate myeloblastic or chronic myeloid leukemia.

▼ DECREASED LEVELS *of neutrophils* may indicate leukemia or aplastic anemia.

▲ INCREASED LEVELS *of eosinophils* may indicate bone marrow cancer, leukemia, pernicious anemia, or lymphadenoma.

▲ INCREASED *myeloid-erythroid ratio* may indicate infection, myeloid leukemia, leukemoid reactions, or impaired hemopoiesis.

▼ DECREASED *myeloid-erythroid ratio* may indicate agranulocytosis, hemopoiesis following hemorrhage, iron deficiency anemia, or polycythemia vera.

████ ACTION ALERT!

Sternal biopsies are associated with sternal fracture, a rare complication that can lead to injury to the heart or great vessels. Assess carefully for signs of shock (faint blood pressure; rapid, thready pulse; and pale, cool, clammy skin).

Interfering Factors

➤ Failure to obtain a representative sample of the marrow.

➤ Fibrotic changes in the marrow due to radiation, chemotherapy agents, or tumors increase the difficulty in entering the bone marrow with a needle and obtaining a representative marrow sample with one try.

➤ Treatment with cytotoxic drugs, folic acid, iron, vitamin B_{12}, and recent blood transfusions may interfere with accurate results.

➤ Failure to use a fixative on a slide or to send specimen immediately to the laboratory.

Contraindications

➤ This test is contraindicated in hemophilia or other bleeding disorders. However, the importance of further information that can be pro-vided through the biopsy is weighed against the risk.

➤ The sternal biopsy site is contraindicated in children due to the possibility of mediastinal and cardiac perforation.

➤ Inability of the client to remain still during the 20–30 minute procedure. Sedation may be required.

Potential Complications

➤ Bleeding, hemorrhage.

➤ Infection of the bone, which may lead to a potentially fatal systemic infection.

➤ Death related to damage to the heart or great vessels with a sternal biopsy.

➤ Damage to bone growth plate can occur if the tibial tubercle is biopsied in children.

NURSING CONSIDERATIONS

Prepare Your Client

➤ Explain that this test is to help discover problems in the forming of blood cells, and if appropriate, how well treatment is working.

➤ Ensure that an informed consent is obtained, because of the possible complications associated with this procedure.

➤ Assess for a history of hypersensitivity to local anesthetics. Novocaine or lidocaine are commonly used.

➤ Check coagulation studies and platelet count prior to the procedure in order to identify coagulopathies, which could increase the risk of hemorrhage.

➤ Take and record vital signs for a baseline assessment.

➤ Administer pain medication or anti-anxiety medications as indicated.

➤ Teach client relaxation techniques and distraction methods for management of the feelings of pressure during aspiration of bone marrow.

➤ Allow verbalization of fears and anxieties associated with the procedure or suspected diagnosis. This is especially true for clients who have experienced this procedure or who have talked with someone who has experienced it.

Perform Procedure

Nurses do not usually perform this procedure but should understand the process to prepare the client and assist the physician.

A needle biopsy or a needle aspiration is performed. The biopsy provides a more representative sample.

Position client depending on site used and age of client. Support with pillows to allow a greater ability to remain still during the procedure. Potential sites include the anterior and posterior iliac crests, sternum, spinous vertebral processes T10–L4, ribs, and tibia. For child, choose site they cannot see, to facilitate cooperation. Prepare area to be biopsied by cleansing with an antiseptic and draping the area as for minor surgery. Inform the client that they will feel slight discomfort with the injection of the local anesthetic. An uncomfortable pressure will be felt upon the needle entering the marrow and during the aspiration of cells. An anesthetic cannot prevent this sensation.

A local anesthetic (novocaine or lidocaine) is injected through the skin and subcutaneous tissues. The periosteum is injected if a needle biopsy is to be performed. The biopsy or aspiration needle and stylet is inserted through the subcutaneous tissue to the periosteum. The bone marrow is entered through the periosteum by using a twisting

motion on the needle. A 10–20 mL syringe is attached to the needle once the stylet is removed.

Needle aspiration: 0.2–0.5 mL of marrow is aspirated and smeared on slides and fixative is applied. Small specks should be visible in aspirate that contains cells.

Needle biopsy: The tissue plug and biopsy needle are removed and placed in a labeled bottle containing an acetic acid solution.

Apply direct pressure for 5–15 minutes. Cleanse site and apply a small, sterile dressing. Apply a pressure dressing to client at risk for bleeding. Instruct the client to lie on the puncture site for 15 minutes to 2 hours after the procedure.

Care After Test

➤ Assess vital signs and biopsy site every 10–15 minutes for 2 hours for bleeding or signs of shock (low blood pressure; weak and rapid pulse; cool, pale, clammy skin).

➤ Assess for pain, respiratory difficulty, and shock after sternal biopsy.

➤ Assist client to lie on biopsy site. Most will be free of restrictions after 15–30 minutes. Pressure to site may be required for as long as 2 hours. Activity restrictions depend on platelet counts and coagulation studies.

➤ Apply ice bags to minimize bleeding and reduce pain.

➤ Apply additional pressure, if indicated, with covered sandbags.

➤ Medicate for pain as indicated.

➤ When this test is performed on a client who has thrombocytopenia (low platelet count), place direct pressure over the biopsy site for 15–30 minutes and maintain bed rest with pressure exerted by positioning client on biopsy site for 1–2 hours. Sandbags are sometimes used to apply additional pressure. A platelet-pheresis transfusion may be indicated prior to the procedure to prevent hemorrhage.

➤ Assess for fever and redness, warmth, swelling, tenderness, and drainage at biopsy site until healed. Infection may lead to death, especially in clients who are immunosuppressed.

➤ Evaluate related tests such as complete blood count (CBC) with differential.

Educate Your Client and the Family

➤ Teach the client and family the signs of infection.

➤ Inform client that discomfort may be felt at the site for several days. It should decrease over time, not increase. Instruct them to report increasing pain.

➤ Educate the client and family about precautions to take if the biopsy shows deficiencies in white blood cells (WBCs), red blood cells (RBCs), or platelets. Examples include:

1. Decrease the risk of infection when WBCs are low by avoiding large crowds, children, and persons with upper respiratory infections.
2. Decrease the risk of bleeding when platelets are low by using an electric razor, soft toothbrush or sponges, wearing shoes, and avoiding injections.
3. Conserve energy when RBCs are low by pacing activities and getting enough sleep.

➤ Teach the client or family to give vitamin B_{12} injections if pernicious anemia is diagnosed.

➤ Educate the client about the need for lifetime B_{12} therapy for pernicious anemia. Research indicates that symptoms will not occur immediately if the B_{12} is stopped, but the pernicious anemia will return in up to 5 years.

➤ Teach the client about the importance of carrying or wearing emergency identification for abnormal bone marrow functioning if the condition is expected to remain abnormal.

Bone Scan

bone • skan
(Bone Radioisotope Scan, Bone Radionuclide Imaging)

Normal Findings
ADULT
No areas of increased or decreased concentration of radioactive material in bone.
NEWBORN
Expected results are the same as for adults.

CHILD AND ADOLESCENT
Sites of high concentration of radioactive material (hot spots) are normal at the epiphysis of growing bone.
ELDERLY
Expected results are the same as for adults. Decalcification of bones from

changes due to aging is common, especially in postmenopausal women.

What This Test Will Tell You

This nuclear scanning test detects early bone disease and metastasis of cancer to bone, and measures the response of bone tissue to therapeutic interventions. Usually the entire skeleton is scanned. Bone abnormalities or tumors may be visualized on the bone scan 3–6 months before standard x-rays can show them. This test may also be used to diagnose degenerative bone disorders and the cause of undetermined bone pain as well as to identify fractures and the abnormal healing of fractures.

The nuclear scan of the bone uses injections of a radioactive tracer compound that concentrates in the bone. The distribution of detectable radiation differs between normal and abnormal tissue relative to bone metabolism. When recorded with a scanning camera on x-ray film, the normal tissue is identified by an equal or uniform gray distribution. "Hot spots" are darker areas of hyperfunction (such as a tumor). The lighter areas of concentration (as seen with decalcified bone) are the "cold spots."

Abnormal Findings

▲INCREASED LEVELS (hot spots) may indicate bone cancer or metastasis, calcification of bone, abnormal healing of bone fractures, or normal and abnormal bone growth.

▼DECREASED LEVELS (cold spots) may indicate degenerative bone disease, bone decalcification, fractures, osteomyelitis, Paget's disease, rheumatoid arthritis, or bone tumors.

Scans revealing sites of high or low concentration may indicate a potential danger for pathological fractures. Safety and environmental precautions should be immediately taken to prevent injury.

Interfering Factors

➤ A distended bladder will decrease visibility of the pubic bone.
➤ Some antihypertensives will interfere with the uptake of radioactive material.
➤ Scanning too soon or too long after the injection of the radionuclide can affect the results.
➤ Dehydration interferes with uptake of radionuclides by tissues.
➤ Interference may occur when two different radionuclides are given in the same day (i.e., two nuclear scans).
➤ Improper injection technique may cause the tracer compound to enter subcutaneous or muscle tissue, producing hot spots.

Contraindications

➤ During pregnancy and breastfeeding, due to exposure of the fetus or baby to radioactive materials
➤ Allergy to the contrast material unless modifications are made

Potential Complication

➤ Allergic or anaphylactic reaction

NURSING CONSIDERATIONS

Prepare Your Client

➤ Explain that this test can find problems in the bones that may not yet be seen on a normal x-ray.
➤ Tell the client that although the insertion of the IV needle causes transient discomfort, the bone scan is not painful. Inform the client that the process will take about 30–60 minutes.

➤ Explain that the client will be alert during the procedure. Small children may be sedated.

➤ Accompany children to the procedure and remain as long as possible in order to reassure them.

➤ Reassure the client that the radiation exposure is less than that of most diagnostic x-rays and that the radioactive material is excreted from the body in 6–24 hours. Be sure they understand they are not exposing family, visitors, or staff to radiation.

➤ Inform the client that there will be a waiting period after the injection of 2–3 hours to allow for absorption of the contrast medium in the bone tissue.

➤ Inform the client that they will need to remain still during the scan. (Sedatives may be used for clients unable to be still.)

➤ Inform the client that there are no food or fluid restrictions.

➤ For a female client, ask the date of her last menstrual cycle and if she believes she could be pregnant.

➤ Assess the client's history for allergies to contrast medium or iodine or any reactions to other types of tests, such as an IVP.

➤ Ensure that an informed consent is obtained, because of the possible complications associated with this procedure.

➤ Have the client remove items containing metal, such as jewelry, glasses, braces, and dental prostheses.

➤ Tell the client to drink 6–8 glasses of water before the scan to help the kidneys get rid of dye that is not being absorbed by the bone tissue. Keep fresh water available.

➤ Have adults and older children void prior to the test to enable better visibility.

Perform Procedure

Nurses do not perform this procedure, but should understand the process to prepare the client. Radioisotope is administered intravenously. The most commonly used radionuclide is a TC-99m-labeled phosphate compound. A wait of 2–3 hours allows the radionuclide to emit energy in the bone. Have the client drink 6–8 glasses of water during this wait in order to facilitate the renal clearance of the radionuclide not picked up by the tissues.

For the scan, a scanning camera moves back and forth over the client's body to transfer detected low-level radiation emitted by the skeleton to an x-ray film. The client may have to be repositioned several times during the procedure.

Care After Test

➤ Monitor injection site for redness or swelling.

➤ Apply warm soaks to injection site if hematoma develops.

➤ Provide support for the client and family if diagnosis is cancer or a metastasis of cancer.

➤ Evaluate the client's pain level and confer with the primary health care provider for medication as indicated.

➤ Provide and encourage fluids in order to facilitate renal clearance of the radionuclide.

➤ Evaluate related tests such as serum and urine calcium levels, serum phosphorus, erythrocyte sedimentation rate (ESR), complete blood cell counts, and bone marrow biopsy.

Educate Your Client and the Family

➤ Encourage the client to drink lots of fluids for the next 24 hours to help excrete the radionuclide.

> If the scan revealed hot or cold spots, teach the client and family to avoid pathological fractures through maintaining proper body alignment when moving or transferring. Also discuss safe walking habits, such as wearing flat, non-skid shoes, keeping walk areas free of clutter, and obtaining support to walk on stairs or hills.

Brain Scan
brane • skan
(Brain Radioisotope Scan, Brain Radionuclide Imaging, Cisternal Scan, Cerebral Blood Flow Scan)

Normal Findings
No abnormal areas of uptake of contrast medium

What This Test Will Tell You
This nuclear scan with isotope imaging identifies abnormalities such as tumors, hematomas, infarctions, and abscesses in the brain associated with headaches, stroke symptoms, seizures, or other neurologic symptoms. Normally the blood-brain barrier limits the amount of radioactive contrast medium injected intravenously that crosses into cerebral circulation. If this natural barrier is compromised, the uptake of the radioactive material is evidenced during the radiologic study and indicates pathologic conditions such as brain lesions, masses, or hemorrhage. The test shows location, size, and shape of the abnormality but it does not provide specific diagnostic data to determine the exact pathologic process. While tumors and abscesses are often found on the initial scan, damage from a cerebrovascular accident may not be evident on scan for 2 weeks.

In addition to the competence of the blood-brain barrier, this test helps evaluate the ventricles and the cerebral spinal fluid (CSF) pathways. The brain scan has mostly been replaced by computed tomography (CT) and magnetic resonance imaging (MRI).

Abnormal Findings
Abnormalities in uptake may indicate intracranial masses (benign or malignant tumors), cerebral abscess, metastatic cancer, head trauma (subdural hematoma, cerebral hemorrhage), cerebral vascular accident (after 3–4 weeks), hydrocephalus, cerebral spinal fluid leakage, and aneurysms.

ACTION ALERT!
Assess clients carefully for allergic reaction to contrast material including dyspnea, itching, urticaria, flushing, hypotension, and shock. Life-threatening anaphylactic reactions can occur and need to be recognized and treated immediately.

Interfering Factors
> Prolonged or insufficient waiting period between time of radioactive contrast media (isotope) and imaging of brain
> Dehydration
> Movement of client during imaging
> Antihypertensives

➤ Injection of more isotope within 24 hours prior to the brain scan may compromise ability to interpret results

Contraindications

➤ Pregnancy, due to radiation exposure to the fetus
➤ Allergy to iodine if the isotope contains radioiodinated human serum albumin (RIHSA)
➤ Clients who are unable to cooperate during the procedure

Potential Complications

➤ Anaphylactic reaction to contrast material

NURSING CONSIDERATIONS

Prepare Your Client

➤ Explain that the test is done to detect various disorders in the brain.
➤ Ensure that an informed consent is obtained, because of the possible complications associated with this procedure.
➤ Assess for a history of allergy to iodine or contrast material.
➤ Explain that the test usually causes no pain and takes less than 1 hour.
➤ Administer blocking agents before the scan. These may be ordered to prevent excessive uptake in the thyroid gland or choroid plexus.
➤ Inform client they must lie still during the procedure. They may be asked to change position. Tell them this should be the only time they move while the pictures are being taken.
➤ Collaborate with the primary health care provider regarding the use of sedatives with agitated client.
➤ Assure the client the amount of radioactive dye used in this test is small and is not a risk to themselves or their family. Tell them the dye leaves the body in approximately 6–24 hours after injection.

Perform Procedure

Nurses do not usually perform this procedure but should understand the process to prepare the client and assist the physician. This procedure is performed in the radiology department.

The contrast medium is injected intravenously. There is a waiting period of 30 minutes to 1 hour between the injection and the scan to allow the medium to accumulate in the area of pathology. Imaging may be repeated several times over a period in the supine, lateral, and prone positions to study the perfusion of the brain. Radioisotope counts occur during the test and are imaged and recorded chronologically as the contrast medium is distributed in the brain.

Care After Test

➤ Encourage fluids to increase excretion of the contrast medium and compensate for the diuretic effect of the contrast material.
➤ Review related tests such as computed tomography (CT), magnetic resonance imaging (MRI), positron-emission tomography (PET), and single-photon emission computed tomography (SPECT) tests.

Educate Your Client and the Family

➤ Tell mothers not to breastfeed or use breast milk to feed infants for 24 hours following the test.

Breast Biopsy

brest • bie op see

Normal Findings

Postpubescent female: Normal breast tissue consists of glandular, ductal, fibrous, and fatty tissue. The appearance is pink with yellow fat globules. Microscopic examination should reveal normal cellular and noncellular breast tissue.

What This Test Will Tell You

This histologic test diagnoses benign and malignant breast lesions. Most abnormal tissue changes in the developed breast occur in females; only 1% of all clients with carcinoma of the breast are male. Breast biopsy is indicated for definitive diagnosis of palpable breast masses, suspicious mammography findings, dimpling, nonlactating nipple discharge including bloody discharge, and persistent external tissue changes or nonhealing lesions. If the tissue biopsy is found to be malignant, an estrogen-receptor and progesterone-receptor assay will also be performed.

Abnormal Findings

➤ *Benign tumors* may reveal fibrocystic disease, fibroadenoma (or adenofibroma), lipomas, or plasma cell mastitis.
➤ *Malignant tumors* may reveal infiltrating ductal carcinoma, invasive lobular carcinoma, medullary or circumscribed carcinoma, cancer in situ (ductal and lobular), Paget's disease, colloid carcinoma, tubular carcinoma, inflammatory carcinoma, adenocarcinoma, or carcinosarcoma.

Interfering Factors

➤ Delay in fixation of slide preparations, resulting in tissue breakdown

➤ Delay in transporting specimen to the laboratory for analysis
➤ Failure to keep the tissue sample refrigerated if transport to a laboratory is not immediate
➤ Refrigeration and/or storage for more than 24 hours
➤ Formaldehyde solution as a preservative if receptor assays are to be conducted
➤ Misplacement of biopsy needle so that abnormal area is not sampled

Contraindications

➤ Coagulopathy

Potential Complications

➤ Possible bleeding or hematoma formation at the surgical site
➤ Possible numbness of the nipple after surgical excision of the mass; should abate in 2 months, but may interfere with sexual arousal

NURSING CONSIDERATIONS

Prepare Your Client

➤ Explain that this test is to find out if problems with the breasts involve cancerous or noncancerous tissue.
➤ Be sure that the client understands why the procedure is being done and what the possible complications are. Recognize that the client may experience a great deal of anxiety related to this test; answer all questions or seek additional information, if needed.
➤ Ensure that an informed consent is obtained, because of the possible complications associated with this procedure.
➤ Explain that the biopsy is done on an outpatient basis in a hospital, surgi-center, or office.

➤ Ask if the client is allergic to iodine, because povidone-iodine (Betadine) may be used for the skin prep prior to the biopsy.

➤ Determine whether the client is allergic to any anesthetics.

➤ Do not restrict food or fluids for client having a local anesthetic.

➤ Explain that a local anesthetic will be administered with a needle and syringe prior to performing the procedure and may cause a stinging or burning sensation.

➤ Instruct client having general anesthesia not to eat or drink anything after midnight on the date of surgery.

➤ Explain that the procedure will take about 20–30 minutes.

➤ Verify with the primary health care provider whether blood analysis, urinalysis, and a chest x-ray are required prior to the biopsy.

Perform Procedure

Nurses assist with this procedure and provide care for the client before, during, and after the procedure. Drape the biopsy site after the skin prep is done to protect the client from infection. Instruct the client not to touch the drapes or the area where the biopsy is being done during the procedure.

For a needle biopsy, a special needle is inserted into the lesion, and tissue and/or fluid is withdrawn into a syringe. Apply pressure after the needle is withdrawn to stop bleeding, then apply a bandage.

For an open biopsy, an incision is made into the breast, and the tissue specimen is removed. Tell the client beforehand that some pulling or tugging may be felt during the procedure, but there should be no sensation of pain. The incision is closed with sutures (stitches) and a tight bandage is applied to prevent bleeding.

Silverman-needle-aspirated fluid is placed in a heparinized tube. Silverman-needle-aspirated tissue is placed in a specimen bottle with normal saline or formaldehyde. Fine-needle-aspirated fluid is placed on a slide with a fixative and undergoes immediate microscopic examination.

In open biopsy, either a portion of the lesion or the total lesion is removed, depending on size, type of lesion (benign or malignant), and whether a lumpectomy is also being done. Frozen sections of tissue being examined for malignancy are done immediately; receptor assays may also be done on this tissue. Tissue not examined immediately may be placed in a formaldehyde solution and sent to the laboratory. Do not place tissue for receptor assays in formaldehyde solution. Label all specimens.

Care After Test

➤ Ice may be applied to control bleeding and promote comfort.

➤ Provide post-anesthesia care if client had general anesthesia.

➤ Observe for bleeding at site.

➤ Provide support, especially if frozen section has demonstrated a malignancy and the client has been informed of the finding. Refer to support groups and the American Cancer Society if a diagnosis of cancer is made.

➤ Explain to client who had general anesthesia that they will not go home until well awake from the anesthesia.

➤ Evaluate related tests such as estrogen-receptor and progesterone-receptor assays.

Educate Your Client and the Family

➤ Instruct the female client to wear a supportive bra 24 hours a day until the site is healed.

➤ If skin sutures were used, instruct the client to return to the primary health care provider's office in 4–5 days for removal.

➤ Instruct the client to notify the primary health care provider if she has any bleeding or drainage from the site or a fever.

➤ Explain that nerves are injured when surgery is done, so the nipple may be numb for a couple of months. This may diminish sexual arousal.

➤ Inform the client that if the lesion is cancerous, additional testing may be done to determine the best treatment option.

➤ Instruct the client to make an appointment with the primary health care provider for follow-up care and to plan for further treatment, if indicated.

➤ If pain medication is prescribed, instruct the client how to take it.

➤ Ensure the client knows how to do a breast self-exam correctly.

B

Bronchoscopy
brong **koss** koe pee

Normal Findings

Normal structure and lining of the larynx, trachea, and bronchi

What This Test Will Tell You

This endoscopic examination is to directly visualize and inspect the larynx, trachea, and bronchi through a rigid metal bronchoscope or a flexible fiber-optic bronchoscope. The rigid bronchoscope permits visualization of large airways. Because the fiber-optic bronchoscope is smaller and flexible, it allows for visualization of the segmental bronchi and has largely replaced use of the rigid bronchoscope.

This procedure has both diagnostic and therapeutic purposes. It is used to diagnose or evaluate airway obstructions, tumors, hemoptysis, unresolved pneumonias, or to take biopsies and brushings for cytologic examinations. Therapeutic uses include aspiration of retained secretions, removal of aspirated foreign bodies, control of bleeding, or laser therapy of bronchial lesions.

Abnormal Findings

Abnormalities may reveal retained secretions, tumors, obstructions, lesions, bleeding sites, pneumonia, inflammation, foreign body, tuberculosis, or atelectasis.

⬛ ACTION ALERT!

Life-threatening complications such as laryngospasm and cardiac arrhythmias may occur during bronchoscopy. Emergency resuscitation equipment must be readily available.

Interfering Factors

➤ Inability of the client to relax and cooperate during the procedure

➤ Failure to properly label and transport specimens to the laboratory immediately

Contraindications

➤ Severe shortness of breath or carbon dioxide retention

Potential Complications

Laryngospasm or bronchospasm
Hypoxemia
Cardiac arrhythmias
Bleeding following biopsy
Pneumothorax
Respiratory failure
Fever

NURSING CONSIDERATIONS

Prepare Your Client

➤ Explain that the procedure is to allow direct inspection of the airways to detect any abnormalities or to remove foreign objects, secretions, etc.

➤ Describe the procedure and tell client that they will be awake, the throat will be anesthetized, and a large tube will be passed into the airway.

➤ Assess for allergies to local anesthetics.

➤ Allow the client to voice concerns and allay the client's anxiety. Inform them they will be given medication to make them sleepy and relaxed during the procedure. (The procedure is occasionally performed under general anesthesia in the operating room.)

➤ Obtain a signed, informed consent because of potential complications associated with this test.

➤ Withhold food and fluids for 4–6 hours prior to the test.

➤ Obtain ordered preprocedure laboratory tests such as arterial blood gases, partial thromboplastin time (PTT), and platelet counts and record baseline vital signs.

➤ Remove dentures, glasses, or contact lenses.

➤ Administer prescribed premedications to decrease respiratory secretions and provide sedation.

➤ Prepare suctioning equipment.

➤ Have emergency resuscitation readily available.

Perform Procedure

Nurses do not usually perform this procedure, but should understand the process to prepare the client and assist the physician. The procedure may be performed in an endoscopy room, at the bedside, or in the operating room. It usually takes about 1 hour. Assist the client to a supine or semi-Fowler's position as indicated. Spray local anesthetic into the nose and throat.

The tube is passed through the mouth or nose or through an endotracheal tube if indicated. More local anesthetic is sprayed into the trachea to inhibit the cough reflex. The trachea and bronchi are examined for abnormalities, secretions are suctioned for pulmonary toilet, foreign bodies may be removed, and biopsy specimens or washings are obtained if pathology is suspected. The tube is withdrawn slowly.

Observe the client during the procedure for signs of respiratory insufficiency or laryngospasm.

Care After Test

➤ Assess respiratory status closely. Notify the physician of dyspnea, wheezing, hemoptysis, bloody sputum, or decreased breath sounds.

➤ Record vital signs every 15 minutes for 1 hour and until stable.

➤ Label collected specimens appropriately and transport to the laboratory immediately.

➤ Observe for the return of the gag reflex by asking the client to swallow or cough. Maintain nothing-by-mouth (NPO) status and assist the client to expectorate saliva into an emesis pan until the gag reflex has returned, usually about 2 hours.

➤ Evaluate related tests such as chest x-ray, computed tomography scans, and sputum cultures.

Educate Your Client and the Family

➤ Tell the client that a sore throat and fever are common for about 24 hours after the test. Inform them that mild analgesics or throat lozenges may be helpful.

➤ Instruct the client not to smoke for 6–8 hours after the test. Smoking may precipitate coughing which could result in bleeding, especially if a biopsy has been taken.

➤ Inform the client that results of cytologic examinations may not be available for 2–3 days.

B

Caloric Study

ka lor ik • stud ee

(Oculovestibular Reflex, Caloric Test, Vestibulo-ocular Reflex, Caloric Reflex, Caloric Ice Water Test, Caloric Test Stimulus, Oculocephalic Testing, Water Caloric Test)

Normal Findings

Normal response is nystagmus (involuntary, rapid eye movement) of both eyes, nausea, vomiting, and dizziness.

What This Test Will Tell You

This reflex test assesses the functioning of the vestibular system, cerebellum, and/or brain stem. The vestibulocochlear nerve (cranial nerve VIII) is a sensory nerve that maintains balance and transmits sounds for hearing. Dysfunction of the vestibular portion results in vertigo, nausea, vomiting, and ataxia.

This test is also part of the clinical evaluation of brain death (death by neurological criteria). Because it tests part of the brain stem, it is a critical component of the clinical assessment for absence of brain function.

Abnormal Findings

Abnormal responses to the stimulus may include dysconjugate eye movement, asymmetric eye movement, or absent eye movement. When cold water is used, the nystagmus usually is observed away from the irrigated ear, while warm water induces nystagmus toward the ear being irrigated. These responses indicate an abnormality of the vestibular system, cerebellum, or brain stem.

Abnormal responses may indicate cerebral gaze palsy, vestibular loss, vestibular neuronitis, cochlear disease, acoustic neuroma, cranial nerve lesion, brain stem dysfunction, or death (brain death or death by neurological criteria).

ACTION ALERT!

After the test, maintain bed rest with the head of bed elevated 45 degrees and side rails up until nausea or vomiting is gone. Maintain safety precautions related to dizziness such as keeping the room free of clutter and the bed in low position. Instruct the client to make position changes slowly.

Interfering Factors

➤ Alcohol, central nervous system depressants, antivertigo agents, hypothermia, and barbiturates may suppress results.
➤ If the client focuses on the dizziness caused by the test, nystagmus results may be accentuated or inconsistent.

Contraindications

➤ Middle ear infections
➤ Blood or fluid collection behind the tympanic membrane
➤ Perforated tympanic membrane unless performed with air instead of water
➤ Acute disease of the labyrinth (Ménière's syndrome)

Potential Complications

➤ Ear infection

NURSING CONSIDERATIONS

Prepare Your Client

➤ Tell client and family that this test is to check how the part of the brain that controls balance and hearing is working.

➤ Inform client and family that water (or occasionally cold air) will be instilled in the ear canal and the primary health care provider will be looking at their eyes for reflex or spontaneous movement.

➤ Teach client that rapid eye movement after the water is instilled is normal. Tell the client that the primary health care provider will be comparing the speed of eye movement and the length of time eye movement continues after water is placed in each ear.

➤ Withhold food and fluids for 4–8 hours prior to the test to minimize the possible side effect of vomiting.

➤ Warn client that dizziness, nausea, and vomiting may be experienced during the procedure.

Perform Procedure

Nurses do not usually perform this procedure but should understand the process to prepare the client and assist the primary health care provider. This procedure is frequently performed in the audiologist's office for screening vestibular abnormalities. Appropriate training is essential to assure consistent test results. A baseline neurologic examination for the presence of nystagmus, postural deviation (Romberg's sign), and past-pointing is performed.

Position client either on their back or seated in a chair. The head is tilted backward and each ear is irrigated separately. The amount of water instilled ranges from 5–10 mL to 30–50 mL. Water temperature may be warm (36°C), cold (20°C), or iced. Water is instilled until symptoms of nystagmus, nausea, vertigo, and/or vomiting are induced or 3 minutes have elapsed, whichever comes first. Usually symptoms occur within 30 seconds. After a rest period of 5–10 minutes, the second ear is irrigated. Observe the client for nausea and vomiting. Assist as necessary.

Care After Test

➤ Maintain a safe environment for the client. Bed rest for 30–60 minutes after the test is recommended to avoid dangers associated with dizziness. Vertigo may have been the reason the client sought medical treatment, so it may occur or even worsen immediately following this test.

➤ Unless contraindicated, a side-lying position is recommended to minimize risks of aspiration.

➤ Offer spiritual and psychosocial support to family members and significant others if test was performed to determine neurological death (brain death).

➤ Evaluate any related tests performed to establish death by neurological criteria. Tests may be of other brain stem reflexes including oculocephalic reflexes and apnea testing, as well as gag and swallowing reflexes.

➤ If the client is declared dead by neurological criteria, consult with an organ procurement coordinator to evaluate the potential for organ and tissue donation.

➤ Evaluate other test results that may suggest reasons for dizziness, such as orthostatic hypotension and decreased cardiac output during the Valsalva maneuver.

➤ Evaluate related tests such as electronystagmography.

Educate Your Client and the Family

➤ Teach client with vertigo to change positions slowly and to become oriented to surroundings before walking to decrease the risk of falls.

- If appropriate, instruct client not to drive or operate equipment.
- If the client is declared dead by neurological criteria, ensure the family is informed by a qualified and trained professional of their right to donate organs or tissues.

Candida Antibody, Serum
kan did ah • an ti bod ee • see rum

Normal Findings
A normal test result is negative for the *Candida* antigen.

What This Test Will Tell You
This blood test helps diagnose candidiasis. The test detects the presence of an antibody to the fungus *Candida albicans* (yeast) in the blood. Infection with *Candida* in humans takes two forms: superficial, involving mucous membranes and skin (vaginal, pharynx, rectal); and deep, involving the bloodstream or organs. Antibody levels are clinically significant only in those clients with the systemic disease. Clients most likely to develop systemic candidiasis are those who are immune suppressed (by cancer, chemotherapy, or chronic disease—especially diabetes, diseases requiring multiple antibiotics, and HIV) or those with long-term intravenous catheters.

Systemic candidiasis can be difficult to diagnose because 50% of blood cultures in infected people are negative for the organism and because the antibody test is subject to a high percentage of false positives and false negatives. For instance, 20%–25% of normal, asymptomatic individuals will test positive. Antibody levels are useful only if the client's history and physical symptoms corroborate them.

Abnormal Findings
▲ INCREASED LEVELS may indicate systemic candidiasis. Titer greater than 1:8 or fourfold increase in titer suggests systemic infection.

Interfering Factors
- False positives: 25% of normal population tests positive.
- False negatives: occur when client is so immunosuppressed that antibodies are not produced.
- Cross reaction on latex agglutination with tuberculosis and cryptococcus.

NURSING CONSIDERATIONS
Prepare Your Client
- Explain that this blood test is to look for evidence of a yeast infection in the blood or internal organs.

Perform Procedure
- Collect 5 cc of venous blood in a red-top tube.

Care After Test
- Monitor temperature patterns. Any fever despite antibiotic therapy may be suggestive of fungal infection.
- Any intravenous or intra-arterial lines must be removed if candidiasis is present. Lines which have been in long term are especially suspect as a source of infection.

➤ Calculate the absolute neutrophil count to ascertain if the client is truly neutropenic. Use the following formula:

% neutrophils of total white blood cell count × (bands + segs) = absolute count

If the absolute count is <1000, then there is a moderate chance of severe bacterial infection. If the absolute count is <500, there is a strong possibility of severe bacterial infection.

➤ Institute precautions for client with neutropenia, which include impeccable handwashing, no rectal temperatures or suppositories, no intramuscular injections, no fresh fruit or flowers in the room, and no visitors or caregivers with upper respiratory tract infections.

➤ If systemic candidiasis is present, prepare for treatment with amphotericin B. Premedicate with steroids, acetaminophen, and diphenhydramine as ordered.

➤ Review related tests such as cerebrospinal fluid analysis, synovial fluid analysis, complete blood count, differential count, absolute neutrophil count, and bronchial washings.

Educate Your Client and the Family

➤ If client is at home with a long-term IV catheter, teach them to inspect site for redness, swelling, and drainage, and to notify the primary health care provider immediately if any of these occur.

➤ If client is neutropenic, ask that family and visitors wash hands carefully before contact. Also review other applicable neutropenic precautions with them.

➤ Teach client and family that *Candida*, unlike other fungal infections, can be transmitted person to person. It can be transmitted between sexual partners, from mother to infant during birth, or to an immunocompromised client on the hands of health care workers.

➤ Explain the side effects of amphotericin B to client and family. Tell them that premedication should help alleviate the worst side effects including kidney problems, fever, low blood pressure, and shaking chills.

Capillary Fragility
cap ih lar ree • frah jil ih tee
(Tourniquet Test, Rumpel-Leed Positive Pressure)

Normal Findings
ALL AGES
0–10 petechiae   Score 1+
Negative test (normal)
10–20 petechiae   Score 2+
Positive test
20–50 petechiae   Score 3+
Positive test

>50 petechiae   Score 4+
Positive test
FEMALES
Decreased estrogen levels, which can occur in premenstrual, menopausal, and postmenopausal women, may produce increases in capillary fragility.

What This Test Will Tell You

This measured pressure test evaluates the relative strength of capillaries in clients with suspected bleeding disorders or platelet dysfunction. The test provides a nonspecific and noninvasive means of evaluating the response of the capillaries and their ability to remain intact with increases in intracapillary pressure. Capillaries typically become more fragile and more likely to rupture under increases in pressure when platelet deficiencies are present.

Abnormal Findings

Increased capillary fragility may indicate thrombocytopenia, thrombasthenia, disseminated intravascular coagulation (DIC), von Willebrand's disease, Cushing's disease, vitamin K deficiency, dysproteinemia, polycythemia vera, chronic renal failure, viral or bacterial infections (such as measles, influenza, or scarlet fever), hypertension, diabetes with associated vascular disease, or estrogen deficiency.

ACTION ALERT!

Strongly positive responses (such as 3+ or 4+) would be considered indicators of a higher degree of capillary fragility and risk for bleeding and hemorrhage. If an individual's response is more pronounced than superficial petechiae, such as the development of severe bruising or hematomas, there may be a severe bleeding disorder involved. In this event, the testing period (5 minutes) should be aborted and the primary health care provider notified immediately.

Interfering Factors

➤ Glucocorticoid therapy may mask evidence of thrombocytopenia by increasing capillary resistance.
➤ Allergies to foods or medications may also produce petechiae and complicate interpretation of the test.

Contraindications

➤ Pronounced petechiae on the forearms prior to the test may be difficult to evaluate.
➤ Vascular compromise to the arms, such as a client with an arteriovenous shunt or fistula, an infant or small child with a Blalock-Taussig shunt, or a client who has undergone a mastectomy.
➤ Skin, vascular or other tissue damage to the forearms, such as burns, fractures, or other trauma.

Potential Complications

➤ Profound platelet deficiencies may lead to extensive bruising or hematoma formation. Since a severe platelet deficiency is easily determined by common laboratory testing, a capillary fragility test is not necessary in individuals known to have severe platelet deficiencies.

NURSING CONSIDERATIONS

Prepare Your Client

➤ Explain that this test helps to identify any bleeding problems in the smallest blood vessels, called capillaries.
➤ Inform the client that some temporary discomfort may be felt in the arm from the pressure of the blood pressure cuff.
➤ Explain that small discolorations of the skin (petechiae) may occur during the test and are what is monitored during this test. These skin discolorations will fade and disappear in a few days and do not pose a danger to the client.
➤ Assess the client's blood pressure to ascertain the *mean* blood pressure.

Perform Procedure

➤ Position the client, sitting or supine, in a position of comfort with the testing arm extended and supported on the bed or table.

➤ Select a 2-inch-diameter area of the testing forearm that is as free of blemishes or pre-existing petechiae as possible. This is ideally a site on the inner aspect of the arm, near the antecubital fossa. The site may be marked prior to the test for valid identification of the test site during the test.

➤ Apply a manual blood pressure cuff to the client's upper arm, in the same manner as for a blood pressure reading. Inflate the cuff to the *mean* blood pressure.

➤ Leave the blood pressure cuff inflated on the client's arm for 5 minutes. Remain with the client during this period to observe for untoward reactions or poor tolerance. Then release the cuff pressure.

➤ Count the number of petechiae present in the test space on the forearm and record the findings.

Care After Test

➤ Instruct the client to open and close the hand a few times to stimulate venous return in the arm.

➤ If the client has developed significant bruising in the test arm, apply cold compresses intermittently for the first 12–24 hours; warm compresses after that time will hasten reabsorption of blood from bruising.

➤ Refrain from using the same arm for capillary fragility testing for a period of 1 week.

➤ Test all body secretions including stool, gastrointestinal aspirate, and tracheal aspirate for occult blood. Closely inspect mucous membranes for bleeding.

➤ Review related tests such as prothrombin time, partial thromboplastin time, bleeding time, and activated clotting time.

Educate Your Client and the Family

➤ Clients with capillary fragility may have prolonged bleeding times. Instruct the client and family on safety measures such as electric razors, non-skid shoes, and soft toothbrushes.

➤ Instruct the client or family to report prolonged or unusual bleeding or bruising.

➤ Significant findings, which indicate a bleeding tendency, require that the client be protected from trauma. Injuries may result in uncontrolled bleeding, which is difficult to manage. Teach family and clients how to evaluate the home environment and increase safety.

➤ Instruct the client or family in diet, activity and/or medication regimens to prevent constipation. Hard stools may be traumatic to anal and rectal mucosa.

➤ Instruct the client with a bleeding tendency to avoid taking medications that prolong bleeding time, such as aspirin and products containing aspirin. Client should be instructed to avoid large quantities of alcohol and its regular use. A written list of products to avoid will provide the client or family with a reference when shopping or selecting home remedies for minor ailments.

Carbon Dioxide Content, Serum

kar bun • die ok side • kon tent • see rum

(CO$_2$ Content, CO$_2$ Combining Power, Total CO$_2$)

Normal Findings

ADULT, ADOLESCENT, ELDERLY, AND PREGNANT

22–30 mEq/L (SI units: 22–30 mmol/L)

NEWBORN

13–22 mEq/L (SI units: 13–22 mmol/L). Newborns normally have low bicarbonate levels. (Premature infants may have even lower reference values.)

CHILD

20–28 mEq/L or mmol/L

What This Test Will Tell You

This blood test for carbon dioxide content, routinely measured as part of the serum electrolytes, is an indirect measure of the serum bicarbonate and is used to determine metabolic acid-base abnormalities in the body. In normal blood plasma, more than 95% of the total CO$_2$ content is contributed by bicarbonate; the other 5% of CO$_2$ is contributed by the dissolved CO$_2$ gas and carbonic acid. The CO$_2$ content reflects the total amount of carbon dioxide in the body and is a general guide to the body's buffering capacity. Total CO$_2$ content is a bicarbonate and base solution that is regulated by the kidneys; therefore, it reflects the metabolic acid-base status of the blood.

Abnormal Findings

▲INCREASED LEVELS may indicate metabolic alkalosis, severe vomiting, gastric suctioning without electrolyte replacement, emphysema, potassium deficit, aldosteronism, or drug use (see Interfering Factors).

▼DECREASED LEVELS may indicate metabolic acidosis, diabetic acidosis, severe diarrhea, acute renal failure, shock, dehydration, starvation, respiratory alkalosis (compensated), or salicylate toxicity.

ACTION ALERT!

A level less than 7 mEq/L may signify life-threatening metabolic acidosis. Decreased CO$_2$ content results in acidosis; increased CO$_2$ content results in alkalosis. Be prepared to treat life-threatening metabolic acidosis with intravenous sodium bicarbonate.

Interfering Factors

➤ Barbiturates, corticosteroids, antacids, mercurial diuretics, loop diuretics, sodium bicarbonate, aldosterone, and ethacrynic acid may increase serum CO$_2$ levels.

➤ Methicillin, tetracycline, nitrofurantoin, acetazolamide, aspirin, thiazide diuretics, and paraldehyde may decrease serum CO$_2$ levels.

➤ Pumping the fist prior to venipuncture may cause falsely elevated results.

➤ High altitudes result in lower values.

➤ Clotted sample or air bubble in sample causes inaccurate results.

➤ Hyperthermia causes an increased CO$_2$ level.

NURSING CONSIDERATIONS

Prepare Your Client

➤ Explain that this test, usually performed with other blood tests, is to determine the acid-base status of the blood.

➤ Instruct the client that it is not necessary to withhold food or fluids.

Perform Procedure

➤ Instruct the client not to clench fist prior to drawing blood because it may cause pooling of the blood, affecting results.

➤ Perform a venipuncture to collect 7–10 mL of blood in a green-topped tube.

➤ Apply pressure to the venipuncture site.

➤ Label the tube and send to the laboratory immediately.

➤ Write the client's temperature on the laboratory requisition if a fever is present.

Care After Test

➤ Assess client with elevated CO_2 content for signs of alkalosis such as shallow breathing. Investigate to determine if the client has been vomiting or had gastric suction for several days.

➤ Assess client with decreased CO_2 levels for signs of acidosis such as deep, rapid breathing or flushed skin.

Suspect acidosis in conditions such as hyperglycemia or shock.

➤ Evaluate related tests such as serum potassium, arterial blood gases, and other electrolytes such as sodium, potassium, and chloride.

Educate Your Client and the Family

➤ Inform the client that acid-base abnormalities may have many causes but that most are related to the kidneys or lungs.

➤ Explain that if results are abnormal, other tests such as blood gases may need to be performed to determine the specific cause.

➤ If metabolic acidosis is present, assess for the cause of this disorder and institute appropriate intervention. Instruct the client on appropriate treatment for diabetes, renal failure, or other metabolic diseases if present.

➤ If metabolic alkalosis is present, assess for drug ingestion or other causes of this disorder. Instruct the client not to ingest large quantities of antacids containing bicarbonate, which could result in alkalosis.

Carboxyhemoglobin, Serum

kar **bok** see **hee** mo **gloe** bin • **see** rum
(Carbon Monoxide, CO, COHb)

Normal Findings

ADULT, PREGNANT, CHILD, AND ADOLESCENT

Nonsmoker: 0%–3% of hemoglobin

Smoker: 2%–5%

Heavy smoker: up to 15%

NEWBORN

Up to 12%. Newborn levels are higher than adult levels because of an

immature respiratory system combined with a more rapid turnover of hemoglobin.

What This Test Will Tell You

This blood test detects carbon monoxide poisoning by measuring the amount of carboxyhemoglobin (COHb) in the blood. Carboxyhemoglobin is formed when inhaled carbon monoxide (CO) combines readily with the hemoglobin molecule. Whereas oxygen's bond with hemoglobin (oxyhemoglobin) is readily reversed, carbon monoxide remains tightly bound to hemoglobin (carboxyhemoglobin). Inhaled carbon monoxide has an affinity for hemoglobin more than 200 times greater than oxygen does. Consequently, with carbon monoxide inhalation, hemoglobin is not available for oxygen transport and tissue hypoxia results.

Arterial blood gases may be measured in conjunction with carboxyhemoglobin. Significant decreases in the oxygen saturation level would be anticipated with elevated carboxyhemoglobin.

Abnormal Findings

▲INCREASED LEVELS may be caused by cigarette smoking (mild elevations), automobile exhaust fumes, intentional inhalation of fumes from combustion of carbon-containing fuels, or defective gas-burning furnaces or appliances.

Interfering Factors

➤ Cigarette smoking, especially heavy smoking, causes elevated results.
➤ Administration of oxygen prior to drawing blood sample will change results.
➤ Lapse of time between carbon monoxide exposure and drawing blood sample may fail to identify CO poisoning.

 ACTION ALERT!

Any value above 20% is critical. High concentrations of oxygen must be administered immediately.
Observe for these symptoms at the following COHb levels:

➤ 20%–30%: headache, dizziness, nausea, vomiting, and loss of judgment
➤ 30%–40%: tachycardia, hyperpnea, hypotension, confusion
➤ 50%–60%: loss of consciousness
➤ Levels greater than 60% are fatal.

NURSING CONSIDERATIONS

Prepare Your Client

➤ Explain to the client and family that the test checks for carbon monoxide poisoning.
➤ Inform the client that the test should be performed as soon as possible after exposure, since carbon monoxide is readily cleared from hemoglobin by breathing room air.
➤ Tell the client that you will need to draw blood from the vein for the test. Describe the venipuncture process clearly.
➤ Obtain client history related to any possible source of carbon monoxide poisoning.
➤ Assess for any symptoms of carbon monoxide poisoning such as dizziness, headache, confusion, tachycardia, hypotension, or decreased level of consciousness. Note color of the skin and mucous membranes.

Perform Procedure

➤ Perform a venipuncture to collect 5–10 mL of blood in a lavender- or blue-top tube.
➤ Apply pressure to the venipuncture site.
➤ Note the color of the blood sample. With carbon monoxide toxicity, the blood is cherry-red to brick-red.
➤ Label the tube and send to the laboratory immediately.

Care After Test

➤ Treat the client with high levels of oxygen as indicated (100% oxygen or

95% oxygen and 5% carbon dioxide) if test results show high levels of carbon monoxide. Often oxygen therapy is initiated prior to receiving results if carbon monoxide inhalation is suspected.

➤ Continue to assess for symptoms of mild to severe carbon monoxide toxicity.

➤ Maintain safety precautions if confusion is present.

➤ Provide emergency resuscitation for severe hypoxia or impending cardiopulmonary arrest.

➤ Closely review client's home environment and health history for risk factors such as a furnace which has not been recently serviced, portable heaters, malfunctioning car muffler, or very heavy smoking.

➤ Review related tests such as arterial blood gases.

Educate Your Client and the Family

➤ Describe the treatment for acute carbon monoxide toxicity.

➤ Obtain additional history related to the source of the carbon monoxide inhalation, if indicated.

➤ Teach client and family about possible sources of carbon monoxide inhalation. Tell them it is a colorless and odorless gas.

➤ Advise client and family not to return home if an improperly functioning furnace is suspected as the source, until repairs are made and the home is cleared of fumes.

➤ Provide appropriate mental health referrals if intentional carbon monoxide poisoning is suspected.

➤ Teach client to take slow, deep breaths to help replace carbon monoxide with oxygen on the hemoglobin molecule.

Carcinoembryonic Antigen

car sin oe em bree on ik • an ti jen
(CEA)

Normal Findings

All ages: <5 ng/mL for nonsmokers (SI units: 0–2.5 μg/L)

What This Test Will Tell You

This blood test monitors the effectiveness of cancer therapy. It measures a glycoprotein that is normally secreted by the gastrointestinal tract epithelium in early fetal life; production stops before birth. The antigen may appear again if a neoplasm develops (malignant or benign) as well as in certain other conditions such as biliary obstruction, alcoholic hepatitis, and chronic heavy smoking.

If serum carcinoembryonic antigen (CEA) levels were elevated before surgical resection, chemotherapy, or radiation therapy, normal levels within 6 weeks of these treatments suggests the therapies were successful. This test is not recommended for screening because the many interfering factors result in a high number of both false positives and false negatives. Serial levels are the most helpful, but the serum level of the initial test may be helpful in staging the cancer and determining the likelihood of recurrence.

Abnormal Findings

▲ INCREASED LEVELS may indicate colon adenocarcinoma, colon polyps, pancreatic cancer, pancreatitis, liver cancer, gastric carcinoma, gastritis, prostatic cancer, breast cancer, bladder cancer, chronic cigarette smoking, inflammatory bowel disease, pulmonary emphysema, benign rectal polyps, benign breast disease, extrahepatic biliary duct obstruction, alcoholic cirrhosis, ulcerative colitis, chronic ischemic heart disease, acute renal failure, neuroblastoma, surgical trauma, peptic ulcer, bronchitis, pulmonary infections, renal failure, or cirrhosis.

▼ DECREASED LEVELS may indicate effective therapy.

Interfering Factors

➤ Chronic cigarette smoking.
➤ Hemolysis of sample.
➤ Use of heparin within 2 days before testing.
➤ Varying laboratory methods to determine results can result in moderate discrepancies in values. Serial testing on the same client should be performed using the same laboratory method.
➤ Tourniquet application for over 1 minute during venous sampling may cause inaccurate results.

NURSING CONSIDERATIONS

Prepare Your Client

➤ Explain that this test detects a special protein that usually appears only when a tumor is present.
➤ Explain that the test will be repeated to monitor the effectiveness of cancer therapy.
➤ If client is on heparin therapy, consult with the primary health care provider about withholding this medication for 2 days prior to venous sampling.
➤ Assess client for presence of other conditions, such as benign hepatic disease, acute pancreatitis, inflammatory bowel disease, pulmonary emphysema, acute renal failure, chronic cigarette smoking, and surgical trauma, that may interfere with interpretation of results.

Perform Procedure

➤ Collect 7 mL of venous blood in a red-top or lavender-top tube. Check with your laboratory for the correct color tube depending upon the method used.
➤ Label the sample and note presence of interfering factors or disease that can affect test results.
➤ Label the sample if heparin was given and not withheld.
➤ Handle specimen gently to avoid hemolysis.

Care After Test

➤ Assess for signs and symptoms of metastatic cancer including bone pain, fatigue, and recurring symptoms of the tumor.
➤ Refer client and family to a cancer support group.
➤ Assess for the client's ability to cope with changes in body image such as weight loss or gain, loss of hair, changes in body functions, decreased sexual function, and role changes.
➤ Refer to social services to assist with the financial and economic impact of cancer.
➤ Consult with a registered dietician for clients with anorexia, weight loss, or special dietary needs.
➤ Assess carefully for chronic and acute pain. Obtain pain management consultation if indicated.

➤ Assess for signs and symptoms of infection such as chills, fever, and drop in the absolute neutrophil count. Institute precautions to protect the client such as no fresh fruits or vegetables. Remove fresh flowers and plants, and enforce good handwashing.

➤ Assess the client for signs and symptoms such as bleeding from injection sites, petechia, or ecchymosis, occult blood, and decreasing platelet count related to increased risk for bleeding.

➤ Clients with impaired bone marrow function may have prolonged bleeding times. Institute safety measures such as electric razors, nonskid shoes, no intramuscular injections, no rectal temperatures, and soft toothbrushes.

➤ Encourage verbalization of fears related to cancer, prognosis, treatment, and death.

➤ Evaluate other diagnostic tests such as computed tomography scan, other tumor markers, alkaline phosphatase, and acid phosphatase levels.

Educate Your Client and the Family

➤ Inform family that the test is most useful in monitoring how well the treatment is working or how much of the tumor the surgery was able to remove.

➤ Instruct client and family on a high-calorie, well-balanced diet, if appropriate.

Carcinoma Antigen 15-3

car si noe mah • an ti jen 15-3
(CA 15-3, Tumor Marker)

Normal Findings

FEMALE
< 22 U/mL

What This Test Will Tell You

This blood test is a tumor marker used to detect recurrence of breast cancer and to monitor response to therapy for metastatic breast cancer. CA 15-3 detects both the membrane antigen against human milk globules and the antigens from a human breast carcinoma. CA 15-3 tumor marker levels correlate more frequently with tumor progression than tumor regression. CA 15-3 is not specific enough to be used as a screening technique in early detection of breast cancer. The major function of this test is to help evaluate metastasis, related to elevated levels, or, to a lesser extent, effectiveness of therapy documented by declining levels. A partial or complete response to treatment results in declining levels, while a persistent rise of CA 15-3 level, despite therapy, strongly suggests progressive disease.

Abnormal Findings

▲ INCREASED LEVELS may indicate breast cancer with metastases, lung cancer, benign breast disease, or benign ovarian disease.

▼ DECREASED LEVELS may indicate response to therapy.

Interfering Factors

➤ Clients with benign breast or ovarian disease may have elevated levels.

➤ Due to lack of specificity this test is not to be used in the surveillance of clients who have had a complete response to therapy.

NURSING CONSIDERATIONS

Prepare Your Client

➤ Explain that this test is most useful in monitoring and/or predicting the spread or recurrence of breast cancer.

Perform the Procedure

➤ Collect 7–10 mL venous blood in a red-top tube.

➤ Observe the venipuncture site closely for hematoma formation or bleeding. Coagulopathies are common in liver disease. Apply a pressure dressing to the venipuncture site.

Care After Test

➤ Assess for signs and symptoms of metastatic cancer including bone pain, fatigue, and recurring symptoms of the tumor.

➤ Refer client and family to a cancer support group.

➤ Assess for the client's ability to cope with changes in body image such as weight loss or gain, loss of hair, changes in body functions, decreased sexual function, and role changes.

➤ Refer to social services to assist with the financial and economic impact of cancer.

➤ Consult with a registered dietician for clients with anorexia, weight loss, or special dietary needs.

➤ Assess carefully for chronic and acute pain. Obtain pain management consultation if indicated.

➤ Assess for signs and symptoms of infection such as chills, fever, and drop in the absolute neutrophil count. Institute precautions to protect the client such as no fresh fruits or vegetables. Remove fresh flowers and plants, and enforce good handwashing.

➤ Assess the client for signs and symptoms such as bleeding from injection sites, petechia, or ecchymosis, occult blood, and decreasing platelet count related to increased risk for bleeding.

➤ Clients with impaired bone marrow function may have prolonged bleeding times. Institute safety measures such as electric razors, nonskid shoes, no intramuscular injections, no rectal temperatures, and soft toothbrushes.

➤ Evaluate other related tests such as carcinoembryonic antigen (CEA), CA 549, and breast biopsy results.

Educate Your Client and the Family

➤ Tell client and family that test results may take 7–10 days.

➤ Explain that greatly elevated levels strongly correlate to the presence or recurrence of disease.

Carcinoma Antigen 19-9

car si noe mah • an ti jen 19-9
(CA 19-9, Tumor Marker)

Normal Findings
All ages: < 37 U/mL

What This Test Will Tell You
This blood test is a tumor marker used in the diagnosis, evaluation of response to treatment, and surveillance of clients with pancreatic or hepatobiliary cancer. CA 19-9 is not widely used because it is elevated in only about 70% of clients with pancreatic carcinoma and 65% of clients with hepatobiliary cancer, and it does not detect tumors early enough to improve prognosis. If this test is combined with a carcinoembryonic antigen (CEA) test, the results are more reliable. The greatest value of CA 19-9 tests is in serial testing to measure the response to therapy.

Abnormal Findings
▲ INCREASED LEVELS may indicate pancreatic carcinoma, gastric cancer, colorectal cancer, hepatobiliary carcinoma, lung cancer, breast cancer, ovarian cancer, pancreatitis, cholecystitis, cirrhosis, inflammatory bowel disease, gallstones, or cystic fibrosis.
▼ DECREASED LEVELS may indicate positive response to therapy.

Interfering Factors
➤ Clients with nonmalignant conditions such as pancreatitis, gallstones, cirrhosis, and cystic fibrosis may have minimally elevated levels of CA 19-9.

NURSING CONSIDERATIONS
Prepare Your Client
➤ Explain that this test is used to help diagnose cancer in the pancreas or liver and gallbladder systems. If appropriate, explain that this test is most useful when repeated tests are done to measure how well the treatment is working, or if the cancer is recurring.

Perform Procedure
➤ Collect 7–10 mL of venous blood in a red-top tube.
➤ Observe the venipuncture site closely for hematoma formation or bleeding. Coagulopathies are common in cancers. Apply a pressure dressing to the venipuncture site.

Care After Test
➤ Assess for signs and symptoms of metastatic cancer including bone pain, fatigue, and recurring symptoms of the tumor.
➤ Refer client and family to a cancer support group.
➤ Assess for the client's ability to cope with changes in body image such as weight loss or gain, loss of hair, changes in body functions, decreased sexual function, and role changes.
➤ Refer to social services to assist with the financial and economic impact of cancer.
➤ Consult with a registered dietician for clients with anorexia, weight loss, or special dietary needs.
➤ Assess carefully for chronic and acute pain. Obtain pain management consultation if indicated.
➤ Assess for signs and symptoms of infection such as chills, fever, and drop in the absolute neutrophil

count. Institute precautions to protect the client such as no fresh fruits or vegetables. Remove fresh flowers and plants, and enforce good handwashing.

➤ Assess the client for signs and symptoms such as bleeding from injection sites, petechia, or ecchymosis, occult blood, and decreasing platelet count related to increased risk for bleeding.

➤ Clients with impaired bone marrow function may have prolonged bleeding times. Institute safety measures such as electric razors, nonskid shoes, no intramuscular injections, no rectal temperatures, and soft toothbrushes.

➤ Evaluate other tumor marker tests such as carcinoembryonic antigen (CEA).

Educate Your Client and the Family

➤ Tell client and family that the test results will take 7–10 days.

➤ If client is being diagnosed, explain that an elevated CA 19-9 can indicate a benign or malignant tumor, and may be used to differentiate pancreatic cancer from pancreatic infection.

➤ If client is being monitored after treatment, explain that a series of tests will be done.

➤ Explain that a decreased level of CA 19-9 will confirm a positive response to treatment.

➤ Tell client and family that a rapid rise in CA 19-9 may indicate a recurrent tumor growth before other symptoms are evident.

Carcinoma Antigen 125

car si noe mah • an ti jen •125
(CA-125, Tumor Marker)

Normal Findings

FEMALE
<35 U/mL
Levels >35 U/mL are highly suggestive of malignancy.
PREGNANT
A mild elevation is found in the third trimester of pregnancy.

What This Test Will Tell You

This blood test detects ovarian cancer, particularly epithelial cell tumors, and determines the extent of disease and response to treatment. CA-125 is a glycoprotein produced by ovarian epithelial neoplasms. Because normal levels do not rule out recurrence or the presence of an extensive tumor, CA-125 tumor marker is not used as a screening test for asymptomatic clients.

CA-125 tumor marker may indicate whether a repeat diagnostic laparotomy is needed. This test does not replace biopsy or pathological examination of tissues. A change in levels from normal to abnormal or a rising titer is most predictive.

Abnormal Findings

▲ INCREASED LEVELS may indicate ovarian cancer, metastatic peritoneal, carcinomatosis, endometriosis, cirrhosis, peritonitis, other gynecological tumor of fallopian tube, cervical cancer, endometrial and vulvar cancer, pregnancy, colon cancer, upper gastrointestinal cancer, pancreatic cancer, lymphoma, or acute pelvic inflammatory disease.

▼ DECREASED LEVELS may indicate positive response to therapy.

Interfering Factors

➤ Pregnancy and menstruation may cause a slight elevation in levels.

➤ Benign peritoneal disease such as peritonitis and cirrhosis may cause slightly elevated levels.

➤ CA-125 test cannot distinguish benign from malignant tumors.

➤ Serum levels may double during menses, especially in clients with endometriosis.

➤ Upper and lower gastrointestinal tract cancer will also elevate levels.

NURSING CONSIDERATIONS

Prepare Your Client

➤ Explain that this test is important to help detect cancer in the ovaries or to help show the response to treatment of that cancer.

➤ Evaluate the client's history for evidence of interfering factors which may alter test results.

Perform Procedure

➤ Perform a venipuncture to collect 7–10 mL of venous blood in a red-top tube.

➤ Observe the venipuncture site closely for hematoma formation or bleeding. Coagulopathies are common in cancer. Apply a pressure dressing to the venipuncture site.

Care After Test

➤ Assess for signs and symptoms of metastatic cancer including bone pain, fatigue, and recurring symptoms of the tumor.

➤ Refer client and family to a cancer support group.

➤ Assess for the client's ability to cope with changes in body image such as weight loss or gain, loss of hair, changes in body functions, decreased sexual function, and role changes.

➤ Refer to social services to assist with the financial and economic impact of cancer.

➤ Consult with a registered dietician for clients with anorexia, weight loss, or special dietary needs.

➤ Assess carefully for chronic and acute pain. Obtain pain management consultation if indicated.

➤ Assess for signs and symptoms of infection such as chills, fever, and drop in the absolute neutrophil count. Institute precautions to protect the client such as no fresh fruits or vegetables. Remove fresh flowers and plants, and enforce good hand-washing.

➤ Assess the client for signs and symptoms such as bleeding from injection sites, petechia, or ecchymosis, occult blood, and decreasing platelet count related to increased risk for bleeding.

➤ Clients with impaired bone marrow function may have prolonged bleeding times. Institute safety measures such as electric razors, non-skid shoes, no intramuscular injections, no rectal temperatures, and soft toothbrushes.

➤ Review related tests such as carcinoma antigen 15-3, carcinoembryonic antigen, parathyroid hormone level, and pelvic ultrasonography results.

Educate Your Client and the Family

➤ Tell client and family that test results may not be available for 7–10 days.

> Explain to client the test may be done in series to monitor response to treatment—falling values indicate a good response to treatment and a better chance for recovery.

> Explain to client that a rise in CA-125 level may be an early sign of the tumor coming back.

> Explain to the client that an elevated CA-125 can indicate benign as well as malignant tumors if being diagnosed for the first time.

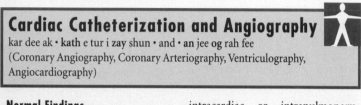

Cardiac Catheterization and Angiography

kar dee ak • **kath** e tur i **zay** shun • and • **an** jee **og** rah fee
(Coronary Angiography, Coronary Arteriography, Ventriculography, Angiocardiography)

Normal Findings

All ages: Normal anatomical structure, intrapulmonary pressures, cardiac output, arterial and venous oxygen saturation, cardiac muscular motion, atrial and ventricular volumes, and patent coronary arteries

What This Test Will Tell You

This radiographic test diagnoses coronary artery occlusive disease, valvular disease, and congenital heart defects. It also investigates causes of chest pain, syncope, abnormal electrocardiograms, and cyanosis or other cardiac symptoms in infants and children. This diagnostic study is performed by inserting arterial and/or venous catheters into the right and/or left sides of the heart under fluoroscopy with contrast material. The structure and function of the chambers, valves, and vessels, as well as hemodynamic pressures, can be determined during the study. Of particular importance in adults is the ability to diagnose coronary artery occlusion. Samples of oxygen saturation can also be obtained during the test to assist in diagnosing intracardiac or intrapulmonary shunting.

This procedure may also be used to treat cardiovascular anomalies. Balloon angioplasty may be done during catheterization to dilate occluded coronary arteries. Balloon catheters may also be used to treat coarctation of the aorta and valvular stenosis. Various stents and umbrella devices may be used to close septal defects as well as occlude collateral vessels or a patent ductus arteriosus. Finally, anti-thrombolytic pharmacologic agents may be infused directly into occluded coronary arteries during catheterization.

Abnormal Findings

> Cardiac abnormalities may indicate coronary artery occlusion, congenital cardiac defects, congenital or acquired septal defects, intracardiac tumors, intracardiac or great vessel aneurysms, ventricular failure, ventricular or atrial thrombi, or valvular stenosis or insufficiency.

> Pulmonary abnormalities may indicate pulmonary emboli, pulmonary hypertension, or anomalous

Pressure and Volume Results During Cardiac Catheterization

Pressure/volume	Normal values: adults	Normal values: pediatric and neonatal
Systemic arterial pressure	90–140/60–90 mm Hg	90–125/50–80 mm Hg (2 years to adolescence) 60–90/20–60 mm Hg (birth to 5 days)
Right atrial pressure	0–5 mm Hg	3 mm Hg
Right ventricular pressure	25/0–5 mm Hg	30/3 mm Hg
Pulmonary artery pressure	15–28/5–20 mm Hg	30/10 mm Hg
Pulmonary artery occlusive pressure	5–15 mm Hg	6–10 mm Hg
Left atrial pressure	5–10 mm Hg	8 mm Hg
Left ventricular pressure	90–140/4–12 mm Hg	100/6 mm Hg
Aortic pressure	90–140/60–90 mm Hg	100/60 mm Hg
Cardiac index	2.8–5.5 L/min/m^2	3.5–4.5 L/min/m^2 (child) 3.5–5.5 L/min/m^2 (newborn)
Cardiac output	3–6 L/min	
Central venous pressure	2–14 cm H$_2$O	2–10 cm H$_2$O

pulmonary venous return.

ACTION ALERT!

Assess client carefully for allergic reaction to contrast material including dyspnea, itching, urticaria, flushing, hypotension, and shock. Life-threatening anaphylactic reactions can occur and need to be recognized and treated immediately.

Interfering Factors

➤ In adults, failure to cooperate with requests, such as to cough and to perform bicycle leg maneuvers, may decrease the information available from the test.

➤ In infants and children, crying may affect accuracy of hemodynamic pressures.

Contraindications

➤ This test should be performed cautiously in clients with severe cardiomegaly because of the danger of serious dysrhythmias and risk of perforation of the heart.

➤ This test would be contraindicated without modifications for clients with an allergy to contrast material.

➤ Contraindicated in pregnancy due to radiation exposure of the fetus.

Potential Complications

➤ Myocardial infarction
➤ Lethal dysrhythmias
➤ Perforation of the heart or great vessels
➤ Thromboemboli
➤ Cerebrovascular accident
➤ Allergic reactions including anaphylaxis
➤ Infection at the catheter insertion site
➤ Endocarditis
➤ Hemopericardium
➤ Hemothorax or pneumothorax
➤ Hemorrhage

NURSING CONSIDERATIONS

Prepare Your Client

➤ Explain to the client or family that this test is to discover if there are any problems in the heart.

➤ Inform client that a local anesthetic is used in the catheterization laboratory to numb the area where the catheters will be inserted. This may produce a brief burning sensation before the area becomes numb.

➤ Explain that catheters (long thin tubes) are threaded through a needle placed in a thigh or arm vein (femoral or subclavian vein). The catheters are threaded through the vein to the heart. Assure client that threading the catheters is not painful.

➤ Tell your client or family that once needles are inserted, the procedure itself is painless, but some pressure may be felt while lines are passed and there may be warmth from the contrast medium.

➤ Ensure that an informed consent is obtained, because of the possible complications associated with this procedure.

➤ Assess for a history of allergy to contrast material or iodine.

➤ Record baseline vital signs.

➤ Confer with the cardiologist about administering cardiac medications while food and fluids are restricted.

➤ Locate peripheral pulses and mark with a pen to assist in monitoring them following the procedure.

➤ Restrict food and fluids for at least 4–12 hours preceding the catheterization.

➤ Administer sedatives or tranquilizers as ordered before the client goes to the cardiac catheterization laboratory.

➤ Confirm that adults and older children have voided before the procedure.

➤ Tell adults that they may be asked to breathe deeply, cough, or do bicycle leg movements during the procedure.

➤ Do not remove glasses, dentures, or hearing aids unless dictated by your hospital policy. The client may need these in order to communicate and cooperate during the procedure.

Perform Procedure

Nurses do not perform this procedure but should understand the process to prepare the client and assist the physician.

Electrocardiogram leads are placed on the chest to monitor for dysrhythmias and the insertion site is cleansed with an antimicrobial agent and/or shaved according to institutional policy. The sites for arterial and venous cannulation are anesthetized with a local anesthetic such as mepivacaine or lidocaine. Percutaneous puncture or a cutdown is performed in the groin or antecubital space to gain arterial and venous access. Fluoroscopy is used to confirm placement of a guide wire introduced through the arterial and venous catheters and to visualize the catheters throughout the procedure as they are advanced through the vessels, valves, and chambers.

Cardiac pressures, volumes, and blood gases are recorded in various vessels and chambers. Films are taken during injection of radiopaque contrast material to visualize the arterial vasculature. Client is asked to perform bicycle movements, or atrial pacing is initiated, to evaluate the heart's function during periods of physiological stress.

Carefully assess the client for signs and symptoms of allergic reaction to contrast material. Apply pressure to the arterial and venous puncture sites after the catheter is removed until bleeding stops. Apply a pressure dressing to the sites.

Care After Test

➤ Monitor vital signs closely until stable; usually every 15 minutes for the first hour, every 30 minutes for the next hour, and then every 4 hours for 24 hours.

➤ Maintain pressure on venipuncture site with either a sandbag or pressure dressing. Ice packs may be used to minimize bleeding.

➤ Maintain bed rest with the extremity extended for 6–12 hours following the procedure to minimize complications of bleeding, hematoma formation, headaches, nausea, and vomiting.

➤ Avoid flexion of the extremity by keeping the bed flat or limiting elevation of the head of the bed to 20 degrees.

➤ Assess the venipuncture site(s) carefully for bleeding and hematoma.

➤ Assess circulation with each vital sign assessment. Assess presence and strength of pulses, capillary refill, color, temperature, and sensation. Report immediately any abnormal findings.

➤ Observe for signs of allergic reaction to the contrast material, which include urticaria, pruritus, conjunctivitis, dyspnea, and apprehension. Delayed reactions usually occur 2–6 hours after the test.

➤ Encourage drinking fluids, because the contrast material has a diuretic effect.

➤ Review related tests such as an electrocardiogram, stress test, chest x-ray, arterial blood gases, and echocardiogram.

Educate Your Client and the Family

➤ Teach client and family a heart healthy diet, including no added salt.

➤ For infants and children with congenital cardiac defects, discuss caloric intake and collaborate with the primary health care provider and dietician to supplement formula and diet as needed.

➤ Tell client to report chest pain (angina) promptly before, during, or after the test.

Cardiac Isotope Imaging

kar dee ak • ie so tope • im aj ing

Normal Findings

All ages: Absence of areas of infarct, normal coronary perfusion without evidence of occlusion, and normal ejection fraction

What This Test Will Tell You

This group of nuclear medicine tests are used primarily to diagnose coronary artery disease and recent myocardial infarction. Cardiac isotope imaging may also be done before and after cardiac surgery to evaluate patency of grafted vessels. A radionuclide is injected intravenously before the scan begins. Several compounds are used. Thallium is injected a few minutes before imaging for thallium scans (perfusion scans), thallium stress testing, and dipyridamole-thallium scans. Infarcted or ischemic areas are easily visualized because thallium is only absorbed by healthy cells. "Cold spots" (areas without thallium) are easily seen during the scan, clearly marking abnormal areas.

Thallium stress testing is particularly helpful in identifying ischemia that only occurs during exercise. Thallium is injected either during exercise (treadmill or bicycle) or during tachycardia induced by pacing. Areas of ischemia that may occur only with exertion are identified as "cold spots" because these sites do not take up the radioactive imaging agent. Scans may be repeated 3–4 hours following exercise or induced tachycardia and again in 18–24 hours to help differentiate ischemic from infarcted areas.

The use of dipyridamole during a thallium scan is common for clients who cannot participate in exercise stress testing. Dipyridamole reproduces dilation of normal coronary arteries that exercise would create and decreases perfusion of occluded vessels, further enhancing the imaging of diseased coronary arteries. Caution is taken with the use of dipyridamole because it may precipitate angina or worsen ischemia and newly infarcted areas.

Technetium-99m pyrophosphate (Tc-99m PYP) is used during cardiac imaging to identify infarcted areas (infarction scan). The radiocompound material is injected 1–3 hours before imaging is begun. Unlike thallium, Tc-99m pyrophosphate is readily taken up by infarcted, not healthy, myocardial cells. Areas of infarct are identified as "hot spots" best visualized in the first 24–72 hours following an infarction.

A newer imaging technique called single-photon emission computed tomography (SPECT) provides a three-dimensional image of the heart and areas of infarction.

Abnormal Findings

Images may reveal coronary artery occlusive disease, myocardial ischemia, myocardial infarction, or blocked coronary artery bypass grafts.

Interfering Factors

➤ Long-acting nitrates may reduce imaging effectiveness.
➤ Unstable angina may give false positive results.

> Recent cardioversion may give false positive results.

> Recent nuclear testing may interfere with imaging of the heart.

Contraindications

> Previous adverse effects with radionuclide studies.

> Pregnancy, due to radiation exposure of the fetus.

> History of reactive airway disease and bronchospasm may contraindicate the use of dipyridamole.

> Angina at rest is a contraindication for dipyridamole-thallium testing.

> Stress testing is contraindicated in clients with right and left bundle branch block, hypokalemia, and left ventricular hypertrophy and clients taking digitalis or quinidine.

Potential Complications

> Myocardial infarction or angina with use of dipyridamole

> Exercise-induced and ventricular dysrhythmias

> Bronchospasm

NURSING CONSIDERATIONS

Prepare Your Client

> Explain that this test is to look for blocked blood vessels in the heart, which can damage the heart's muscle.

> Ensure that an informed consent is obtained.

> Check the chart to be sure the client has no history of problems with radiopharmaceuticals.

> Reassure the client and family that there is no significant danger to them associated with these small levels of radiation that have short half lives (disintegrate rapidly).

> Record baseline vital signs.

> Check institutional policy regarding fasting before thallium scans. Generally a minimum of 2 hours' fasting is required.

> Check with the primary health care provider to determine if medications should be administered while the client is fasting. Long-acting nitrates should be discontinued 8–12 hours before testing.

> Confirm that adult or older child has voided before the procedure.

> Do not remove glasses, dentures, or hearing aids unless dictated by your institution's policy. The client may need these in order to communicate and cooperate during the procedure.

Perform Procedure

Nurses do not perform this procedure but should understand the process to prepare the client and assist the physician. Client is assisted to a supine position on a special x-ray table with a scanner (camera) over their chest. The camera moves to take pictures from different angles. Depending upon which test is being done, they may be required to ride a stationary bicycle or walk on a treadmill. Tell client that imaging may not begin until 15 minutes to 4 hours following injection of the radionuclide. (See *Stress Exercise Testing* for more information.)

Care After Test

> Monitor vital signs closely until stable.

> Assess the venipuncture site(s) carefully for bleeding and hematoma.

> Encourage fluids to help eliminate the radioactive imaging agent and replace fluids lost due to the diuretic effect of the contrast media.

➤ Review related tests such as cardiac enzymes, electrocardiogram, echocardiogram, and stress exercise tests.

Educate Your Client and the Family

➤ Teach client and family a heart-healthy diet, including no added salt.
➤ Review medications taken for angina and coronary artery disease with the client or family.

➤ Discuss signs and symptoms of myocardial infarction and instruct client and family to report these to their nurse or physician immediately.
➤ Encourage all family members to take a course in cardiopulmonary resuscitation.

Carotid Duplex Scanning

ka **rot** id • **doo** pleks • **skan** ing
(Duplex Scan, Doppler Studies)

Normal Findings

Normal carotid artery anatomy
Absence of atherosclerotic plaques and stenosis
Absence of arterial aneurysms
Less than 15% occlusion

What This Test Will Tell You

This ultrasonic test diagnoses carotid artery disease by using ultrasound and Doppler technology to image the carotid arteries in the neck noninvasively. The test is performed by placing a probe/transducer on the skin and positioning the transducer to produce the best image on an accompanying monitor. A two-dimensional (2-D) image of the carotid arteries is produced using ultrasound waves (duplex scanning), which can identify narrowing or aneurysmal areas. The Doppler study component of this test records blood flow velocities that are generally abnormal in stenotic and partially occluded areas.

Abnormal Findings

Abnormalities may reveal carotid artery aneurysms or carotid artery occlusive disease:

16%–49% occlusion signifies mild stenosis.
50%–75% occlusion signifies moderate stenosis.
>75% occlusion signifies severe stenosis.

Interfering Factors

➤ Large neck may make probe positioning and imaging difficult.

Contraindications

➤ Back problems, restlessness, confusion, and anxiety may make it difficult for the client to lie still for the duration of the test (15–30 minutes).

NURSING CONSIDERATIONS

Prepare Your Client

➤ Explain that this test is used to find any blockages in the blood vessels (arteries) in the neck.
➤ Assure your client that the test is painless.

Perform Procedure

Nurses do not usually perform this

procedure but should understand the process to prepare the client and assist the physician. A colorless gel is placed on the neck to improve conduction of sound waves. A transducer, which resembles a microphone, is then placed on the neck to transmit and receive the sound waves. Patency of the vessel is verified by hearing and measuring blood flow.

Care After Test

➤ Assess for signs and symptoms of carotid artery disease including transient ischemic events.

➤ Remove transducer gel with soap and water.

➤ Review related tests such as blood lipid studies and cerebral perfusion scans.

Educate Your Client and the Family

➤ Teach your client and family a heart-healthy diet if there is evidence of atherosclerotic disease.

Catecholamines, Serum

cat eh kole ah meens, see rum
(Serum Epinephrine, Serum Norepinephrine, Serum Dopamine)

Normal Findings

All ages

Epinephrine:

> *Supine*: 0–110 pg/mL (SI units: 0–600 pmol/L)
> *Standing*: 0–140 pg/mL (SI units: 0–900 pmol/L)

Norepinephrine:

> *Supine*: 70–750 pg/mL (SI units: 0.4–4.4 nmol/L)
> *Standing*: 200–1,700 pg/mL (SI units: 1.2–10 nmol/L)

Dopamine:

> *Supine*: 0–30 pg/mL (SI units: 0–150 pmol/L)
> *Standing*: 0–30 pg/mL (SI units: 0–150 pmol/L)

What This Test Will Tell You

This blood test measures levels of circulating catecholamines, to determine the cause of hypertension or to detect an adrenal medullary or

neural tumor. Norepinephrine has major effects on the vascular system and epinephrine affects metabolic processes. They are important hormones in preparing the body for the "fight or flight" response. Heart rate, respiratory rate, and blood pressure as well as blood flow to the skeletal and heart muscles are increased in response to the release of these hormones. Additional effects include pupil and bronchial dilation, decreased visceral blood flow, and increased breakdown of glucose and fat stores for energy.

It is more common to assess the catecholamines by a 24-hour urine collection than by serum analysis because of varying levels throughout the day.

Abnormal Findings

▲ INCREASED LEVELS may indicate

pheochromocytoma, tumor of the adrenal medulla, ganglioneuroma, ganglioblastoma, or neuroblastoma.

▼DECREASED LEVELS may indicate autonomic nervous system dysfunction.

Interfering Factors

➤ Any delay from the time the blood is drawn until the lab test is run may significantly alter levels.

➤ Repeated venipunctures can alter levels. If multiple testing is needed, blood should be drawn through a central line or heparin lock.

➤ Levels may be increased by epinephrine, amphetamines, levodopa, decongestants, tricyclic antidepressants, chlorpromazine, and sympathomimetic drugs.

➤ Levels may be decreased by reserpine and cholinergic medications.

➤ Amine-rich substances including bananas, cheese, coffee, tea, cocoa, beer, and avocados affect levels.

➤ Stress, fever, anxiety, and hypothermia can elevate levels.

➤ Radioactive scan within 1 week of serum levels testing will interfere with radioimmunoassay determination of levels.

➤ Smoking may increase levels.

➤ Levels vary greatly throughout a 24-hour period.

NURSING CONSIDERATIONS

Prepare Your Client

➤ Explain that the purpose of this test is to check levels of certain hormones that help the body during times of stress.

➤ Withhold food and fluids for 10–12 hours before blood specimen is drawn.

➤ Instruct client to refrain from nicotine and caffeine for 24 hours prior to the test.

➤ Ensure the client has not had amine-rich foods or beverages for at least 48 hours.

➤ Collaborate with the primary health care provider regarding restrictions of prescribed medications which may affect test results.

➤ Check that client is calm and without fever or infection.

➤ Keep client warm and lying down for at least 45–60 minutes before the blood is drawn.

Perform Procedure

➤ Collect 10 mL of blood into a chilled purple-top tube between 6 A.M. and 8 A.M.

➤ If ordered, draw a second sample after the client has been standing for 10 minutes.

Care After Test

➤ Evaluate physical and emotional stressors in the client's environment. Refer for counseling and initiate community referrals as necessary.

➤ Assess for end organ damage if hypertension is present by evaluating renal function studies, visual acuity, signs or symptoms of transient ischemic attacks.

➤ Review related tests such as urine catecholamine levels, vanillylmandelic acid, and homovanillic acid levels.

Educate Your Client and the Family

➤ Explain the clinical significance of the catecholamines.

➤ If the possible diagnosis is pheochromocytoma, discuss the treatment of the disease. Teach client and family to monitor blood pressure carefully.

Cerebral Angiography

seh **ree** bral • **an** jee **og** rah fee
(Cerebral Arteriography)

Normal Findings

Normal cerebral vascular anatomy

What This Test Will Tell You

This radiographic test with contrast is performed to visualize cerebral circulation and diagnose abnormalities in the blood vessels. The contrast medium allows visualization of both the arteries and veins, including the carotid artery, vertebral artery, large blood vessels of the circle of Willis, and small cerebral arterial branches. Leakage of blood from the circulatory system and blockage of vessels may be detected. Nonvascular masses such as tumors and abscesses may also be identified by the distortion of the normal vascular locations.

Abnormal Findings

Abnormalities may indicate cerebral aneurysm, cerebral vessel occlusion, hematoma, tumors, cerebral plaques, cerebral vessel spasms, cerebral fistula, atherosclerotic cerebral vascular disease, cerebral vascular malformations, arteritis, abscess, arterial dissection, or fibromuscular dysplasia.

ACTION ALERT!

Assess client carefully for allergic reaction to contrast material including dyspnea, itching, urticaria, flushing, hypotension, and shock. Life-threatening anaphylactic reactions can occur and need to be recognized and treated immediately.

Interfering Factors

➤ Movement of the client during the test

Contraindications

➤ Allergies to iodine or shellfish without modifications in the test
➤ Pregnancy and lactation, due to exposure of the fetus or infant to radiation
➤ Atherosclerosis, due to risk of embolus
➤ Coagulopathies

Potential Complications

➤ Dysphagia and respiratory distress if a carotid artery was used
➤ Transient ischemic attack (TIA)
➤ Allergic or anaphylactic reaction to contrast medium
➤ Hemorrhage, hematoma, or infection at arterial access site
➤ Embolism
➤ Infection

NURSING CONSIDERATIONS

Prepare Your Client

➤ Explain that this test is used to see the blood vessels in the brain and to find if there is blockage or leakage in the vessels.
➤ Assess the client's history for an allergy to contrast media or iodine.
➤ Explain to the client or family that a local anesthetic is used to numb the area where the catheter will be inserted. This may produce a brief burning sensation before the area becomes numb.
➤ Explain that the catheter (long thin tube) is threaded through a needle placed in a thigh or arm artery (femoral or brachial artery). The catheter is threaded through the

artery to the part of the body the physician needs to see. Assure the client that threading the catheter is not painful.

➤ Tell your client or family that once the needle is inserted, the procedure itself is painless, but some pressure may be felt while lines are passed and there may be warmth from the contrast medium.

➤ Ensure that an informed consent is obtained, because of the possible complications associated with this procedure.

➤ Record baseline vital signs.

➤ Document baseline peripheral pulse evaluations.

➤ Administer sedative, narcotic, and prophylactic allergy premedications as ordered.

➤ Restrict food and fluids for 8–12 hours before the test.

➤ Ensure anticoagulant therapy is discontinued before the test. Review with the primary health care provider laboratory work such as prothrombin time (PT), partial thromboplastin time (PTT), or activated clotting time (ACT) before the test.

Perform Procedure

Nurses do not perform this procedure but should understand the process to prepare the client and assist the physician.

Place the client on an x-ray table while maintaining body alignment. Use safety measures since clients are usually sedated. Instruct the client to remain very still during the procedure, because movement may cause inaccurate findings.

The arterial access site is prepared by scrubbing with an antimicrobial solution and/or removing hair, according to institutional policy. The site is numbed with a local anesthetic and the catheter is inserted and followed to the desired artery by fluoroscopy. Radiopaque contrast material is injected. Inform client that they may feel a warm, flushed sensation immediately after the dye is injected. This sensation passes within 1 or 2 minutes.

Serial x-ray films are taken showing the arterial and venous cerebral circulation. The catheter is removed and a pressure dressing is applied.

Care After Test

➤ Monitor the client's vital signs as ordered. Frequency is usually every 15 minutes, increasing to every hour. Be aware of changes in vital signs such as decreasing blood pressure and increasing pulse rate, which may indicate bleeding.

➤ Evaluate pulse volume, skin color, sensation, capillary refill, and skin temperature in the involved limb with each set of vital signs. Report changes from baseline immediately.

➤ Assess for vasovagal response. The client's blood pressure and pulse rate will decrease. The skin will be cool, clammy, and pale. This reaction lasts about 15 minutes. Treatment includes IV fluids and atropine.

➤ Explain the importance of minimizing activity in the involved limb. Limiting activity will decrease the risk of bleeding.

➤ Assess the injection site for swelling and hematoma formation.

➤ Assess for dysphagia and respiratory distress when the carotid artery is used for the test.

➤ Assess for transient ischemic attacks (TIAs). Changes in mental status, sensation, or speech may indicate a TIA.

➤ Assess for signs of allergic reaction

which include tachycardia, dyspnea, skin rash, and urticaria. Delayed reaction usually occurs within 2–4 hours.

➤ Encourage fluids to facilitate excretion of dye and to prevent dehydration from the diuretic effects of the contrast material.

➤ Evaluate related tests such as computed tomography scan and magnetic resonance imaging.

Educate Your Client and the Family

➤ Instruct your client in behaviors that modify risk factors for stroke, such as controlling hypertension through medication and/or diet, refraining from smoking, getting regular exercise, controlling diabetes through diet and medication, and limiting alcohol, caffeine, and nitrite consumption.

Cerebrospinal Fluid Analysis
seh **ree** broe **spie** nal • floo id • ah **nal** ah sis
(CSF, Spinal Fluid, Encephalospinal Fluid)

Normal Findings
Fluid: Clear, colorless, sterile
TOTAL CELL COUNT
(LEUKOCYTES)
Adult: 0–8/mm^3
Child: 0–8/mm^3
Premature infant: 0–20/mm^3
Infant: 0–19/mm^3
GLUCOSE
Adult: 40–80 mg/dL
Child: 35–75 mg/dL
Premature infant: 24–63 mg/dL
Infant:122 mg/dL
The CSF glucose value should be 50%–80% of serum glucose.
TOTAL PROTEIN
Adult: 15–45 mg/dL
Child: 14–45 mg/dL
Infant: 30–200 mg/dL
Elderly: 15–60 mg/dL
GRAM STAINS AND CULTURES
No growth on culturing, because CSF is normally sterile.

What This Test Will Tell You
This fluid analysis test diagnoses spinal cord and brain diseases. Cere-

brospinal fluid (CSF) is produced in the lateral ventricles of the brain and circulates around the brain and spinal cord to protect the central nervous system from trauma. Normally the brain produces 400–600 mL of CSF daily. Much of this is reabsorbed into the bloodstream, resulting in a total circulating volume of 100–160 mL.

Abnormal color of pink to red indicates bleeding. The red hues may result from a traumatic spinal puncture that contaminated the sample, subarachnoid hemorrhage, or cerebral hemorrhage. Xanthochromia (yellow color) indicates a high protein count (>150 mg/dL), previous subarachnoid bleeding, or bilirubin >6 mg/dL associated with liver disease. The discoloration may remain for 3 weeks.

Lymphocytes are normally the only cells in the total cell count. White blood cell (WBC) counts of 200–300/mm^3 will cause cloudiness of the CSF. An increase in the number of cells in CSF causes the sample to be cloudy to turbid. This may be due to the presence of a brain abscess, acute or purulent meningitis, and organisms such as bacteria, fungi, and amoebae.

CSF glucose levels vary directly with serum glucose levels. A change in serum glucose will be evidenced in CSF glucose levels 2–4 hours later. Serum and CSF glucose levels should be compared to determine if an abnormal result is due to a physiologic variation or a pathologic cerebrospinal variation such as bacterial infection.

Disintegration of red blood cells (RBCs) and WBCs will elevate the CSF protein value. CSF protein electrophoresis (immunoelectrophoresis) may be done to differentiate protein bands and aid in diagnosis of disorders. Oligoclonal bands are an abnormal finding resulting from antibodies produced in the central nervous system and indicate an infectious process (meningitis) or immunologic process (multiple sclerosis).

Abnormal Findings

▲ INCREASED LEVELS *in total cell count* may indicate acute pyrogenic meningitis, bacterial meningitis, tuberculosis, viral infections, brain abscess, parasites, neoplasms, multiple sclerosis, or neurosyphilis.

▲ INCREASED LEVELS *in glucose* may indicate hyperglycemia, cerebral trauma, or hypothalamic lesions.

▼ DECREASED LEVELS *in glucose* may indicate bacterial infections, fungal infections, tuberculosis, encephalitis, subarachnoid hemorrhage, brain abscess, or protozoa infections.

▲ INCREASED LEVELS *in protein* may indicate bacterial meningitis, cerebral hemorrhage, traumatic spinal tap, cord tumor with spinal blockage, polyneuritis, brain tumor, or Guillain-Barré syndrome.

▼ DECREASED LEVELS *in protein* may indicate hyperthyroidism or benign intracranial hypertension.

ACTION ALERT!

If an organism is identified by Gram stain, the primary health care provider should be notified immediately so treatment may be started.

Interfering Factors

➤ A traumatic spinal tap may result in the presence of blood in the specimen leading to inaccurate results.

➤ Serum protein values need to be within normal limits for accurate interpretation of CSF total protein results.

➤ Serum glucose levels are reflected in CSF glucose results; therefore hyperglycemia could increase CSF glucose values.

➤ Medications such as acetophenetidin, chlorpromazine, salicylates, streptomycin, and sulfonamides can all cause a false elevation of protein levels.

Contraindications

➤ Do not perform this when increased intracranial pressure is suspected. A rapid decrease in intracranial pressure secondary to the lumbar puncture and removal of cerebrospinal fluid may cause the brain to shift downward (herniate) into the spinal column. The herniation could cause serious damage to the vital centers in the medulla and result in neurological damage or death.

➤ Do not perform this test on a client with primary clotting defects such as thrombocytopenia because of the risk of extradural or subdural hematoma formation.

Potential Complications
➤ Bleeding into the spinal canal
➤ Neurologic injury including herniation
➤ Infection
➤ Headache, nausea, dizziness, neck pain

NURSING CONSIDERATIONS

Prepare Your Client
➤ Explain that the test will measure specific substances in the cerebrospinal fluid to assist the physician in making a diagnosis.
➤ Explain that the physician will place a needle into the lower back and withdraw spinal fluid.
➤ Assure your client that the needle is inserted below where the spinal cord is so there is no danger of damage to the nerves.
➤ Review the potential complications of the procedure and be sure the client has signed an informed consent.
➤ Tell your client there is no need to restrict food or fluids before the procedure.

Perform Procedure
Nurses do not usually perform this procedure but should understand the process to prepare the client and assist the physician.

Position the client in a side-lying position with knees drawn to chest

and chin tucked down. Assist the physician during collection of the CSF. Approximately 3–5 mL of fluid will be collected in a series of tubes which must be numbered sequentially. Tube 1 may be contaminated with blood and may need to be discarded. Tube 2 is usually sent to the lab for analysis of glucose, protein, and cell count. Tube 3 is used for microbiology tests such as culture and smears. Send tubes to the lab immediately.

Care After Test
➤ Position the client flat in bed for up to 12 hours to decrease the risk of a headache. Assess for pain and administer analgesics for headache and discomforts as ordered.
➤ Observe your client for complications of lumbar puncture including changes in vital signs, numbness and tingling of the lower extremities, neck rigidity, and changes in level of consciousness.
➤ Keep the environment quiet and the lighting dim to decrease headache.
➤ Evaluate related tests such as lumbar puncture and immunofixation cerebrospinal fluid.

Educate Your Client and the Family
➤ Teach importance of compliance with pharmacological treatment to prevent any relapses in conditions such as infection, multiple sclerosis, and syphilis.

Ceruloplasmin

seh **roo** loe **plaz** min
(Serum Copper)

Normal Findings

ADULT, CHILD, ADOLESCENT,
ELDERLY
17–43 mg/dL
NEWBORN AND EARLY
INFANCY
Levels are decreased.
PREGNANT
Levels are increased.

What This Test Will Tell You

This test assesses nutritional status
and detects the hereditary liver disorder Wilson's disease. Blood levels of
the plasma protein ceruloplasmin,
which carries 90%–95% of copper in
the blood, are used as a measure of
body copper status. Although the
roles of ceruloplasmin are not fully
understood, functions include
hemoglobin synthesis and red blood
cell formation, bone formation, healing processes, and thought processes.
Low levels of ceruloplasmin result in
increased intestinal absorption of
copper. The excess copper is then
deposited on the corneas, brain, liver,
and kidneys, leading to their destruction. Copper toxicity may also result
from ingestion of copper-contami-
nated solutions, use of copper
intrauterine devices (IUDs), or exposure to copper fungicides.

Abnormal Findings

▼DECREASED LEVELS may indi-
cate Wilson's disease, gastrointestinal
disease (sprue), cystic fibrosis,
Menkes' syndrome, iron deficiency,
burns, nephrotic syndrome, or protein malnutrition.
▲INCREASED LEVELS may indicate infection and inflammation,
pregnancy, leukemia, biliary cirrhosis, Hodgkin's disease, small bowel
disease, total parenteral nutrition,
scleroderma, lupus erythematosus,
viral hepatitis, ankylosis, spondylitis,
neonatal transfusions, sickle-cell disease, thalassemia, myocardial infarction, cystic fibrosis, hemochromatosis, pulmonary tuberculosis, anemia,
rheumatic fever, or cancer of the
bone, breast, cervix, stomach, lung,
or hemopoietic system.

Interfering Factors

➤ Oral contraceptives, estrogen
agents, phenobarbital, phenytoin,
antacids, carbamazepine, and recent
exercise may limit the information
available from the test.
➤ Ceruloplasmin blood levels for
African-Americans are 8%–12%
higher than for Caucasians.
➤ Pregnancy will elevate levels.

NURSING CONSIDERATIONS

Prepare Your Client

➤ Explain that this test is used to
measure the amount of copper in the
blood.
➤ Consult with primary health care
provider about withholding medications containing estrogen for 24
hours prior to the test.

Perform Procedure

➤ Collect 5 mL of venous blood in a
red-top tube.

Care After Test

➤ Assess nutritional status for clues
to disorders that cause changes in

ceruloplasmin levels.

➤ Observe for clinical manifestations of low ceruloplasmin level, such as weakness, skin lesions, and alterations in respiratory status.

➤ Observe for clinical manifestations of a high ceruloplasmin level, such as nausea, vomiting, headache, diarrhea, and abdominal pain.

➤ Evaluate other nutritional function tests such as electrolytes, serum albumin, urine copper levels, and complete blood count.

Educate Your Client and the Family

➤ For client with Wilson's disease, stress the importance of avoiding foods high in copper, such as molasses, nuts, organ meats, raisins, and seafood.

➤ Teach client safety measures to protect against injury related to impaired vision (e.g., keep walking areas free of clutter).

Cervical Mucus Test

sur vi kal • myoo kus • test
(Fern Test)

Normal Findings

At time of ovulation: Cervical mucus forms a fern or palm-leaf pattern when dried on a glass slide. Seven days later, no ferning should occur. Also at ovulation, cervical mucus is clear, thin, demonstrates elasticity or spinnbarkheit, and has the appearance and stretchability of raw egg white. Its pH is 7.0–7.5, more alkaline than at other times to favor sperm survival.

What This Test Will Tell You

This fluid analysis assists in determining the presence or absence of ovulation. During the proliferative phase of the menstrual cycle, as the time of ovulation approaches, estrogen levels increase. Under the influence of estrogen, ferning, or crystallization, of the cervical mucus secretions occur through the interaction of salt and water with glycoproteins.

Abnormal Findings

Absence of ferning in pregnancy, infertility, and premenopausal anovulation

Interfering Factors

➤ Use of tap water to wash glass slides. Electrolytes in tap water may cause ferning; use distilled water.

➤ Lubrication of vaginal speculum or moistening it with tap water.

➤ Tissue trauma with bleeding; blood inhibits ferning.

➤ Deficient estrogen production.

➤ Cervicitis.

NURSING CONSIDERATIONS

Prepare Your Client

➤ Explain, as appropriate, that this test helps check whether the ovaries are releasing eggs, determines whether conditions are favorable for the male sperm so that pregnancy can occur, and evaluates hormone production.

> Tell the client that results are usually available before she leaves the office and the primary health care provider will discuss them with her.

> Tell the client there is no need to restrict food or fluids prior to this test.

> Instruct the client not to use vaginal lubricants or douches or have intercourse for at least 2 days prior to this test.

> Tell the client there should be no pain associated with this test.

Perform Procedure

> The procedure is explained to the client as it is performed.

> The slide will be examined microscopically by the examiner; spinnbarkheit and pH may also be evaluated.

> The test will be done in an office or clinic in approximately 20 minutes.

> Position the client as for a vaginal exam (lithotomy position).

> The vaginal speculum is inserted. Next, a cotton-tipped applicator is inserted into the cervical canal and turned gently to obtain the mucus.

Care After Test

> Tell client her activities are not restricted.

> Instruct the client to return in 1 week so the test can be repeated to determine changes in hormone production.

> Review related tests such as the spinnbarkheit test. It is conducted by placing cervical mucus between two glass slides and lifting the top slide away from the bottom slide; the mucus should stretch 5–6 cm or longer.

Educate Your Client and the Family

> Explain that additional tests will be conducted to find out why she is unable to get pregnant.

> Teach client how to do a spinnbarkheit test by obtaining mucus from high in the vagina with clean fingers and stretching it between her fingers for ongoing monthly evaluation and to help determine the optimum time for pregnancy to occur. Tell her the mucus looks like raw egg white and will stretch to 2 or more inches.

> If applicable, provide information about infertility support groups.

> Teach client and partner about influences on fertility, including basal body temperature, alcohol and drug intake, stress, and environmental conditions.

Cervical Punch Biopsy

sur vi kal • punch • bie op see

Normal Findings

Normal cervical tissue is a light pink color and consists of columnar and squamous epithelial cells with no abnormal cell growth.

What This Test Will Tell You

This histologic examination diagnoses cervical lesions and cancer. When an abnormal Pap smear is reported and/or when the examiner observes suspicious lesions, the tissue is biopsied for definitive diagnosis. The procedure is done in an office or clinic 1 week after the menses to ensure that the client is not pregnant and when the cervix is the least vascular. Visualization of cervical lesions is facilitated by use of a colposcope and/or a Schiller's iodine test. The colposcope or colpomicroscope is a magnifying glass with a high-intensity light source to illuminate the cervix, allowing the examiner to define the site, size, and character of cervical lesions. Schiller's iodine solution may be applied to the cervix with a long applicator stick. Glycogen, a component of normal cervical epithelial cells, absorbs iodine, whereas abnormal cells without glycogen do not. Tissues that are not stained brown are selected for biopsy.

Abnormal Findings

Abnormalities may reveal cervical dysplasia, mild to severe; carcinoma in situ; invasive carcinoma; low-grade squamous intraepithelial lesion; or high-grade squamous intraepithelial lesion.

Interfering Factors

➤ Failure to place each specimen in a 10% formaldehyde solution immediately after obtaining the tissue
➤ Failure of examiner to obtain tissue from all areas of suspicion
➤ Failure to send specimen to laboratory immediately

Contraindications

➤ Diagnosed infections such as chlamydia and gonorrhea need to be treated prior to performing a biopsy.
➤ Coagulopathies.

Potential Complications

➤ Excessive bleeding

➤ Infection

NURSING CONSIDERATIONS

Prepare Your Client

➤ Explain that the cervix will be examined and tissue removed from it to check for cell changes that may need to be stopped.
➤ Ensure that an informed consent is obtained, because of the possible complications associated with this procedure.
➤ Recommend that the client have a family member or friend drive her home after the test.
➤ Ask the client if she is allergic to iodine, as a Schiller's iodine solution may be applied to the cervix to better identify abnormal tissue.
➤ Explain that the biopsy is done on an outpatient basis in an office or clinic.
➤ Instruct the client to urinate before the test.

Perform Procedure

Nurses do not usually perform this procedure but should understand the process to prepare the client and assist the primary health care provider. Medication may be given about 30 minutes before the procedure to inhibit uterine cramping that may occur when tissue is removed from the cervix. Tell the client she may feel pressure, but no pain, from tissue removal as the cervix is sensitive to pressure but not to cutting.

Place the client on an exam table in the same position as for a vaginal exam (lithotomy position). A vaginal speculum is inserted. A colposcope to magnify the tissue will be inserted through the speculum for the examiner to visualize the cervix. Some offices have the colposcope hooked up to a camera and an overhead video monitor so the client can observe the procedure as it is being performed. Schiller's iodine solution may be applied to identify abnormal tissue.

The site(s) to be biopsied is cleansed with a cotton-tipped swab moistened with a 3% acetic acid solution. Forceps are used to pinch off the tissue. Silver nitrate may be applied to control bleeding and/or a tampon may be inserted for pressure control of bleeding.

Each tissue specimen is placed in a labeled specimen bottle containing a 10% formaldehyde solution and sent to the laboratory immediately. The procedure normally takes less than 30 minutes.

Care After Test

➤ Have client rest for a short while before leaving.

➤ Check client for excessive bleeding before she leaves.

➤ Review related tests such as the Papanicolaou smear.

Educate Your Client and the Family

➤ Instruct client to remove packing, if in place, within 12–24 hours.

➤ Instruct client not to insert any tampons and to avoid douching and sexual intercourse for 2 weeks or as directed.

➤ Tell her to avoid heavy lifting and strenuous exercise for 24 hours.

➤ Explain that when the report is in, an appointment will be made to discuss the results.

➤ Explain to client that a gray-green vaginal discharge with an unpleasant odor may occur for up to 3 weeks after the test.

Chest X-Ray

chest • eks ray
(CXR, Chest Radiography)

Normal Findings

All ages: Normal chest and surrounding structures, including bony thorax, soft tissues, mediastinum, lungs, pleura, heart, and great vessels

What This Test Will Tell You

Chest x-rays identify various abnormalities of the lungs and structures in the thorax, including the heart, great vessels, ribs, or diaphragm. Chest x-ray may be used as a general screening tool or for a specific diagnostic purpose, including identifica-

tion of pulmonary diseases or orthopedic abnormalities. Serial chest x-rays may be used to evaluate the status of respiratory abnormalities or cardiac conditions. General uses include confirming placement of central venous lines, pulmonary artery catheters, pacemaker leads, or endotracheal tubes.

Various chest x-ray views may be ordered. A posterioranterior (PA) view is often taken with the client standing. Anteriorposterior (AP) views are taken with the client sitting or lying down. Lateral or decubitus (recumbent lateral) views may be ordered, with the x-ray passing through the client's side. Oblique views are rays slanted at an angle rather than perpendicular such as AP and lateral films. Lordotic views may be ordered to specifically view the apices of the lungs, omitting the normal visual interference of the clavicles.

When evaluating x-rays, the darkest (blackest) areas are usually air filled. Dark gray areas usually represent fat and lighter gray areas are fluid filled. The lightest or whitest areas of all are generally bone.

Abnormal Findings

Abnormalities may indicate pneumonia, chronic obstructive pulmonary disease, congestive heart failure, atelectasis, kyphosis, scoliosis, lordosis, lung tumors, rib fractures, pneumothorax or hemothorax, pleurisy, pericarditis, adult respiratory distress syndrome (ARDS), pericardial effusion, lung abscess, tuberculosis, cystic fibrosis, aortic aneurysm, or diaphragmatic hernia.

Interfering Factors

➤ Client movement obscures the clarity of the picture.
➤ The client's inability to take and hold a deep breath limits the quality of the film.
➤ Portable chest x-rays do not demonstrate lung structures as reliably as PA films performed in the radiology department.
➤ Obesity may prevent adequate viewing of lower thoracic structures.
➤ Heavy breast tissue or breast implants in female clients may prevent optimal visualization of chest structures.

Contraindications

➤ Pregnancy or potential pregnancy, due to radiation exposure of fetus

Potential Complications

➤ Exposure of a developing fetus, particularly during the first trimester, may cause congenital anomalies.
➤ Exposure of the genital organs (testicles in males, ovaries in females) may cause chromosomal mutations that could lead to congenital anomalies in offspring.

NURSING CONSIDERATIONS

Prepare Your Client

➤ Explain to the client that the test is used in evaluating the lungs and the heart. If the x-ray is ordered for a specific purpose (e.g., to check fluid levels), describe this to the client.
➤ Routinely ask any woman of childbearing age if there is any possibility she could be pregnant before performing x-ray studies. X-rays on pregnant women are performed only if it is deemed the benefits outweigh the risks.
➤ Inform the client whether they will be transported to the radiology department or have the x-ray done at the bedside (portable CXR).
➤ Instruct the client to remove clothing to the waist and to put on an x-ray gown. Necklaces, long earrings, or other metal objects should be removed.
➤ Explain the procedure of taking a deep breath, holding it, and remaining motionless during the x-ray.
➤ Cover the testicles or ovaries with a lead shield or apron to prevent exposure.
➤ Tell the client the test will take only a few minutes and is painless.

Perform Procedure

➤ For PA views, position the client sitting or standing in front of the x-ray machine and place the x-ray film against the anterior chest.

➤ For lateral views, position the client standing with arms elevated above the head and place the film against the right or left side of the chest.

➤ For portable x-rays, position the client in high Fowler's position, place the x-ray machine in front of the chest, and position the film behind the back and chest.

➤ Upright films of the chest are extremely important to demonstrate fluid levels. Assist client to sit upright if portable chest x-rays are done in bed.

➤ Ask the client to hold very still, take in a deep breath, and hold it. The radiology technician takes the x-ray on full inspiration unless otherwise indicated. Be sure to tell the client when to exhale.

➤ Provide a lead apron for any personnel who must hold the client during the procedure.

Care After Test

➤ Provide extra blankets for client chilled from exposure during chest x-ray.

➤ Assess respiratory status of client (rate, depth, lung sounds, and color).

➤ Evaluate related tests such as previous chest x-rays, computed tomography scans, bronchoscopy, or lung scans.

Educate Your Client and the Family

➤ Inform client that the x-ray will be interpreted by the radiologist and the results conveyed to their physician.

➤ Allow client to express concerns about impending results of the procedure.

➤ Tell client that serial x-rays may be needed to follow the status of their condition.

➤ Teach client with respiratory difficulty about their needs for nutrition and rest, including pacing activities.

Chlamydia Antibodies

klah mih dee ah • an ti bod ees

Normal Findings

Titer < 1:5 indicates no detectable antibodies to chlamydia.

Titer of 1:5–1:160 suggests recent chlamydia infection.

Titer > 1:640 suggests recent systemic chlamydia infection.

What This Test Will Tell You

This blood test detects antibodies that indicate a recent chlamydia infection related to symptoms of cervicitis, urethritis, or respiratory tract infections. The chlamydial organism is an obligate intracellular parasite that is classified into three species: *Chlamydia psittaci, Chlamydia pneumoniae,* and *Chlamydia trachomatis.* Two serum tests are used to detect antibodies to chlamydia. The single-antigen indirect immunofluorescence test assays antibodies that develop following *C. trachomatis, C. pneumoniae,* and *C. psittaci* infections.

Lower-level titers are associated with genitourinary and eye infections. Higher titers are associated with pneumonia, pelvic inflammatory disease, and lymphogranuloma venereum.

Abnormal Findings

➤ *Chlamydia trachomatis* antibodies may reveal nongonococcal urethritis (NGU), mucopurulent cervicitis, endometritis, salpingitis, pelvic inflammatory disease, epididymitis, prostatitis, proctitis, neonatal conjunctivitis, neonatal pneumonitis, inclusion conjunctivitis, trachoma, or lymphogranuloma venereum.

➤ *Chlamydia psittaci* antibodies may reveal psittacosis.

➤ *Chlamydia pneumoniae* antibodies may reveal a respiratory tract infection.

Interfering Factors

➤ Hemolysis of blood sample.

➤ Refrigeration of sample, which prevents proper clotting for serum retrieval.

➤ Failure to send serum to a laboratory immediately. If delay is unavoidable, serum may be stored at 39.2°F for up to 2 days or frozen (–4°F) if delay is more than 2 days.

NURSING CONSIDERATIONS

Prepare Your Client

➤ Explain that this test is to check for a current or recent infection.

➤ Tell the client they can continue taking food, fluid, and medication before the test.

Perform Procedure

➤ Collect 5 mL of venous blood in a 10-mL red-top tube.

➤ Allow blood to clot for 1 hour at room temperature; then transfer serum to a sterile vial and submit to a laboratory immediately or freeze specimen.

Care After Test

➤ If *Chlamydia trachomatis* is found, encourage testing for other sexually transmitted diseases. Instruct client to have their sexual partner(s) tested as well.

➤ If *Chlamydia psittaci* is found, inquire about the presence of pet birds and explain the need to consult a veterinarian for evaluation of the pet.

➤ Review related tests such as those for other sexually transmitted diseases, urinalysis, and chest x-rays.

Educate Your Client and the Family

➤ Provide an opportunity for client to ask questions. Recognize that client may be sensitive about having a sexually transmitted disease and may be concerned about partner relationships.

➤ If *Chlamydia trachomatis* is found, instruct the client on this sexually transmitted disease organism and the use of condoms during sexual contact.

➤ Explain that if no antibodies are found, a chlamydia infection has not occurred. If antibodies are found, it suggests but does not prove a chlamydia infection.

➤ Explain that in the event that antibodies are found, further testing may be done by collecting a specimen from the area most likely infected.

➤ Explain that if an infection is present, an antibiotic that is effective in the treatment of chlamydia infections will be prescribed and should be taken until gone.

➤ Inform clients that sex is to be

avoided until the client and the partner(s) are cured.

➤ Reinforce that another exam should be done 5–7 days after all of the antibiotic has been taken.

➤ Instruct the client to call the primary health care provider right away if symptoms continue after all of the antibiotic has been taken.

Chlamydia trachomatis Amplicor
klah mih dee ah • tray koe may tis • am plih kor

Normal Findings
A450 reading < 0.2A is interpreted as presumptive negative for *C. trachomatis* plasmid DNA.

What This Test Will Tell You
This microbiologic analysis test detects chlamydia infections by identifying *Chlamydia trachomatis* plasmid DNA in endocervical specimens from females and in urethral and urine specimens from males. *C. trachomatis* is currently recognized as the agent responsible for the most prevalent sexually transmitted disease (STD) in the United States. Various tests may be used to confirm a chlamydia infection. The cell tissue culture method is the standard for diagnosis, as other tests may give false positives. However, in clinical studies the *Amplicor C. trachomatis* test was equal to or better than the tissue culture method in identifying endocervical infections in females and urethral infections in males and provides easier diagnosis in males.

Abnormal Findings
Positive results may indicate non-gonococcal urethritis (NGU), mucopurulent cervicitis, endometritis, salpingitis, pelvic inflammatory disease, epididymitis, prostatitis, proctitis, neonatal inclusion conjunctivitis, or neonatal pneumonitis.

A450 reading > 0.5A is interpreted as positive for *C. trachomatis* plasmid DNA. A450 reading 0.2A–0.5A is considered equivocal; duplicate repeat testing is required before reporting outcome to client. 0.25A is used as the cutoff for determining results. If 2 of the 3 readings (original and duplicate repeats) are < 0.25A, the test is interpreted as presumptive negative for *C. trachomatis* plasmid DNA. If 2 of the 3 readings are > 0.25A, the test is interpreted as positive for *C. trachomatis* plasmid DNA.

Interfering Factors
➤ The test does not detect plasmid-free variants of *C. trachomatis*. Negative results do not exclude infection, as reliable results depend on correct specimen collection techniques and absence of inhibitors. Only standard cell tissue culture methods should be used for medico-legal concerns including evaluation of suspected sexual abuse.

➤ Antibiotic therapy may yield a false negative result.

➤ Presence of spermicide in excess of 1%.

➤ Presence of surgical lubricant in excess of 10%.

➤ Presence of mucus in cervical samples has not been shown to adversely affect test; however, to ensure test performance, a mucus-free specimen is preferred.

➤ Leaving the endocervical or urethral sample collection swab in the specimen transport medium tube.

➤ Failure to swirl swabs vigorously in specimen transport medium prior to removal.

➤ Storing the specimen at room temperature for more than 24 hours; should be stored at test site at 2–8°C.

➤ Not processing swab specimens within 10 days of collection and urine specimens within 4 days of collection.

➤ Collection of urine in cup with preservatives.

➤ Males voiding within 2 hours of urine collection sample and within 1 hour of urethral swab.

Contraindications

➤ Do not collect cervical specimen during menstruation.

NURSING CONSIDERATIONS

Prepare Your Client

➤ Explain that this test is performed to see if there is an infection called chlamydia.

➤ Explain that this test can only check for cervical (portion of womb that opens into vagina) infections in the female and urethral (opening through which urine passes) infections in the male.

➤ Explain that the laboratory may request further specimens for study if the results are inconclusive.

➤ Instruct female client not to douche or insert spermicidal contraceptive products (creams, foams, jellies, suppositories, sponges) into vagina for 24–48 hours prior to test.

➤ Instruct male not to urinate for at least 1 hour prior to obtaining swab

sample or for at least 2 hours prior to collecting urine sample.

Perform Procedure

Nurses do not usually perform this procedure but should understand the process to prepare the client and assist the primary health care physician. Assemble appropriate specimen collection equipment: For urine collection, obtain a clean specimen collection cup without preservatives. For swab, obtain a swab specimen collection kit that contains 2 large (female) swabs or 1 small (male) swab and 1 tube of specimen transport medium. Position client appropriately.

Assist with procedure for female cervical sample: Provide light and vaginal speculum without surgical lubricant. Provide large swab for removal of mucus from the exocervix; discard swab. Provide large swab for insertion into the endocervical canal; swab will be inserted into canal until tip is no longer visible and then rotated for 3–5 seconds. Swab is withdrawn, avoiding contact with vaginal surfaces, and placed in the specimen transport medium tube. Swirl or agitate swab vigorously in liquid for 15 seconds. Express liquid from swab by pressing against side of tube. Collect excess mucus in sample on swab and express residual liquid from mucus by pressing against side of tube. Remove swab with excess mucus collected on it and discard. Place cap on tube.

Assist with procedure for male urethral sample: Provide small swab for insertion of 2–4 cm into urethra. Rotate swab in urethra for 3–5 seconds, withdraw, and place in specimen transport medium tube. Swirl or agitate swab vigorously in liquid

C

for 15 seconds. Express liquid from swab by pressing against side of tube. Remove swab and discard. Place cap on tube.

Collect male urine sample: Provide client with a clean, empty urine specimen collection cup without preservatives. Instruct client to begin specimen collection as soon as urine starts to flow (first catch urine). Collect 10–50 mL of urine. Cap specimen.

Label specimens appropriately and send specimens to test site without delay; specimens may be at room temperature for up to 24 hours.

Care After Test

➤ Provide an opportunity for client to ask questions. Recognize that clients may be sensitive about having a sexually transmitted disease and may be concerned about partner relationships.

➤ Review related tests such as the *Chlamydia trachomatis* culture.

Educate Your Client and the Family

➤ Explain to the client that the report should be available within 2–3 days. (Test requires only 4–5 hours to complete; time needed to receive report will depend on specimen transport time and lab schedule.)

➤ Explain that if an infection is present, an antibiotic effective in the treatment of chlamydia infections will be prescribed and should be taken until gone. This could be a medication taken one time only (very expensive) or a medication taken for a longer period (less expensive).

➤ Explain that the sexual partner(s) must also be treated. Teach client that there are usually no symptoms accompanying this infection, so the partner may be unaware of having the infection.

➤ Instruct the client to avoid sex until the client and the partner(s) are cured. An exam should be done on both the client and the client's partner(s) 5–7 days after all of the antibiotic has been taken.

➤ Instruct the client to notify the primary health care practitioner if any problems arise when taking the antibiotic.

➤ Explain to the client that the use of condoms will prevent future infections.

Chlamlydia trachomatis, Culture
klah **mih** dee ah • **tray** koe **may** tis • **kul** chur

Normal Findings
Cell culture negative for *C. trachomatis*
Inclusions detected by FITC-MoAb specific to *C. trachomatis*.

What This Test Will Tell You
This culture test diagnoses chlamydia infections. Positive cell cultures and detection of inclusions are definitive proof for diagnosis of a chlamydia infection. The chlamydial organism is an obligate intracellular parasite that is classified into three species: *Chlamydia psittaci, Chlamydia pneumoniae,* and *Chlamydia trachomatis.*

Various tests are used to confirm a chlamydia infection, but the cell tissue culture is considered the standard for diagnosis as other tests may give a false positive. To culture cells for the diagnosis of *C. trachomatis*, epithelial cells are obtained from the infected site. The culture may require up to 6 days.

Abnormal Findings

Positive results may reveal nongonococcal urethritis (NGU), mucopurulent cervicitis, endometritis, salpingitis, pelvic inflammatory disease, epididymitis, prostatitis, proctitis, neonatal conjunctivitis, neonatal pneumonitis, inclusion conjunctivitis, trachoma, or lymphogranuloma venereum.

Interfering Factors

➤ Menses discharge in the specimen
➤ Douching or tub baths if the specimen site is the cervix
➤ Use of lubricants on the vaginal speculum
➤ Medications specific to the treatment of *C. trachomatis* such as tetracycline, erythromycin, and sulfa drugs
➤ Voiding within 3–4 hours of obtaining a urethral specimen
➤ Failure to use the correct medium for the specimen

NURSING CONSIDERATIONS

Prepare Your Client

➤ Explain that this test is conducted in an office or clinic to look for an infection.
➤ Explain that a swab will be rubbed in the infected area by the primary health care provider to obtain the specimen.
➤ Explain that the procedure takes a short time to complete.
➤ Explain that there will be mild discomfort, but the swabbing should not be painful.

Perform Procedure

Nurses do not usually perform this procedure but should understand it to prepare the client and assist with the process. Position the client appropriately for the sample being taken (female: lithotomy for cervical and urethral; male: supine for urethral; knee-chest for rectal; Fowler's for eye and upper respiratory). The sample is collected from involved tissue by scraping epithelial cells with a swab from infected site: conjunctiva, urethra, cervix, rectum. Epithelial cells must be collected directly from the surface of the involved tissue and not from discharges. Aspirates are collected from the nasopharynx and tracheobronchial area. Place specimen in labeled container with medium provided by lab; it may be an antibiotic medium or sucrose phosphate (2SP) transport medium.

Assist client to a sitting or standing position and with dressing if needed. Submit specimen to lab without delay. 2SP transport medium can be frozen if the time between collection and cell culture inoculation exceeds 24 hours.

Care After Test

➤ If *Chlamydia psittaci* is found, inquire about the presence of pet birds and explain the need to consult a veterinarian for evaluation of the pet.
➤ Review related tests such as chlamydial smear, which is conducted by swabbing the infected site, usually the cervix or urethra, and submitting the secretions for culture. Also review direct fluorescent antibody (DFA) tests where epithelial

cells are obtained from the infected site, placed on slides specific for the test, and submitted to a laboratory. The test uses a monoclonal antibody that is labeled with a fluorescent dye to detect *C. trachomatis*. The antibody attaches to chlamydia organisms on the slide and appears fluorescent green under the microscope. The test takes several hours to run and is subject to error.

Educate Your Client and the Family

➤ Explain to client that the report will not be available for at least 1 week; when it is received, an appointment should be made to review the report.

➤ Provide an opportunity for client to ask questions. Recognize that client may be sensitive about having a sexually transmitted disease and may be concerned about partner relationships.

➤ Explain that if an infection is present, an antibiotic that is effective in the treatment of chlamydia infections will be prescribed and should be taken until gone.

➤ Inform client that their sexual partner(s) must also be treated.

➤ Instruct client to avoid sex until the client and the partner(s) are cured.

➤ Make an appointment for another examination 5–7 days after all of the antibiotic has been taken.

➤ Instruct client to call the primary health care provider right away if symptoms continue after all of the antibiotic has been taken.

➤ Teach the client that the use of condoms will help prevent future infections.

Chloride, Serum

klore ide • see rum
(Cl, Cl⁻, Serum Chloride)

Normal Findings

ADULT, PREGNANT, ADOLESCENT, AND ELDERLY
90–110 mEq/L (SI units: 95–110 mmol/L)
INFANT
96–110 mEq/L (SI units: 96–110 mmol/L)
NEWBORN
94–112 mEq/L (SI units: 96–106 mmol/L)
CHILD
95–106 mEq/L (SI units: 98–105 mmol/L)

What This Test Will Tell You

This blood test helps diagnose disorders of acid-base and water balance. Chloride is predominantly an extracellular anion (negatively charged particle). Chemically it combines with sodium to form sodium chloride and with hydrogen to form hydrochloric acid. Therefore, it is responsible for maintaining water balance and cellular integrity through its influence on osmotic pressure. Chloride and sodium levels closely relate to each other. In a critically ill client, all electrolytes (sodium, potassium, bicarbonate, chloride) need to be measured. Chloride is generally the least important of the electrolytes.

Abnormal Findings

▲INCREASED LEVELS may indicate dehydration, hypernatremia, hyperventilation, eclampsia, anemia, cardiac decompensation, renal tubular acidosis, excessive intravenous (IV) saline (0.9% NaCl), Cushing's syndrome, hyperaldosteronism, or metabolic acidosis.

▼DECREASED LEVELS may indicate severe vomiting, epigastric suctioning, severe diarrhea, ulcerative colitis, severe burns, diabetic acidosis, Addison's disease, or acute infection.

ACTION ALERT!

➤ Serum chloride values <80 mEq/L or >120 mEq/L indicate a severe electrolyte disturbance that can rapidly deteriorate to cardiopulmonary arrest. Carefully monitor cardiac and pulmonary function.
➤ Treatment of electrolyte imbalances may result in shifts of fluids causing cerebral edema. Infants, children, and the elderly are at greatest risk.

Interfering Factors

➤ Medications that may increase chloride levels include androgens, estrogens, non-steroidal anti-inflammatory drugs, cholestyramine, methyldopa, guanethidine, cortisone medications, chlorothiazide, acetazolamide, excessive saline intravenous fluids, prolonged use of triamterene, ion exchange resins, boric acid, and ammonium chloride.
➤ Medications that may decrease chloride levels include thiazide diuretics, furosemide, ethacrynic acid, bicarbonates, aldosterone, corticosteroids, cortisone, and hydrocortisone.

NURSING CONSIDERATIONS

Prepare Your Client

➤ Explain that this test is used to measure the amount of a chemical in the body called chloride.

Perform Procedure

➤ Collect 5–15 mL of venous blood in a red-top tube.

Care After Test

➤ Assess for signs of hypochloremia tetany, twitching, tremors, mental status changes, headache, drowsiness, confusion, hyperexcitability of the nervous system and muscles, slow and shallow breathing, and hypotension. Notify the primary health care provider immediately of these findings.
➤ Assess for signs and symptoms of hyperchloremia including weakness, lethargy, and deep, rapid breathing if the blood chloride value is high. Notify the primary health care provider immediately of these findings. Institute seizure precautions by placing client on bed rest, padding side rails, and having an oral airway at the bedside.
➤ Take measures to protect client with mental status changes.
➤ Client with alterations in breathing pattern or irregular pulses should be immediately placed on continuous cardiac monitoring and closely observed while treatment is determined and initiated.
➤ Notify the primary health care provider if the client is receiving intravenous fluids containing normal saline. Sodium causes water

retention. Assess the client for signs of overhydration including dyspnea, hepatomegaly, and neck vein engorgement.

➤ Monitor intake and output and weight daily to assess fluid retention or dehydration.

➤ If a client is being rapidly rehydrated, watch for signs and symptoms of cerebral edema including headache, nausea, seizures, and changes in mental status. Notify the primary health care provider immediately and be prepared to protect the client's airway and prevent injuries.

➤ Evaluate other electrolyte tests such as sodium, potassium, magnesium, calcium, glucose, and bicarbonate levels.

Educate Your Client and the Family

➤ Teach the client to avoid drinking plain water if there is a serum chloride deficit. Encourage fluids containing both sodium and chloride such as cola and tomato juice. Encourage foods rich in chloride such as milk, meat, and eggs unless contraindicated.

➤ Teach the client to avoid eating salty foods, table salt, or salt substitute if the chloride value is high.

➤ Instruct the client and family on reading labels to identify foods that contain calcium chloride or potassium chloride.

➤ Consult with a registered dietician to assist the family and client in meeting special dietary needs.

➤ Teach client at risk for chloride deficit, such as athlete or outdoor laborer, to drink fluids with electrolytes instead of plain water.

Chloride, Urine
klore ide • yur in
(Chlorides, Cl, Cl⁻, Urine Chloride, Quantitative Urine Chloride)

Normal Findings
ADULT, PREGNANT, ADOLESCENT, ELDERLY
110–254 mEq/24 hours (SI units: 110–254 mmol/24 hours)
INFANT
2–10 mEq/24 hours (SI units: 2–10 mmol/24 hours)
CHILD
15–40 mEq/24 hours (SI units: 15–40 mmol/24 hours)

What This Test Will Tell You
This urine test evaluates renal function, acid-base balance, effectiveness of low-salt diets, and hydration status, and is used to adjust fluid and electrolyte therapy. Chloride is the most abundant extracellular anion (negatively charged particle). Normal acid-base and fluid and electrolyte balance are maintained through the excretion of chloride by the kidney. Chloride values correlate with sodium and fluid changes.

Abnormal Findings
▲ INCREASED LEVELS may indicate dehydration, starvation, acute renal failure, toxemia of pregnancy,

or salicylate toxicity.

▼DECREASED LEVELS may indicate malabsorption syndrome, prolonged gastric suctioning, diarrhea, diaphoresis, emphysema or other chronic respiratory disorders, Addison's disease, syndrome of inappropriate antidiuretic hormone secretion, shock, hyperaldosteronism, or congestive heart failure.

███████ ACTION ALERT!

Metabolic alkalosis or acidosis frequently accompany chloride imbalances. Closely monitor respiratory status for hypoventilation and cardiovascular status for irregularities in the heart rhythm. Notify the primary health care provider of any abnormal findings, institute continuous cardiac monitoring, and closely observe the client while therapy is being instituted.

Interfering Factors

➤ Failure to include all urine voided for 24 hours will give a falsely low result.

➤ Ingestion of bromides may cause elevations of urine chloride levels.

➤ Mercurial and chlorothiazide diuretics increase urinary levels of chloride because passive excretion of chloride occurs with sodium or potassium.

➤ Glucocorticoids may increase results due to passive reabsorption of chloride with sodium.

➤ Dietary salt intake and urine volume cause urinary chloride levels to vary.

➤ Hypovolemia and dehydration will decrease urine sodium levels due to retention of sodium and, passively, chloride.

NURSING CONSIDERATIONS

Prepare Your Client

➤ Explain that this test is important to help understand how well the kidneys and acid-base system are working in the body.

➤ Instruct the client on how to collect a 24-hour urine sample.

Perform Procedure

➤ Obtain 3-L container without preservatives.

➤ Follow protocol for collection of a 24-hour urine sample. If the client is catheterized, keep the drainage bag on ice and empty urine into collection device hourly.

➤ Indicate diuretics or glucocorticoids on lab requisition slip.

Care After Test

➤ Note the urine quantity collected and compare with the urine output documented on the 24-hour urine output collection sheet. If the urine quantity collection is less than the urine output documented for 24 hours some urine may have been discarded, invalidating the specimen.

➤ Evaluate the client's state of hydration by monitoring intake and output, daily weights, skin turgor, and the appearance of the tongue and the urine.

➤ Review related tests such as serum electrolytes, urine electrolytes, plasma aldosterone levels, arterial blood gases, and anion gap.

Educate Your Client and the Family

➤ Instruct client and family on sodium and chloride dietary restrictions if indicated by urine chloride value.

Cholangiography, Intravenous

kow lan jee og rah fee • in trah vee nus
(Cholangiography, IVC, Cholangiogram)

Normal Findings

ALL AGES

Patent biliary, hepatic, and common bile ducts

Absence of common bile duct dilatation: less than 1 cm in diameter

What This Test Will Tell You

This radiographic test detects strictures, stones, or tumors in the biliary system. Intravenous cholangiography (IVC) visualizes the biliary tree (hepatic ducts within the liver, common hepatic duct, cystic duct, and common bile duct) by using an intravenous contrast medium with radiographic and tomographic methods. This 2–8 hour test is used rarely because endoscopic retrograde cholangiopancreatography (ERCP) and percutaneous transhepatic cholangiography are more accurate and efficient.

Abnormal Findings

Abnormalities may indicate obstruction of biliary ducts within the liver; obstruction of common hepatic duct, cystic duct, or common bile duct; cholelithiasis; strictures of a bile duct; tumor within the biliary system; or malformation of the biliary system.

Interfering Factors

➤ Movement of client during required films may limit the clarity of images.

➤ Obesity or presence of stool or barium in the intestine may decrease the clarity of x-ray films.

Contraindications

➤ Allergy to contrast media, unless the test is modified

➤ Pregnancy, due to radiation exposure of fetus

Potential Complications

➤ Allergic reaction, including anaphylaxis

NURSING CONSIDERATIONS

Prepare Your Client

➤ Explain that this test is to look inside the gallbladder to see if there are any problems with stones or the drainage of bile.

➤ Explain that the test will be performed in the x-ray department. An intravenous infusion (IV) will be started to administer the contrast medium.

➤ Check to be sure the client has no allergy to contrast material or iodine.

➤ Ensure that an informed consent is obtained, because of the possible complications associated with this procedure.

➤ Restrict food and fluids for 8 hours prior to the test.

➤ Consult with the primary health care provider about the need for bowel cleansing (laxatives or enemas) the night before and/or morning of the examination to prevent shadows on the x-rays.

➤ Confirm that adults and older children have voided before the procedure.

Perform Procedure

Nurses do not perform this procedure, but should understand the process to prepare the client. First, a baseline x-ray is taken of the upper right quadrant of the abdomen. An IV is started to administer the contrast medium. X-rays are taken every 15–30 minutes until the common bile duct is visualized for a total time of 2–8 hours. Tomography, radiographic studies that can look at layers or slices of tissue at differing depths, is also frequently done to improve imaging.

Observe for side effects of contrast media administration such as nausea, vomiting, hypertension, rash, and flushing.

Care After Test

➤ Observe for signs of allergic reaction up to 6 hours after the test in reaction to the contrast material, including urticaria, pruritus, fever, and dyspnea.

➤ Consult with a registered dietician to assist the family and client in meeting special dietary needs.

➤ Encourage a liberal fluid intake unless otherwise contraindicated to help eliminate contrast material in the urine. Inform client that some discomfort upon urination may occur when the dye is being excreted.

➤ Review related tests such as serum lipase levels, serum bilirubin, percutaneous transhepatic cholangiography, intravenous cholangiography, endoscopic retrograde cholangiopancreatography (ERCP), intravenous cholecystography, abdominal x-ray, and cholangiogram.

Educate Your Client and the Family

➤ Instruct overweight client on a low-calorie, low-fat, weight reduction diet with the assistance of a registered dietician.

Cholecalciferol
koe leh kal sif eh rol
(Vitamin D$_3$)

Normal Findings

ALL AGES

10–55 ng/mL (SI units: 25–135 nmol/L)

PREGNANT

Values are decreased.

What This Test Will Tell You

This blood test measures the level of cholecalciferol (vitamin D$_3$) to determine adequacy of calcium metabolism, screen for some skeletal diseases, and detect vitamin D toxicity.

Produced in skin exposed to ultraviolet rays and added as a dietary supplement in commercially processed milk, vitamin D$_3$ is important to promote intestinal absorption of calcium and stimulate bone reabsorption. Parathyroid hormone is critical in the regulation of vitamin D$_3$.

Abnormal Findings

▲INCREASED LEVELS may indicate vitamin D$_3$ toxicity (more common in infants and children than adults), sarcoidosis, hyperparathyroidism, or hypercalcemia.

▼ DECREASED LEVELS may indicate rickets in children, osteomalacia in adults, malnutrition, malabsorption, biliary or portal cirrhosis, thyrotoxicosis, renal failure, decreased exposure to sunlight, pancreatic insufficiency, inflammatory bowel disease, or bowel resection.

███████ ACTION ALERT!

Elevated or decreased levels of calcium may be associated with abnormal cholecalciferol levels. Derangements in serum calcium can lead to seizures, cardiopulmonary arrest, and death. Assess for abnormal patterns of respiration, cardiac dysrhythmias, and neuromuscular dysfunction.

Interfering Factors

➤ Aluminum hydroxide, cholestyramine, colestipol, glucocorticoids, isoniazid, mineral oil, phenobarbital, phenytoin, and rifampin can lower serum levels of cholecalciferol.

➤ Excessive exposure to sunlight can raise serum levels of cholecalciferol.

NURSING CONSIDERATIONS

Prepare Your Client

➤ Explain that this test is important to measure the level of vitamin D_3 in the blood, to see if there may be too much or too little.

➤ Confer with the primary health care provider to determine if any anticonvulsant or steroid medications should be withheld for 24 hours prior to the test.

Perform Procedure

➤ Collect 5 mL of venous blood in a 10–15 mL red-top tube.

Care After Test

➤ Assess the client's nutritional status for disorders that could cause changes in vitamin D_3 levels.

➤ Assess for symptoms of vitamin D_3 toxicity, which are more common in infants and children than adults. Symptoms include hypercalcemia, hypercalciuria, vomiting, constipation, anorexia, nausea, and growth and mental retardation.

➤ For client with a low vitamin D_3 level, watch for signs of hypocalcemia, such as muscle twitching and muscle spasms.

➤ Assess and provide for safety needs of client with osteomalacia related to vitamin D_3 deficiency, since fractures are common and heal slowly when they occur.

➤ Administer calcitonin and glucocorticoids as ordered to treat vitamin D_3 toxicity.

➤ Review related tests such as parathyroid hormone levels, serum calcium, serum phosphorus, alkaline phosphatase, serum albumin, electrolytes, blood urea nitrogen (BUN), serum creatinine, and complete blood count.

Educate Your Client and the Family

➤ Teach the client with renal failure to take vitamin D_3 supplements in order to raise the calcium level.

➤ If the client has renal failure, stress the importance of taking calcium supplements and avoiding foods high in phosphates, such as spinach, rhubarb, and asparagus, which decrease calcium absorption.

➤ Explain to the client with renal failure that aluminum-containing antacids may also be given to bind phosphates and increase calcium utilization.

➤ Teach the client with a low vitamin D_3 level the importance of ingesting foods high in calcium, such as milk and green leafy vegetables.

➤ Educate client with excess vitamin D about the dangers of overexposure to the sun (vitamin D excess and skin cancer). Teach them to keep skin covered and to limit time in the sun.

Cholecystography
koe leh sis **tog** rah fee
(Gallbladder Series, GB Series, Gallbladder Radiography, Oral Cholecystogram)

Normal Findings
All ages: Normal size, filling, and structure of gallbladder and absence of gallstones.

What This Test Will Tell You
This radiographic test detects gallstones, inflammatory disease of the gallbladder, or presence of a tumor of the gallbladder. This test allows for visualization of gallbladder stones, which usually cannot be seen on x-rays without contrast material. While useful in visualizing gallbladder stones, the procedure is time-consuming and not as sensitive as a gallbladder ultrasound.

Abnormal Findings
Abnormalities may indicate cholelithiasis (gallstones), cholecystitis (inflammation of the gallbladder), obstruction of the cystic duct, tumor of the gallbladder, polyps, gallbladder carcinoma, or cholesterosis.

ACTION ALERT!

Assess clients carefully for rare allergic reaction to oral contrast material including dyspnea, itching, urticaria, flushing, hypotension, and shock. Life-threatening anaphylactic reactions can occur and need to be recognized and treated immediately.

Interfering Factors
➤ Movement of client during required films may limit the clarity of images.

➤ Obesity or presence of stool or barium in the intestine may decrease the clarity of x-ray films.

➤ Failure to ingest all dye tablets at indicated time or consumption of a high-fat meal prior to the examination will interfere with results.

➤ The presence of liver disease may interfere with the excretion of radiopaque dye.

➤ Thyroid scans, ^{131}I uptake, and protein-bound iodine tests must be performed before cholecystography so as not to impair imaging.

➤ Cholecystography should be performed before or 2–4 days after barium studies.

➤ Diarrhea or vomiting may interfere with absorption of radiopaque dye.

➤ Liver disease or elevated bilirubin levels may inhibit visualization.

Contraindications
➤ This test would be contraindicated unless modified in clients with an allergy to contrast media, seafood, or iodine.

➤ This test is contraindicated in pregnancy, due to radiation exposure of fetus.

➤ Known hepatic dysfunction or bilirubin >2 mg/dL.

➤ Known abdominal inflammatory disease or infection.

➤ Diarrhea, vomiting, or malabsorption syndromes.

Potential Complications

➤ Rarely, allergic reaction including anaphylaxis

NURSING CONSIDERATIONS

Prepare Your Client

➤ Explain that this test will help diagnose problems in the gallbladder.

➤ Assess for allergy to iodine, shellfish, or contrast material.

➤ Instruct the client on how to take the radiopaque contrast tablets orally.

➤ The day before the examination, start the client on a fat-free diet until after dinner that evening. Then restrict all food and fluids except sips of water until the test. A high-fat meal prior to the test will cause the gallbladder to empty and expel the contrast material prematurely.

➤ Administer the radiopaque dye tablets 2 hours after the fat-free dinner: give 1 tablet every 5 minutes until the complete dose is taken. These tablets should each be taken with an 8-ounce glass of water. There are several different preparations of radiopaque dye available. Follow the specific instructions for the preparation used at your institution.

➤ After the radiopaque dye is taken, restrict all intake except for water until the studies are completed.

➤ Instruct the client to report signs of allergic reaction to dye immediately, including rash, hives, elevated temperature, difficulty breathing, or dizziness.

➤ Some radiology departments require that a saline enema be given the morning of the examination. Follow your institution's procedure.

➤ Instruct the client or family to notify the nurse or primary health care provider of vomiting or diarrhea after the radiopaque dye is taken. This could cause the dye not to be absorbed, so the test would need to be rescheduled.

➤ Explain to client or family that sometimes a second part of the study is performed to see how well the gallbladder empties. If this is ordered, the fasting x-rays are completed, then the client eats a high-fat meal, usually in liquid form, followed by additional x-rays until the gallbladder is empty.

Perform Procedure

Nurses do not perform this procedure, but should understand the process to prepare the client. The client ingests radiopaque dye tablets the night before the exam. The dye is concentrated in the gallbladder 12–14 hours after ingestion. X-rays of the gallbladder are taken at this time. Observe for side effects of contrast media administration; however, allergic reactions with oral administration are rare.

Care After Test

➤ Observe for signs of allergic reaction to the contrast material, including urticaria, pruritus, fever, and dyspnea.

➤ Assess for dysuria, which some clients experience because the contrast material is excreted through the kidneys and urine. Encourage a liberal fluid intake unless otherwise contraindicated.

➤ Consult with a registered dietician to assist the family and client in meeting special dietary needs.

➤ Review related tests such as serum lipase levels, serum bilirubin, percutaneous transhepatic cholangiography, intravenous cholangiography, endoscopic retrograde cholangiopancreatography (ERCP), intravenous cholecystography, abdominal x-ray, and cholangiogram.

Educate Your Client and the Family

➤ Instruct overweight client on a low-calorie, low-fat, weight reduction diet with the assistance of a registered dietician.

Cholesterol, Serum
koe les te rol • see rum

Normal Findings

ADULT
Values are often higher in males and postmenopausal women. See data at bottom of page.

PREGNANT
Values are increased during pregnancy, but should return to normal following delivery.

NEWBORN
53–175 mg/dL

CHILD
70–200 mg/dL

ADOLESCENT
120–200 mg/dL

ELDERLY
140–200 mg/dL, though higher values may be individually acceptable.

What This Test Will Tell You

This blood test evaluates blood lipids and assesses the risk of cardiovascular disease, specifically atherosclerotic coronary artery disease. Serum cholesterol levels may also be used to evaluate liver and thyroid function.

This test measures the blood levels of cholesterol, carried predominantly by low-density lipids (LDLs), very low density lipids (VLDLs), and high-density lipids (HDLs). Cholesterol has both positive and negative biologic activity. It is an important component in cell membrane structure, steroid hormones, and bile salts. Excessive cholesterol, as LDL, can have negative biologic effects; for example, its deposition on arterial walls leads to atherosclerosis. Some theories, however, suggest that HDL may be beneficial through its action as a carrier to remove excess cholesterol. VLDLs do not have a strong correlation with increased risk of cardiovascular disease, but generally are not viewed positively because of their high triglyceride concentration.

Abnormal Findings

▲ INCREASED LEVELS may indicate hypercholesterolemia, hyperlipidemia, pregnancy, atherosclerotic

Total cholesterol	LDL	HDL	VLDL
140–200 mg/dL	60–160 mg/dL	male: ≥45 mg/dL female: 55 mg/dL	25%–50%
<6.5 mmol/L	≤3.2 mmol/L	≥0.1 mmol/L	

heart disease, liver disease, hypothyroidism, pancreatic disease, heart disease, hepatitis, biliary disease, or obstructive jaundice.

▼DECREASED LEVELS may indicate malnutrition, malabsorption, anemia, liver disease, hyperthyroidism, cortisone therapy, sepsis, acquired immune deficiency syndrome (AIDS), or cholesterol-reducing medications.

ACTION ALERT!

Any value greater than 240 mg/dL may indicate serious risk of cardiovascular disease. Because of natural fluctuations day to day, and within each 24-hour period, this test should be repeated if the initial result is elevated.

Interfering Factors

➤ Birth control pills, pregnancy, and salicylates may elevate total cholesterol levels.

➤ Estrogen may lower cholesterol levels.

➤ Many other medications may either lower or raise levels.

➤ Alcohol consumed within 24 hours of the test.

➤ Any change in normal dietary habits over the previous 14 days.

NURSING CONSIDERATIONS

Prepare Your Client

➤ Explain that this test will help determine the risk of heart disease or hardening of the arteries and heart attacks.

➤ Check to see if the primary health care provider wants to withhold lipid-lowering drugs prior to the test if client is taking them.

➤ Ensure the client has had no alcohol for at least 24 hours prior to the test.

➤ Explain to the client that this test will reflect dietary intake for at least the last 14 days. Ask if there were any significant changes from their normal diet during that time.

➤ Explain that you will need to draw blood from the vein for the test. Explain the venipuncture process clearly.

➤ Check with your laboratory to see if overnight fasting is required for this test. If so, water still is allowed.

Perform Procedure

➤ Seat the client at least 5 minutes before the venipuncture is performed to reduce fluctuations in serum levels associated with postural changes.

➤ Perform a venipuncture to collect 5–10 mL of venous blood in a red-top tube. For pediatric or neonatal clients, draw blood from a heel or finger stick, or use a smaller pediatric-size red-top tube.

➤ Apply pressure or a pressure dressing to the venipuncture site.

➤ Label the sample and note any interfering factors or medications.

➤ Send the sample to the lab immediately.

Care After Test

➤ Evaluate the client's dietary patterns for the amount of saturated and unsaturated fat intake.

➤ Evaluate the client's history for coronary and vascular disease. Especially note pain in the legs with walking, chest pain, and family deaths from heart attacks.

➤ Investigate other risk factors such as smoking, diabetes mellitus, and obesity.

➤ Evaluate other tests such as triglycerides and lipoproteins.

Educate Your Client and the Family

➤ Teach the client with elevated cholesterol the need to reduce fat intake from animal sources such as meat. Total fat intake should not be more than 30% of the required daily calories. Refer to a registered dietician as indicated.

➤ Emphasize foods that are part of a heart-healthy diet, rather than dwelling on foods that are not.

➤ Stress the importance of regularly scheduled exercise, which may help reduce serum cholesterol.

➤ Assist the client who weighs more than the ideal body weight to choose a reduced fat and calorie diet that incorporates personal food preferences. Be particularly attuned to including ethnic foods the client may value.

➤ Emphasize to the client that there are risk factors for heart disease that can be controlled such as diet, exercise, weight, and smoking. Risk factors such as gender, family history, and diabetes cannot be eliminated, but can be minimized by addressing controllable risk factors.

Cholinesterase, RBC or Plasma

koe lin es tur ase • RBC • or • plaz mah
(RBC: Acetylcholinesterase; True Cholinesterase; E Acetylcholinesterase; Erythrocyte Acetylcholinesterase; Plasma: Pseudocholinesterase; Serum Cholinesterase; PCHE; Nonspecific: CHE; Cholinesterase)

Normal Findings

ADULT, ADOLESCENT, ELDERLY
0.5–1.0 U/mL (SI units: 8-18 U/L)

NEWBORN
Level is low at birth and first 6 months of life, then begins to increase as the nervous system matures.

PREGNANT
Values decrease in late pregnancy.

CHILD
Level is 30%–50% above adult values until age 5, then gradually decreases until reaching adult levels by adolescence.

What This Test Will Tell You

This blood test monitors levels of exposure to phosphorus insecticides and screens surgical clients for ability to metabolize succinylcholine anesthesia. Cholinesterase is an enzyme that breaks down acetylcholine at the nerve endings. There are two types of cholinesterase: acetylcholinesterase, which is found at nerve endings and in erythrocytes, and pseudocholinesterase, which is found in the serum.

Adult values of cholinesterase (CHE) range widely, so workers who risk exposure to phosphorus insecticides should have a baseline test. A decrease of 30%–50% from baseline indicates toxicity even when values are within normal ranges. Clients with genetically predisposed low cholinesterase levels may experience prolonged sedation and apnea after succinylcholine anesthesia because the body metabolizes the drug inefficiently.

Abnormal Findings

▲ INCREASED LEVELS may indicate nephrotic syndrome, diabetes mellitus, hyperthyroidism, or type IV hyperlipoproteinemia.

▼ DECREASED LEVELS may indicate insecticide exposure, genetic succinylcholine sensitivity, hepatitis, cirrhosis, hepatic congestion of heart failure, metastatic carcinoma of liver, malnutrition, anemias, acute infections, pulmonary emboli, muscular dystrophy, or conditions with low serum albumin (malabsorption, exfoliative dermatitis).

ACTION ALERT!

➤ Monitor for severe neurologic impairment in clients with industrial exposure to pesticides. Symptoms include headache, visual disturbances, nausea, vomiting, confusion, seizures, pulmonary edema, respiratory paralysis, and coma. Levels should return to 75% of normal before returning to work. RBC cholinesterase is replenished at a rate of 1% per day (25% every 7–10 days in plasma cholinesterase).

➤ When a client with a low cholinesterase level is given succinylcholine anesthesia be prepared to give respiratory support. Do not give neurologic depressants (such as morphine or other narcotics) until awake and alert.

Interfering Factors

➤ Hemolysis of blood specimen may cause false elevated values.

➤ Medications may cause decreased values: muscle relaxants, oral contraceptives, neostigmine, quinine, estrogens, phenothiazines, and radiographic agents (iopanoic acid).

NURSING CONSIDERATIONS

Prepare Your Client

➤ Explain that the test is used to determine the levels of a particular chemical, cholinesterase, in the body.

➤ Tell the client who is being prepared for surgery the screening is done to determine if the body produces enough of the chemical cholinesterase for the anesthesia to work safely.

➤ Inform the client who has been exposed to phosphorus insecticides that the test helps pinpoint poisonous levels.

➤ Explain that blood will be drawn from the client's vein.

➤ Assure the client there is no reason to restrict foods or fluids before the test.

Perform Procedure

➤ Collect 5–10 mL of blood in a red-top tube for the pseudocholinesterase (plasma) test.

➤ Collect 5–10 mL of blood in a green-top tube for the true cholinesterase (RBC) test.

➤ Label the specimen container and send to the lab. Specimen is stable for 6 hours at room temperature, for 1 week at 4°C, and for 6 months at –70°C.

Care After Test

➤ Assure a complete history for pesticide exposure has been explored and obtained.

➤ Instruct the client on follow-up appointments for future blood draws if the test is being done to monitor toxic levels of phosphorus insecticides.

➤ Evaluate client for neurological changes associated with phosphorus poisoning.

➤ Evaluate related tests such as complete blood count, liver function test, renal function tests, and serum glucose.

Educate Your Client and the Family

➤ Tell client that if relatives have had episodes of slow recovery from anesthesia, there may be a family tendency (recessive genetic predisposition) to slowly rid the body of some anesthesias (slow metabolism of succinylcholine anesthesia).

➤ Stress the importance of protection such as masks and protective clothing to prevent toxic contact with the chemicals to the client who works with phosphorus insecticides.

➤ Instruct the client or family to keep insecticides and toxic substances out of reach of children.

➤ The client with an industrial exposure to phosphorus insecticides should not return to work until cholinesterase levels return to 75% of normal. RBC cholinesterase increases at a rate of about 1% per day. Return to baseline takes about 5–7 weeks. Serum cholinesterase increases at a rate of about 25% in 7–10 days and returns to baseline in about 4–6 weeks.

Chorionic Villus Sampling

core ee on ik • vil us • sam pling
(CVS, Chorionic Villus Biopsy, CVB)

Normal Findings

PREGNANT CLIENT
Absence of chromosomal, DNA, and biochemical abnormalities in developing embryo/fetus

What This Test Will Tell You

This microscopic analysis examines cells from the chorionic villi to diagnosing genetic disorders during the first trimester of pregnancy. Alterations from normal will alert clients and caregivers to chromosomal defects, hemoglobinopathies, biochemical abnormalities, and possible sex-linked disorders in the developing fetus. Chorionic villus samples are obtained from weeks 7–12 of gestation, with the optimum time being weeks 8–9, when there is a more equal distribution of trophoblastic villi over the periphery of the chorion. This test can be conducted earlier than an amniocentesis and can provide the same information except for neural tube defects. Initial results of the diagnostic test are available in 24 hours, with the complete analysis available in 1–2 weeks.

Abnormal Findings

▲ INCREASED NUMBER OF AUTOSOMES may indicate trisomy 21 (Down syndrome), secondary mosaicism (Down syndrome), trisomy 18, or trisomy 13. *Increased number of sex chromosomes* may indicate Klinefelter syndrome (extra X in male), Triple X (XXX) syndrome, or XYY syndrome.

▼ DECREASED NUMBER OF AUTOSOMES may indicate autosomal monosomy (absence of a chromosome), resulting in 45 chromosomes, which is incompatible with life. *Decreased number of sex chromosomes* may indicate Turner syndrome (only one X chromosome in female).

Abnormalities of chromosome structure include translocations, partial deletion, inversion, abnormal splitting, and breakage and reunion of ends. These may indicate 14/21 unbalanced translocation (Down syndrome), deletion of long arm of 18 (microcephaly, motor retardation), deletion of short arm of 5 (*cri du chat,* or cat cry, syndrome), translocation of long arm of 22—often to 9 (confirms chronic myelogenous leukemia), aneuploidy—usually of 8 and 12 (acute myelogenous leukemia), Prader-Willi syndrome, Bloom's syndrome, Fanconi's syndrome, or telangiectasia.

Approximately 200 other disorders can be diagnosed with this test. These include hemoglobinopathies such as sickle-cell anemia and thalassemia; phenylketonuria and $alpha_1$- antitrypsin deficiency; Duchenne's muscular dystrophy; and lysosomal storage disorders such as Tay-Sachs disease.

ACTION ALERT!

Clients with a history of incompetent cervix are at high risk for a spontaneous abortion.

Interfering Factors

➤ Contamination of fetal cells with maternal cells can give false results.
➤ Chemotherapy can cause structural damage to chromosomes.
➤ Contamination of specimen with bacteria, viruses, or fungi interferes with cell culture.
➤ Cervix of primigravida client may be resistant to passage of catheter to obtain specimen.
➤ Contamination of specimen with perineum and vaginal preparation solution—povidone-iodine is destructive to cells and interferes with cell culture.

Contraindication

➤ Client with history of fetal loss due to incompetent cervix

Potential Complications

➤ Spontaneous abortion—risk is approximately 1% greater than for amniocentesis
➤ Bleeding
➤ Infection
➤ Intrauterine death
➤ Rh isoimmunization
➤ Hematoma
➤ Amniotic fluid leakage
➤ Possible fetal limb reduction defects when sampling at <10 weeks gestation

---

NURSING CONSIDERATIONS

Prepare Your Client

➤ Explain to the client and family that this test is to help discover or rule out certain problems in the developing baby.
➤ Ensure that an informed consent is obtained, because of the possible complications associated with this procedure.
➤ Tell the client that there are no restrictions on food or fluid prior to the test.
➤ Ask the client if she is allergic to iodine, as a povidone-iodine (betadine) skin prep may be done prior to the test.
➤ Ask client the date of her last menstrual period.
➤ Obtain family history of genetic disorders, if any.
➤ Have the client void before the procedure; however, with an anteverted uterus, a full bladder may be preferred to support the uterus in an optimal position.
➤ Take baseline vital signs before the procedure.

Perform Procedure

Nurses do not perform this procedure, but need to understand it so that it can be explained to clients. Ultrasound is used to guide the procedure so that the specimen can be obtained from the optimal location.

Place the client in a supine position with her legs in stirrups (lithotomy position). Tell the client that the procedure takes about 5 minutes. Cleanse the area around the vagina (vulva and perineum) with an antiseptic solution to prevent contamination of the specimen. Tell the client that she may experience the same type of feeling as when a Pap smear is done.

A sterile speculum is inserted in the vagina. The upper vagina (vaginal vault) and cervix are cleansed with the same antiseptic solution. A flexible tube (aspiration catheter) is inserted through the cervix to the specimen site; placement is guided by ultrasound observation. Remove the obturator used for guiding the catheter.

Gentle suction is used to obtain the specimen. The sample is placed in a petri dish with an appropriate culture medium. The catheter and speculum are removed. Label specimen and take to the laboratory immediately.

Gonorrhea and chlamydia cultures may be done to help diagnose infection. If a transcervical approach is contraindicated or not successful, a transabdominal approach, similar to conducting an amniocentesis, may be used.

Care After Test

➤ Assess and record client vital signs; report deviations from normal to primary maternity care provider.

➤ Assess the client for rupture of membranes after the procedure by looking for a leak of fluid from the vagina.

➤ Determine whether or not the Rh-negative client has had her prenatal injection of Rh_o (D) immune globulin (RhoGAM); if not, the primary maternity care provider will prescribe it at this time to prevent Rh sensitization.

➤ Explain to the client that it takes approximately 2 weeks before the results of the test are available.

➤ Help the client to understand that negative results do not assure a normal baby, but rather that the baby does not have any of the conditions that can be detected by this test.

➤ Encourage client to rest on her back or left side for a short time after the procedure.

➤ Schedule the client for an ultrasound within 5 days after sampling to assure that no fetal harm has occurred.

➤ Review related tests such as amniocentesis and fetal ultrasound.

Educate Your Client and the Family

➤ Explain that an appointment will be made to review the test results, that questions about the results will be answered, and that referrals will be made, if indicated, to provide for the best care possible.

➤ Instruct the client that after the procedure she should notify her primary maternity care provider if she has abdominal pain or cramping, her water breaks, she has bleeding from the vagina, or she has chills and a fever.

Chromium, Serum

kroe mee um • see rum

(Blood Chromium)

Normal Findings

ADULT, CHILD, ADOLESCENT

0.18–0.85 ng/mL (SI units: 4–17 nmol/L)

INFANT

High levels at birth may be normal, but should demonstrate a steady decline with increasing age.

ELDERLY

Values decline with age, related to loss of muscle mass. Decline may contribute to glucose intolerance.

What This Test Will Tell You

This blood test assesses lipid and carbohydrate metabolism and insulin activity, and it screens for chromium toxicity. Chromium, a trace element in the body, aids in the transport of amino acids to the heart and liver and is an essential component of the organic complex glucose tolerance factor. This factor forms a "bridge" between the insulin molecule and the cell membrane to potentiate the action of insulin. Chromium also lowers serum cholesterol and low-density lipoprotein (LDL) cholesterol, while it elevates high-density lipoprotein (HDL) cholesterol. Chromium toxicity may occur from industrial exposure.

Abnormal Findings

▲INCREASED LEVELS may indicate chromium toxicity related to exposure in the tanning, electroplating, steel and metal, photography, paint, dye, and explosives industries as well as chromium-tainted water.

▼DECREASED LEVELS are often associated with deficiencies from total parenteral nutrition; impaired ability to metabolize glucose as in atherosclerosis, pregnancy, and diabetic children; stress; acute infectious diseases; and congestive heart failure.

███████ ACTION ALERT!

Any value greater than 0.47 ng/mL may indicate chromium toxicity. Carefully assess renal and liver function, as they may be impaired in the presence of chromium toxicity.

Interfering Factors

➤ Recent diagnostic tests in which radioactive chromium was injected will invalidate test results.

➤ Test measurement with metal or stainless steel instruments will result in false positive findings.

NURSING CONSIDERATIONS

Prepare Your Client

➤ Explain that this test is used to determine how well the client's body uses fats, carbohydrates, and insulin, or to look for high levels of a material called chromium.

➤ Assess for industrial exposure to chromium.

Perform Procedure

➤ Collect 5 mL of venous blood in a metal-free (sometimes navy blue) tube. Check with your laboratory for a special collection kit.

Care After Test

➤ Assess for industrial exposure by investigating work history for employment in high-risk industries.

➤ Assess nutritional status if the

client has a chromium deficiency. Look for signs of altered carbohydrate metabolism, including impaired growth, peripheral neuropathy, and negative nitrogen balance.
➤ Consult with a registered dietician to assist the family and client in meeting special dietary needs.
➤ Evaluate related tests such as alanine aminotransferase (ALT), aspartate aminotransferase (AST), blood urea nitrogen (BUN), serum creatinine, serum cholesterol, low-density lipoprotein (LDL) cholesterol, high-density lipoprotein (HDL) cholesterol, and creatinine clearance.

Educate Your Client and the Family

➤ If chromium toxicity is detected, explain that additional diagnostic tests will be done to assess for liver and kidney impairment.
➤ If chromium level is low, instruct client and family on nutritional sources high in chromium, such as brewer's yeast and whole grains.
➤ Instruct client and family that body chromium can be conserved by using table sugar. Sucrose consumption increases insulin levels.

Chromosome Analysis
kroe mah some • ah nal ah sis

Normal Findings
46 chromosomes in a normal cell with 22 pairs of autosomes and 1 pair of sex chromosomes

What This Test Will Tell You
This test identifies genetic abnormalities that might be the underlying cause of fetal malformation, or of the client's maldevelopment or disease. Tissue cells, usually leukocytes and/or fibroblasts, are obtained for culture, and various chemical processes are used to stimulate and arrest cell division or mitosis at the metaphase, the ideal phase of division for study. The cell is stained, examined microscopically, and may be photographed to provide a photomicrograph of chromosome groupings (the karyotype) arranged according to size in descending order with the sex chromosomes being last. Usually 20 to 30 cells are examined and a representative sample photographed. For definitive diagnosis it may be necessary to study at least two different cell lines; that is, both leukocytes and fibroblasts should be examined.

Examination of chromosomes in a cell will reveal whether or not there are abnormalities in the number of chromosomes (less than or more than 46) and the location of these deviations. In addition, any structural alterations in the chromosomes, which result from chromosome breakage, will be revealed.

Abnormal Findings
▲ INCREASED NUMBER OF AUTOSOMES may indicate trisomy 21 (Down syndrome), secondary mosaicism (Down syndrome), trisomy 18, or trisomy 13. *Increased number of sex chromosomes* may indicate Kline-

felter syndrome (extra X in male), Triple X (XXX) syndrome, or XYY syndrome.

▼ DECREASED NUMBER OF AUTO-SOMES may indicate autosomal monosomy (absence of a chromosome), resulting in 45 chromosomes, which is incompatible with life. *Decreased number of sex chromosomes* may indicate Turner syndrome (only one X chromosome in female).

ABNORMALITIES OF CHROMOSOME STRUCTURE include translocations, partial deletion, inversion, abnormal splitting, and breakage and reunion of ends. These may indicate 14/21 unbalanced translocation (Down syndrome), deletion of long arm of 18 (microcephaly, motor retardation), deletion of short arm of 5 (*cri du chat*, or cat cry, syndrome), translocation of long arm of 22—often to 9 (confirms chronic myelogenous leukemia), aneuploidy—usually of 8 and 12 (acute myelogenous leukemia), Prader-Willi syndrome, Bloom's syndrome, Fanconi's syndrome, or telangiectasia.

███████ ACTION ALERT!

Obtaining specimens by amniocentesis can result in fetal morbidity or mortality. Specimens obtained by bone marrow biopsy can result in bleeding and shock. All methods of obtaining specimens can result in severe bleeding or infection.

Interfering Factors

➤ Preparation of a skin biopsy site with a povidone-iodine solution is destructive to cells and interferes with the cell culture.

➤ Contamination of fetal cells with maternal cells can give false results.

➤ Chemotherapy can cause structural damage to chromosomes.

➤ Contamination of specimen with bacteria, viruses, or fungi interferes with cell culture.

➤ Placement of a blood sample in a non-heparinized tube can damage cells.

➤ For postmortem or aborted specimens, a time since death greater than 2 days affects results.

➤ Freezing of specimen; refrigeration is indicated if not taken immediately to lab after collection.

Contraindications

FOR AMNIOCENTESIS

➤ Anteriorly placed placenta that prohibits access without placental disruption.

➤ Abruptio placenta.

➤ History of premature labor.

➤ Incompetent cervix.

FOR BONE MARROW BIOPSY

➤ Hemophilia or other bleeding disorders. However, the importance of further information that can be provided through the biopsy is weighed against the risk.

➤ The sternal biopsy site is contraindicated in children due to the possibility of mediastinal and cardiac perforation.

➤ Inability of the client to remain still during the 20–30 minute procedure. Sedation may be required.

Potential Complications

FOR AMNIOCENTESIS

➤ Trauma to the fetus, umbilical cord, or placenta.

➤ Maternal bleeding.

➤ Abruptio placenta.

➤ Rh sensitization from fetal bleeding into maternal circulation.

➤ Leak of amniotic fluid.

➤ Infection.

➤ Spontaneous abortion.

➤ Premature labor.

➤ Amniotic fluid embolism.

➤ Accidental puncture of bladder or intestines.

FOR BONE MARROW BIOPSY

➤ Bleeding, hemorrhage.

➤ Infection of the bone, which may lead to a potentially fatal systemic infection.

➤ Death related to damage to the heart or great vessels with a sternal biopsy.

➤ Damage to bone growth plate can occur if the tibial tubercle is biopsied in children.

Note: Appropriate precautions must be taken when obtaining specimens from clients with acute coagulation disorders.

NURSING CONSIDERATIONS
Prepare Your Client

➤ Explain that this test is done to evaluate the genes and genetic makeup of a person to help diagnose problems or the potential to pass on problems from generation to generation. For example: (1) Explain that the test will help to determine whether or not the developmental problem, malformation, or other health deficit experienced by the client is related to inherited traits. (2) Explain that the test will help to determine whether or not a couple has the potential to transmit genetic disorders to their natural children. (3) Explain that the test aids in the diagnosis of a particular type of leukemia (acute and chronic myelogenous leukemia). (4) Explain that the test (amniocentesis) helps to diagnose whether or not the developing fetus (baby) has any chromosomal abnormalities.

Perform Procedure

➤ For blood sample, perform venipuncture and collect 5–10 mL of blood in a sterile, green-top, heparinized tube.

➤ Apply pressure dressing to venipuncture site.

➤ For bone marrow and amniotic fluid specimens, follow procedures indicated in those sections, obtaining 1 mL of bone marrow and at least 20 mL of amniotic fluid; place in sterile containers.

➤ When a skin specimen is obtained, the skin will be cleansed with an antiseptic agent and a local anesthetic injected so that the area will be numb. The skin specimen will be removed with a sharp instrument and some bleeding may occur.

➤ Apply a sterile dressing.

➤ See *Amniocentesis* and *Bone Marrow Biopsy* for information to tell the client when those procedures are being done to obtain the specimen.

➤ The specimen will be placed in a sterile container.

➤ Label specimen, providing reason for test and a brief client history.

➤ Transport specimen to laboratory immediately; if delay is unavoidable, refrigerate specimen.

Care After Test

➤ Inspect skin specimen site for bleeding.

➤ See amniocentesis and bone marrow biopsy for care after test.

➤ Review related tests such as developmental testing and amniocentesis.

Educate Your Client and the Family

➤ Tell client and family when results should be available: (1) for blood sample 3–4 days, (2) for other specimens several weeks.

➤ Explain that the specimen obtained will be studied microscopically and that pictures will be made of what is seen through the microscope to show the number and structure of chromosomes in a body cell.

➤ Instruct client and family to make an appointment to review the test results, have their questions about the results answered, and receive referrals, if indicated, to provide for the best care possible.

➤ Tell a client who had a tissue specimen taken that the adhesive dressing can be removed in 24 hours and regular bathing can take place.

➤ Teach client and family any special wound care which the primary health care provider may order, and let them know it can usually be discontinued after 1 week.

➤ Instruct client and family to notify the primary health care provider if there are any signs of infection at the specimen site.

➤ See *Amniocentesis* and *Bone Marrow Biopsy* for additional information to teach client.

Cisternal Puncture
sis tur nal • punk chur

Normal Findings
Fluid: Clear, colorless, sterile

What This Test Will Tell You
This cerebrospinal fluid (CSF) analysis test is used to obtain CSF when a lumbar puncture is contraindicated due to infection at the lumbar puncture site or a lumbar deformity, and to visualize an upper cord lesion. This is an infrequently used test to obtain cerebrospinal fluid for analysis or to relieve an increase in pressure. Its role in visualizing lesions is minimal because less invasive methods, such as computed tomography and magnetic resonance imaging, are usually effective. This procedure may be used to introduce contrast material or air for myelography or encephalography.

Abnormal Findings
▲ INCREASED SPINAL FLUID PRESSURE may indicate meningitis, subarachnoid hemorrhage, brain or spinal cord tumors, lesions, cerebral edema or hemorrhage, brain abscess, encephalitis, viral infections, multiple sclerosis, impaired CSF resorption, hepatic encephalopathy, syphilis, or Reye's syndrome.

▼ DECREASED SPINAL FLUID PRESSURE may indicate leakage of CSF, dehydration, hypovolemia, or complete spinal subarachnoid block.

ACTION ALERT!
This test should not be performed when increased intracranial pressure is suspected. A rapid decrease in intracranial pressure secondary to the cisternal puncture and removal of CSF may cause the brain to shift downward (herniate) into the spinal column. The herniation could cause serious damage to the vital center in the medulla and result in neurological damage or death.

Contraindications
➤ Increased intracranial pressure.
➤ Infection at or near the puncture site.
➤ Lack of cooperation of client. This

is a hazardous procedure because the needle is in very close proximity to the brain stem.

➤ Abnormalities in anatomy at the level of the foramen magnum.

➤ Lesions suspected in the cisterna magna.

Potential Complications

➤ Brain stem injury

➤ Infection: meningitis or local infection

➤ Bleeding into the cisterna cerebro medullaris

➤ Neurologic injury or death from herniation

NURSING CONSIDERATIONS

Prepare Your Client

➤ Explain that this procedure is performed to look at fluid from the brain (CSF) and to measure pressure inside the head and brain.

➤ Ensure that an informed consent is obtained, because of the possible complications associated with this procedure.

➤ Tell the client the procedure takes 20–60 minutes.

➤ Instruct the client to remain very still during the procedure.

➤ Tell your client there is no need to restrict fluids or foods before the procedure.

➤ This procedure is usually described as uncomfortable or painful. Assure the client that health care professionals will be there for support.

Perform Procedure

Nurses do not perform this procedure; however, the physician frequently needs nursing assistance during the procedure. Position the client in the side-lying position with the neck flexed forward so the chin touches the chest. Assure the client you will help hold the head in the correct position during the procedure. The physician may prefer to have the client in the sitting position with neck flexed forward. The back of the head (occipital area) is shaved and cleansed with antiseptic according to institutional policy. The neck region will be anesthetized before placing the cisternal puncture needle. Maintain sterile technique throughout the procedure.

The spinal needle is inserted between the first cervical vertebra and the rim of the foramen magnum. A manometer is attached to the needle when the obturator is removed and the opening pressure is measured. Prior to recording the pressure, the client is asked to straighten and relax the legs in order to reduce intra-abdominal pressure. Reassure the client throughout the procedure. Encourage the client to breathe slowly and deeply. Stress the importance of remaining still.

Three sterile test tubes are used to collect 5–10 mL of CSF. Label the tubes 1, 2, and 3 in the order collected. The closing pressure is then measured. A dry dressing is applied. Send tubes to the lab immediately.

Care After Test

➤ Instruct the client to lie flat for 2–3 hours. Activities can be resumed if no complications occur.

➤ Evaluate the puncture site for redness, edema, bleeding, and drainage.

➤ Headaches are usually not experienced after this procedure.

➤ Assess the client carefully for changes in neurological status such as headache or neck stiffness, altered level of consciousness, and widening pulse pressure.

➤ Carefully assess for changes in respiration or cardiac arrhythmias, which could indicate damage to the brain (medulla).

➤ Encourage intake of fluids to prevent dehydration.

➤ Review related tests such as CSF analysis, computed tomography, magnetic resonance imaging, brain scan, cerebral angiography, and electroencephalography.

Educate Your Client and the Family

➤ Instruct the client to remain flat for several hours after the puncture to decrease the risk of CSF leakage from the puncture site.

➤ Teach client with impaired sensory function or mobility safety measures and methods to compensate for losses.

➤ Teach family of client with headaches to keep environment dim and quiet.

Clostridial Toxin Assay

kloe **strid** ee ahl • **tok** sin • a **say**

(Pseudomembranous Colitis Toxin Assay, Antibiotic-Associated Colitis Assay, Assay for *Clostridium difficile*, Assay for *C. diff*)

Normal Findings

All ages: No growth of *Clostridium difficile*

What This Test Will Tell You

This fecal culture measures the presence of *Clostridium difficile* (*C. diff*) and diagnoses clostridial enterocolitis. *C. diff* is an infection of the gastrointestinal tract that most commonly occurs in clients who are immunosuppressed, immunocompromised, or receiving broad spectrum antibiotic therapy.

Abnormal Findings

Positive results may reveal the presence of clostridial enterocolitis.

NURSING CONSIDERATIONS

Prepare Your Client

➤ Explain that this test is important to see if an unhealthy bacteria is growing in the gut (gastrointestinal tract).

➤ Instruct the client to defecate directly into a clean container with a lid. Emphasize that toilet paper and urine cannot be mixed with the sample.

Perform Procedure

➤ Obtain a 25–50 gram stool sample in a clean container with a lid.

➤ Refrigerate the stool sample only if transportation to the laboratory is delayed.

➤ Label the sample and note the time of suspected exposure to *Clostridium botulinum*.

Care After Test

➤ Observe the client for signs and symptoms of *C. diff* including cramping, diarrhea, and intolerance of feeding.

➤ Discontinue broad spectrum

antibiotic therapy and initiate specific antibiotic therapy with vancomycin and metronidazole as ordered.

➤ Carefully assess fluid and electrolyte balance for dehydration and electrolyte derangements.

➤ Review related tests such as stool culture, serum electrolytes, and intestinal biopsy.

Educate Your Client and the Family

➤ Explain that different medicine (antibiotic therapy) is required to get rid of abnormal germs (bacteria) in the gut (intestinal tract).

➤ For immunocompromised client, explain the role of the immune system in keeping a normal balance of healthy and disease-producing germs in the intestinal tract.

Clot Retraction
klot • ree trak shun

Normal Findings

All ages: 50% retraction in 1 hour; 100% retraction by 24 hours

What This Test Will Tell You

This blood test provides a gross estimate of the intrinsic clotting mechanism for clients with suspected or actual bleeding/coagulation disorders. The test helps to evaluate platelet adequacy as well as utilization of fibrinogen in the normal clotting cascade.

Abnormal Findings

▲ INCREASED *clot retraction* may indicate anemia or hypofibrinogenemia.

▼ DECREASED *clot retraction* may indicate thrombocytopenia, von Willebrand's disease, polycythemia, thrombasthenia, disseminated intravascular coagulation (DIC), Waldenström's macroglobulinemia, or secondary fibrinolysis.

ACTION ALERT!

Failure of a clot to form, slow or incomplete clot retraction, or a soft, poor-quality clot formation, as observed at 1, 2, and 4 hours, is indicative of conditions that can result in severe bleeding disorders. Observe the client closely for overt and occult signs of hemorrhage and shock.

Interfering Factors

➤ Aspirin and aspirin-containing products as well as a platelet count <100,000/mm^3 may interfere with the test by prolonging clot retraction.

➤ Anticoagulant therapy (heparin or warfarin), administration of nonsteroidal anti-inflammatory medications, abnormal hematocrit value, abnormal fibrinogen levels, and uremia may interfere with accurate results.

➤ Improper handling of the sample may influence the test results: use only plain glass blood collection tubes; perform the venipuncture with care to avoid traumatic acquisition of the sample; handle the sample gently to avoid hemolysis of the sample.

Contraindications

➤ Low platelet counts
➤ Hypofibrinogenemia

➤ Anticoagulation or aspirin therapy

NURSING CONSIDERATIONS

Prepare Your Client

➤ Explain that this test helps to evaluate how well the blood can clot.

Perform Procedure

➤ Collect 5–7 mL of venous blood in a plain, red-top *glass* collection tube (some laboratories use three small red-top tubes and compare the results of all three samples).

➤ The sample is transported to the laboratory as soon as possible. The sample *must* reach the lab in less than 1 hour.

➤ Handle the sample with care to avoid hemolysis of the specimen or disturbing a forming clot.

Care After Test

➤ Assess client for unusual bruising or prolonged bleeding from venipuncture site. Delayed clotting is a complication of many conditions for which this test is ordered.

➤ Avoid intramuscular (IM) injections, if possible. If it is not possible to avoid injections, use the smallest possible needle for the injection. Rotation of the injection sites allows healing time for these sites. Pressure rather than massage after injection may reduce the potential for the development of a hematoma at the injection site.

➤ Test all body secretions including stool, gastrointestinal aspirate, and tracheal aspirate for occult blood.

Closely inspect mucous membranes for bleeding.

➤ Review related tests such as prothrombin time, partial thromboplastin time, bleeding time, and activated clotting time.

Educate Your Client and the Family

➤ Clients with impaired clotting have prolonged bleeding times. Instruct the client and family on safety measures such as electric razors, non-skid shoes, and soft toothbrushes.

➤ Instruct the client or family to report prolonged or unusual bleeding or bruising.

➤ Significant delays in clotting indicate a bleeding tendency which requires that the client be protected from trauma. Injuries may result in uncontrolled bleeding, which is difficult to manage. Teach family and clients how to evaluate the home environment and increase safety.

➤ Instruct the client or family in diet, activity, and/or medication regimens to prevent constipation. Hard stools may be traumatic to anal and rectal mucosa.

➤ Instruct the client with a bleeding tendency to avoid taking medications that prolong bleeding time, such as aspirin and products containing aspirin. Client should be instructed to avoid large quantities of alcohol and its regular use. A written list of products to avoid will provide the client or family with a reference when shopping or selecting home remedies for minor ailments.

Coagulation Factors Assay, Intrinsic and Extrinsic

koe ag yu lay shun • fak turs • a say • in **trin** sik • and • eks **trin** sik

Normal Findings

INTRINSIC ASSAY

Adult, child, adolescent, and elderly:

Factor VIII 55%–145% of the control value (SI units: .55–1.45 μmol/L)

Factor IX 60%–140% of the control value (SI units: .60–1.40 μmol/L)

Factor XI 65%–145% of the control value (SI units: .65–1.45 μmol/L)

Factor XII 60%–160% of the control value (SI units: .60–1.60 μmol/L)

Pregnant: Factor VIII is normally elevated during pregnancy.

Newborn: Factors XI and XII deficiencies may occur in newborns as transient phenomena.

EXTRINSIC ASSAY

All ages:

Factor V 50%–150% of the control value (SI units: .50–1.50 μmol/L)

Factor VII 65%–135% of the control value (SI units: .65–1.35 μmol/L)

Factor X 45%–155% of the control value (SI units: .45–1.55 μmol/L)

Factor II 225%–290 U/mL (SI units: 2.25–2.90 μmol/L)

(1 unit of Factor II equals 1 unit of thrombin that clots 1 mL of standard fibrinogen in 15 seconds.)

What This Test Will Tell You

This collection of blood tests identifies coagulation disorders of the intrinsic and extrinsic coagulation pathways. The intrinsic system is activated by injury to blood, and the extrinsic system is activated by injury to tissues or blood vessels. See the section on coagulation cascade for further information.

Abnormal Findings

INTRINSIC ASSAY

▼DECREASED *Factor VIII* may indicate hemophilia A, von Willebrand's disease, Factor VIII inhibitor (post-transfusion), disseminated intravascular coagulation (DIC), or fibrinolysis.

▼DECREASED *Factor IX* may indicate hemophilia B (Christmas disease), hepatic disease, Factor IX inhibitor (post-transfusion), vitamin K deficiency, or warfarin therapy.

▼DECREASED *Factor XI* may indicate plasma thromboplastin antecedent deficiency (PTA) or a transient deficiency in newborns.

▼DECREASED *Factor XII* may indicate Hageman trait, nephrosis, or a transient deficiency in newborns.

EXTRINSIC ASSAY

▼DECREASED *Factor II* may indicate hypoprothrombinemia, hepatic disease, or vitamin K deficiency.

▼DECREASED *Factor V* may indicate parahemophilia, hepatic dysfunction, fibrinolysis, or disseminated intravascular coagulation.

▼DECREASED *Factor VII* may indicate congenital Factor VII deficiency, hepatic disease, or vitamin K deficiency.

▼DECREASED *Factor X* may indicate Stuart factor deficiency, hepatic disease, disseminated intravascular coagulation, or vitamin K deficiency.

ACTION ALERT!

Deficiencies in clotting factors indicate an increased risk for bleeding and hemorrhage. Closely observe the client for signs and symptoms such as frank bleeding, hypotension, tachycardia, apprehension, dyspnea, pale and cool skin, and anxiety. Be prepared to transfuse with blood products, including appropriate clotting factors.

Interfering Factors

➤ Hemolysis.

➤ Delay in the transport of the specimen to the laboratory, or failure to stabilize the sample by transporting on ice may affect test reliability.

➤ Warfarin therapy for anticoagulation will reduce levels of Factors II, VII, IX, and X.

➤ Pregnancy elevates Factor VIII.

NURSING CONSIDERATIONS

Prepare Your Client

➤ Explain that this test helps find any problems with clotting of the blood.

➤Withhold administration of oral anticoagulants prior to drawing the blood sample for this test.

Perform Procedure

➤ Collect 7 mL of venous blood in a blue-top tube.

Care After Test

➤ Assess client for unusual bruising or prolonged bleeding from venipuncture site. Delayed clotting is a complication of severely impaired clotting.

➤ Test all body secretions including stool, gastrointestinal aspirate, and tracheal aspirate for occult blood. Closely inspect mucous membranes for bleeding.

➤ Review related tests such as prothrombin time, partial thromboplastin time, bleeding time, and activated clotting time.

Educate Your Client and the Family

➤ Clients with abnormal coagulation may have prolonged bleeding times. Instruct the client and family on safety measures such as electric razors, non-skid shoes, and soft toothbrushes.

➤ Instruct the client or family to report prolonged or unusual bleeding or bruising.

➤ Significant findings that indicate a bleeding tendency require that the client be protected from trauma. Injuries may result in uncontrolled bleeding, which is difficult to manage. Teach family and clients how to evaluate the home environment and increase safety.

➤ Instruct the client with a bleeding tendency to avoid taking medications that prolong bleeding time, such as aspirin and products containing aspirin. Client should be instructed to avoid large quantities of alcohol and its regular use. A written list of products to avoid will provide the client or family with a reference when shopping or selecting home remedies for minor ailments.

➤ Provide information to parents about support groups for families with children with coagulation disorders.

COAGULATION CASCADE

Activation of the coagulation process occurs through two systems of interactions and responses. These systems, called the **intrinsic** and **extrinsic** pathways, eventually form a common path that terminates in the formation of a stable fibrin clot.

The **intrinsic** pathway is initiated when the blood itself is traumatized

COAGULATION CASCADE

Intrinsic Pathway evaluated by partial prothrombin time (PTT)	**Extrinsic Pathway** evaluated by prothrombin time (PT)
↓	↓
Activation event	Activation event
↓	↓
Factor XII	Factor III or tissue thromboplastin
↓	↓
Factor XI with calcium ions	Factors III + VII* with calcium ions
↓	
Factor IX*	
↓	
Factors VIII + IX	

Common Pathway

Factor X*

↓

Factor II*† (prothrombin) → Thrombin

↓

Factor I (fibrinogen)†

↓

Fibrin

Factor XIII →   ↓

Stable fibrin clot

↓

Activators

↓

Plasminogen→plasmin →   Clot
deterioration

↓

Fibrin degradation products

*Warfarin works by depressing these factors, which are vitamin K dependent.
†Heparin works by preventing conversion of fibrinogen to fibrin, and
prothrombin to thrombin.

in some way. This event stimulates Factor XII. Activated Factor XII then causes the activation of Factor XI. Factor XI, in the presence of calcium ions, activates Factor IX. Factor IX, or Christmas factor, is synthesized in the liver in a vitamin K–related process. (Factor IX is the deficient factor in hemophilia B, or Christmas disease.) Factor IX converts to Factor VIII in the presence of plasma phospholipid. Factor VIII forms a complex with activated Factor IX that is a major force in the activation of Factor X. Factor VIII is also important in promoting platelet adhesiveness. (Factor VIII is the deficient coagulation factor in hemophilia A).

The extrinsic pathway is activated by trauma to the endothelium of the vessel wall, or to other tissues, which causes the release of Factor III. Factor III interacts with Factor VII in the presence of calcium ions. The sequence of this pathway concludes with the activation of Factor X, at which point the extrinsic and intrinsic pathways combine to form a common path.

The common or shared pathway begins with Factor X. Factor X, with stimulation from both the intrinsic and extrinsic pathways, reacts with Factor V, again in the presence of calcium ions and phospholipid. The result of this interaction is a pro-thrombin-converting complex. Prothrombin (Factor II) is converted to thrombin. Thrombin serves as an enzyme to convert fibrinogen (Factor I) into fibrin threads. These fibrin threads intertwine to form a soluble plug. Thrombin also activates Factor XIII, which strengthens the fibrin polymer and results in a stable, insoluble clot.

Colonoscopy
koe lon oss koe pee
(Lower Gastrointestinal Endoscopy, Proctosigmoidoscopy)

Normal Findings
Absence of bleeding, mass lesions, and strictures/stenoses
Normal intestinal mucosa and structure

What This Test Will Tell You
This endoscopic test evaluates active or occult lower gastrointestinal (GI) bleeding, and monitors the presence of neoplasms in clients with risk factors for colon cancer. Direct visualization of the entire colon from the anus to the cecum using a long flexible endoscope allows the colonoscopist to assess mucosal vascular patterns for abnormalities such as bleeding sites or inflammation, and to detect small mass lesions such as polyps or tumors. Specimens of tumors, polyps, and inflamed areas can be taken through the colono-

scope for analysis.

This procedure may also be used therapeutically, to treat disorders of the lower GI tract. Polypectomy, balloon dilatation of strictures or stenoses, bowel decompression, removal of foreign bodies, and treatment of bleeding sites may all be performed during colonoscopy.

Abnormal Findings
Abnormalities may indicate lower GI tract ulceration/bleeding, inflammatory bowel disease, precancerous and cancerous polyps, colon cancer, arteriovenous malformation (angiodysplasia), and diverticulosis.

ACTION ALERT!
Monitor for rare but life-threatening complications of this procedure, which include intestinal perforation, hemorrhage, and

cardiopulmonary arrest. Evaluate vital signs for tachycardia, dysrhythmias, weak and thready pulses, hypotension, and cold, clammy skin. Assess for signs of perforation which include rigid abdomen, pain, and fever.

Interfering Factors
➤ Stool, blood, or barium in the colon can prevent adequate visualization of the lower GI tract.

Contraindications
➤ Recent myocardial infarction or pulmonary embolism, shock, and any condition which results in unstable cardiovascular status, because of the danger of cardiorespiratory compromise and arrest
➤ Suspected bowel perforation, peritonitis, or infectious bowel disease, since the insufflation of air during the procedure may blow out a confined perforation to freely communicate with the peritoneal cavity
➤ Fulminant ulcerative colitis, acute ischemic colitis, acute radiation colitis, and/or severe diverticulitis, since colonic wall distention during the procedure can worsen hemorrhage and colonic ischemia, and increase the risk of perforation and bacteremia
➤ Active lower intestinal bleeding because blood may cover the colonoscope lens, thus preventing adequate visualization
➤ Third trimester of pregnancy, because of the risk of inducing labor

Potential Complications
➤ Bowel perforation
➤ Hemorrhage
➤ Medication reactions which induce cardiorespiratory depression, resulting from intravenous sedation given prior to the procedure
➤ Medication reactions which induce cardiac arrhythmias, resulting from intravenous medications to decrease bowel spasms given during the procedure
➤ Vasovagal reactions
➤ Hypotension related to dehydration of at-risk patients during bowel preparation
➤ Cardiac failure related to overhydration of at-risk patients during bowel preparation

---

NURSING CONSIDERATIONS
Prepare Your Client
➤ Explain that this test is used to visualize the lower gut (GI tract), in order to see if any problems exist.
➤ Ensure that an informed consent is obtained, because of the possible complications associated with this procedure.
➤ Inform the client or family that the client will remain awake during the procedure, but that intravenous sedation will be given to promote comfort and relaxation.
➤ Advise the client that the procedure is uncomfortable, but should not be painful. As the colonoscope is being inserted, a pressure sensation may be felt. Tell the client to notify the nurse if severe abdominal pain is felt.
➤ Tell client that they may be asked to breathe deeply or change positions in order to help the colonoscope pass smoothly into the colon.
➤ Administer the bowel preparation. In adults, this is usually about 1 gallon of an iso-osmolar electrolyte lavage solution, either orally or via a nasogastric tube over a 4-hour period. The bowel preparation should be given 6–12 hours before the procedure. Some institutions use a bowel preparation protocol con-

sisting of 2–3 days of liquid diets, cathartics, and enemas.

➤ Administer the appropriate bowel preparation for pediatric client. The solution is usually magnesium citrate, 30 mL per year of age to a maximum of 300 mL given the day before the procedure, along with saline enemas the night before and the morning of the procedure. A clear, liquid diet for 48 hours before the procedure is recommended.

➤ Have the client urinate before the procedure.

➤ Give the client preoperative sedation. General anesthesia may be used in certain pediatric clients.

➤ Establish intravenous access before the test begins.

Perform Procedure

Nurses do not perform this procedure, but should understand the process to prepare the client and to assist the colonoscopist in obtaining the best results from the procedure.

A long flexible endoscope is used to visualize the entire lower GI tract. The colonoscope is equipped with suction to remove secretions. It also has air controls that distend the bowel lumen for safe passage through the abdominal structures, and water controls which keep the fiber-optic tip of the instrument clean. The physician inserts the instrument into the rectum, and insufflates a small amount of air to help dilate the bowel lumen. The colonoscope is then passed through the splenic flexure, the transverse colon, the hepatic flexure, the ascending colon, and the cecum.

Assist the client into a left lateral decubitus position and instruct the client to breathe slowly and deeply as the colonoscopist inserts the colono-scope into the rectum. Apply pressure to areas of the client's abdomen as needed, to assist with passage of the colonoscope through the lower GI tract. Assess the client's vital signs, oxygenation status, level of abdominal distention, level of consciousness, vagal response, and pain tolerance during the procedure. Administer atropine or glucagon as needed to decrease bowel spasms and/or motility. Monitor for the cardiovascular side effects of these drugs including tachycardia and hemodynamic changes.

Care After Test

➤ Monitor vital signs every 15–30 minutes until the client is stable.

➤ Observe for signs of complications, such as bleeding, vomiting, change in vital signs, severe abdominal pain and/or distention, and abdominal rigidity.

➤ Encourage drinking more fluids to counteract any dehydration related to the bowel preparation.

➤ Review related tests such as barium enema, fecal occult blood, hemoglobin, hematocrit, and carcinoembryonic antigen.

Educate Your Client and the Family

➤ Inform client that they will feel some abdominal discomfort following the procedure, due to the air inflated into the bowel lumen during the procedure. Getting up and walking around can help get rid of the air and minimize the discomfort.

➤ Advise client to avoid strenuous activities for 24 hours after colonoscopy.

➤ Teach client and family an anti-cancer diet, including the need for adequate fluid and fiber intake.

➤ Instruct client at high risk for colon cancer that this test should be performed yearly in order to diagnose and treat early any malignancy.

Reinforce that colon cancer is often asymptomatic.

Colposcopy
kahl **pah** skah pee

Normal Findings
Normal vaginal and cervical tissue

What This Test Will Tell You
Colposcopy is a visual examination of vaginal and cervical tissue through an instrument (colposcope or colpomicroscope) with a light and magnifying lens to evaluate abnormal tissue changes. Photographs of lesions and tissue biopsies may also be performed to facilitate diagnosis. Depending upon the instrument used, magnification of 10–400 times with a three-dimensional view permits evaluation of tissue and identification of the boundaries of a lesion so that a representative specimen can be obtained for tissue analysis. With the advent of this procedure, cone biopsies of the cervix following positive Pap smears have decreased as affected tissue can be identified and obtained for laboratory analysis. This procedure is also used to monitor treatment of lesions and to monitor daughters of women who received diethylstilbestrol during pregnancy, who have an increased incidence of precancerous and cancerous lesions of the vagina and cervix. Abnormal tissue findings will undergo analysis to differentiate between infections, dysplasia, neoplasia, and cancer.

Abnormal Findings
Abnormal tissue may indicate cervical erosion, infections including condyloma, cervical dysplasia, cervical intraepithelial neoplasia, carcinoma in situ, or invasive carcinoma.

Interfering Factors
➤ Creams, medications, mucus, cervical secretions, and seminal fluid not cleansed from the cervix by the examiner can interfere with visualization of tissue.
➤ Menses.

Contraindication
➤ Moderate to heavy menses

Potential Complications
In the event of a biopsy:
➤ Bleeding from biopsy site; preferable to schedule exam 1 week after menses due to increased cervical vascularity before and immediately following menses
➤ Infection at biopsy site

NURSING CONSIDERATIONS
Prepare Your Client
➤ Explain that this test will help identify the cause of an abnormal Pap smear.
➤ Ensure that an informed consent is obtained, because of the possible complications associated with this

procedure.

➤ Do not restrict food or fluids prior to the test.

➤ Tell the client that the test will be conducted in an office or clinic.

➤ Inform the client that anesthetics are not required as little or no discomfort will be experienced. If biopsies are anticipated, some practitioners may administer ibuprofen prior to the procedure to ease cramping.

➤ Have the client void before the procedure.

Perform Procedure

Physicians and advanced practice nurses perform this procedure; other nurses need to understand it so that it can be explained to clients. Place the client in a supine position with her legs in stirrups (lithotomy position). Tell the client that the procedure takes about 10–20 minutes.

A sterile vaginal speculum is inserted into the vagina. The upper vagina (vaginal vault) and cervix are cleansed with a long cotton-tipped applicator (swab) to remove any secretions. Special solutions are applied with a long cotton-tipped applicator (swab) to facilitate visualization of the tissue (saline to visualize vascular patterns; 3% acetic acid to produce color changes in cervical epithelium and enhance identification of abnormal tissue).

Photographs may be taken of the tissue. Some practitioners have equipment attached to a video monitor so that client can view procedure as it is being done. A biopsy of abnormal tissue may be done. Some cramping may occur when the tissue sample is removed. An endocervical curettage (scraping inside the cervix) is occasionally done for analysis of tissue that cannot be visualized.

Any bleeding from biopsy site will be controlled by pressure or cautery. A tampon may be also inserted by some health care providers for pressure or alternately, silver nitrate may be applied to control bleeding. Tissue specimens are placed in a biopsy bottle with a preservative. Pap smears must be sprayed with a fixative. Label specimen(s), if any, and send to the laboratory.

Care After Test

➤ Assess client for any unusual vaginal bleeding. Report immediately bright red blood.

➤ Provide a perineal pad for client if a tampon was not inserted.

➤ Review related tests such as Pap smear and cervical biopsy.

Educate Your Client and the Family

➤ Explain to client that a small amount of bleeding or spotting from biopsy site may occur for several hours.

➤ Instruct client who had a biopsy to wear a sanitary pad (or tampon if recommended by the primary health care provider) until bleeding ceases.

➤ Tell her to notify her primary health care provider if she experiences heavy bleeding not associated with a menstrual period, a foul-smelling vaginal discharge, and/or chills and fever.

➤ Instruct her to abstain from intercourse and insert nothing into the vagina (other than a tampon if allowed) for at least 1 week or as directed by care provider until biopsy site has healed.

➤ If silver nitrate was used, explain to client that she may have a slight gray vaginal discharge.

➤ Inform client that she will be notified when the results are available. If the test is positive, an appointment will be made to discuss the findings and treatment options.

Complement Assay

kom ple ment • a say
(C1, C1Q, C1r, C1s, C2, C3, C4, C5, C6, C7, C8, C9, C1 Esterase Inhibitor, C'1 Esterase Inhibitor, C'1 INH, CH50)

Normal Findings

➤ Total complement: 25–90 hemolytic units/mL
➤ C1 esterase inhibitor: 16–33 mg/dL (160–330 mg/L)
➤ C3, males: 70–252 mg/dL (700–2500 mg/L)
➤ C3, females: 70–206 mg/dL (700–2100 mg/L)
➤ C4, males: 10–72 mg/dL (100–720 mg/L)
➤ C4, females: 10–75 mg/dL (100–750 mg/L)
➤ C'1 esterase inhibitor: 8–33 mg/dL

What This Test Will Tell You

This analysis of synovial, pericardial, or pleural fluid or blood is used to diagnose diseases of the immune system, including congenital defects and autoimmune diseases. Complement assay includes a series of about 20 serum proteins that play an important role in noncellular immunity by assisting in the destruction and disposal of invaders or antigens. These proteins are consumed and replaced in the normal formation of antigen-antibody immune complexes. Complement levels rise normally in response to an antigen. Decreases in levels are the most clinically significant because they may signal an inability to fight infection. Complement levels are decreased during excessive complex formation, inadequate replacement, or from an inborn deficiency. The CH50 is a measure of the total hemolytic complement's functional ability to hemolyze or destroy invaders. If CH50 is normal, the complement system is functional. Ch3 is a vital component of the complement system, crucial to the pathway that regulates formation of antigen-antibody complexes and to the pathway that destroys bacteria. C4 plays a role in the clearance of immune complexes from the body. C1 esterase inhibitor is associated with hereditary angioedema.

Abnormal Findings

▲INCREASED LEVELS may indicate thyroiditis, acute rheumatoid arthritis, myocardial infarction, ulcerative colitis, obstructive jaundice, diabetes mellitus, cancer, or rheumatic fever.

▼DECREASED LEVELS in serum may indicate systemic lupus erythematosus (SLE), glomerulonephritis, serum sickness, rheumatoid arthritis, hereditary angioedema, autoimmune hemolytic anemia, cirrhosis of the liver, myeloma, subacute bacterial endocarditis, cryoglobulinemia, transplant rejection, medication reactions, disseminated intravascular coagulation (DIC), hypogammaglobulinemia, or septicemia.

▼ DECREASED LEVELS in synovial, pleural, or pericardial fluid may indicate rheumatoid arthritis.

████ ACTION ALERT!

Clients with depressed C3 levels are susceptible to serious recurrent bacterial infections. Special precautions to avoid infection are critical, including scrupulous handwashing and avoiding contact with crowds and people who are known to be ill. Clients with depressed C4 levels have an increased incidence of rheumatic diseases.

Interfering Factors

➤ Failure to promptly transport the specimen to the laboratory or place it in cold storage may result in rapid deterioration of the sample and inaccurate results.

➤ Heparin interferes with accuracy.

Prepare Your Client

➤ Explain that this test helps detect how well the body is able to fight infections or whether the immune system is causing problems.

➤ Explain that a blood or other fluid sample will be drawn and sent to the lab for immediate processing.

➤ Ensure that an informed consent is obtained with removal of synovial, pleural, or pericardial fluid because of the possible complications.

Perform Procedure

BLOOD COLLECTION

➤ Collect 10 mL of venous blood in a red-top tube.

➤ Label specimen and note if client has had recent heparin therapy.

➤ Handle specimen carefully to avoid hemolysis and send specimen to laboratory immediately.

SYNOVIAL, PERICARDIAL, OR PLEURAL FLUID COLLECTION

Nurses do not usually perform this procedure but should understand the process to prepare the client and assist the physician. See *Pericardiocentesis, Pleural Fluid Analysis,* and *Synovial Fluid Analysis* tests.

Care After Test

➤ Evaluate the client's joints for inflammation and range of motion to assess improvement or deterioration if client suffers from rheumatic disease. Careful inspection of joints is indicated if synovial fluid has been withdrawn.

➤ Assess parameters of renal function such as blood urea nitrogen (BUN), creatinine, edema, and urine output in a client with glomerulonephritis or other immune-mediated diseases that affect renal function.

➤ Monitor for signs of infection such as rising of subnormal temperature or purulent drainage or sputum in a client with C3 deficiencies.

➤ Review related tests such as the white blood cell count.

Educate Your Client and the Family

➤ Explain that complement levels are not definitely diagnostic of any particular disease, but are suggestive and can confirm if the problem lies with the complement system. Complement assay can also be used to indicate if treatment is successful in a client with known immune-mediated disease.

➤ Explain that other blood tests will be drawn, such as to assist in an accurate diagnosis.

➤ Teach the client and family the symptoms of infection and instruct them to contact the primary health care provider immediately when they occur.

➤ Teach the client and family the importance of proper hygiene.

Computed Tomography of Abdomen

kum pyoo ted • toe mah grah fee • uv • ab doe men
(CT Scan of the Abdomen, CAT Scan of the Abdomen, Computerized Axial Tomography of the Abdomen, EMI Scan)

Normal Findings

Absence of inflammation, infection, abscesses, stones, abnormal fluid collections, and/or mass lesions

What This Test Will Tell You

This radiologic test evaluates and diagnoses a large number of clinical conditions of the abdomen with x-rays taken at multiple and various angles throughout the abdominal cavity. Computed tomography (CT) uses a radiologic scanning machine depicting differences in tissue density as differing shades of gray; it provides a noninvasive yet three-dimensional view of the abdominal structures. Intravenous injection of radiopaque contrast material, oral ingestion of a contrast agent, or rectal administration of a contrast medium may be used during CT scanning to better visualize the organs and structures of the abdomen.

The CT scan allows the physician to assess abdominal organs and structures for a variety of abnormalities such as inflammation, abscesses, and mass lesions or tumors. Computed tomography can provide radiologic images of the abdominal vasculature, such as the aorta, renal arteries, and splanchnic circulations, in addition to the abdominal organs. CT scanning is also used to characterize the source of intra-abdominal and pelvic fluid collections, since it can help to differentiate between blood, ascites, bile, and/or pus as the type of intra-abdominal fluid accumulation. Finally, CT scanning is used to detect mass lesions, cancers, or tumors of the peritoneal cavity, and to stage various types of cancers for abdominal lymph node metastases.

Abnormal Findings

Gallbladder abnormalities may include common bile duct calculi, bile duct dilatation, tumors, or traumatic injury. *Kidney abnormalities* may include calculi, obstructions of the collecting system, cysts, traumatic injury, congenital anomalies, or tumors. *Liver abnormalities* may include abscess, tumor, or traumatic injury. *Lymph abnormalities* may include Hodgkin's disease. *Pancreas abnormalities* may include pancreatitis, pseudocyst, tumor, or bleeding. *Spleen abnormalities* may include traumatic injury such as hematoma and laceration, or a tumor. *Vascular structure abnormalities* may include abdominal aortic aneurysm, abdominal aortic dissection, renal artery stenosis, abnormalities of the mesentery vasculature, or celiac bypass graft occlusion. *Other abnormalities* include abscesses, ascites, appendicitis, mesentery disease, or cancer.

ACTION ALERT!

➤ Clients with pre-existing renal problems have an increased risk of nephrotoxicity if radiopaque dye is used during the test.
➤ Assess clients carefully for allergic reaction to contrast material, including dyspnea, itching, urticaria, flushing, hypotension, and shock. Life-threatening anaphylactic reactions can occur and need to be recognized and treated immediately.

Interfering Factors

➤ Barium in the stomach and/or small intestine can prevent adequate visualization of abdominal structures.
➤ Internal metal objects such as surgically placed wires or clips or abdominally placed pacemaker generators.
➤ Obesity makes visualization of internal structures difficult.
➤ Contents of bowel including fecal material or air.

Contraindications

➤ Uncooperativeness, combativeness, or inability to lie still on the examination table.
➤ Absence of gag or cough reflex, endotracheal intubation, and impending general anesthesia are contraindications for oral contrast medium.
➤ Pregnancy, due to radiologic exposure of fetus.
➤ Renal impairment is a relative contraindication to the use of contrast medium.
➤ Allergy to iodine, contrast material, or shellfish.
➤ Gross obesity.
➤ Unstable vital signs requiring frequent monitoring and intervention.

Potential Complications

➤ Reactions to intravenous radiopaque contrast dye given prior to the procedure can include anaphylactic shock, vasovagal reaction, and/or thromboembolism.
➤ Nephrotoxicity may result from intravenous radiopaque contrast dye given prior to the procedure.

NURSING CONSIDERATIONS

Prepare Your Client

➤ Explain that this test is used to look at the organs and structures of the entire abdomen, in order to see if any problems exist.
➤ Check to see if the client has an allergy to iodine or to seafood if an intravenous contrast agent is to be used.
➤ Withhold food and fluids for at least 4 hours prior to the procedure.
➤ Assess client for claustrophobia since they will need to remain motionless inside a scanner, which can seem tunnel-like to clients. If client exhibits this fear, consult with the primary health care provider for a sedation order, or evaluate appropriateness of continuing with testing.
➤ Inform the client and family that the test will take approximately 15–30 minutes (30–60 minutes if a contrast agent is used), and that the client will remain awake during the procedure unless sedation is ordered to produce a light sleep.
➤ Advise the client that the procedure is painless, but that lying motionless on the flat examination table while the x-ray pictures are

being taken may be uncomfortable.

➤ Ensure that an informed consent is obtained if contrast material is to be used, because of the possible complications associated with this procedure.

➤ Inform the client that when the radiopaque dye is injected intravenously, a flushed, warm sensation may be felt.

➤ Instruct the client to notify the nurse if severe pain or distress is felt.

Perform Procedure

Nurses do not perform this procedure, but should understand the process to prepare the client and to assist the physician in obtaining the best results from the procedure. Assist the client into a supine position and ensure safe positioning on the examination table. The client is moved inside the body scanner, which encircles the body. Numerous pictures are taken at varying angles throughout the procedure. Instruct client to hold their breath at varying times throughout the procedure while radiographic images are being taken. Technicians and/or the radiologist move the table and the scanner throughout the testing period to obtain various images. Assess the client's vital signs, oxygenation status, level of abdominal distention, level of consciousness, vagal response, and pain tolerance during the procedure.

➤ Watch the client for signs of allergy to the contrast agent, such as nausea, vomiting, palpitations, dyspnea, or dizziness.

Care After Test

➤ Observe for complications of the client's underlying disease process, such as bleeding, vomiting, change in vital signs, severe abdominal pain and/or distention, and abdominal rigidity.

➤ Assess for any manifestations of allergy and/or nephrotoxicity.

➤ Encourage drinking fluids to flush the contrast agent out of the system.

➤ Evaluate specific tests related to the organ system being targeted for the CT imaging.

Educate Your Client and the Family

➤ Instruct client in a balanced diet, including fiber and plenty of fluids.

➤ Warn client that the oral contrast material may cause diarrhea, and to increase oral fluids if this occurs.

Computed Tomography of the Adrenals

kom **pyoo** ted • toe **mog** rah fee • uv • the • ah **dree** nals

(CT Scan of the Adrenals, Computed Axial Tomography of the Adrenals, CAT Scan of the Adrenals, CATT Scan of the Adrenals)

Normal Findings

Presence of adrenal glands bilaterally. Normal shape and size. Absence of hemorrhage, tumors, cysts, or other abnormalities.

What This Test Will Tell You

This radiographic test diagnoses congenital or acquired abnormalities of the adrenal glands, especially tumors and hemorrhage. Computed tomography (CT) of the adrenals can detect even very small tumors or masses (pheochromocytoma and adenoma). It can also detect hemorrhage, hyperplasia, or hypoplasia of the adrenal gland. The test may be done with or without contrast material.

Abnormal Findings

Abnormalities may indicate adenoma, pheochromocytoma, hemorrhage, congenital absence of adrenals, or cancer of the adrenal glands.

ACTION ALERT!

Assess clients carefully for allergic reaction to contrast material, including dyspnea, itching, urticaria, flushing, hypotension, and shock. Life-threatening anaphylactic reactions can occur and need to be recognized and treated immediately.

Interfering Factors

➤ Pacemakers, skeletal traction, or large metal implants (for hip replacement, etc.) may not be able to be scanned. Metal cannot go into the CT machine. Call the x-ray department for specific information on the type and amount of metal allowed.
➤ Barium in the intestines from previous studies.
➤ Stool or gas in the bowel.

Contraindications

➤ Pregnancy, due to potential damage to the fetus
➤ Allergy to iodinated dye or shellfish if using contrast dye
➤ Severely claustrophobic clients
➤ Clients that are unable to lie on their backs for 15 minutes to 1 hour
➤ Obese clients whose body girth may exceed the size of the machine opening
➤ Highly anxious/restless clients
➤ Instability of vital signs and client's status

Potential Complications

➤ Allergic reaction to contrast material
➤ Renal failure related to contrast material

NURSING CONSIDERATIONS

Prepare Your Client

➤ Explain that this test is performed to look at two important glands in the body called the adrenals. These glands are important in controlling adrenaline and other hormones.
➤ Tell clients that they must lie still for 30–60 minutes during the test.
➤ Ensure that an informed consent is obtained if contrast material is used, because of the possible complications associated with this procedure.
➤ Ask about dye allergies, even if the client is only having a non-contrast CT scan. If they are allergic to intravenous (IV) dye or shellfish, notify the radiologist, as sometimes the non-contrast CT does not visualize the area well enough and IV contrast is needed when not planned for.
➤ If the client is extremely restless, notify the radiologist to obtain a sedative.
➤ Check with institutional policy about restricting food and fluids for 4–8 hours prior to the test. This is especially indicated when administration of contrast material is anticipated.

Perform Procedure

Nurses do not perform this procedure but should understand the process to prepare the client and assist the physician. This test is performed by an x-ray technologist or radiologist. The client is taken to the CT scanner and placed on the CT table. The table is then brought into the scanner, where an overhead camera takes multiple pictures at various angles. The client must lie still for 30 minutes to 1 hour. To combat feelings of claustrophobia, many scanners have music speakers within the scanner tunnel. The client is asked to pick music or a radio station that they want to listen to. There are also speakers within the CT tunnel for the technologist and client to speak to each other.

If intravenous contrast dye is used to improve imaging of the kidneys, the client may feel a transient hot flush. They may also feel nauseated during the dye injection. Contrast material may be administered orally to improve imaging of the adrenal glands in relation to the intestinal tract.

Care After Test

➤ Encourage the client to drink increased amounts of fluids after the test because contrast material has a diuretic effect.

➤ Monitor for delayed allergic reaction to the dye. This may occur up to 6 hours after dye injection.

➤ For client with suspected pheochromocytoma, assess for tachycardia, diaphoresis, tremor, pallor, flushing, anxiety, and hyperglycemia, which may signal a crisis.

➤ Review related tests including abdominal ultrasound, magnetic resonance imaging, and serum and urine catecholamines.

Educate Your Client and the Family

➤ Teach the client with suspected or confirmed pheochromocytoma about drug therapy, specifically alpha-blocking agents, and the need for surgery as definitive treatment for the tumor.

➤ Inform family members of client with confirmed pheochromocytoma that they need to be evaluated as well.

Computed Tomography of Kidney

kum pyoo ted • toe mah grah fee • uv • kid nee

(EMI [Electric Music Industries] Scan, CT Scan, Computerized Axial Tomography [CAT] scan, Computerized Transaxial [Transverse] Tomography [CTT] Scan, Computer-Assisted Transaxial Tomography [CATT] scan)

Normal Findings

ADULT

Negative; no tumor or pathologic conditions

PREGNANT

Slight to moderate hydronephrosis; right kidney larger than left kidney

ELDERLY

Kidneys are smaller in size as a result of progressive loss of whole nephrons and renal mass.

INFANT AND CHILD

Presence of all structures; no congenital or acquired abnormalities. Complete maturity of the kidney occurs during the latter half of the second year.

What This Test Will Tell You

This radiographic scanning test diagnoses an early stage of disease or congenital anomalies of the kidney. X-rays are taken at varying angles to produce a picture of the contents of the kidney based on differences in densities and composition of the organ tissue. Contrast dye may be used to enhance imaging. The varying densities measured are translated by a computer into varying shades of gray to produce high-quality pictures of the urinary system. Computed tomography (CT) scans are not useful for evaluating blood flow, perfusion, or metabolic function of organs and tissues.

Abnormal Findings

Abnormalities may indicate renal tumors, renal calculi, renal cysts, strictures or other obstructions, congenital anomalies, perirenal hematomas, or perirenal abscesses.

ACTION ALERT!

Assess client carefully for allergic reaction to contrast material including dyspnea, itching, urticaria, flushing, hypotension, and shock. Life-threatening anaphylactic reactions can occur and need to be recognized and treated immediately.

Interfering Factors

➤ Body movement of the client may compromise image quality.
➤ Radiopaque objects such as snaps, zippers, or jewelry obscure kidney visualization.
➤ Barium sulfate can obscure abdominal organ visualization. Barium studies should be completed 4 days prior to or following the CT scan.
➤ Excessive flatus or stool in the intestinal tract may cause client discomfort and inaccurate results.

Contraindications

➤ Clients who are unable to lie still
➤ Allergy to contrast material, unless modifications are made

➤ Pregnancy, due to radiation exposure to the unborn fetus
➤ Obesity, usually greater than 300 pounds

Potential Complications

➤ CT scan with contrast:
➤ Dehydration
➤ Headache
➤ Nausea
➤ Vomiting
➤ Acute renal failure
➤ Allergic reactions/anaphylaxis

NURSING CONSIDERATIONS

Prepare Your Client

➤ Explain that this test is to discover any problems there may be in the kidneys or other parts of the urinary system.
➤ Ensure that an informed consent is obtained when contrast medium is used, because of the possible complications associated with this procedure.
➤ Remove radiopaque objects such as jewelry, snaps, and electrocardiographic leads.
➤ Check the chart and interview the client and family to be sure the client has no allergy to contrast material, iodine, or shellfish.
➤ If contrast media is ordered and the client is allergic to iodine products, steroids or other antihistamines may be given several days before the scan or may be given intravenously during the scan.
➤ Withhold food and fluids for at least 4 hours before the procedure if contrast dye is used.
➤ Inform client the CT scan takes 30 minutes to 1 1/2 hours.
➤ Explain that the procedure is painless, but a feeling of warmth from the contrast medium (if used) may be

felt. Sometimes mild nausea may also be experienced.

► If ordered, insert an indwelling urethral catheter or rectal catheter as a landmark prior to the procedure.

► Assess the client for claustrophobic tendencies. Discuss with the primary health care provider the need for and benefit of sedation.

Perform Procedure

Nurses do not perform this procedure, but should understand the process to prepare the client. Assist the client into a supine position with head secured and resting on a head rest on a motorized handling table. Remind client to lie still as the table slowly advances through the circular opening of the scanner. Advise client they will hear loud banging or clicking noises as the scanner revolves to take pictures at different angles.

Contrast media is injected (if required) after one set of pictures is taken, and the scan is repeated. Observe client for anaphylaxis (rash, respiratory difficulty, hypotension, tachycardia, anxiety). Assure suction and an emesis basin are available if vomiting should occur.

Care After Test

► Observe for signs of delayed allergic reaction (if contrast dye is used) such as skin rash, urticaria, headache, or vomiting. Administer oral antihistamines if ordered. Allergic reactions may occur up to 6 hours after the procedure.

► Remove catheters from bladder and bowel if indicated.

► Encourage drinking fluids to counteract diuretic effect of contrast media (if indicated).

► Evaluate related tests such as serum creatinine, blood urea nitrogen (BUN), magnetic resonance imaging (MRI), serum and urine uric acid levels, and x-ray of kidney, ureters, bladder (KUB).

Educate Your Client and the Family

► Teach client the importance of adequate fluid intake, unless otherwise contraindicated, to help eliminate contrast material.

Computed Tomography Scan of Brain

kom pyoo ted • toe mog rah fee • skan
(CT Scan, CT, Computerized Axial Tomography, CAT, Computerized Transaxial Tomography, CTT, CATT, EMI [Electric Music Industries, Ltd.] Scan)

Normal Findings

Normal brain structure and blood flow

What This Test Will Tell You

This computer-assisted x-ray test provides three-dimensional images of the brain showing alterations in cerebral blood flow, breaks in the blood-brain barrier, and structural abnormalities of the brain. The scan is capable of producing images with greater detail than conventional x-rays. Soft tissues and organs are particularly well visualized with a computed tomography (CT) scan. It is the primary diagnostic test for stroke and is used for assessing the size, type, location, and extent of the lesion. This test is also important in diagnosing tumors, aneurysms, abscesses, ischemia, hematomas, and arteriovenous malformations, as well as abnormalities of the ventricles and cortex of the brain. Serial CT scans are helpful in monitoring pathology progression or healing.

CT angiography is being used experimentally, especially when intra-arterial angiography is contraindicated.

Abnormal Findings

Abnormalities may indicate stroke, infarction, hemorrhage, hematoma, tumor, cyst, edema, hydrocephalus, or brain atrophy.

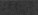 ACTION ALERT!

Assess client carefully for allergic reaction if contrast material is used for angiography. Symptoms include dyspnea, itching, urticaria, flushing, hypotension, and shock. Life-threatening anaphylactic reactions can occur and need to be recognized and treated immediately.

Interfering Factors

➤ Client movement during the scan will diminish quality of the images.
➤ Metal objects such as hairpins and clips, jewelry, glasses, and dental bridges will hinder visualization of the brain during the scan.

Contraindications

➤ Pregnancy, due to radiation exposure of the fetus
➤ Iodine or shellfish allergies unless alterations are made, such as antihistamines or steroid therapy several days before the procedure and/or during the procedure

➤ Unstable clients who may have sudden changes in their condition that make being inside the CT scanner dangerous
➤ Claustrophobia
➤ Extreme obesity (>300 pounds)

Potential Complications

➤ Allergic reaction, anaphylaxis
➤ Hypovolemia from diuresis associated with contrast material
➤ Renal failure related to contrast material

NURSING CONSIDERATIONS

Prepare Your Client

➤ Explain that this test is done to take excellent pictures of the brain to locate any problem areas if they exist.
➤ Assess the client for allergies to iodine, seafood, and contrast medium.
➤ Evaluate the client for restlessness. Clients unable to remain still 30–90 minutes during the scan may need a sedative.
➤ Ensure an informed consent has been obtained if contrast medium is used.
➤ Remove metal objects such as jewelry, hairpins, glasses, and dental bridges from the head and neck before the procedure.
➤ Restrict food and fluids for 8 hours before the scan if contrast medium is injected.
➤ Do not restrict food, fluids, or medications when contrast medium is not used for the scan.

Perform Procedure

Nurses do not perform this procedure, but should understand the process to explain it to the client. The CT scanner is a large cylinder with a table in the center. The client will be strapped to the table and the cylindrical scanner will revolve around them. Advise client that clicking noises will be heard during the scan. The client is placed supine on a table with the head stabilized securely. The x-ray scanner takes multiple images at different angles during the test. Assure client that radiology personnel will be in a control room where they can observe and talk to the client throughout the procedure.

Inform the client that a contrast medium to enhance the images may be injected through an intravenous (IV) line. Warn client that when the contrast medium is injected, they may experience a warm, flushed feeling, a salty or metallic taste, or nausea for 1–2 minutes. Administer the IV contrast medium through the IV. Observe for allergic reaction such as nausea, vomiting, palpitations, dyspnea, dizziness, tachycardia, hypotension, or itching.

Care After Test
➤ Assess the client for delayed allergic reactions to the contrast medium such as skin rash, itching, headache, dyspnea, and vomiting. An oral anti-histamine may be given for mild reactions.
➤ Encourage drinking fluids to prevent dehydration resulting from the diuretic effect of the contrast medium.
➤ Observe the IV site for redness, tenderness, and edema.
➤ Assess the client for pain. Neck and back pain may be aggravated by lying on the table during the scan. A pain medication may be administered after the scan if needed.
➤ Evaluate related tests such as magnetic resonance imaging (MRI), x-rays, cerebral angiography, and radiologic studies.

Educate Your Client and the Family
➤ Explain that this procedure takes a series of black-and-white pictures of the brain at different angles to evaluate all the parts of the brain, looking for both normal and abnormal structures.
➤ Hypertension is the most important risk factor for stroke. Educate your client to take antihypertensive medications if this is a risk factor for them.

Contraction Stress Test
kun trak shun • stress • test
(CST, Oxytocin Challenge Test, OCT, CST with Breast Self-Stimulation Test, BSST, Nipple Stimulation Contraction Stress Test, NSCST)

Normal Findings
PREGNANT CLIENT
Fetal heart rate should increase. An unchanged or decreased rate is an abnormal finding.

What This Test Will Tell You
This electrodiagnostic contraction stress test monitors high-risk pregnancies. The test measures the placental oxygen and carbon dioxide

exchange that occurs during a contraction when uterine blood flow is diminished. If the respiratory function is adequate, placental-fetal oxygen transfer will not be compromised. A positive test indicates possible compromised placental reserves, increasing the risk of perinatal morbidity and mortality.

During the test, uterine contractions are stimulated by a strictly controlled infusion of oxytocin. An alternative method is manual nipple stimulation, which signals the hypothalamus to trigger the release of oxytocin from the posterior pituitary gland. This may be attempted before oxytocin infusion. An electronic fetal monitor is used to record uterine activity and fetal heart rate (FHR). Contractions are stimulated until the client experiences three contractions in a 10-minute period with each contraction lasting 40–60 seconds. During the contraction, the fetal heart rate is observed for late or Type II decelerations; that is, the fetal heart rate decreases significantly after the peak of the contraction and does not recover until 15 seconds or more following the contraction. This finding is indicative of uteroplacental insufficiency with placental reserve being inadequate to prevent hypoxic insult to the fetus during the contraction.

This is not a routine test for all pregnant clients, but is used in the event of certain maternal disorders, including diabetes mellitus, hypertensive disorders, hemoglobinopathies, heart disease, Rh isoimmunization, hyperthyroidism, and chronic renal disease. It may also be prescribed for evaluation of fetal intrauterine growth retardation (IUGR), postmature fetus (>40 weeks gestation), abnormal estriol values, and women with a history of stillbirths.

Abnormal Findings

Positive results (persistent and consistent late decelerations of the FHR which occur with more than 50% of the contractions) may indicate fetoplacental inadequacy.

Suspicious results (late decelerations of the FHR which occur with less than 50% of the contractions following establishment of desired contraction pattern) may also indicate fetoplacental inadequacy.

Hyperstimulation (late deceleration of FHR with excessive uterine activity—contractions < every 2 minutes, lasting > 90 seconds or persistent increase in uterine tone) may indicate fetoplacental inadequacy.

Unsatisfactory results are contraction patterns that are inadequate or FHR tracings that are too poor to interpret; the test may be repeated later.

ACTION ALERT!

Decelerations of fetal heart rate must be reported to the primary health care provider immediately and warrant other studies such as amniocentesis or fetal ultrasound to determine if delivery should be hastened.

Interfering Factors

➤ Morbid obesity can interfere with monitoring.

➤ Hypotension can cause a false positive.

➤ Vena cava compression due to maternal supine position can cause hypotension.

➤ Excessive maternal or fetal activity can interfere with monitor recording.

➤ Polyhydramnios can interfere with monitoring.

➤ Maternal medications that depress sympathetic and parasympathetic nervous system can depress the FHR.

Contraindications

➤ History of vertical or classical cesarean section(s), due to threat of uterine rupture
➤ Incompetent cervix
➤ Less than 32–34 weeks gestation
➤ Multiple pregnancy
➤ Partial placental abruption(s); evidence of transplacental bleeding as Rh isoimmunization
➤ Placenta previa
➤ Premature rupture of the membranes

Potential Complications

➤ Premature labor
➤ Uterine hyperstimulation (uterine contractions lasting more than 90 seconds or more frequent than every 2 minutes)
➤ Abruptio placenta
➤ Premature delivery resulting in fetal morbidity

NURSING CONSIDERATIONS

Prepare Your Client

➤ Explain that this test is done to see how well the baby is supplied with oxygen through the mother's blood system and the umbilical cord.
➤ Ensure that an informed consent is obtained, because of the possible complications associated with this procedure.
➤ The client may be advised to eat lightly or not at all in case labor is stimulated.
➤ Tell the client that the test will be conducted on an outpatient basis in a birthing center or a labor and delivery unit in case labor is stimulated. Tell the client that the procedure takes about 1.5–2 hours.

➤ Have the client void before the procedure.
➤ Take vital signs and FHR for baseline data.
➤ Encourage breathing and relaxation techniques during contractions to control any discomfort.
➤ Encourage client to avoid moving and frequent turning, especially during a contraction.

Perform Procedure

➤ The test is conducted by nurses prepared to administer a CST or NSCST and to use a fetal monitor.
➤ Instruct the client to disrobe from the waist down with a sheet for cover.
➤ Place the client during the procedure in a semi-Fowler's position and slightly to her left side to prevent interference with circulation. A reclining chair or birthing bed may be used.
➤ Attach a fetal monitor to record the FHR and contractions. Place a transducer on the abdomen over the fetal back or chest to record the FHR and a tocodynamometer at the uterine fundus to record uterine activity.
➤ Record the FHR and uterine activity for 20–30 minutes for baseline data. If three spontaneous uterine contractions lasting 40–60 seconds occur during this period, oxytocin stimulation will not be needed.
➤ Apply fundal pressure toward the client's feet to check for cord compression. This technique, the Hillis procedure, will cause cord compression as the fetal chin pushes against the chest. The FHR will drop and then return to normal when pressure is released; if cord compression does not occur, there will be no change in FHR.
➤ Prepare for possible vaginal exam to check for cervical effacement and

dilatation.

➤ Instruct the client to gently massage a breast nipple for 15–30 minutes. The desired duration, frequency and intensity (moderate) of uterine contractions usually will occur within 15 minutes; nipple stimulation should cease during a contraction and continue after 5 minutes. The process continues until desired number of contractions have occurred. If not successful with one breast, stimulation of the alternate breast is attempted.

➤ Perform a venipuncture for administration of an intravenous infusion and oxytocin via infusion pump if NSCST is not used or not effective. The oxytocin will be increased in small increments every 15–30 minutes according to hospital protocol until desired duration, frequency, and intensity of uterine contractions occur.

➤ Monitor blood pressure recording every 10 minutes for hypotension.

➤ The physician, certified nurse-midwife (CNM), or other advanced practice nurse will be advised of the outcome of the test.

➤ Place the graphic monitor strip in the client's prenatal record.

Care After Test

➤ Continue monitoring fetal heart rate for 30 minutes after test is completed and nipple stimulation or oxytocin administration has been discontinued to observe for uterine contractions until oxytocin is metabolized by the body.

➤ Discontinue IV, if used, and assess site.

➤ In the event that premature labor is stimulated, client may be admitted to labor and delivery unit for labor care or administered tocolytic drugs to inhibit labor.

➤ In the event the test is positive, the physician or advanced practice nurse will decide whether to conduct additional diagnostic tests and/or to proceed with delivery of the fetus, vaginally or by cesarean section.

➤ Review related tests such as the fetal movement count, biophysical profile, estriol level, and cord pH.

Educate Your Client and the Family

➤ Explain to the client that the test may be repeated weekly, if indicated, until the end of the pregnancy.

➤ If the test is negative, instruct the client to notify her primary health care provider if she experiences labor contractions or pains that occur at regular intervals and increase in intensity or amount of pain, her water breaks, or she has sudden intense abdominal pain.

➤ If the test is positive, explain to the client that the primary health care provider will meet with her to discuss the options that are best for her and her baby.

Coombs' Test, Direct and Indirect

kooms • test • di rekt • and • in di rekt

(Direct and Indirect Antiglobulin Test, Cross-Matching)

Normal Findings

Negative, or without agglutination

What This Test Will Tell You

The direct Coombs' test identifies the presence of antibodies against red blood cells to make a differential diagnosis of anemia or to confirm transfusion reactions. The indirect Coombs' test is used to cross-match blood for transfusion, identify sensitization in an Rh-negative mother, or diagnose a transfusion reaction and hemolytic anemia. Antibodies against red blood cells (RBCs) may cause a hemolytic anemia. The direct Coombs' test mixes the client's washed RBCs with Coombs' serum. Coombs' serum contains antibodies against RBC antibodies. The indirect test involves mixing donor with recipient blood. If RBC antibodies form, the Coombs' serum reacts with them, resulting in agglutination.

Abnormal Findings

Positive results (direct test: trace to 4+, indirect test: titer > 1:10) may reveal hemolytic disease in newborns (HDN, or erythroblastosis fetalis), autoimmune hemolytic anemia, lymphoma, sepsis, systemic lupus erythematosus, mycoplasmal infection, infectious mononucleosis, or transfusion reaction.

ACTION ALERT!

➤ Positive agglutination in a pregnant woman who is Rh-negative may indicate that the fetus is Rh-positive. Assessment of the fetus with ultrasound, amniocentesis, or delta optical density testing may provide information about fetal well-being. Treatment for a compromised pregnancy may include intrauterine transfusions to the fetus, early delivery, and exchange transfusion of the neonate after delivery.

➤ Moderately or strongly positive test results in a newborn may be indicative of hemolytic disease in newborns (HDN). Transfusion with compatible Rh-negative blood may be necessary to prevent a life-threatening anemia. The fetus or neonate with Rh incompatibility is also at risk for congestive heart failure, fetal hydrops (ascites and subcutaneous edema), hydramnios, and for the fetus, intrauterine death.

➤ If a transfusion reaction is suspected, stop the transfusion immediately. Maintain patency of the venous line by infusing normal saline at least at a minimal rate.

➤ The Rh-negative (Rh–) client with evidence of fetal Rh-positive (Rh+) blood in her circulatory system will need an injection of $Rh_o(D)$immune globulin (RhoGAM) within 72 hours of delivery to prevent maternal isoimmunization.

Interfering Factors

➤ Trauma during venipuncture or rough handling of the specimen may produce RBC hemolysis and interfere with test results.

➤ Some medications that may cause false positive results are ampicillin, dipyrone, diphenylhydantoin, hydralazine, indomethacin, isoniazid, insulin, methyldopa, phenytoin, procainamide, captopril, cephalosporins, chlorpromazine, melphalan, mefenamic acid, quinidine, rifampin, streptomycin, sulfonamide, and tetracycline.

➤ Delay in testing of the sample may result in erroneous results. For accuracy, the Coombs' test must be performed within 24 hours of obtaining the blood sample.

NURSING CONSIDERATIONS

Prepare Your Client

➤ As indicated, explain that this test is to diagnose a lack of red blood cells called anemia, a blood reaction between the mother and baby, a reaction to donated and transfused blood, or to check compatibility with donated blood.

➤ Explain to new parents that a Coombs' test is performed on the newborn by obtaining a sample of blood from the umbilical cord, just minutes after birth. Explain to parents that this is not painful to the baby.

Perform Procedure

➤ Collect 7–10 mL of venous blood in each of two red-top tubes.

➤ If the client is a neonate, collect a sample from the umbilical cord after the cord has been clamped and cut. Collect the cord blood in either a red-top or lavender-top tube.

Care After Test

➤ Observe the client for signs and symptoms of anemia including pallor, dyspnea, chest pain, and fatigue.

➤ Encourage rest periods for client experiencing fatigue related to anemia.

➤ Evaluate client's ability to perform activities of daily living.

➤ Obtain a dietary consult to assist the client and family in choosing a well-balanced diet, including foods high in iron and vitamin B_{12}.

➤ Monitor closely for signs and symptoms of blood incompatibility including chills, fever, urticaria, tachycardia, dyspnea, nausea, vomiting, tightness in the chest, chest and back pain, hypotension, bronchospasm, angioedema, pulmonary edema, congestive heart failure, and shock. If a transfusion reaction is suspected, maintain a patent venous line for medication and fluid administration if necessary.

➤ Administer Rh_o (D) immune globulin to the Rh-negative (Rh–) client with evidence of fetal Rh-positive (Rh+) blood in her circulatory system within 72 hours of abortion or delivery.

➤ Apply an umbilical clamp to the umbilical cord immediately after obtaining a cord blood sample from a neonate.

➤ Review related tests such as hemoglobin, hematocrit, reticulocyte count, red blood cell indices, hemoglobin electrophoresis, ferritin level, total iron-binding capacity (TIBC), bone marrow and liver biopsies, and iron absorption and excretion studies.

Educate Your Client and the Family

➤ Explain to the client or family that positive test results will likely require additional testing for more definitive diagnosis or monitoring of the identified anemia.

➤ If treatment for an anemia or hemolytic process identified by Coombs' testing is to include transfusion of blood components, explain to the client or family why blood transfusion is indicated in this case.

➤ If a hemolytic process is identified, explain other treatments or assessments the client will receive.

Copper, Urine
cop pur • yur in

Normal Findings
15–60 µg/24 hours (SI units: 0.2–1.0 µmol/24 hours)
Values are the same for all ages.

What This Test Will Tell You
This urine test is used primarily to diagnose Wilson's disease, an autosomal recessive disorder. This test measures the urine level of copper, which is an essential trace element. Small amounts of free copper are present in urine and plasma. Most copper in plasma is bound to and transported by ceruloplasmin, which is a plasma protein. Wilson's disease is an inborn error in metabolism, an inherited disorder, characterized by decreased ceruloplasmin, increased urinary excretion of copper, and accumulation of copper in the interstitial tissues of the liver and brain.

Abnormal Findings
▲ INCREASED LEVELS may indicate Wilson's disease, chronic active hepatitis, biliary cirrhosis, rheumatoid arthritis, or nephrotic syndrome.
▼ DECREASED LEVELS may indicate protein malnutrition.

ACTION ALERT!
If one family member has been diagnosed with Wilson's disease, all members of the family should be screened for possible diagnosis.

Interfering Factors
➤ Failure to collect all urine during the 24-hour collection period.
➤ Urine must be collected in a metal-free container or levels will be falsely increased.

➤ Administration of D-penicillamine causes elevated urine levels of copper.

NURSING CONSIDERATIONS
Prepare Your Client
➤ Explain that this test measures levels of copper in the urine and is used to diagnose Wilson's disease, a disease that one is born with and that can be passed on in families.
➤ Explain the procedure for collecting a 24-hour urine specimen.
➤ Obtain a 24-hour urine collection container, metal-free.

Perform Procedure
➤ Closely follow the procedure for 24-hour urine collection, using a metal-free container.
➤ If collection is performed on an infant, observe the urine collection bag frequently to assure patency of device so that urine is not lost from the collection.

Care After Test
➤ For collections involving infants, remove collection bag carefully at the end of the collection and assess the perineal area thoroughly for breakdown. Treat area accordingly.
➤ Client diagnosed with Wilson's disease is started on chelating therapy with either D-penicillamine or trientine to reduce copper levels. These agents remove excess copper from the body. Vitamin B_6 should be administered along with these agents to prevent vitamin deficiency.
➤ Client who does not respond to chelating therapy may be considered for liver transplantation.

> Review related tests such as liver enzyme levels and liver biopsy results.

Educate Your Client and the Family

> Explain that a liver biopsy may be needed to confirm the diagnosis.

> If diagnosis of Wilson's disease is confirmed, stress importance of screening other family members and compliance with medical therapy to prevent complications. Lifelong follow-up with a gastroenterologist specializing in treatment of this disease is required.

> Instruct family and client on the lifelong need for medication therapy to prevent accumulation of copper.

> Instruct family to avoid foods high in copper such as shellfish, nuts, liver, chocolate, and mushrooms.

Cortisol, Serum

kore ti zahl • see rum
(Hydrocortisone, Blood Serum)

Normal Findings

ADULT AND ELDERLY
8 A.M. 6–28 µg/dL (SI units: 170–760 nmol/L)
4 P.M. 2–18 µg/dL (SI units: 50–490 nmol/L)
PREGNANT
Increased cortisol levels
NEWBORN
1–24 µg/dL (SI units: 30–670 nmol/L)
CHILD
8 A.M. 15–25 µg/dL (SI units: 450–750 nmol/L)
4 P.M. 5–10 µg/dL (SI units: 150–300 nmol/L)

What This Test Will Tell You

This blood test helps diagnose Cushing's disease, Cushing's syndrome, Addison's disease, and secondary adrenal insufficiency. The test measures the function of the adrenal cortex, which makes glucocorticoids. Cortisol, the most potent of the glucocorticoids, inhibits the effects of insulin and decreases the rate of glucose use by the cells. Cortisol also helps the body respond to stress and regulates the immune system.

Normal cortisol levels show a biphasic pattern with the early morning level being $1/2$ to $2/3$ higher than the 4 P.M. level. Persons with Cushing's syndrome and/or those under stress lose this biphasic pattern. If the client is a night-shift worker and sleeps during the day, these times may not be accurate.

Abnormal Findings

▲INCREASED LEVELS may indicate Cushing's syndrome, adrenal adenoma, ectopic ACTH-producing tumor, obesity, stress, hyperthyroidism, hyperpituitarism, or liver disease.

▼DECREASED LEVELS may indicate Addison's disease, hypopituitarism, or hypothyroidism.

Interfering Factors

> Some medications such as glucocorticoids, androgens, and phenytoin may decrease cortisol levels.

➤ Some medications such as estrogens, oral contraceptives, and spironolactone may elevate levels.

➤ Stress and recent exercise may increase levels even in the absence of disease.

➤ Recent radioisotope scan (within 1 week of blood sampling).

➤ Hemolysis of sample.

NURSING CONSIDERATIONS

Prepare Your Client

➤ Explain that this test is given to make sure that the glands responsible for making cortisol are functioning properly. Explain that cortisol helps regulate the immune system, helps convert proteins, carbohydrates, and fats into forms the body can use, and helps the body handle stress.

➤ Instruct client to maintain normal salt intake for at least 3 days before the test.

➤ Tell client not to exercise, but to limit activity for 12 hours prior to testing.

➤ Assess for emotional stress from life events.

➤ Consult with the primary health care provider about withholding medications such as estrogens, androgens, and phenytoin for 48 hours before the test. If these must be administered, note them on the lab slip.

➤ Keep the client free of stress and lying down for at least 30 minutes prior to sampling.

➤ Report infections, colds, and other acute illnesses to primary health care provider, as these may affect results.

Perform Procedure

➤ Delay the blood collection if the client was unable to receive adequate sleep during the prior night.

➤ Perform a venipuncture at 8 A.M. and place 7–10 mL of venous blood in a red- or green-top tube.

➤ Perform a venipuncture at 4 P.M. and place 7–10 mL of venous blood in a red- or green-top tube.

Care After Test

➤ Refer client to counseling or social services for problems in their lives which are causing undue stress.

➤ For obese client, refer to a registered dietician for weight-loss diet.

➤ Assess for other signs and symptoms of endocrine imbalance, including weight change, Cushingoid features, hyperglycemia, poor wound healing, and thin, shiny skin.

➤ Obtain dietary consult from a registered dietician to optimize nutritional status and minimize complications associated with altered function of the integumentary system and weight gain.

➤ Evaluate related tests such as ACTH levels, liver function tests, and thyroid function tests.

Educate Your Client and the Family

➤ Discuss the effects of too much cortisol, including altered body weight, altered body shape, moon-face, elevated blood sugar, slow healing, and skin thinning.

➤ Teach client relaxation techniques.

Cortisol, Urine Free
kor ti zahl • yur in • free

Normal Findings
ADULT AND ELDERLY
10–100 µg/24 hours (SI units: 26–260 nmol/24 hours)
PREGNANT
Increased cortisol levels
CHILD
2–27 µg/24 hours (SI units: 5–67.5 nmol/24 hours)
ADOLESCENT
5–55 µg/24 hours (SI units: 12–137 nmol/24 hours)

What This Test Will Tell You
This 24-hour urine test is one of the best tools for diagnosing Cushing's syndrome. The test measures the function of the adrenal cortex, which makes glucocorticoids. Cortisol, the most potent of the glucocorticoids, inhibits the effects of insulin and decreases the rate of glucose use by the cells.

Normal cortisol levels show a biphasic pattern with the early morning level being $1/2$ to $2/3$ higher than the 4 P.M. level. Persons with Cushing's syndrome and/or those under stress lose this biphasic pattern. The advantage of measuring urine-free cortisol levels is that the diurnal variations are eliminated and an average determination can be assessed.

Abnormal Findings
▲INCREASED LEVELS may indicate Cushing's syndrome, adrenal adenoma, ectopic ACTH-producing tumor, stress, hyperthyroidism, or hyperpituitarism.

Interfering Factors
➤ Some medications such as steroid therapy, reserpine, phenothiazines, morphine, amphetamines, oral contraceptives, and spironolactone may increase free cortisol levels.
➤ Stress, pregnancy, and recent exercise may increase levels even in the absence of disease.

NURSING CONSIDERATIONS
Prepare Your Client
➤ Explain that this test is given to make sure that the glands responsible for making cortisol are functioning properly. Explain that cortisol helps regulate the immune system, helps convert proteins, carbohydrates, and fats into forms the body can use, and helps the body handle stress.
➤ Obtain 24-hour urine container, with preservative.
➤ Caution the client to urinate into a urinal or other collection device. Urinating directly into the container may make the urine splash out.
➤ Instruct client to maintain normal salt intake for at least 3 days before the test.
➤ Tell client not to exercise, but to limit activity during urine collection period.
➤ Assess for emotional stress from life events.
➤ Consult with the primary health care provider about withholding medications which may affect results. If these must be administered, note them on the lab slip.

➤ Encourage client to consume adequate fluids.

Perform Procedure
➤ Closely follow procedure for 24-hour urine collection. Keep the urine collection on ice or refrigerated throughout the collection period.

Care After Test
➤ Refer client to counseling or social services for problems in their lives which are causing undue stress.
➤ For obese client, refer to a registered dietician for weight-loss diet.
➤ Assess for other signs and symptoms of endocrine imbalance, including weight change, Cushingoid features, hyperglycemia, poor wound healing, and thin, shiny skin.
➤ Obtain dietary consult from a registered dietician to optimize nutritional status and minimize complications associated with altered function of the integumentary system and weight gain.
➤ Evaluate related tests such as ACTH levels, liver function tests, and thyroid function tests.

Educate Your Client and the Family
➤ Discuss the effects of too much cortisol, including altered body weight, altered body shape, elevated blood sugar, slow healing, and skin thinning.
➤ Teach client relaxation techniques.

C-Reactive Protein
see • ree ak tiv • proe teen
(CRP)

Normal Findings
Negative: less than 0.8 mg/dL

What This Test Will Tell You
This blood test is a nonspecific marker of tissue inflammation or injury used to diagnose various inflammatory processes. CRP is produced in the liver and rapidly released in response to inflammation or tissue destruction. It is absent from the blood of healthy clients. CRP levels rise in response to bacterial infections, but are lower in viral infections. Levels fall as inflammation disappears and injured tissues heal.

CRP is most useful in detecting flare-ups of rheumatic fever and rheumatic arthritis before severe symptoms and tissue damage occurs. Falls in CRP herald improvement. CRP may also be useful in detecting occult surgical wound infection or transplant rejection. In uncomplicated postoperative cases, levels normally fall in 4 days.

CRP and erythrocyte sedimentation rate (ESR), both nonspecific markers of inflammation, are usually drawn together. CRP levels rise more quickly than the ESR, within 4–20 hours of tissue inflammation or damage, and fall more rapidly when the client improves. Unlike the ESR, the CRP level is not influenced by changes in the hematocrit.

Abnormal Findings

▲ INCREASED LEVELS may indicate bacterial infections, pneumococcal pneumonia, rheumatic fever, rheumatic arthritis, systemic lupus erythematosus, myocardial infarction, cancer, wound infection, tuberculosis, Crohn's disease, or transplanted organ rejection.

▼ DECREASED LEVELS may indicate positive response to therapy.

███████ ACTION ALERT!

A rise in CRP indicates tissue damage or inflammation.

Interfering Factors

➤ Levels decrease and may disappear with administration of steroids and salicylates.

➤ Pregnancy, oral contraceptives, and intrauterine devices can cause false elevations.

NURSING CONSIDERATIONS

Prepare Your Client

➤ Tell your client that this test will help detect inflamed or damaged tissue in the body.

➤ Withhold food and all fluids except water for 4–12 hours before venous sampling. Check with your laboratory for specific guidelines based on methods used.

➤ Collaborate with the primary health care provider regarding restrictions of medications that may affect test results.

Perform Procedure

➤ Collect 7–10 mL of venous blood in a red-top tube.

➤ Protect from heat, which can damage specimen.

Care After Test

➤ Monitor temperature and white blood cell count for signs of an infection.

➤ Assess client for joint pain, redness, swelling, or limited mobility.

➤ Carefully assess surgical incisions and wounds for erythema, swelling, induration, or purulent drainage.

➤ Review chart for recent steroid or salicylate administration.

➤ Evaluate related tests such as the ESR, which will remain elevated even after the CRP decreases.

Educate Your Client and the Family

➤ Teach your client and the family that CRP rises as an inflammatory process worsens and falls as healing occurs. It is helpful in monitoring success of therapy.

➤ Ask client to avoid taking aspirin (salicylates) or other anti-inflammatory drugs such as ibuprofen and even acetaminophen, which may lower levels, unless they have been specifically prescribed by the primary health care provider. Tell them that many over-the-counter drugs contain these anti-inflammatory medications, so they shouldn't take any medication without first consulting with their primary health care provider.

Creatinine Clearance

kree **at** in in • **kleer** ens

(12- or 24-hour Urine Creatinine Clearance, Cr-Cl)

Normal Findings

ADULT

Varies according to lean body mass, so muscular people are found at higher limits of ranges.

Male:

70–150 mL/minute

90 mL/minute/1.73 m^2 of body surface (SI units: 1.50 mL/second/1.73 m^2)

Female:

85–130 mL/minute

84 mL/minute/1.73 m^2 (SI units: 2.04 mL/second/1.73 m^2)

PREGNANT

150–200 mL/minute

Glomerular filtration rate may increase up to 50%.

INFANT

40–65 mL/minute

ADOLESCENT AND CHILD

84–90 mL/minute

Values tend to increase with growth, because values reflect muscle mass.

ELDERLY

Values tend to decline up to 30% even in the absence of renal disease. This is reflective of declining glomerular filtration rate, 6.5 mL/minute/decade after age 50.

What This Test Will Tell You

This urine and serum test evaluates renal function and quantifies the degree of any impairment. This test is the most specific determinant of renal function. The creatinine clearance rate is equivalent to the glomerular filtration rate (GFR) because all the creatinine filtered over a defined period appears in the urine. By definition, "clearance" is the amount of creatinine removed from the blood in 1 minute, independent of the urine flow rate. Thus, this test requires the measurement of the serum creatinine level, the urine creatinine level, and the urine volume. The urine volume is collected over 12 or 24 hours.

The creatinine clearance test detects renal impairment earlier than the serum creatinine test because serum creatinine levels remain normal until the creatinine clearance is less than half of normal.

Abnormal Findings

▲ INCREASED LEVELS may indicate hypertension (renovascular), hypothyroidism, or strenuous exercise.

▼ DECREASED LEVELS may indicate mild to severe renal impairment, acute tubular necrosis, glomerulonephritis, pyelonephritis, shock (cardiogenic or hypovolemic), amyotrophic lateral sclerosis (ALS), renal artery obstruction, renal vein thrombosis, nephrotoxic drug toxicity, dehydration, polycystic kidney disease, congestive heart failure, renal tuberculosis, hyperthyroidism, or muscular dystrophy.

ACTION ALERT!

A creatinine clearance less than 10 mL/min indicates severe renal impairment. Creatinine clearance levels should be checked **prior** to administering any nephrotoxic, anticancer, or antibiotic drugs.

Interfering Factors

➤ Phenacetin, androgens, anabolic steroids, and thiazide diuretics reduce creatinine clearance.

➤ Strenuous physical exercise and/or a high-protein diet may increase creatinine excretion.

➤ Inaccurate urine collection will falsify test results.

➤ Ascorbic acid, steroids, chemotherapeutic agents, cimetidine, amphotericin B, thiazide diuretics, furosemide, aminoglycosides, cephalosporins, clonidine, dextran, doxycycline, and levodopa may increase creatinine clearance.

➤ Creatinine will decompose if the urine specimen is not refrigerated during the collection period.

➤ Blood, feces, toilet paper, and stool in the urine will invalidate the results.

NURSING CONSIDERATIONS

Prepare Your Client

➤ Explain that this test is important to help understand how well the kidneys are working.

➤ Instruct the client to avoid excessive exercise and meat, poultry, and fish consumption for 8 hours before the test and during the collection period.

➤ Unless otherwise indicated, encourage client to drink plenty of fluids.

➤ Explain how to correctly save urine during the timed collection period.

Perform Procedure

➤ Obtain a clean, 3-L, 12- or 24-hour urine bottle.

➤ Carefully follow guidelines for timed urine collection testing.

➤ Keep the urine specimen refrigerated or the urine drainage bag (for catheterized client) on ice.

➤ Offer fluids except caffeinated beverages regularly to encourage adequate urine output.

➤ Collect 7 mL of venous blood for serum creatinine in a red-top tube the same day as the 12- or 24-hour urine collection is completed.

Care After Test

➤ Compare urine specimen quantity in collection container with urine output recorded for the test period. If the specimen quantity is less than the urine amount recorded, the test results are invalid.

➤ Document quantity of urine output, starting and ending times of urine collection, and any interfering factors on the lab requisition.

➤ Consult with a registered dietician to assist the family and client in meeting special dietary needs.

➤ Evaluate all medications of client who has renal impairment for possible nephrotoxicity or the danger of failure to metabolize and excrete drugs. Collaborate with the primary health care provider as needed to evaluate and modify pharmacologic therapy.

➤ Evaluate other renal tests such as blood urea nitrogen (BUN), serum and urine uric acid levels, cyclic adenosine monophosphate (cAMP), serum and urine electrolytes, and urea clearance.

Educate Your Client and the Family

➤ If the client is in end-stage renal failure, explain that eating large quantities of fish, meat, and poultry can increase serum creatinine levels.

➤ If the client is in end-stage renal failure, stress the importance of regularly scheduled exercise. Regular exercise minimizes fluctuations in serum creatinine levels that occur with increased muscle work from heavy exercise.

➤ Educate client and family on foods that are high in restricted electrolytes or protein, if renal impairment exists.

Creatinine Phosphokinase
kree at in in • fos foe kin ase
(CPK, Creatine Kinase, CK)

Normal Findings
(Note: different methods give different ranges. Check with your laboratory.)
ADULT
Levels are for total CPK.
Male: 40–175 U/L
Female: 30–140 U/L
PREGNANT
Levels are low early in pregnancy, but rise during last trimester.
NEWBORN
68–580 U/L
CHILD
Male: 56–185 U/L
Female: 35–145 U/L
ADOLESCENT
Male: 35–185 U/L
Female: 20–100 U/L

Isoenzymes: CPK-MM (CPK$_3$): 100% or 5–70 U/L
CPK-MB (CPK$_2$): 0% or 0–7 U/L
CPK-BB (CPK$_1$): 0% or undetectable

What This Test Will Tell You
This blood test helps in the diagnosis of muscular diseases or trauma as well as myocardial infarction (MI). Less often it is used to monitor therapy in prostate, breast, and lung cancer. The test measures the blood levels of CPK as well as its three isoenzymes. CPK is an enzyme found mostly in skeletal muscle, heart muscle, and brain tissue, where it plays an important role in energy production inside cells. If cells are damaged by injury or disease, these enzymes are released and can be detected in the blood. Specific isoenzymes reflect specific tissues. Because CPK and its isoenzymes are found almost exclusively in only a few tissues, elevations in levels are helpful in diagnosing diseases and trauma to muscles, the brain, and the heart. Small amounts of CPK-BB is found in the brain, lungs, gastrointestinal and genitourinary systems.

Elevated CPK-MB isoenzyme levels are highly diagnostic of myocardial infarctions and cardiac trauma. These levels do not rise with non-ischemic chest pain, angina, or congestive heart failure.

Abnormal Findings
▲ INCREASED TOTAL LEVELS may indicate acute myocardial infarction, hypokalemia, cerebral vascular accident and infarction, alcoholism, chest trauma, head trauma, muscular dystrophy, polymyositis, cardioversion or electrical shock, or pulmonary infarction.
▼ DECREASED TOTAL LEVELS may indicate early pregnancy.
▲ INCREASED LEVELS *of CPK-MM*

Use of CPK-MB in Detection and Diagnosis of Myocardial Infarction

Enzyme	Detectable in serum	Peak	Duration
CPK-MB	2–6 hours following onset of myocardial infarction	12–36 hours following onset of myocardial infarction	24–72 hours

may indicate surgery, muscular dystrophy, multiple trauma associated with crush injuries, electrical shock, electroconvulsive therapy, hypokalemia, hypothyroidism, dermatomyositis, hemophilia, or recent intramuscular injection.

▲INCREASED LEVELS *of CPK-MB* may indicate myocardial infarction 4–6 hours after injury, cardiac surgery, cardioversion, cardiopulmonary resuscitation, Reye's syndrome, poliomyositis, malignant hyperthermia, or rhabdomyolysis.

▲INCREASED LEVELS *of CPK-BB* may indicate pulmonary infarction, chest trauma, biliary atresia, head trauma, cerebrovascular accident, severe shock syndrome, seizures, brain cancer, lung cancer, breast cancer, or prostate cancer.

ACTION ALERT!

Elevations in CPK-MB and CPK-BB isoenzymes can signify serious injuries or disease processes involving heart or brain tissues. More than 5% CPK-MB 4–24 hours following cardiac symptoms may be diagnostic of a myocardial infarction.

Interfering Factors

➤ Increased relative muscle mass
➤ Vigorous exercise
➤ Intramuscular injections
➤ Hypothermia accompanied by prolonged shivering
➤ Convulsions
➤ Recent surgery
➤ Cardioversion
➤ Lung disease/infection accompanied by severe coughing
➤ Alcohol
➤ Pregnancy
➤ Childbirth
➤ Medications such as antibiotics, anticoagulants, morphine, aspirin, and lithium
➤ Hemolysis of sample
➤ Refrigeration of blood sample
➤ Timing of sampling if it misses rises in isoenzymes

NURSING CONSIDERATIONS

Prepare Your Client

➤ Explain that this test is important in the diagnosis of diseases of the muscles and brain, as well as heart damage. Tailor this explanation to the specific reason the test was ordered for your client.

➤ Determine as exactly as possible the onset of chest pain in client being evaluated for myocardial infarction.

➤ Explain that you will need to draw blood from the vein for the test. Explain the venipuncture process clearly.

➤ Tell the client there is no need to restrict fluid or food before the test, but there should be no strenuous exercise for 24 hours preceding the test.

➤ If this test is being done to evaluate CPK-MB isoenzymes for myocardial infarction, explain that multiple blood samples over time will be necessary to follow the rise and fall of the blood levels.

Perform Procedure

➤ Perform a venipuncture to collect 7 mL of venous blood in a red-top tube.

➤ Send the sample to the laboratory immediately. Do not refrigerate.

➤ If serial isoenzymes are being evaluated for myocardial infarction, be sure that blood is drawn strictly by the schedule and sent for evaluation immediately.

➤ If the client has received an intramuscular injection within 24–48 hours of drawing enzymes, note this on the laboratory slip.

Care After Test

➤ Evaluate the client's history for coronary and vascular disease if the test is being done to help diagnose a myocardial infarction.

➤ Assess and collaborate with the primary health care provider to relieve the client's chest pain.

➤ Carefully evaluate vital signs and cardiovascular function if the client is being evaluated for heart disease.

➤ Evaluate other tests such as lactic dehydrogenase (LDH) and aspartate aminotransferase (SGOT or AST).

Educate Your Client and the Family

➤ Instruct client with suspected heart disease to notify the nurse or primary health care provider immediately if chest pain should occur or worsen.

Creatinine, Serum

kree **at** in in • see rum
(Serum Creatinine, Cr-bld)

Normal Findings

ADULT

Male: 0.6–1.5 mg/dL (SI units: 45–132 µmol/L)

Female: 0.5–1.1 mg/dL (SI units: 44–97 µmol/L)

Values tend to be greater in males because of greater muscle mass.

PREGNANT

Values are reduced, because creatinine clearance is often increased by as much as 50%.

NEWBORN

0.3–1.2 mg/dL (SI units: 26–105 µmol/L)

Creatinine crosses all membranes permeable to water, including placenta; therefore, serum creatinine levels in the mother and fetus are identical.

INFANT

0.2–0.4 mg/dL (SI units: 18–35 µmol/L)

CHILD

0.3–0.7 mg/dL (SI units: 26–61 µmol/L)

ADOLESCENT

0.5–1.0 mg/dL (SI units: 44–88 µmol/L)

Slight increases with age are proportional to body mass.

ELDERLY

Values are decreased, due to decreased muscle mass. A "normal" adult value may indicate renal impairment.

What This Test Will Tell You

This blood test is essential in the evaluation of renal function. The continuous breakdown of the high-energy compound creatinine-phosphate creates creatinine as a nonprotein waste product in skeletal muscle. Creatinine is constantly excreted by the kidneys. A significant increase in this value is only seen when a large number of kidney nephrons have been destroyed, resulting in impaired creatinine excretion.

Abnormal Findings

▲ INCREASED LEVELS may indicate impaired renal function, gigantism, acromegaly, essential hypertension, diabetic nephropathy, rhabdomyolysis, nephritis, urinary obstruction, shock, acute myocardial infarction, cancer, severe congestive heart failure, scleroderma, systemic lupus erythematosus, or testosterone therapy.

▼ DECREASED LEVELS may indicate pregnancy toxemia, muscular dystrophy, or myasthenia gravis.

ACTION ALERT!

Any value exceeding 4 mg/dL creatinine in blood may indicate serious impairment in renal function.

Interfering Factors

➤ A diet very high in meat products and fish may produce elevated levels.
➤ Medications that may elevate levels include cimetidine, chemotherapeutic drugs, cephalosporins, and aminoglycosides.
➤ Elevated levels may be associated with high levels of ascorbic acid, diuretics, lithium, barbiturates, some antibiotics, and methyldopa.
➤ Clients with early chronic renal failure may have normal results.

➤ Values are 20%–40% higher in late afternoon.
➤ Marijuana may decrease levels.
➤ Athletes with exceptionally high muscle mass may have elevated levels of creatinine and normal renal function.
➤ A phenolsulfonphthalein (PSP) test may increase the results if done within the preceding 24 hours.
➤ A bromosulfophthalein (BSP) test may decrease serum creatinine levels if done within the preceding 24 hours.
➤ Hyperglycemia and ketonuria may elevate results.

NURSING CONSIDERATIONS

Prepare Your Client

➤ Explain that this test is important to help understand how well the kidneys are working.

Perform Procedure

➤ Collect 5–7 mL of venous blood in a red-top tube (for newborn, draw blood from a heel stick).

Care After Test

➤ Assess fluid and nutritional status of client for clues of renal impairment and other diseases causing changes in creatinine levels.
➤ Continuously monitor fluid balance through daily weights and intake and output recordings.
➤ Evaluate for increased fluid volume manifested by edema, decreased urine output, neck vein distention, dyspnea, and hepatomegaly.
➤ Initiate safety precautions such as night lights for uremic client (creatinine greater than 7 mg/dL), because cognitive function may be impaired.
➤ For client with oliguria, carefully assess for cardiac dysrhythmias

because hyperkalemia is common. Institute continuous cardiac monitoring if serum potassium levels are elevated or dysrhythmias are noted.

➤ Consult with a registered dietician to assist the family and client in meeting special dietary needs.

➤ Evaluate other renal tests such as blood urea nitrogen (BUN), serum electrolytes, intravenous pyelogram, creatinine clearance, serum and uric acid levels, and urea clearance.

Educate Your Client and the Family

➤ If the client is in end-stage renal failure, explain that eating large amounts of fish, meat, and poultry can increase serum creatinine levels.

➤ If the client is in end-stage renal failure, stress the importance of regularly scheduled exercise. Regular exercise minimizes fluctuations in serum creatinine levels that occur with increased muscle work from heavy exercise.

Creatinine, Urine
kree at in in • yur in

Normal Findings

ADULT

Males: 0.8–2.0 g/24 hours (SI units: 6–14 mmol/24 hours)
Females: 0.6–1.8 grams/24 hours (SI units: 5–14 mmol/24 hours)
Values tend to be higher in males because of their greater muscle mass.

PREGNANT

Value may be elevated related to an increase in glomerular filtration rate.

NEWBORN

8–20 mg/kg/24 hours
The glomerular filtration rate reaches 30% of adult value within the first 2 days of extrauterine life.

CHILD

8–22 mg/kg/24 hours
The glomerular filtration rate attains full adult value about age 2.

ADOLESCENT

8–30 mg/kg/24 hours
Values tend to increase with growth, because values are proportional to muscle mass.

ELDERLY

Glomerular filtration rate decreases approximately 10% every 10 years after age 50. Values are also decreased due to the decreased muscle mass.

What This Test Will Tell You

This urine collection test measures kidney function and assesses renal impairment. Creatinine is a normal component of blood and urine which develops from metabolism of creatine in muscles. Serum levels are positively related to total body muscle mass. Plasma removal of creatinine occurs through glomerular filtration, resulting in a relatively constant day-to-day rate of excretion in the urine. Reduced urine creatinine levels indicate a decreased glomerular filtration rate. Both peak and trough levels of creatinine are captured in the 24-hour urine sample.

Abnormal Findings

▲INCREASED LEVELS may indicate tissue catabolism, strenuous exercise, or fever.

▼DECREASED LEVELS may indicate renal disease, urinary tract obstruction, acute or chronic glomerulonephritis, chronic bilateral pyelonephritis, polycystic kidney disease, muscle atrophy, nephrotoxic drugs, or hypovolemic shock.

■ ACTION ALERT!

➤ Creatinine levels should be checked prior to administering nephrotoxic chemotherapeutic agents such as cisplatin, cytoxin, methotrexate, and mithramycin.
➤ Monitor for drug toxicity when levels are decreased, because the kidneys may be unable to excrete medications sufficiently. Confer with the primary health care provider to determine if drug or dosage modifications are indicated.

Interfering Factors

➤ Values are 20%–40% higher in the afternoon than in the morning.
➤ Elevations occur in athletes with high muscle mass and following extremely strenuous exercise. The elevation may exist without renal impairment.
➤ High consumption of beef, fish, and poultry may elevate levels because of their high creatinine content.
➤ Failure to add all urine voided over 24 hours causes a falsely low result.
➤ Lack of specimen refrigeration causes a falsely low result.
➤ Feces, menstrual blood, and toilet paper will interfere with accurate results.
➤ Medications that may affect urinary creatinine levels include gentamicin, aminoglycosides, cimetidine, chemotherapeutic agents, cephalosporins, tetracyclines, diuretics, corticosteroids, androgens, and amphotericin B.

NURSING CONSIDERATIONS
Prepare Your Client

➤ Explain that this test is important to help determine how well the kidneys are working.
➤ Explain the 24-hour urine collection method.
➤ Teach the client not to eat excessive amounts of meat, tea, and coffee and not to exercise strenuously during the 24-hour collection period.

Perform Procedure

➤ Obtain a clean 3-L, 24-hour urine container with preservative.
➤ Follow 24-hour urine collection guidelines closely.
➤ Keep the specimen on ice or refrigerate it during the collection period.
➤ Offer fluids other than coffee or tea hourly to ensure adequate urinary output unless otherwise indicated.

Care After Test

➤ Compare urine output recorded over 24 hours with urine quantity collected in specimen container. If urine is less than recorded amount discard specimen and begin a new 24-hour urine specimen collection.
➤ Assess fluid and nutritional states of the client for indications of renal impairment if urine creatinine levels are low and serum creatinine levels are high.
➤ Encourage fluid consumption unless contraindicated.
➤ Evaluate for increased fluid volume as noted by neck vein distention, dyspnea, edema, reduced urine output, and hepatomegaly.

- Initiate safety precautions such as side rails up for client with uremia (serum creatinine greater than 7 mg/dL), because cognitive function may be altered.
- Consult with a registered dietician to assist the family and client in meeting special dietary needs.
- Evaluate other renal tests such as blood urea nitrogen (BUN), creatinine clearance, serum and urine uric acid levels, serum electrolytes, and urea clearance.

Educate Your Client and the Family

- If the client is in end-stage renal failure (ESRD), explain that eating large amount of fish, meat, and poultry can further affect urine creatinine results.
- If the client is in ESRD, stress the importance of regularly scheduled exercise to balance fluctuating creatinine levels.
- For client in ESRD, teach them to avoid foods high in potassium, sodium, and protein.

Cryoglobulin, Serum

crie oe glob yoo lin • see rum

Normal Findings

Negative. If cryoglobulins precipitate, they are analyzed to identify the protein complexes.

What This Test Will Tell You

This blood test detects the presence of cryoglobulins, the antigen-antibody complexes in the blood responsible for inflammatory disorders. These proteins precipitate out when cooled and then dissolve when rewarmed. The cryoglobulin test is an inexpensive screening tool to detect the presence of these immune complexes, which form in multiple disorders.

Abnormal Findings

▲INCREASED LEVELS may indicate systemic lupus erythematosus, multiple myeloma, primary cryoglobulinemia, rheumatoid arthritis, hepatitis, polyarthritis nodosa, Hodgkin's disease, cirrhosis, lymphocytic leukemia, Waldenström's macroglobulinemia, infectious mononucleosis, sarcoidosis, glomerulonephritis, hemolytic anemia, bacterial endocarditis, or Hansen's disease.

NURSING CONSIDERATIONS

Prepare Your Client

- Tell your client that this test is given to determine if there are abnormal proteins in the body which could be causing problems. Explain that the test will involve chilling, then rewarming a sample of blood, and then checking the sample for particles.
- Explain that the test results take a few days to come back.
- Withhold food and fluids for 4–8 hours before venous sampling.

Perform Procedure

- Collect 15 mL of venous blood in a red-top tube warmed to 37°C.
- Observe the venipuncture site

closely for hematoma formation or bleeding. Coagulopathies may be associated with many disorders for which this test is ordered. Apply a pressure dressing to the venipuncture site.

➤ Keep specimen at room temperature.

Care After Test

➤ Palpate cervical, axilla, and inguinal area for enlarged lymph nodes characteristic of leukemias and Hodgkin's disease.

➤ Evaluate complete blood count and differential for leukocytosis, bands, anemia, and neutropenia.

➤ Monitor temperature and fever patterns.

➤ Assess joints and client's mobility. Note any redness, deformity, stiffness, or swelling characteristic of rheumatoid arthritis.

➤ Assess client for symptoms of renal insufficiency, elevated creatinine, proteinuria, oliguria, or hematuria. Cryoglobulins may indicate renal impairment.

➤ Collaborate with the primary health care provider to encourage use of salicylates or non-steroidal inflammatory drugs when indicated. Remind the client to take these drugs with food and notify the primary health care provider if gastric distress occurs.

➤ Review related tests such as the erythrocyte sedimentation rate, C-reactive protein level, urinalysis, serum complement, blood cultures, serum and urine creatinine, complete blood count, and tissue biopsies.

Educate Your Client and the Family

➤ Warn your client to avoid cold temperatures if client tests positive for primary cryoglobulinemia.

➤ Tell your client that the cryoglobulin test is a valuable tool for screening for problems. If results are positive, other diagnostic tests will need to be performed.

➤ If client suffers from joint disease secondary to immune complex formation, encourage the use of moist heat and moderate exercise for painful joints.

➤ If steroid therapy is prescribed, inform client of side effects including weight gain, moon-face, increased appetite, increased bruising, and gastric irritation. Instruct them to avoid any other medications such as salicylates and anti-inflammatory medications that may further increase gastric irritation. If client is diabetic, warn them that steroid therapy can make glucose control more difficult. Mood swings, personality changes, bone fragility, and muscle weakness are also potential side effects of steroid therapy.

Cryptococcus Antigen and Antibody, Cerebrospinal Fluid

krip toe kok us • an ti jen • and • an ti bod ee • seh ree broe spie nal • floo id

Normal Findings

All ages:

Negative for antibodies and antigens.

Normal antigen titer is >1:8.

An antigen titer of 1:4 is suggestive of disease.

What This Test Will Tell You

This analysis of cerebrospinal fluid is used to diagnose cryptococcosis, an infection that primarily affects the central nervous system. Cryptococcosis is an infection found throughout the world and is caused by a fungus called *Cryptococcus neoformans.* Most commonly, this organism has been isolated in pigeon droppings. Infections with this fungus are on the rise because they sometimes occur in immunosuppressed people such as those with AIDS, malignancies, sarcoidosis, and organ transplants and those undergoing steroid therapy.

Antigen titers show the extent of the infection; the greater the titer, the greater the extent of the disease. A negative antigen titer does not rule out infection, however, because the antigen level may be too low to detect in early stages of infection. If infection is suspected and a negative titer is found, serologic antigen studies are useful to determine increasing antigen titer levels. Cerebrospinal fluid (CSF) glucose levels are decreased and lymphocytic cells are found in the CSF in this infection.

Abnormal Findings

▲INCREASED LEVELS may indicate cryptococcosis, meningitis, aseptic meningitis, or acquired immune deficiency syndrome (AIDS).

Interfering Factors

➤ Infection with other fungi may cause a false positive.

➤ Early infection may cause a false negative due to low concentration of the antigen.

➤ Contamination of the specimen with a fungus.

Contraindications

➤ Contraindications are those associated with a lumbar puncture to obtain a CSF sample.

➤ Increased intracranial pressure. A rapid decrease in intracranial pressure secondary to the lumbar puncture and removal of cerebrospinal fluid may cause the brain to shift downward (herniate) into the spinal column. The herniation could cause serious damage to the vital centers in the medulla and result in neurological damage or death.

➤ Primary clotting defects such as thrombocytopenia because of the risk of extradural or subdural hematoma formation.

Potential Complications

Complications associated with lumbar puncture:

➤ Infection
➤ Headache
➤ Nausea
➤ Dizziness
➤ Bleeding into the spinal column
➤ Neurologic injury or death from herniation

NURSING CONSIDERATIONS

Prepare Your Client

➤ Explain that this test is important to help diagnose an infection in the nervous system.

➤ Explain that the physician will place a needle into the lower back and withdraw spinal fluid.

➤ Ensure that an informed consent is obtained, because of the possible complications associated with this procedure.

➤ Assure the client that the needle is placed far below any spinal nerves into an empty space filled with fluid, not nerves.

➤ Explain that the physician will numb the lumbar region of the back before placing the lumbar puncture needle.

Perform Procedure

Nurses do not perform the procedure, but should understand the process to explain it to the client and assist the physician. Sterile technique must be maintained throughout the procedure. Place the client in the fetal position, and reassure the client throughout the procedure. Encourage the client to breathe slowly and deeply.

After the lumbar puncture needle is in the subarachnoid space, the client will need to straighten both legs for the initial pressure reading. The reading is taken with a manometer, provided in the lumbar puncture tray, that is attached to the needle via a three-way stopcock.

Approximately 3–5 mL of fluid will be collected in a series of tubes, which must be numbered sequentially. Tube 1 may be contaminated with blood and may need to be dis-

carded. Tube 2 is usually sent to the lab for analysis of glucose, protein, and cell count. Tube 3 is used for microbiology tests such as culture and smears. Send tubes to the lab immediately.

Care After Test

➤ Place a sterile dressing over the puncture site.

➤ Maintain client in a flat position for several hours after the lumbar puncture.

➤ Assess vital signs for elevated systolic pressure, widened pulse pressure, and respiratory depression, which can signal increased intracranial pressure. Decreased blood pressure may indicate shock.

➤ Report a persistent severe headache to the primary health care provider because this may require a blood patch, or injection of the client's blood into the epidural space to act as a fibrin patch for CSF leakage.

➤ Assess for pain and medicate as ordered.

➤ In head-injured client, ensure any nasal drainage is evaluated for cerebrospinal fluid content. Do not suction nasally.

➤ Encourage drinking fluids to assist the body in replacing CSF loss.

➤ Assess for signs and symptoms of complications including changes in mental status, changes in sensory perception of lower extremities, and neck rigidity.

➤ Evaluate related tests such as cerebrospinal fluid analysis.

Educate Your Client and the Family

➤ Instruct your client to remain flat for several hours after the lumbar puncture. Loss of spinal fluid during the lumbar puncture and potential leakage of CSF from the puncture site may cause headaches. Risk of CSF leakage is minimized when the client remains in a recumbent position.

➤ If increased intracranial pressure is present, instruct client on importance of avoiding the Valsalva maneuver by not coughing, sneezing, straining with bowel movements, or bending. Instruct the client to use stool softeners, sneeze with mouth open, and avoid lifting.

➤ Evaluate related tests such as blood culture and sensitivity, CSF culture and sensitivity, cerebrospinal fluid analysis, and serum cryptococcus antigen.

Cryptococcus Antigen, Serum
krip toe kok us • an ti jen • see rum

Normal Findings
All ages:
Normal: Titer >1:8 (negative)
Titer of 1:4 is suggestive of disease.

What This Test Will Tell You
This blood test diagnoses cryptococcosis, a fungal infection that primarily affects the central nervous system. This test screens for *Cryptococcus neoformans* antigens when infection is suspected. Cryptococcosis is a systemic fungal infection that may affect the lungs, skin, or other body organs. It disseminates to the brain and meninges. An increasing antigen titer level indicates progressing disease. The antigen titer will decrease with therapeutic levels of medications. A cryptococcus antibody test may be done at the same time as the antigen test, especially when antigen tests are negative and the client is showing evidence of infection. See *Cryptococcus Antigen and Antibody, Cerebrospinal Fluid*, for additional information.

Abnormal Findings
▲INCREASED LEVELS may indicate pulmonary infection, organ abscess, or meningitis.

Interfering Factors
➤ IgM rheumatoid factor will cause a false positive test result.
➤ Infection with other fungi may cause a false positive.
➤ Early infection may cause a false negative due to low concentration of the antigen.
➤ Contamination of the specimen.

NURSING CONSIDERATIONS
Prepare Your Client
➤ Explain that this test is important to determine the presence of a fungal infection by detecting the cryptococcal antigen.
➤ Explain that you will need to draw blood from the vein for the test. Explain the venipuncture procedure.
➤ Tell your client there is no need to restrict food, fluid, or medication before the test.

Perform Procedure
➤ Collect 7–10 mL of venous blood in a red-top tube.

Care After Test
➤ Monitor client's temperature for

fever.

➤ Assess neurologic status. Cryptococcal meningitis causes headache, dizziness, vertigo, stiffness of neck muscles and, in final stages, coma and respiratory failure.

➤ Assess for pain and medicate as ordered.

➤ Evaluate related tests such as blood culture and sensitivity, CSF culture and sensitivity, cerebrospinal fluid analysis, and cerebrospinal fluid cryptococcus antigen.

Educate Your Client and the Family

➤ Instruct a client who is taking steroids or immunosuppression medications or has an immunocompromising disease to wear a mask when exposed to pigeon feces.

➤ Instruct your client to get assistance when getting up if experiencing dizziness or vertigo.

➤ Instruct infected client to avoid persons with impaired immune system such as those with leukemia, diabetes, organ transplants, or AIDS.

Culdoscopy
kul doss koe pee

Normal Findings

Normal female reproductive organs
Absence of tumors, cysts, inappropriately located endometrial tissue, or other pathology

What This Test Will Tell You

This endoscopic examination provides direct visualization of the uterus, fallopian tubes, ovaries, broad ligaments, uterosacral ligaments, rectal wall, sigmoid colon, and small intestines. A small incision is made in the vaginal posterior fornix and the culdoscope, an instrument equipped with optical devices and a light, is inserted through the cul-de-sac of Douglas between the rectum and the uterus into the peritoneal cavity. This procedure permits the examiner to visualize deviations from normal in the surrounding tissue. With the advent of laparoscopic techniques, culdoscopy is used less frequently than in the past. However, it may be used for endoscopic exami-

nations of morbidly obese women as well as for performing tubal ligation for these clients. The laparoscopic approach is more difficult in these women due to excessive adipose tissue.

Abnormal Findings

Visualization may reveal abnormal fallopian tube(s), ectopic pregnancy, ovarian cysts or tumors, fibromyoma, or a pelvic mass.

ACTION ALERT!

Perforation of the intestines, rectum, or other abdominal and pelvic organs can occur with this procedure, resulting in hemorrhage or infection. Acute abdominal pain, elevated temperature, tachycardia, and hypotension can signal these complications and require immediate medical intervention.

Interfering Factors

➤ Physical impairment that prevents client from assuming a knee-chest position

➤ Adhesions from prior surgery, especially if bowel adheres to the cul-de-sac
➤ Menses

Contraindications
➤ Peritonitis
➤ Pelvic inflammatory disease
➤ Pelvic adhesions
➤ Labial and vaginal infections
➤ Mass in the cul-de-sac

Potential Complications
➤ Infection
➤ Hemorrhage
➤ Perforation of rectum and intestines

NURSING CONSIDERATIONS

Prepare Your Client
➤ Explain as appropriate that this test is to help find out why pregnancy has not occurred or to help diagnose problems in the female organs.
➤ Be sure that the client understands that immediate surgery will be needed if an ectopic pregnancy is found, since this could critically endanger the woman's health.
➤ Ensure that an informed consent is obtained, because of the possible complications associated with this procedure.
➤ Restrict food and fluids for at least 8 hours before the test is performed.
➤ Instruct the client that the procedure will be performed in a day surgery.
➤ Instruct client to bathe prior to admission.
➤ Ask client if she is allergic to iodine, as a povidone-iodine (beta-dine) skin prep may be done prior to surgery and she may be directed to take a betadine douche the night

before the surgery.
➤ Instruct client to take medication and/or a Fleet's enema the night before surgery as directed by the primary health care provider to evacuate bowel.

Perform Procedure
Nurses do not perform this procedure, but need to understand it so that it can be explained to client. Administer preoperative medication before surgery as ordered. Consult with the physician regarding the need for an intravenous infusion or an indwelling urinary catheter prior to arriving in the operating room.

Epidural, spinal, or general anesthesia is administered depending on decision made by client with her primary health care provider and anesthesiologist. Assist the client to a knee-chest position on the operating table with the head lowered to displace bowel from reproductive organs. The vagina and surrounding area is cleansed with a disinfecting solution such as a povidone-iodine (betadine) solution. A sterile instrument is placed into vagina to retract tissue to visualize posterior fornix. An incision is made, the culdoscope is inserted, and the examination is made.

The culdoscope is removed and the incision sutured depending on preference of surgeon. The perineal area is cleansed and a perineal pad applied. Clients generally are transferred to the post-anesthesia room prior to discharge to home or transfer back to the unit. Explain to client that procedure takes about 1 hour from entering operating room until transferring to post-anesthesia room.

Care After Test

➤ Monitor vital signs closely until stable; usually every 15 minutes for the first hour, every 30 minutes for the next hour, and then every 4 hours for 24 hours or until discharge.

➤ Assess vaginal discharge for frank bleeding. Report any immediately.

➤ Review related tests such as complete blood count, Pap smear, and ultrasound.

Educate Your Client and the Family

➤ Instruct the client that it takes 1–2 weeks for the vaginal incision to heal. During that time she is not to have sex, douche, or insert anything into her vagina, including tampons.

➤ Tell the client that she may wear a sanitary pad for any bleeding or discharge, which should be minimal. For her menstrual period, a sanitary pad should be worn until incision heals, approximately 2 weeks from the surgery date.

➤ Tell client to notify the primary health care provider if she has excessive vaginal bleeding not associated with her period, chills and fever, or a foul-smelling vaginal discharge.

➤ Instruct client to take mild analgesics as prescribed by the primary health care provider for discomfort.

➤ Instruct client to make an appointment with the primary health care provider for postoperative checkup to be sure incision has healed and to discuss findings.

Cyanocobalamin

sie ah noe koe bal ah min

(Vitamin B$_{12}$, Extrinsic Factor, Antipernicious Anemia Factor)

Normal Findings

ADULT, CHILD, ADOLESCENT
100–1300 pg/mL (SI units: 75–960 pmol/L)

PREGNANT
Values are decreased, due to higher demand to meet the needs of the fetus and lactation.

NEWBORN
160–1300 pg/mL

ELDERLY
Values may be decreased due to fewer marrow cells with aging.

What This Test Will Tell You

This blood test is used in the diagnosis of megaloblastic anemia and central nervous system diseases related to demyelination. The test measures the blood levels of cyanocobalamin, also known as vitamin B$_{12}$, which is essential in normal red blood cell production, myelination of nerves, and other important tissue synthesis. Vitamin B$_{12}$ is a cobalt-containing compound that is synthesized by bacteria and molds and is required for normal differentiation and maturation of bone marrow cells. It cannot be synthesized by the body, but is furnished in the diet by foods of animal origin. For vitamin B$_{12}$ to be absorbed, intrinsic factor produced by the gastric mucosa is necessary. To prevent deficiency, approximately 5 micrograms of the vitamin is needed daily.

Abnormal Findings

▼DECREASED LEVELS may indicate pernicious anemia, Zollinger-Ellison syndrome, hypothyroidism, loss of gastric mucosa (e.g., gastrectomy), macrocytic anemia, disorders of folate and/or vitamin B_{12} metabolism, malabsorption, alcoholism, dietary deficiencies, parasitic infections, intestinal disease, malignancies, chemotherapeutic agents, or human immunodeficiency virus (HIV) infection.

▲INCREASED LEVELS may indicate myeloproliferative disorders, hepatocellular disorders, or polycythemia vera.

Interfering Factors

➤ Aminoglycosides, neomycin, colchicine, extended-release potassium preparations, aspirin, phenytoin, phenobarbital, primidone, oral contraceptives, tranquilizers, cholestyramine, cimetidine, and ranitidine can lower serum level of cyanocobalamin.

➤ Pregnancy and oral contraceptives may elevate levels.

➤ Radionuclides may invalidate results.

NURSING CONSIDERATIONS

Prepare Your Client

➤ Explain that this test is important to help understand the amount of vitamin B_{12} in the blood, in order to see if abnormalities exist.

➤ If the test is being performed to rule out malabsorption, draw the sample prior to performing the Schilling test.

➤ Restrict food and fluids for 8 hours prior to the test if required by your laboratory.

Perform Procedure

➤ Collect 5 mL of venous blood in a red-top tube.

Care After Test

➤ Assess for signs and symptoms of B_{12} deficiency including dyspnea, pallor, angina, congestive heart failure, anorexia, alterations in bowel and bladder elimination patterns, weight loss, thick and red tongue, paresthesia in extremities, gait disturbances, and changes in personality or mentation.

➤ For client with neurological dysfunction, institute safety precautions to prevent injury.

➤ Encourage rest periods for client experiencing fatigue related to anemia.

➤ Evaluate client's ability to perform activities of daily living.

➤ Refer to community health care services as needed if client is unable to perform basic daily needs.

➤ Obtain a dietary consult to assist the client and family in choosing a well-balanced diet, including foods high in iron and vitamin B_{12}.

➤ Review related tests such as hemoglobin, hematocrit, reticulocyte count, red blood cell indices, hemoglobin electrophoresis, ferritin level, total iron binding capacity (TIBC), bone marrow and liver biopsies, folic acid level, the Schilling test for vitamin B_{12} absorption, and iron absorption and excretion studies.

Educate Your Client and the Family

➤ If the client has a low cyanocobalamin level due to a dietary deficiency, explain that eating beef, fish, milk, eggs, and poultry may increase levels because they are high in vitamin B_{12}.

➤ If the client has a low cyanocobalamin level due to pernicious anemia and lack of intrinsic factor, stress the importance of taking replacement B_{12} therapy on a lifelong basis. Explain the need for regular checkups and screening for gastric carcinoma, since gastric cancer risk is higher in people with pernicious anemia.

➤ If the client has a low cyanocobalamin level due to nutritional deficiencies seen in alcoholism, explain the need to refrain from alcoholic beverages, and refer the client to support groups such as Alcoholics Anonymous.

Cyclic Adenosine Monophosphate
sie klic • ah den oe seen • mon oe fos fate
(cAMP, Cyclic AMP)

Normal Findings
URINE
All ages: 3–4 μmol/g creatinine (SI units: 0.4–0.5 μmol/mmol creatinine)
An increase of 10–20 times with parathyroid infusion
SERUM
All ages: 5.6–10.9 ng/mL

What This Test Will Tell You
This urine test is used in the differential diagnosis of a rare inherited disorder called type I pseudohypoparathyroidism where there is diminished response to the parathyroid-stimulating hormone. Cyclic adenosine monophosphate (cAMP) is produced in the renal tubules in response to parathyroid-stimulating hormone (PSH) and controls the protein synthesis rate within cells, increases renal reabsorption and gastrointestinal absorption of calcium, and enhances the release of calcium from bone, increasing serum calcium levels. In pseudohypoparathyroidism, the body's resistance to the effects of parathyroid hormone causes hypocalcemia, hyperphosphatemia, and skeletal anomalies. Commonly, the serum and urine levels of cAMP are compared to determine how much cAMP is being excreted by the renal tubules. The urinary excretion of cAMP is measured indirectly by the creatinine levels.

Abnormal Findings
➤ *Failure to respond to parathyroid infusion* may indicate type I pseudohypoparathyroidism.
➤ *Response to parathyroid infusion* may indicate type II pseudohypoparathyroidism.

ACTION ALERT!
Hypocalcemia is a common complication of hypoparathyroidism and may result in life-threatening laryngospasm. Assess for Chvostek's sign (spasm of facial muscle with tapping of facial nerve) and Trousseau's sign (carpopedal spasm when blood pressure cuff is inflated) as an indication of neuromuscular irritability. Ensure that an airway is at the bedside and intubation as well as other resuscitation equipment is readily available.

Interfering Factors
➤ Radioisotope scans less than 1 week prior to test will alter results.
➤ Allowing specimen to sit will alter

results.

Contraindications

➤ Hypercalcemia or digitalis therapy, because PSH stimulates calcium reabsorption

---

NURSING CONSIDERATIONS

Prepare Your Client

➤ Explain that this test is used to see if a hormone called parathyroid hormone is being properly used by the body.

➤ Explain urine collection technique to client undergoing urinary cAMP evaluation.

Perform Procedure

SERUM

➤ Collect 5 mL of venous blood into a red-top tube.

URINE

Parathyroid hormone is administered intravenously over 15 minutes. Begin the urine collection when the infusion begins. Keep the collection bag and/or urine samples on ice or refrigerated. Collect the urine sample 3–4 hours after infusion.

Care After Test

➤ Monitor for signs and symptoms of hypoparathyroidism including hypocalcemia, which may result in lethargy, anorexia, nausea, vomiting, dysrhythmias, abdominal cramping, diarrhea, uncontrolled spasms, muscular hyperexcitability, tetany, and dizziness.

➤ Strain urine for renal calculi, which may accompany hypocalcemia.

➤ Review related tests such as serum calcium, phosphorus, and magnesium.

Educate Your Client and the Family

➤ Teach client signs and symptoms of hypocalcemia and instruct them to report these to the primary health care provider immediately.

➤ Instruct client with hypocalcemia how to follow a high-calcium and phosphorus-restricted diet.

➤ Teach client to limit whole grains in diet, as they block calcium absorption.

➤ Instruct client on the importance of regular monitoring of calcium levels.

Cystine, Urine
sis teen • yur in

Normal Findings

ADULT, ADOLESCENT, ELDERLY, AND CHILD OLDER THAN 8 YEARS
Qualitative sample: Negative
Quantitative sample: 10–100 mg/24 hours

INFANT AND CHILD YOUNGER THAN 8 YEARS
Qualitative sample: Negative
Quantitative sample: 2–13 mg/24 hours

Limited tubular reabsorption may cause inappropriate loss of amino acids in the glomerular filtrate.

What This Test Will Tell You

This urine test determines the presence of cystinuria, a hereditary metabolic disorder. Cystine is a sulfur-containing amino acid produced through the action of acids on proteins that contain cystine. It is an essential source of sulfur in metabolism. Normally there is no cystine in the urine. A genetic defect may result from inborn errors of metabolism, related to the absence of certain enzymatic activity. This may cause cystine and other amino acids to appear in plasma and in urine if the renal threshold is exceeded. In conditions causing cystinuria, over 300 mg/24 hours of cystine may be excreted, and clients are at risk of forming waxy, cystine stones in the kidney that may be passed in the urine. A positive random urine specimen result is confirmed by a 24-hour quantitative test.

Abnormal Findings

▲ INCREASED LEVELS may indicate congenital cystinuria, nephrolithiasis, cystinosis, nephrotoxicity, pyelonephritis, renal tubular acidosis, or Wilson's disease.

Interfering Factors

➤ Penicillamine may cause false negative results.
➤ Intravenous pyelogram that precedes urine sampling.
➤ If a newborn has not ingested dietary protein, results are not valid.
➤ Failure to transport the specimen to the laboratory immediately.

NURSING CONSIDERATIONS

Prepare Your Client

➤ Explain that this test looks for a problem in how the body uses and processes protein.
➤ Tell the client that this test requires a urine specimen.
➤ Instruct the client on the urine collection procedure for the random qualitative or 24-hour quantitative collection.
➤ Instruct the client to avoid getting urine, stool, or menses in the specimen.

Perform Procedure

RANDOM SAMPLING FOR QUALITATIVE STUDY
➤ Collect 20 mL of urine into a specimen container for a qualitative study.
24-HOUR URINE COLLECTION FOR QUANTITATIVE STUDY
➤ Collect a 24-hour urine specimen in a 3-L container with a preservative. Follow general guidelines for collection for a 24-hour specimen.

Care After Test

➤ If the client has cystinuria, assess diet for food products that enhance kidney stone formation.
➤ Consult with a registered dietician to assist the family and client in meeting special dietary needs.
➤ If cystine renal calculi are present or suspected, strain all urine for stones.
➤ Evaluate other related tests such as blood and 24-hour urine quantitative column chromatography to identify specific amino acid abnormalities.

Educate Your Client and the Family

➤ If the client has cystine stones, instruct them to drink more than a gallon (4 L) of fluids a day, if not contraindicated.
➤ If the client has cystine stones,

teach them an alkaline ash diet (no carbonated drinks, chocolates, nuts, dried fruits) to raise the urinary pH to 7.5.

Cystography

sis **tog** rah fee

(Cystogram, Retrograde Cystography, Retrograde Cystogram, Diagnostic Cystography, Diagnostic Cystogram, Cystourethrography, Cystourethrogram, Voiding Cystography, Voiding Cystogram, Voiding Cystourethrography, Voiding Cystourethrogram)

Normal Findings

ALL AGES

The urethra, bladder, and ureteral orifices are normal in appearance and intact.

Bladder location is normal. Bladder is free of fistula, tumors, or ruptures.

What This Test Will Tell You

This x-ray test diagnoses structural bladder defects as well as bladder dysfunction. This test is also used in male infants when excretory urography has not adequately visualized the bladder. The study can determine the structure and function of the bladder, ureters, and urethra. In the elderly, this test is particularly helpful in differentiating between neurogenic and non-neurogenic incontinence. It may also detect changes in bladder and urethral flow during urination. Stones, ruptures, fistulas, or tumors in the bladder may be identified.

Abnormal Findings

Abnormalities may indicate calculi, space-occupying lesions, neurogenic bladder, non-neurogenic bladder, hypertonic bladder, origin of urinary tract infection, vesicular trabeculae, diverticula, blood clots, vesico-ureteral reflux, prostatic hyperplasia, or origin of hematuria.

ACTION ALERT!

Assess clients carefully for allergic reaction to contrast material, including dyspnea, itching, urticaria, flushing, hypotension, and shock. Life-threatening anaphylactic reactions can occur and need to be recognized and treated immediately.

Interfering Factors

➤ Feces, gas in the bowel, and residual barium from diagnostic tests may interfere with test results by causing cloudy radiographic pictures.

Contraindications

➤ Pregnancy
➤ Recent bladder surgery
➤ Urethral obstruction
➤ Acute phase of urinary tract infection
➤ Urethral evulsion
➤ Urethral transection

Potential Complications

➤ Urinary sepsis
➤ Urinary tract infection
➤ Hematuria
➤ Extravasation of contrast medium into general circulation or pelvis
➤ Urinary retention

➤ Allergic reaction to contrast material

NURSING CONSIDERATIONS
Prepare Your Client
➤ Explain that this test is used to determine if the bladder is working properly.

➤ Inform the client that the test takes 30–60 minutes.

➤ Administer laxatives as ordered the night before the test to clear the intestinal system and improve visualization of the bladder.

➤ Ensure that a clear liquid diet is consumed the day of the test.

➤ Ensure that an informed consent is obtained, because of the possible complications associated with this procedure.

➤ Instruct the client to disrobe below the waist or wear a gown.

➤ Check the chart to make sure the client has no allergy to contrast material or iodine.

➤ Record baseline vital signs.

➤ Administer sedatives or tranquilizers as ordered before the client leaves for the test.

➤ Do not remove glasses, dentures, or hearing aids unless dictated by your hospital policy. The client may need these in order to communicate during the procedure.

Perform Procedure
Nurses do not perform this procedure, but should understand the process to prepare the client. Assist the client to a supine position on the radiographic table. A baseline kidney-ureter-bladder (KUB) x-ray is taken. A urinary catheter is inserted and 200–300 mL (50–100 mL for infants) of contrast medium is inserted by gravity or gentle syringe injection. The catheter is clamped and the client assisted to several different positions for radiographic examination of the bladder and surrounding structures. The catheter is unclamped and the bladder fluid is allowed to drain. One additional x-ray is taken to detect fistulas or dye extravasation.

Lead shields can be used to protect male testes during this test. Shielding of female gonads is not possible; it would block bladder visualization.

Care After Test
➤ Monitor vital signs every 15 minutes for the first hour, every 30 minutes for the second hour, then every 2 hours for up to 24 hours.

➤ If fluids are not contraindicated, encourage fluid intake to promote removal of the contrast medium from the bladder and prevent urinary tract infection.

➤ Observe for signs of allergic reaction to the contrast material, including urticaria, pruritus, dyspnea, and apprehension.

➤ Record time of voiding, and color and volume of urine. Note hematuria. If it continues after the third voiding, notify the primary health care provider.

➤ Observe for signs of urinary sepsis or signs associated with extravasation of contrast medium into the systemic circulation (chills, fever, rapid pulse, dyspnea, and hypotension). Notify the primary health care provider.

➤ Evaluate related tests such as cystoscopy, KUB, diagnostic cystometry, or voiding cystogram.

Educate Your Client and the Family
➤ Inform the client that a slight

burning sensation when voiding for the first or second day after the procedure is considered normal.

➤ If the client has stress incontinence, teach pelvic floor exercises (Kegel exercises) to retrain the muscles of the pelvic floor.

➤ If the client has established incontinence, begin instruction on bladder retraining or behavior modification.

Cystometry
sis **tom** eh tree
(Cystometrogram, CMG)

Normal Findings

ALL AGES

Normal bladder sensation of fullness, heat, and cold. Normal filling pattern. Absence of residual urine.

ADULT, ADOLESCENT, AND ELDERLY

Normal adult bladder capacity is 250–750 mL. Normal first desire to void at 175–250 mL. Normal sensation of fullness at 300–500 mL. Detrusor muscle reflex contraction suppressed upon command, and pressure is < 10 cm H_2O. Normal maximal flow of 25 mL/second reached in 5 seconds. Normal intravesical pressure with an empty bladder is < 40 cm H_2O.

NEWBORN

Normal newborn capacity is 30–50 mL. Normal child capacity at 1 year is up to 100 mL.

CHILD

Normal bladder capacity at 5 years is up to 200 mL.
Normal bladder capacity at 10 years is up to 300 mL.

What This Test Will Tell You

This x-ray test determines bladder function, capacity, sensation, pressure, and the presence of residual urine in the bladder. This test assesses neuromuscular function of the bladder following the instillation of measured quantities of fluid and/or air. Neurologic sensations of heat and cold can be determined. The detrusor muscle reflex and intravesical (within the bladder) pressure and capacity can be evaluated. Voiding flow patterns can detect if abnormalities causing involuntary bladder contractions are present.

Abnormal Findings

Abnormalities may indicate neurogenic bladder differentiation, uninhibited neurogenic bladder, reflex neurogenic bladder, autonomous neurogenic bladder, sensory paralytic bladder, motor paralytic bladder, stress incontinence, hypotonic bladder muscle, hypertonic bladder muscle, obstruction, infections, or loss of vesicle reflex.

    ACTION ALERT!

In clients with a cervical spinal cord lesion, carefully monitor for autonomic dysreflexia (bradycardia, life-threatening hypertension, and flushing), which may occur during air or fluid instillation. This response may be prevented by intravenous administration of propantheline bromide.

Interfering Factors

➤ Antihistamines may interfere with bladder function by causing relaxation of the detrusor muscle.

➤ Movement during the procedure may interfere with bladder reflexes.

➤ Inability to void in a supine position may alter test results.

➤ Clients requiring surgery for spinal cord injury should wait 6–8 weeks after surgery for this test to avoid inconclusive test results.

Contraindications

➤ Acute urinary tract infections or urethral obstructions

➤ Recent bladder surgery

Potential Complications

Sepsis
Pyelonephritis
Hematuria
Urinary retention
Urinary tract infection
Bladder spasms
Autonomic dysreflexia

NURSING CONSIDERATIONS

Prepare Your Client

➤ Explain that this test looks at how well the bladder is working, including the feeling of needing to urinate and the ability to wait to urinate.

➤ Ensure that an informed consent is obtained, because of the possible complications associated with this procedure.

➤ Ask the client to urinate just prior to the procedure.

➤ Do not remove dentures, glasses, or hearing aids unless dictated by your hospital policy. The client may need these in order to communicate and cooperate during the procedure.

➤ Record baseline vital signs.

Perform Procedure

Nurses do not usually perform this procedure, but should understand the process to prepare the client. The client is assisted to a supine position on the examining table. An appropriate size of indwelling catheter is placed into the bladder. Residual urine is measured.

The client's thermal sensation is tested through the instillation of 30 mL of room-temperature, sterile, 0.9% saline or distilled water into the bladder. Next, 30 mL of warm, sterile, 0.9% saline or distilled water is instilled into the bladder. The client is asked to describe the sensations that are felt (need to urinate, warmth, discomfort). The client's bladder is then drained.

A cystometer is connected to the urinary catheter, and measured amounts of sterile, distilled water; sterile, 0.9% saline; or carbon dioxide are instilled into the bladder. Bladder volume and pressure are measured, and the client's statements of the first urge to void, of feeling unable to go any longer without voiding, or of discomfort are recorded. The instillation is stopped when the client describes discomfort or feeling full, or is unable to sense filling of the bladder. The client is then asked to void the fluid, and any residual is drained from the bladder. If necessary, the cystometer procedure is repeated with the client in a sitting or standing position. Bladder tone stimulants such as bethanechol chloride are administered if needed.

Care After Test

➤ Monitor fluid intake and urine output for 24 hours.

➤ Notify the primary health care provider if hematuria persists after the third voiding.

➤ Administer analgesics as ordered for bladder spasms.

➤ Notify the primary health care

provider if the client develops signs of septic shock (such as fever, hypotension, tachycardia, or chills).

➤ Encourage oral fluid intake if not contraindicated.

➤ Assess voiding patterns including difficulty initiating urination, weak stream, dribbling, incontinence, straining, and hesitancy.

➤ Review related tests such as the voiding cystourethrogram, the cystourethrogram, and the excretory urogram.

Educate Your Client and the Family

➤ Inform the client that a slight burning sensation when voiding for the first or second day after the procedure is considered normal.

➤ If the client has stress incontinence, explain pelvic floor exercises (Kegel exercises) to retrain the muscles of the pelvic floor.

➤ If the client has established incontinence, begin instruction on bladder retraining or behavior modification.

Cystoscopy
sis **tos** koe pee
(Cystourethroscopy, Endourology)

Normal Findings
ALL AGES
Normal structure and function of the bladder, urethra, urethral orifices, and male prostate.

What This Test Will Tell You
This endoscopic test diagnoses bladder, ureteral, and prostatic impairment. The study can determine structure and function of the bladder, urethra, and male prostate. The cystoscope, a fiber-optic light source, is used to evaluate and differentiate disorders of the lower urinary tract such as unexplained hematuria, recurrent urinary tract infections, or urinary symptoms of undetermined origin (such as dysuria, frequency, hesitancy, or urgency).

This procedure may also be used as a therapeutic procedure to treat lower urinary tract anomalies. Cystoscopy may be done to remove calculi, to obtain a tissue biopsy, or to resect lesions from the bladder, urethra, or prostate gland. Cystoscopy is also used to irrigate the bladder and to perform a transurethral resection of the prostate gland. In addition, a ureteral catheter may be inserted to the renal pelvis for pyelography (radiographic visualization of the bladder and ureters with contrast dye). Kidney-ureter-bladder radiography (KUB) and excretory urography usually precede cystoscopy. Cystography, the instillation of contrast dye into the bladder through a catheter, may be helpful when radiographs are necessary and cystoscopy is contraindicated.

Abnormal Findings
➤ *Bladder abnormalities* may reveal cancer, calculi, vesicle neck stenosis, inflammation, diverticula, abnormally large or small bladder capacity, or polyps.

➤ *Ureteral abnormalities* may reveal

ureteral reflux, ureteroceles, duplicate ureteral orifices, or urinary fistulas.

➤ *Urethral abnormalities* may reveal urethral strictures or dysfunctional urethral valves in children.

➤ *Prostatic abnormalities* may reveal prostatic hyperplasia/hypertrophy, prostatitis, or cancer.

Potential Complications

➤ Acute manifestations of prostatitis, cystitis, or urethritis, because the instrumentation may cause sepsis

➤ Hematuria or blood clots in the urine

➤ Urinary retention

➤ Bacteremia

➤ Sepsis

➤ Urinary tract infection

➤ Bladder spasms

➤ Dysuria

➤ Bladder perforation

NURSING CONSIDERATIONS

Prepare Your Client

➤ Explain that this test is used to evaluate and diagnose problems with the bladder and urethra.

➤ If a local anesthetic is used, restrict food for 8 hours and give large amounts of clear liquids to promote urine flow during the procedure. If a general anesthetic is used, restrict food and fluids for 8 hours prior to the test.

➤ Make sure that an informed consent is obtained, because of the possible complications associated with this procedure.

➤ Check the chart to be sure the client has no allergy to contrast material or iodine if pyelography is also to be performed.

➤ Record baseline vital signs.

➤ Administer sedatives, tranquilizers, and/or bladder antispasmodics as ordered before the client goes to the cystoscopy room.

➤ Do not remove glasses, dentures, or hearing aids unless dictated by your hospital, or unless client is receiving general anesthesia. If local anesthesia is used the client may need these in order to communicate and cooperate during the procedure.

➤ Explain that slight burning on urination is not unusual following this test.

➤ Instruct the client to urinate before leaving for the test, to disrobe below the waist, and to wear a hospital gown.

Perform Procedure

Nurses do not perform this procedure but should understand the process to prepare the client. The client is assisted to a supine lithotomy position. The external genitalia are cleansed and draped for the examination.

Local anesthesia is instilled and the urethra is visually examined. The cystoscope is inserted, moving toward the bladder through the urethra. Urine specimens are obtained for culture or cystography if needed, and residual urine is measured. The bladder is filled with irrigating solution. The cystoscope is then rotated with magnification to examine the entire bladder wall surface and the ureteral orifices. The bladder is inspected for tumors, calculi, diverticuli, strictures, or obstructions. Small tumors, calculi, or tissue from the bladder or ureters may be excised if necessary. A transurethral resection of prostate (TURP) may be performed if prostatic hypertrophy is present. As the cystoscope is removed, the bladder neck and the urethral sphincters are examined.

Care After Test

➤ Monitor vital signs closely until stable; usually every 15 minutes for the first hour, every 30 minutes for the next hour, and then every 4 hours for 24 hours.

➤ Encourage the client to drink fluids liberally, if not contraindicated, to provide adequate urinary flow. This can help promote expulsion of any bacteria that may have been introduced.

➤ Administer prescribed analgesics and bladder antispasmodics for discomfort.

➤ Monitor client intake and output for 24 hours, and note bladder distention to assess for possible urine retention.

➤ Observe for signs of urinary tract infection, which include fever, chills, flank pain, dysuria, and hematuria. Report findings to primary health care provider.

➤ Note any hematuria. Report frank bleeding or clotting to the primary health care provider. Pink-tinged urine is usually seen initially.

➤ Administer prescribed antispasmodics for bladder spasms if necessary.

➤ Observe for signs of allergic reaction to the contrast material such as urticaria, pruritus, or dyspnea if dye is used during the test.

➤ Assist the client to stand after the procedure since they may experience dizziness or fainting from orthostatic hypotension.

➤ Evaluate related tests such as kidney, ureter, and bladder (KUB) radiograph or retrograde pyelography.

Educate Your Client and the Family

➤ If a urethral dilation was done, instruct the client to rest and increase fluid intake.

➤ Teach the client that slight burning on urination is common immediately following the test. If burning, urgency, chills, fever, and/or hesitancy are noted the client should notify the primary health care provider. These are signs of a urinary tract infection.

➤ If the procedure is done on an outpatient basis inform the client to arrange for transportation.

➤ Teach the client not to strain during defecation. For several days following this test, straining may initiate bleeding in the urinary tract.

➤ Unless otherwise indicated, collaborate with the primary health care provider about instructing the client to use laxatives or bowel softeners for the first 3–5 days.

Cytomegalovirus Antibody Screen, Serum

sie toe **meg** ah loe **vie** russ • an ti **bod** ee • screen • see rum
(CMV, Cytomegalovirus, Rapid Monoclonal Test, Shell Vial Assay)

Normal Findings

ADULT AND CHILD
Negative titers
CMV less than 1:5 indicates no previous exposure to CMV.
NEWBORN
Negative
Presence of IgM antibody at birth indicates in utero infection.
MOTHER
Negative antibody in mother rules out congenital infection.

What This Test Will Tell You

This blood test confirms infection with the cytomegalovirus by detecting and measuring titers or levels of antibody to CMV. Diagnosis of CMV is difficult when based on viral cultures, which are unreliable and can take weeks to grow. Because antibody to CMV is common in the general population, diagnosis must be made by a rise in serial antibody titers.

Conventional testing for CMV by tube cell cultures can take up to 9 days for results. The rapid monoclonal test can yield results in 16 hours.

Abnormal Findings

CMV titer > 1:8 indicates an acute infection.
Suspect acute infection with a fourfold rise in serial titer.
▲ INCREASED LEVELS may indicate positive CMV infection, atypical infectious mononucleosis, Guillain-Barré, viral myocarditis, or viral pneumonia.

Interfering Factors

➤ 20% false positives and false negatives in newborns
➤ Administration of antiviral medications before sampling occurs

NURSING CONSIDERATIONS

Prepare Your Client

➤ Explain that this test will determine whether there is a virus (cytomegalovirus) in the body that could cause problems.
➤ Tell your client that if the first test is positive serial titers will be drawn.

Perform Procedure

➤ Collect 5–7 mL of venous blood in a red-top tube.
➤ *For the rapid monoclonal test for CMV*: Collect specimen from throat, urine, cerebrospinal fluid, or blood or by bronchoalveolar lavage. Ensure sample is collected and transported in a sterile container.

Care After Test

➤ Check the client's CMV antibody status. Use filters on blood to avoid transmitting the virus to seronegative, vulnerable clients.
➤ Obtain client's recent infection history.
➤ Ensure that client with negative serum titers receives only CMV-negative blood products and organs from CMV-negative donors.

Educate Your Client and the Family

➤ If infection resembles mononucleosis, recommend bed rest, fluids, and antipyretics.

➤ Offer support and obtain counseling for the parents and other family of a positive newborn.

Daily Fetal Movement Count

day lee • fee tal • moov ment • kownt

(DFMC, Fetal Kick Count, Cardiff-Count-To-Ten, DFMR, Daily Fetal Movement Record)

Normal Findings

This test is performed on pregnant clients only. Ten or more movements in 10 hours is normal.

What This Test Will Tell You

This fetal assessment test evaluates fetal well-being by assessing daily fetal activity. Fetal activity in utero reflects fetal well-being. Decreased activity in a fetus that has been active may be a sign of a problem. Daily fetal movement increases until about week 32 and then gradually decreases until delivery. Women with low-risk pregnancies should begin daily fetal movement counting (DFMC) at 34–36 weeks. Women with high-risk pregnancies should begin DFMC at 28 weeks.

Abnormal Findings

Decreased activity may indicate fetal demise or fetal distress.

ACTION ALERT!

Any significant decrease in fetal movement should be reported to the primary health care provider immediately. This may be a sign of a problem with the fetus.

Interfering Factors

➤ Gestational age, since DFM increases with gestational age up to week 32 and then decreases gradually.
➤ Glucose loading and decreased glucose levels decrease activity.
➤ Smoking.
➤ Time of day; some fetuses are more active at certain times of day.
➤ Fetal sleep states.

➤ Decreased maternal perception.

NURSING CONSIDERATIONS

Prepare Your Client

➤ Explain that this is a simple test that is performed at home each day to help see how well the baby is doing and if there could be any problems with the baby's health.
➤ Explain to the client that all that is needed is a watch, pencil, and paper.
➤ Instruct the high-risk client to begin DFMC at 28 weeks and the low-risk client to begin at 34–36 weeks of gestation.

Perform Procedure

➤ Instruct the client to select a convenient time of day to count fetal movements, and to allow up to 10 hours.
➤ Instruct the client to count how long it takes to feel 10 movements. Write on paper if necessary.
➤ Do the procedure at the same time every day if possible.

Care After Test

➤ Ask the client if she is taking her prenatal vitamins as ordered by her primary health care provider. Stress the importance of supplemental vitamins in providing good nutrition and normal growth and development of her baby.
➤ Assess the client's knowledge of prenatal care including diet, activity, rest, signs and symptoms of labor, and danger signs in pregnancy. Provide instruction as indicated.

➤ Assess mother's readiness to meet parental role functions by reviewing infant care knowledge, methods of infant feeding, and ability to obtain needed supplies. Provide instruction and/or community health service referrals as indicated.

➤ Assess the client's ability to provide adequate nutrition for the fetus. Refer to social services and Women, Infants, and Children program (WIC) for assistance.

➤ Refer to a registered dietician if dietary deficiencies are suspected.

➤ Assess the client for use of cigarettes, tobacco products, alcohol, over-the-counter medications, and street drugs. Instruct the client as necessary to avoid these substances as they may cause intrauterine growth retardation.

➤ If the client reports decreased fetal movements, assess recent maternal history for maternal activity and relationship to fetal movement. Assess also her recent consumption of food or fluids and its relationship to fetal movement. Consult with the primary health care provider about instructing the client to eat, drink, and then rest. During rest, tell her to concentrate on fetal movements for 1 hour. Three fetal movements in 1 hour are reassuring.

➤ Review related tests such as amniocentesis, nonstress test, nipple stimulation test, and biophysical profile.

Educate Your Client and the Family

➤ Tell the client to call the primary health care provider if she detects less than 10 movements in 10 hours for 2 days, if she feels less than 3 movements in 1 hour, or if she feels no movements at all. Instruct her to notify the primary health care provider if it takes longer and longer each day to feel 10 movements.

➤ Instruct the client about normal signs of labor such as a gush of fluid, bloody show, and contractions that increase in frequency, intensity, and duration.

➤ Instruct the client about danger signs in pregnancy such as a gush of fluid more than 2 weeks before her due date, vaginal bleeding, abdominal pain, temperature elevation, dizziness, blurred vision, persistent vomiting, severe headache, edema, muscular irritability, difficult urination, or decreased/absent fetal movements.

➤ Teach the client the signs of preterm labor such as abdominal cramping with or without diarrhea, uterine contractions every 10 minutes or less, menstrual-like cramps in the lower abdomen, low backache, increase or change in vaginal discharge, or pelvic pressure.

➤ Advise the client to lie down on her side and notify the primary health care provider if preterm labor is suspected.

D

Digital Subtraction Angiography

(Transvenous Digital Subtraction, Digital Venous Subtraction Angiography, Digital Radiography, DSA, DVSA, TDS)

Normal Findings

Normal anatomical structure, normal and patent arteries and/or veins

What This Test Will Tell You

This radiographic test is used primarily to diagnose arterial and venous vascular disease or anomalies. The study is performed by inserting a catheter into a vein or an artery and injecting contrast material to produce a highly specific and sensitive picture of the vasculature. Before the contrast material is injected, an x-ray image is taken to serve as a baseline picture of the targeted area. Following injection, another x-ray image is taken that highlights the arteries or veins. The first picture, which may include bony structures, the outline of organs, and other images, is "subtracted" from the second picture by computer-assisted imaging. The resulting picture, the digitally subtracted image, is therefore an excellent image of the vasculature because interfering images have been removed. This test is especially useful in imaging the carotid arteries and vasculature of the brain. Digital subtraction angiography is also commonly used to image the aorta, renal vasculature, vertebral arteries, and peripheral vessels, as well as to visualize tumors.

Abnormal Findings

Abnormalities may reveal peripheral vascular disease; arterial occlusion from thrombus formation, embolus, or other stenosis; aneurysm; tumor; congenital arterial malformation; cerebrovascular accident; meningioma; pheochromocytoma; thoracic outlet syndrome; vascular parathyroid adenoma; or subclavian steal.

ACTION ALERT!

Assess clients carefully for allergic reaction to contrast material, including dyspnea, itching, urticaria, flushing, hypotension, and shock. Life-threatening anaphylactic reactions can occur and need to be recognized and treated immediately.

Interfering Factors

➤ Movement and swallowing during imaging may interfere with clear imaging.

Contraindications

➤ A history of contrast allergy contraindicates or requires caution with this test.
➤ Renal failure requires caution in proceeding.
➤ Pregnancy is a contraindication due to radiation exposure of the fetus.

Potential Complications

➤ Hemorrhage
➤ Thrombus or embolus resulting in arterial and/or venous occlusion in the extremity
➤ Allergic reactions including anaphylaxis
➤ Infection

NURSING CONSIDERATIONS

Prepare Your Client

➤ Explain that this test is to find any problems with arteries and veins (blood vessels).

➤ Ensure that an informed consent is obtained, because of the possible complications associated with this procedure.

➤ Check the chart to be sure the client has no allergy to contrast material or iodine.

➤ Record baseline vital signs.

➤ Explain to the client or family that a local anesthetic is used to numb the area where the catheter will be inserted. This may produce a brief burning sensation before the area becomes numb.

➤ Explain that the catheter (a long thin tube) is threaded through a needle placed in an artery of the thigh or arm. The catheters are threaded from the needle in the artery to the part of the body the physician needs to see. Assure the client that threading the catheters is not painful.

➤ Tell your client or family that once needles are inserted, the procedure itself is painless, but the client may feel pressure while lines are passed and warmth from the contrast medium.

➤ Locate peripheral pulses and mark with a pen to assist in monitoring them following the procedure.

➤ Review with client the need to hold their breath intermittently during the test.

➤ Restrict food and fluids for 2 hours prior to the test.

➤ Confirm that adults and older children have voided before the procedure.

➤ Do not remove glasses, dentures, or hearing aids unless dictated by your hospital policy. The client may need these in order to communicate and cooperate during the procedure.

Perform Procedure

Nurses do not perform this procedure but should understand the process to prepare the client and assist the physician. The client is placed on a special x-ray table in the catheterization laboratory. Local anesthetic is instilled subcutaneously over the arterial vascular access site. A catheter is inserted through the arterial vascular access site to the targeted area of the body. Fluoroscopy throughout the examination helps guide placement. Contrast material is inserted through the catheter. Warn the client that a warm, flushed feeling may occur. By computer, the image is improved by "subtracting" adjacent structures that might interfere with imaging. The catheter is removed and pressure applied to the site to stop bleeding and prevent hematoma formation.

Care After Test

➤ Monitor vital signs closely until stable; usually every 15 minutes for the first hour, every 30 minutes for the next hour, and then every 4 hours for 24 hours.

➤ Maintain pressure on the arterial puncture site with either a sandbag or pressure dressing.

➤ Observe for complications such as bleeding, hematoma formation, headaches, nausea, and vomiting.

➤ Assess any arterial puncture site(s) carefully for bleeding and hematoma.

➤ Assess circulation distal to the arterial puncture site, with each vital sign assessment. Assess presence and strength of pulses, capillary refill, color, temperature, and sensation. Report immediately any abnormal findings.

➤ Observe for signs of allergic reaction to the contrast material, which include urticaria, pruritus, conjunctivitis, dyspnea, and apprehension. These may occur as late as 2–6 hours following the test.

➤ Encourage drinking fluids to counteract the diuretic effect of the contrast material.

➤ Evaluate related tests such as cardiac catheterization, arteriography of the extremities, and echocardiogram.

Educate Your Client and the Family

➤ Teach client and family a heart-healthy diet, including no added salt, if there is evidence of atherosclerotic vessel disease.

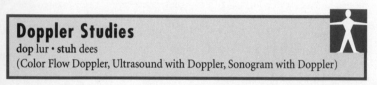

Doppler Studies
dop lur • stuh dees
(Color Flow Doppler, Ultrasound with Doppler, Sonogram with Doppler)

Normal Findings

Normal anatomical structure of arteries and veins, normal and patent arteries and veins, normal cardiac structure and function

What This Test Will Tell You

This ultrasound test is used primarily to diagnose arterial and venous disease as well as anatomical abnormalities in vessels, vascular grafts, and the heart. In venous Doppler studies, ultrasound beams are bounced off moving red blood cells to measure velocity or flow of blood through the veins. The returning sound waves from the Doppler transducer are transformed into sounds for the examiner to evaluate. These sounds may be picked up using a simple Doppler stethoscope through earphones, or directly from such ultrasound as an echocardiogram machine. In the presence of partial or complete occlusion of the vein, the sound and/or image are altered and abnormal flow can be documented.

Doppler stethoscopes are also used to assess the flow in arterial grafts following surgery; this evalua-

tion can be performed at the bedside with little training.

Doppler studies are an important part of an echocardiogram. They are able to provide critical information on blood flow through the heart, especially concerning valvular function. Both stenosis and regurgitation of valves as well as flow through prosthetic shunts and conduits can be demonstrated using Doppler technique during an echocardiographic study.

Abnormal Findings

Abnormalities may reveal peripheral vascular disease, arterial occlusion from thrombus formation or embolus, arterial aneurysms, congenital arterial malformations, venous occlusion from thrombus formation or embolus, thrombosis of prosthetic venous or arterial grafts, thrombosis of prosthetic vascular shunts, or cardiac valvular dysfunction.

Interfering Factors

➤ Vasoconstrictive medications or cigarette smoking can result in inaccurate information about arterial patency.

NURSING CONSIDERATIONS

Prepare Your Client

➤ Explain that this test is to evaluate blood vessels in the body or the heart and its structures for blockages or other problems.

➤ Assure the client that the test is painless and tell them where it will be done. Venous and arterial studies and echocardiograms are generally not done at the bedside, but rather in radiology or cardiology and average 30–60 minutes.

➤ If the procedure is simply using the Doppler stethoscope at the bedside to identify flow through native or grafted vessels, tell the client and family that this special stethoscope can actually hear blood flow.

➤ Instruct the client to refrain from smoking for at least 1 hour prior to the test.

➤ Do not remove glasses, dentures, or hearing aids unless dictated by your hospital policy. The client may need these in order to communicate and cooperate during the procedure.

Perform Procedure

Nurses do not perform this procedure but should understand it to prepare the client and assist with the process. The ultrasound gel is applied to the skin wherever they will be using the transducer to locate venous or arterial blood flow. Arteries and veins are identified anatomi-cally. The Doppler transducer is applied over these areas and patency of the vessel is established by hearing blood flow. With arterial studies, blood pressure cuffs are placed proximal to the transducer and flow is verified as pressure in the blood pressure cuff is released.

Care After Test

➤ Clean the skin of any conduction gel that may be on the chest or extremities.

➤ If results are abnormal, adjust nursing care plan and activities of client appropriately.

➤ Review related tests such as venous and arterial plethysmography, peripheral angiography, and digital subtraction angiography.

Educate Your Client and the Family

➤ Teach client and family a heart-healthy diet, including no added salt, if there is evidence of peripheral vascular disease.

➤ Educate the client on ways to promote arterial and venous blood flow through the vessels, such as wearing properly fitting shoes, avoiding constrictive clothing, and elevating the legs when possible.

➤ Teach client to protect affected extremities from injury and infection, because wound healing depends on adequate blood supplies.

Duodenal Contents, Culture

doo **od** en al • **con** tents

(Duodenal Parasites Test)

Normal Findings

All ages:

Bacteria count < 100,000

Absence of parasites

Only small amounts of polymorphonuclear leukocytes and epithelial cells

What This Test Will Tell You

This microscopic examination of aspirated duodenal contents diagnoses infectious and/or parasitic disorders of the small intestine. It may also be performed to evaluate the efficacy of antibiotic or antiparasitic medications. After the test, the tube may be left in place to provide intestinal decompression, prevent nausea, vomiting and abdominal distention, and/or to prepare the intestinal tract for surgery.

Abnormal Findings

▲ INCREASED LEVELS *of leukocytes or epithelial cells* may indicate pancreatitis, inflammation of the hepatobiliary system, or cholelithiasis.

▲ INCREASED *bacterial count* may indicate infection with *Escherichia coli, Vibrio cholerae, Bacillus cereus, Clostridium perfringens, Staphylococcus aureus, Salmonella, Shigella,* or *Yersinia enterocolitica.*

Presence of parasites may indicate giardiasis, ascariasis, coccidiosis, strongyloidiosis, or cryptosporidiosis.

ACTION ALERT!

Intubation of the gastrointestinal tract can result in perforation of tissues or organs. Assess for signs and symptoms of perforation, which include pain in the shoulder or upper gastric region, dyspnea, dysphagia, tachycardia, and fever.

Interfering Factors

➤ The presence of barium within the gastrointestinal tract may limit the information available from the test.

➤ Failure to fast for at least 12 hours prior to sampling.

➤ Contamination of specimen during collection.

Contraindications

➤ Acute pancreatitis or cholecystitis

➤ Esophageal varices

➤ Pregnancy

➤ Neoplasms

➤ Diverticula

➤ Prior gastric hemorrhage

➤ Aortic aneurysm

Potential Complications

➤ Pulmonary complications may occur, due to the client's inability to cough effectively with the nasoenteric tube in place.

➤ Otitis media, although rare, may occur from nasoenteric tubal irritation of the eustachian tube.

➤ Rare complications of nasoenteric intubation include pressure necrosis with perforation of the intestine, rupture of esophageal varices, and intussusception.

➤ Indwelling nasoenteric tubes can result in reflux esophagitis, inflammation of the nose or mouth, and nasal and/or laryngeal ulceration.

NURSING CONSIDERATIONS

Prepare Your Client

➤ Explain that the test is used to

examine the fluid inside the stomach and intestines to tell if any infection is present.

➤ Explain the nasoenteric intubation procedure and tell how mouth breathing, panting, and swallowing will help in passing the tube.

➤ Advise the client that although the intubation may be uncomfortable, it should not be painful. Talk with the client to decide upon a signal to use, such as raising the hand, to indicate "wait a few moments" because of discomfort.

➤ Withhold food and fluids for at least 12 hours prior to gastric intubation.

Perform Procedure

Nurses do not usually perform this procedure, but should understand the process to prepare the client. The specific type and size of nasoenteric tube is chosen based on the size of the client's nostrils and the length of time the tube will be in place. Several types of nasoenteric tubes may be used for the test. Nasoenteric tubes have a balloon or rubber bag at one end which is filled with air, mercury, or water to stimulate peristalsis and facilitate passage of the tube through the pylorus into the intestinal tract. The tubes should be inserted and maintained according to manufacturer's instructions.

Place the client in semi-Fowler's position and apply a local anesthetic spray to the nostril or back of the throat. The tip of the nasoenteric tube is positioned from the client's nose to the earlobe and extended down to the xiphoid process, in order to determine the length of tube required to reach the stomach. The tube is inserted into the nose and guided into the stomach. Stomach contents are aspirated with a syringe to confirm placement of the tube in the stomach.

After tube position in the stomach is verified, the client is placed in a left side-lying position and then in an upright position, to help the tube pass into the duodenum. Once the nasoenteric tube has been inserted the necessary distance into the duodenum, its position is confirmed by x-ray. Duodenal contents are aspirated with a syringe and sent to the laboratory for culture and detection of microorganisms.

Care After Test

➤ Check tube patency and adequacy of suction at least every 2 hours while the nasoenteric tube is in place.

➤ Perform frequent respiratory assessments to detect pulmonary complications which may occur from tube placement.

➤ Observe for fluid and electrolyte imbalance and document intake and output. Note color, amount, consistency, and odor of any drainage.

➤ Give frequent mouth care and nostril care to minimize discomfort and avoid complications.

➤ Withdraw the tube slowly by removing only 6 inches every 10–15 minutes until it reaches the esophagus. Once the tube has reached this level, clamp it and remove quickly.

➤ Advance the client's diet gradually after the nasoenteric tube is removed, progressing from fluids to a regular diet. Initial feedings should be small.

➤ Evaluate additional diagnostic tests used to assess small intestine and hepatobiliary function, such as the stool for ova and parasites, stool culture, small intestine biopsy, cholecystography, cholangiography, serum amylase, urine urobilinogen, and white blood cell count with differential.

Educate Your Client and the Family

➤ Teach a client with bacterial or parasitic disease of the small intestine not to discontinue antimicrobial therapy when they feel better. To be effective, medication must be taken as prescribed.

➤ Instruct a client with bacterial or parasitic disease of the small intestine to eat a variety of foods and drink plenty of fluids to maintain nutritional status and avoid dehydration.

➤ Teach client the importance of handwashing, especially after bowel and bladder elimination, to avoid transmitting any microorganisms.

➤ Inform client and family not to eat raw eggs, which may harbor salmonella, and to always wash hands when preparing food.

D-Xylose Absorption

dee • zie lose • ab sorp shun
(Xylose Tolerance Test)

Normal Findings

SERUM
Adult: 25–40 mg/dL between 1 and 2 hours after ingestion of D-xylose (SI units: 1.7–2.7 mmol/L)
Child: 1–10 years: 10%–33% of the dose ingested, or >30 mg/dL (SI units: >2.0 mmol/L)
>10 years: 16% of 25-g dose
URINE
Adult: >80%–95% excreted in 5 hours, >5 g excreted in 24 hours
Child: 16%–33% excreted in 5 hours

What This Test Will Tell You

These urine and blood tests help differentiate malabsorption syndromes caused by pancreatic disorders from those caused by intestinal disorders. The tests measure absorption of the pentose sugar D-xylose to evaluate small-intestinal absorption capacity. Serum and urine levels are measured after the ingestion of D-xylose. D-xylose is used to test intestinal absorption because it is not metabolized by the body.

Normally the urine is collected over a 5-hour period, but a 24-hour test may be indicated for an older adult with minor renal dysfunction. These clients may have a normal 24-hour level with a low 5-hour level.

Abnormal Findings

▼ DECREASED LEVELS may indicate intestinal malabsorption syndromes related to lymphatic obstruction, celiac disease, Crohn's disease, sprue, enteropathy, or Whipple's disease; small intestinal bacterial overgrowth; *Giardia lamblia* infection; hookworm; lymphoma; amyloidosis; scleroderma; or gastroenteritis.

Interfering Factors

➤ Renal failure may give falsely low urine xylose levels.
➤ Incomplete urine collections, ascites, and indomethacin may result in falsely low levels of urine xylose.

➤ Non-steroidal anti-inflammatory drugs such as aspirin and indomethacin as well as atropine may affect test results by decreasing xylose absorption in the intestine.

➤ Vomiting, dehydration, and alcoholism may decrease levels.

➤ Increased physical activity may decrease measured levels.

➤ Foods high in pentose (fruits, jellies, jams, and pastries) can elevate urine and serum levels.

Contraindications

➤ Dehydration
➤ Renal impairment

Potential Complications

➤ Nausea, vomiting, diarrhea

NURSING CONSIDERATIONS

Prepare Your Client

➤ Explain that this test is used to see how well the intestines absorb food to use as it passes through, and identify problems with absorption.

➤ Restrict food and fluids except water for 6–8 hours (4–6 hours for children) before the test. Tell client to avoid jellies, jams, fruits, and pastries for 24 hours prior to the test.

➤ Instruct the client on proper 5- or 24-hour urine collection.

➤ Keep the client recumbent or in quiet activity during the test, as physical activity can affect results.

Perform Procedure

➤ The client swallows a 25-g dose of D-xylose mixed in water, and the amount of D-xylose excreted in the urine over a 5-hour period is measured. Serum levels of D-xylose are also measured 1 hour after consuming the D-xylose. The D-xylose dose for infants is 14.5 g/m^2 orally, and for

children 5 g/kg of D-xylose in 100 mL of water.

➤ Maintain a food-and-fluid fast throughout the collection period.

➤ Keep the client on bed rest during the test because activity may interfere with the results.

➤ Collect 1–7 mL of venous blood in a red-top tube 1 hour after D-xylose dose is consumed (for neonates, a heel stick may be used to collect a smaller sample). Generally, adult venous samples are collected after 2 hours, and children's venous samples are collected after 1 hour. Sampling may occur at 30, 60, and 120 minutes after ingestion of D-xylose.

➤ Label the sample and note any interfering factors or medications.

➤ Save all urine during the 5- or 24-hour testing period. Instruct the client to void at the end of the 5-hour period and include this amount.

Care After Test

➤ Evaluate the client's nutritional status. Consult with a registered dietician for assistance in evaluation and treatment plan.

➤ Ensure the client is allowed to resume eating and drinking as condition allows.

➤ Assess the client for nausea, vomiting, and diarrhea, which can be side effects of D-xylose ingestion.

➤ Evaluate other tests of intestinal absorption such as the fecal fat, upper gastrointestinal series, endoscopic examinations and biopsies, and Schilling test for vitamin B$_{12}$ absorption.

Educate Your Client and the Family

➤ Teach client with malabsorption to consume a high-calorie diet with plenty of fruits and vegetables that contain fat-soluble vitamins A, D, E, and K.

➤ Instruct client to eat small, frequent meals and to drink between meals instead of with meals to decrease symptoms.

Echocardiogram

eh koe **kar** dee oe gram

(Cardiac or Heart Ultrasound, Cardiac or Heart Sonogram, M-mode Echocardiogram, 2-D Echocardiogram, Echo with Doppler, Echo, Transesophageal Echocardiogram, TEE)

Normal Findings

All ages:
Normal anatomical structure and position
Normal and patent arteries and/or veins of the heart
Normal valve structure
Normal blood flow within the heart
Normal ventricular function
Absence of thrombi or bacterial vegctations
Absence of pericardial effusions

What This Test Will Tell You

This ultrasonic test diagnoses abnormalities in anatomy and valvular function within the heart. As in other ultrasound tests, sound waves are bounced off the heart using a transducer to image the heart in motion as well as its valves and vessels. Echocardiographic imaging of the heart, vessels, valves, and blood flow may actually replace the need for angiography.

M-mode echocardiography provides information about both structure and function, but does not produce as true a visual image of the heart as does two-dimensional echocardiography. Echocardiograms can also be performed during stress testing to provide additional information about cardiac function.

This test can also be performed invasively by passing a transducer down the esophagus for imaging. This test is called a *transesophageal echocardiogram (TEE)* and usually requires sedation.

Abnormal Findings

Abnormalities may indicate mitral valve prolapse, valvular stenosis, valvular insufficiency or regurgitation, ventricular dysfunction, congenital cardiac defects, intracardiac thrombus, bacterial endocarditis, pericardial effusion, ventricular or atrial septal defects, or aneurysms.

Interfering Factors

➤ Movement or failure to lie still during testing
➤ Obesity
➤ High-pressure mechanical ventilation
➤ Chronic pulmonary obstructive disease
➤ Dysrhythmias
➤ Chest wall; interference can be reduced by using the transesophageal approach (TEE)

Contraindications

➤ For TEE, previous history of gastroesophageal disease

Potential Complications

➤ None for echocardiogram
➤ Bradycardia, emesis, and aspiration related to TEE
➤ For TEE, complications may include those associated with sedation and oral-gastric intubation. Most frequently these complications are chipped or loose teeth, gagging, vomiting, aspiration, respiratory depression, and apnea.

NURSING CONSIDERATIONS

Prepare Your Client

➤ Explain to the client or family that this test is performed by placing a clear gel on the chest wall, and then placing a transducer (microphone) on the gel to send and receive painless soundwaves.

➤ Tell the client that an electrocardiogram (EKG, ECG) will also be taken during this test. (See *Electrocardiogram*.)

➤ Inform the client and family that the test is usually done in a cardiac imaging laboratory and takes about 30–45 minutes. The room is usually darkened for the technician to better see the screen. Occasionally during the test, a loud swishing sound of the heart beating may be heard.

➤ For TEE, explain that medication will be used to make the client sleepy and a tube will be passed down their esophagus (the tube going to the stomach, not the windpipe) to better see the heart.

➤ Assure the client there is no pain with an echocardiogram.

➤ For a TEE, some discomfort from having the esophageal probe passed may be experienced. Topical analgesia should provide relief.

➤ Do not remove glasses, dentures, or hearing aids unless dictated by your hospital policy. The client may need these in order to communicate and cooperate during the procedure.

➤ For TEE, administer any preprocedure sedation that is ordered. Carefully assess history for respiratory disease, current respiratory infection, or previous adverse reactions to sedation.

Perform Procedure

Nurses do not perform this procedure but should understand the process to prepare the client and assist the physician.

TRANSTHORACIC ECHOCARDIOGRAPHY

An ultrasound gel is applied to the chest wall where the transducer is placed. A variety of angles are obtained using different placement and angles of the transducer. These commonly include short axis, parasternal long axis, suprasternal, subcostal, and four-chamber views.

TRANSESOPHAGEAL ECHOCARDIOGRAPHY

For transesophageal echocardiography, client is usually sedated before the transducer, built into an esophageal probe, is passed down the esophagus. Imaging is done from inside the body rather than across the chest wall.

Care After Test

➤ No special care is required after transthoracic imaging.

➤ After TEE, careful observation for recovery from sedation is indicated. Assessments should include return of gag and swallow reflexes as well as adequate chest wall movement (excursion) during respirations.

➤ Review related tests such as electrocardiogram, cardiac enzymes, chest x-ray, and stress test.

Educate Your Client and the Family

➤ Teach client and family a heart-healthy diet, including no added salt.

➤ Encourage family and significant others to learn cardiopulmonary resuscitation.

➤ If indicated, teach client methods to conserve energy, such as pacing activities, not overeating, and reducing stress.

Electrocardiogram

ee lek troe kar dee oe gram

(EKG, ECG, Electrocardiography)

Normal Findings

Normal sinus rhythm

Normal conduction patterns

Absence of areas of infarct or ischemia

What This Test Will Tell You

This electrophysiologic test is used primarily to screen for and diagnose a variety of cardiac conditions as well as to monitor the heart's response to therapy. The electrocardiogram (ECG) is frequently used to diagnose abnormal heart rhythms, conduction disturbances, hypertrophy of cardiac chambers, myocardial infarction and ischemia, and pericarditis. An ECG measures electrical flow through the heart by using electrodes applied painlessly to the chest wall and limbs.

Electrical flow through the heart's conduction system causes the heart to mechanically contract to pump blood. The impulse begins in the sinoatrial (SA) node and travels across the atria to the atrioventricular (AV) node, where it pauses briefly. From the AV node, the impulse travels toward the ventricles by flowing down the bundle of His (His bundle) to the Purkinje fibers and throughout the ventricular tissue. Each of these key points in the conduction system can be analyzed by examining different waveforms that are created. See the table on page 268. The electrocardiogram can record the electrical flow of each impulse from a variety of *leads*, or positions, which helps the health care provider pinpoint locations of problems within the heart.

In addition to diagnosing prob-

lems and abnormalities in cardiac function, the ECG can help monitor clients' responses to therapy. The ECG is used to monitor pacemaker function and the effectiveness of medications such as digoxin, fibrinolytics, and antidysrhythmics.

Abnormal Findings

Abnormalities may reveal myocardial infarction, myocardial ischemia, dysrhythmias, ventricular hypertrophy, conduction defects, heart block, Wolff-Parkinson-White syndrome, pericarditis, or atrial hypertrophy.

ACTION ALERT!

Diagnostic indications of myocardial ischemia, myocardial infarction, and second- or third-degree heart blocks with accompanying symptoms all require immediate medical attention and intervention. These conditions may be associated with a high incidence of cardiopulmonary arrest.

Interfering Factors

➤ Improperly grounded recording equipment can distort electrical tracings.

➤ Improper placement of electrodes.

➤ Electrodes without adequate amounts of conduction gel.

➤ Dried conduction gel on electrodes.

➤ Movement of client.

➤ Heavy chest hair.

➤ Anxiety or fear may cause sinus tachycardia during the test only.

NURSING CONSIDERATIONS

Prepare Your Client

➤ Explain that this test is performed

Electrocardiogram Waveforms

ECG component	What it means to normal heart function	Normal findings
P wave	Represents depolarization of the atria. This should also represent contraction of the atria. If normal in appearance and upright, it usually indicates a rhythm originated by the sinoatrial (SA) node (sinus rhythm).	0.10 second in duration 2.5 mm in height/amplitude
PR interval	Measures time for conduction to travel from the SA node throughout the atria, to the atrioventricular (AV) node, to the ventricles to initiate depolarization there. Measured from the start of the P wave to the beginning of the QRS complex.	0.12–0.20 second in duration
QRS complex	Represents depolarization of the ventricles. This should also represent contraction of the ventricles. It may normally appear upright or deflected downward. This complex is measured from the start of the Q wave to the end of the S wave.	Less than 0.12 second in duration
T wave	Represents repolarization of the ventricles. This complex is normally upright.	1–5 mm in height/amplitude
R to R interval	Represents the time between generation of each impulse. It should also represent the time between each contraction of the heart. This interval should be regular.	Normal heart rate for age and condition
U wave	Believed to represent repolarization of the Purkinje fibers (conduction system within the ventricles).	1.5 mm in height/amplitude. 0.24 second in duration

by placing small discs or strips that stick to the skin on the chest, arms, and legs. Tell them they will have to lie still on their back while the ECG machine is recording the heart's activity.

➤ Explain that although the test is used to look at how the body's own natural electrical system in the heart is working, the machine does not permit electricity to enter the body nor is there any sensation of electrical shock. By looking at the heart's own natural flow of current, the primary health care provider can get information on how well the heart is pumping and receiving blood.

➤ Inform the client and family that the test is usually done in a cardiac imaging laboratory and takes about 5–10 minutes.

➤ Assure the client there is no pain

with this test.

➤ Inform client with heavy chest hair that small areas may need to be shaved or clipped to assure adequate electrode-to-skin contact.

➤ Note any medications the client is taking for hypertension or cardiac disease and inform the professional interpreting the ECG.

➤ Do not remove glasses, dentures, or hearing aids unless dictated by your hospital policy. The client may need these in order to communicate and cooperate during the procedure.

➤ Explain that the chest will need to be exposed during electrode placement. Drape female client as much as possible during placement.

Perform Procedure

Nurses may perform this procedure and need to understand the process to prepare the client and assist the physician or technician. Electrodes are placed on the chest wall and connected by wires to an electrocardiographic machine, which records the electrical activity of the heart.

Care After Test

➤ Wipe off electrode paste or jelly.

➤ Review exercise tolerance and cardiac rehabilitation program in client if results indicate cardiac disease.

➤ Evaluate related tests such as an echocardiogram, cardiac enzymes, cardiac stress test, and cardiac catheterization.

Educate Your Client and the Family

➤ Teach client and family a heart-healthy diet, including no added salt, if there is evidence of atherosclerotic vessel disease.

Electroencephalography

ee lek troe en sef ah log rah fee
(EEG, Electroencephalogram)

Normal Findings
Normal brain wave patterns

What This Test Will Tell You

This electrophysiologic test records brain wave activity and is especially useful in diagnosing seizure disorders and in monitoring cerebral blood flow during surgical procedures where the carotid artery is temporarily occluded. Electrical impulses produced by brain cells are sensed by surface electrodes placed on the client's scalp. Wires connect the scalp electrodes to the electroencephalogram machine, which produces tracings of brain wave activity on graph paper. This test not only helps detect abnormal electrical activity in seizure disorders, but may also be useful in locating tumors and assessing cerebral blood flow patterns by its sensitivity to hypoxia.

This test is occasionally used in establishing death by neurologic criteria (brain death), but is not required and is considered by medical experts to be of minimal value.

Occasionally client may be asked to go to bed late and awaken early to stimulate abnormal brain waves or enhance sleep during testing.

Abnormal Findings

Abnormal patterns may indicate epilepsy, seizure activity, brain tumors, brain abscesses, brain lesions, intracranial hemorrhage, encephalitis, Alzheimer's disease, brain trauma, cerebral infarct, narcolepsy, cerebral death, or coma.

███████ ACTION ALERT!

Assess for possible seizure activity and maintain safety precautions.

Interfering Factors

➤ Dirt, oil, gel, or hair spray on the scalp interferes with transmission of electrical impulses.

➤ Any medications affecting central nervous system function such as sleeping pills, tranquilizers, stimulants, alcohol, cigarettes, coffee, tea, and colas can change brain wave activity.

➤ Sleep deprivation may cause abnormal brain wave patterns.

➤ Hypoglycemia can cause changes in brain wave patterns.

➤ Manipulation of the electrodes and electrical interference from equipment can cause inaccurate tracings. This is especially important in critical care settings.

➤ Fasting may cause hypoglycemia and alter brain wave patterns.

➤ Movement of the body or eyes can cause disruptions in brain wave patterns.

NURSING CONSIDERATIONS

Prepare Your Client

➤ Explain that this test is used to measure activity of different parts of the brain by measuring brain waves.

➤ Check that the client has clean hair and scalp to ensure accurate results of the test. No oil, gels, or hairspray

should be placed on the hair after it is shampooed the night before the test.

➤ Stress the importance of getting a restful sleep the night before the test unless the primary health care provider wishes to restrict sleep for the study.

➤ Tell client that the test will take $1^1/2$ to 2 hours. The client will be lying down or sitting in a reclining chair.

➤ Verify that client has taken only those medications the primary care provider has approved before the test. Some medications are normally discontinued the night before to ensure accurate tracings. Medications such as sleeping pills, tranquilizers, sedatives, and stimulants as well as alcohol will cause changes in the brain wave activity and should generally not be taken.

➤ Confirm that client has not been drinking caffeinated beverages such as coffee, tea, and colas before the test. Other foods and drinks are not restricted. Client needs to eat a full meal before the test.

➤ Tell client that the EEG (electroencephalogram) is not painful and will not send any electrical impulses to the brain. This is *not* shock therapy.

➤ Verify that any changes in normal sleep patterns ordered by the primary care provider have occurred.

Perform Procedure

Nurses do not usually perform this procedure. They need to understand the process to explain it to the client or to assist in the procedure. This procedure is usually performed in a controlled environment to decrease the risk of interfering stimuli. Electrodes are applied to the scalp in specifically designated areas. If the procedure is performed at the bedside, keep the environment as quiet as possible. Avoid manipulating the client, wires, or electrodes during the test. Observe for seizures. If seizures occur during the test, describe the activity and the length of time activity lasted. Tracings are collected while client is awake, drowsy, sleeping, and being stimulated (hyperventilating, flickering lights, sounds).

Care After Test

➤ Clean the paste from the scalp.

➤ The client may resume normal activity.

➤ Protect client at risk for seizure activity by padding side rails of the bed, keeping the bed in a low position, and assuring an oral airway is available immediately.

➤ Evaluate the client's skin for pressure areas if prolonged lying in one position was necessary during the test.

➤ Evaluate related studies such as computed tomography scan, mag-

netic resonance imaging, cerebral perfusion studies, and skull x-rays.

Educate Your Client and the Family

➤ Help client and family to understand that a normal EEG does not always rule out neurologic pathology. Some conditions do not alter brain wave activity. If the EEG is done between seizures, abnormal activity may not be traced.

➤ Instruct client in safety measures such as wearing helmets to prevent head trauma that may be associated with seizure activity.

➤ Stress the importance of prenatal care to decrease the risk of fetal hypoxia and trauma that may lead to seizure activity.

➤ Teach the family safety measures to protect the client during seizures, such as moving furniture and large objects away, and not restraining a person having a seizure.

E

Electromyography

ee lek troe mie og rah fee
(EMG, Electromyogram)

Normal Findings

At rest: Minimal or no electrical activity

Voluntary muscular activity: Increased electrical activity

ELDERLY

Electrical activity may be decreased in some elderly people.

What This Test Will Tell You

This electrophysiologic test differentiates between diseases of muscles (myopathies) and nerves (neu-

ropathies). Myopathies are associated with diseases of skeletal muscle fibers, whereas neuropathies involve disruption of lower motor neurons, which innervate muscle. This test helps diagnose neurologic and/or muscular diseases.

Abnormal Findings

➤ Myopathy may indicate muscular dystrophy, myasthenia gravis, multiple sclerosis, polymyositis, or myotonia.

➤ *Neuropathy* may indicate diabetic neuropathy, alcoholic neuropathy, poliomyelitis, segmental motor neuron lesions, lower motor neuron lesions, and amyotrophic lateral sclerosis, Guillain-Barré syndrome, or nerve loss associated with trauma.

Interfering Factors

➤ Drugs that affect neurotransmission such as muscle relaxants, anticholinergics, and cholinergics.
➤ Caffeinated beverages may contribute to tremors, which may invalidate the test.
➤ Pain may invalidate the results.
➤ Peripheral edema.
➤ Obesity.

Contraindications

➤ Anticoagulation therapy
➤ Skin infection

Potential Complications

➤ Infection and hematoma at insertion sites

NURSING CONSIDERATIONS

Prepare Your Client

➤ Explain that this procedure measures the electrical activity of the muscle fibers to help diagnose problems with nerves and/or muscles.
➤ Ensure that an informed consent is obtained, because of the possible complications associated with this procedure.
➤ Verify that client has refrained from drinking caffeinated beverages and from smoking for 2–3 hours before the test.
➤ Ask the primary care provider about withholding medications that may affect the test, such as muscle relaxants, anticholinergics, and cholinergics. If medications cannot

be withheld, schedule the test when medications will have the least effect on test results.
➤ Warn client that the needles may cause some discomfort during insertion. However, if pain persists, the client needs to tell the technician performing the test. The electrodes may need to be repositioned.
➤ Explain that amplified noises of neuromuscular activity will be heard during the procedure. Electrical activity will be recorded on a screen like a computer (cathode-ray oscilloscope).
➤ Advise client on how to relax and contract certain muscles during the test. Stress the importance of following the instructions in order to obtain accurate test results.
➤ Check orders for blood tests. If serum enzyme tests are ordered, draw blood before or 5–10 days after the procedure. Stimulation of muscle may affect SGOT (serum glutamic-oxalacetic transaminase), CPK (creatinine phosphokinase), and LDH (lactic dehydrogenase) results.

Perform Procedure

Nurses do not usually perform this procedure, but should understand the process to explain the test to the client. Surface electrodes are placed on the skin near the area being tested. A reference electrode is placed on the skin surface near the area to be tested. The client is asked to keep that muscle at rest. Electrodes (recording) are inserted into the specific muscles to be tested and the client is positioned depending upon the part of the body being tested. An oscilloscope screen displays the electrical response of the area as the client is asked to slowly contract or relax a specific muscle or muscle group.

Care After Test
➤ Medicate the client as needed for muscle aches.
➤ Observe for bruising or infection at electrode needle insertion sites.
➤ Help client and family to identify effective strategies to cope with changes in ability to perform activities of daily living.
➤ Stress the importance of continuing to remain as independent as possible despite limited or decreasing functioning.

➤ Evaluate related tests such as evoked potential studies.

Educate Your Client and the Family
➤ Teach client, as indicated by findings, energy-conserving activities to pace activities and strengthen muscles.
➤ Instruct the client and family on home safety related to weakness or dysfunction of affected muscle groups.

E

Electroneurography
ee lek troe noo rog rah fee
(ENoG, ENOG)

Normal Findings
Normal stimulus response. Conduction velocity is decreased in the elderly.

What This Test Will Tell You
This electrophysiologic measurement test assesses peripheral nerve function that may be impaired from either injury or disease. The test measures electrical changes and nerve conduction velocities of peripheral nerves and can determine whether sensory or motor nerves are involved. The test also measures the time it takes for an electrical stimulus to cause a muscle contraction. Normal values are established by comparing affected and unaffected sides.

Abnormal Findings
Abnormal response may indicate malnutrition, alcoholism, metabolic disorders, diabetic neuropathy, trauma, myasthenia gravis, acoustic neuromas, facial nerve paralysis, muscular dystrophy, carpal tunnel syndrome, Guillain-Barré syndrome, facial nerve degeneration, intraoperative localization of conduction abnormality, or Bell's palsy.

Interfering Factors
➤ Primary muscle disorders
➤ Pain

Contraindications
➤ Inability of the client to cooperate with the test

NURSING CONSIDERATIONS
Prepare Your Client
➤ Explain that the test is used to diagnose problems with the body's nerves.
➤ Warn the client that small electrical shocks may be felt during the test. They are not harmful, but may be uncomfortable.

➤ Prepare client to lie very still during the test.

Perform Procedure

Nurses do not usually perform this procedure, but should understand the process to prepare the client and assist the physician. The test can be performed at the bedside or in a special laboratory.

Electrodes are placed over the areas to be tested. They serve as stimulating and receptive sites. The electrodes are attached to specialized equipment that measures the time of impulse transmission.

Care After Test

➤ Evaluate other electrophysiologic tests such as electromyography and visual evoked potentials.

➤ Obtain referrals to occupational and physical therapy for client with significant neural dysfunction.

➤ For client with metabolic disorders, malnutrition, alcoholism, or diabetic neuropathy, obtain nutritional consults.

Educate Your Client and the Family

➤ Assist the client in understanding the disorder that may be diagnosed and how to best minimize long-term nervous system effects.

➤ Educate client with sensory loss on how to protect extremities from injury. Instruct them to wear shoes that fit well to prevent foot injury, to test bath water carefully before stepping in, and to protect against other situations of temperature extremes.

Electronystagmography (ENG)
ee lek troe nis tag mog rah fee

Normal Findings

Normal vestibular-ocular reflex response
Nystagmus with turning of the head

What This Test Will Tell You

This electrophysiologic test is used in the differential diagnosis of conditions involving the vestibular system and muscles controlling eye movement. Nystagmus is a normal response to head movement and requires normally functioning ocular and vestibular systems for the vestibular-ocular reflex to occur. The vestibular system attempts to maintain visual fixation during head rotation, causing involuntary back-and-forth movement of the eyes. This test

studies three conditions: lesions in the brain stem and cerebellum, unilateral hearing loss of unknown origin, and vertigo, dizziness, or tinnitus.

Abnormal Findings

Abnormal response may indicate cerebellar lesion; brain stem lesion; peripheral lesion due to head trauma, drugs, increased age; ototoxicity; eighth cranial nerve tumor; demyelinating disease; or congenital disorders.

ACTION ALERT!

Irrigating the ear with water should not be performed in client with perforated eardrum unless tympanic membrane is protected with a finger cot, due to risk of serious infections.

Interfering Factors

➤ Inability of the client to cooperate with instructions.

➤ Poor vision.

➤ Improperly applied electrodes.

➤ Stimulants, tranquilizers, sedatives, alcohol, and antivertigo drugs may cause false positive test results.

➤ Client anxiety may cause false positive results.

➤ Large amounts of ear wax may interfere with caloric study portion of the test.

➤ Blinking of eyes.

Contraindications

➤ Contraindications for including the caloric study are middle ear infections, blood or fluid behind the tympanic membrane, tympanic membrane tubes, and perforated membrane. If the client has a perforated eardrum, a finger cot may be used to protect the middle ear from water irrigation.

➤ Client with pacemaker. Electrical equipment may interfere with pacemaker function.

➤ Client with known back or neck pathology may experience exacerbation of symptoms. Consult the primary health care provider about deleting some of the positional changes.

Potential Complications

➤ Ear infection

NURSING CONSIDERATIONS

Prepare Your Client

➤ Explain that the purpose of the test is to help find the cause of symptoms such as vision and dizziness problems.

➤ Assure the client there is no pain with this test.

➤ Instruct the client that medication restrictions include sedatives, tranquilizers, and antivertigo drugs. Suggested times for refraining from these medications vary from 2–5 days before the test.

➤ Instruct the client to refrain from drinking caffeinated and alcoholic beverages for 2 days before the test.

➤ Advise the client to refrain from eating solids for 8 hours before the test since nausea and vomiting may be experienced.

➤ Tell the client to take prescription glasses, if they wear any, to the test.

➤ Tell the client to refrain from wearing makeup and facial oils to the test.

Perform Procedure

Nurses normally do not perform this test but need to understand the procedure to explain it to the client.

The test takes place in a darkened room. The client may be sitting in a chair or lying on a table. Provide the client with an emesis basin and moist washcloth. Five electrodes are placed on the forehead and around the eyes to measure eye movement during the test. The client will be asked to look at moving lights/objects, fixed lights/objects, and to open and close eyes on cue. The client will be asked to change positions quickly. Stress the importance of following all instructions in order to get accurate test results.

A caloric study is the final phase of the test. This is an irrigation of the ear with cold or warm water for 3 minutes or until nystagmus occurs or nausea and dizziness are experienced. The test usually takes 60–90 minutes.

Care After Test

➤ Monitor for signs and symptoms of ear infection if caloric study was included.

➤ Provide a quiet, calm environment for at least 1 hour. The client will be tired. Vertigo, weakness, and nausea are often present for some time following the test.

➤ If balance is severely impaired due to underlying condition, arrange for occupational health, physical therapy, and home nursing consultations as indicated.

➤ Review related tests such as electroencephalogram and computer tomography.

Educate Your Client and the Family

➤ Teach safety precautions if symptoms of vertigo are present, including keeping a night light on, wearing non-skid shoes, and using railings or a walker for balance.

Electrophysiology Study
ee lek troe fiz ee ol oe jee • stuh dee
(EPS, EP Study, HIS Bundle Procedure, Cardiac Mapping)

Normal Findings
All ages: Normal conduction patterns, refractory periods, and recovery times with no dysrhythmias

What This Test Will Tell You
This electrophysiology test is used primarily to diagnose dysrhythmias and abnormal conduction of impulses through the heart. Through the same basic procedure as a cardiac catheterization (see *Cardiac Catheterization* test), electrode catheters are placed into the atria and ventricles that pace and stimulate the heart. The test maps normal and abnormal conduction pathways and evaluates the normal recovery and refractory periods of the heart's own pacing mechanism. The procedure diagnoses and accurately locates areas of abnormalities, and then evaluates effectiveness of pharmacologic therapy.

This procedure may also be used therapeutically to treat abnormal cardiac rhythms and conduction pathways. Destruction of abnormal conduction tissue can be accomplished during the electrophysiology study (EPS) by using laser or cryotherapy, or during surgery with excision of abnormal tissue or severing of accessory pathways.

Abnormal Findings
Abnormalities may reveal an acquired or congenital conduction defect, Wolff-Parkinson-White syndrome, sick sinus syndrome, a heart block, or an accessory pathway.

ACTION ALERT!

➤ Cardiopulmonary arrest is a high risk associated with this procedure. Constant monitoring of heart rhythm, vital signs, systemic circulation, and level of consciousness is critical.
➤ Assess client carefully for allergic response to contrast medium, including dyspnea, urticaria, flushing, hypotension, itching, and shock. Life-threatening anaphylactic reactions can occur and need to be recognized and treated immediately.

Interfering Factors

➤ In confused or uncooperative adults as well as preverbal infants and children, it may be difficult to monitor the level of consciousness during EPS. This is important in determining the clinical response to dysrhythmias, abnormalities in conduction, and response to treatment.

➤ Tranquilizers and sedatives may also interfere with test results.

Contraindications

➤ Pregnancy, due to radiation exposure of the fetus.

➤ Acute myocardial infarction.

➤ Medications client is currently taking, such as calcium channel blockers, beta blockers, other antidysrhythmics, and antihypertensive agents, may affect the ability to induce and map abnormalities.

➤ Acute pulmonary embolism.

➤ Coagulopathy.

➤ This test should be performed cautiously in clients with severe cardiomegaly because of the danger of serious dysrhythmias and risk of perforation of the heart.

Potential Complications

➤ Cardiopulmonary arrest

➤ Lethal dysrhythmias such as ventricular tachycardia or ventricular fibrillation

➤ Perforation of the heart or great vessels

➤ Thromboemboli

➤ Cerebrovascular accident

➤ Allergic reactions including anaphylaxis

➤ Infection

➤ Hemopericardium

➤ Hemothorax

➤ Hemorrhage

NURSING CONSIDERATIONS

Prepare Your Client

➤ Explain that this test is to help diagnose the spot in the heart that is causing abnormal heartbeats. If possible, medications will be tested to control the problem, or the abnormal spot will be destroyed.

➤ Ensure that an informed consent is obtained, because of the possible complications associated with this procedure.

➤ Obtain a potassium level and electrocardiogram prior to the EPS.

➤ Inform your client they may experience lightheadedness, dizziness, nausea, palpitations, or chest pain and should inform the personnel in the EPS laboratory immediately.

➤ Review with adult client actions they may be asked to perform: breathe deeply, cough, or do bicycle leg movements.

➤ Record baseline vital signs.

➤ Locate peripheral pulses and mark with a pen to assist in monitoring them following the procedure.

➤ Restrict food and fluids (NPO) for at least 4 hours before the procedure.

➤ Check with the primary care provider to determine if medications should be administered while the client is NPO.

➤ Do not administer sedatives or tranquilizers before the client goes to the cardiac catheterization laboratory. It is important to be able to judge the level of consciousness during this study.

➤ Confirm that adults and older children have voided before the procedure.

➤ Do not remove glasses, dentures, or hearing aids unless dictated by your hospital policy. The client may need these in order to communicate and cooperate during the procedure.

Perform Procedure

Nurses do not perform this procedure but should understand the process to prepare the client and assist the physician. A local anesthetic is used in the catheterization laboratory to numb the area where the needle will be inserted in the femoral or subclavian vein. This may produce a brief burning sensation before the area becomes numb. Catheters are threaded through the needle and vein to the heart. Assure client that threading the catheters is not painful. They may feel some pressure and warmth from the contrast medium while lines are passed. See *Cardiac Catheterization* for other details.

Care After Test

➤ Monitor vital signs every 15 minutes for 1 hour, then hourly for 4 hours, then every 4 hours for a total of 24 hours.

➤ Continuously monitor the client's electrocardiogram using telemetry or bedside monitoring.

➤ Maintain pressure on venipuncture site with either a sandbag or pressure dressing.

➤ Maintain bed rest with the extremity extended for 6–12 hours following the procedure to minimize complications of bleeding, hematoma formation, headaches, nausea, and vomiting.

➤ Assess the venipuncture site(s) carefully for bleeding and hematoma.

➤ Assess circulation at least every 30 minutes for 4 hours, then hourly for 24 hours, including presence and strength of pulses, capillary refill, color, temperature, and sensation. Compare to pretest assessment.

➤ Occasionally an indwelling catheter electrode is left in place for additional studies. This should be covered with a sterile dressing and checked daily by the electrophysiology or cardiac catheterization nurse. These catheters may also require flushing to remain patent, and should only be flushed by specially trained personnel.

➤ Evaluate related tests such as Holter recording, 12-lead electrocardiogram, and exercise stress test.

Educate Your Client and the Family

➤ Teach client and family a heart-healthy diet, including no added salt.

➤ For infant or child with congenital cardiac defects, discuss caloric intake and collaborate with the primary health care provider and dietician to supplement formula and diet as needed.

➤ Encourage family and significant others to learn cardiopulmonary resuscitation.

➤ Teach client to conserve energy by pacing activities, not overeating, and learning methods to relax and reduce stress.

Endometrial Biopsy

en doe mee tree uhl • bie op see

Normal Findings

Secretory phase endometrium found 3–5 days prior to menses

Absence of pathology

What This Test Will Tell You

This test for fertility disorders is a microscopic examination of the endometrial lining of the uterus to determine ovarian function and adequacy of circulating progesterone levels or proper function of progesterone receptors in the endometrium. It also diagnoses endometrial hyperplasia, polyps, carcinoma, and tuberculosis. Evaluation of the proliferative phase and the secretory or luteal phase of the menstrual cycle is useful in the diagnosis of fertility disorders. In the event of anovulation, a proliferative, rather than secretory, phase endometrium will be present at the time of the test, 3–5 days pre-menses. Luteal phase dysfunction is evidenced when a discrepancy of ±4 (plus or minus 4) days exists between the pathologist's estimation of ovulation upon examination of the secretory phase endometrium and indication of ovulation on a basal body temperature (BBT) chart. Decreased amounts of secretory type tissue also indicate inadequate progesterone levels or endometrial progesterone receptors.

Endometrial biopsy is also useful in investigating and diagnosing the cause of postmenopausal bleeding and premenopausal recurrent metrorrhagia. It may be done prior to the initiation of postmenopausal estrogen replacement therapy to rule out endometrial carcinoma.

Abnormal Findings

➤ *Fertility abnormalities* may include abnormal findings during the luteal phase such as anovulation, decreased levels of progesterone, or abnormal functioning of the progesterone receptors in the endometrium. Fertility abnormalities also include decreased level of circulating progesterone, or impaired endometrial progesterone receptors.

➤ *Pathological abnormalities* may include inflammatory disorders, polyps, hyperplasia, carcinoma, or tuberculosis.

ACTION ALERT!

This is an invasive procedure that can potentially result in perforation of the uterus, hemorrhaging, or severe infection.

Interfering Factors

➤ Menses
➤ Pregnancy (early conception rarely disturbed by procedure)

Contraindications

➤ Vaginal or cervical infections (chlamydia, gonorrhea, moniliasis, trichomoniasis)
➤ Abnormal positioning of cervix preventing visualization

Potential Complications

➤ Bleeding
➤ Infection
➤ Perforation of the uterus
➤ Dislodging an embryo

NURSING CONSIDERATIONS

Prepare Your Client

➤ Explain, depending on client's case, that this test is done to get information about how the body is releasing eggs, how the womb is preparing for pregnancy, or why abnormal bleeding may be occurring.

➤ Inform the client that the procedure takes about 15–30 minutes.

➤ Ensure that an informed consent is obtained, because of the possible complications associated with this procedure.

➤ Do not restrict food or fluid prior to the test.

➤ Have the client void before the procedure.

Perform Procedure

Nurses do not perform this procedure, but need to understand it so that it can be explained to clients. Place the client in a supine position with her legs in stirrups (lithotomy position). Premedication with a prostaglandin inhibitor such as naproxen sodium may be given to prevent uterine cramping. Usually no anesthetics are administered; however, a paracervical block may be used upon primary health care provider evaluation of client's condition. If a local anesthetic is not administered, explain that cramping will be experienced as the tissue is removed, but that cramps should be reduced by the medication taken.

A pelvic examination is performed to determine the uterine position. A vaginal speculum is inserted. The vagina and cervix are visualized and cleaned with an antiseptic solution. A uterine sound to determine uterine depth is inserted following dilatation of the cervix, if required. A curette or aspirator is introduced into the uterus and specimens are obtained from four quadrants. In the event of early pregnancy, small specimens will be removed only from the side wall of

the fundus to avoid dislodging the embryo. An alternative method of cervical dilatation is inserting laminaria 4–24 hours before the procedure. These small, packed seaweed inserts expand with moisture and dilate the cervix. They are removed at the beginning of the procedure.

Place tissue specimens in a biopsy bottle with a 10% formalin solution. Label specimens and send to lab for histologic examination.

Care After Test

➤ Monitor vital signs closely until stable; usually every 15 minutes for the first hour, every 30 minutes for the next hour, and then as indicated or at least once more before discharge.

➤ Assess client for excessive bleeding.

➤ Provide client with a sanitary pad.

➤ Review related tests such as a Pap smear and cervical biopsy.

Educate Your Client and the Family

➤ Explain to client that a small amount of bleeding may occur from biopsy site and that she may experience cramping for several days.

➤ Instruct client to wear a sanitary pad until bleeding stops.

➤ Tell client to notify the primary health care provider if excessive bleeding occurs (soaks a sanitary pad in an hour).

➤ Warn the client to notify her primary health care provider if she has a foul-smelling vaginal discharge and/or chills and fever.

➤ Instruct the client to abstain from intercourse (no sex) and douching, and to insert nothing into vagina for 3 days or as directed by the primary health care provider.

> Inform client that resting for 24 hours and avoiding strenuous exercise or heavy lifting are important to prevent excessive bleeding.

> Tell the client that she will be notified when the results are available. For fertility investigation, an appointment will be made to discuss the results. For diagnosis of pathology, if the test is positive, an appointment will be made to discuss other diagnostic tests and/or treatment options.

E

Endoscopic Retrograde Cholangiopancreatography

en doe **skop** ik • **reh** troe grade • kole **an** gee oe **pan** kree ah **tog** rah fee
(ERCP, ERCP of the Pancreatic and Biliary Ducts)

Normal Findings

> Presence and normal size of biliary and pancreatic ducts
> No obstructions, tumors, or masses present
> No abnormalities in filling of ducts

What This Test Will Tell You

This radiographic, endoscopic test helps diagnose jaundice and specific disorders of the pancreas, bile ducts, and gallbladder. The test allows for direct visualization of the biliary tree and pancreatic duct at the duodenal papilla (ampulla of Vater, the duodenal end of the drainage system for the pancreas and common bile duct). It aids in the diagnosis of pancreatitis, obstruction of bile duct, presence of cholelithiasis, carcinoma, and sclerosing cholangitis. This test is especially helpful in inspecting the biliary tree when elevated bilirubin levels are present. The procedure may also be used therapeutically to place stents into ducts to aid in drainage of the bile system.

Abnormal Findings

Visualization may reveal stricture of pancreatic duct; pancreatic tumor; obstruction of bile duct by tumors, strictures, or gallstones; obstruction of pancreatic duct by tumors, strictures, pseudocysts, or inflammation; cholelithiasis; sclerosing cholangitis; cysts; or congenital malformations of the biliary tree and pancreatic ducts.

ACTION ALERT!

> Assess client carefully for allergic reaction to contrast material including dyspnea, itching, urticaria, flushing, hypotension, and shock. Life-threatening anaphylactic reactions can occur and need to be recognized and treated immediately.

> Sedation used for this procedure may result in respiratory depression or respiratory arrest progressing to death. Naloxone or other antagonist medication should be readily available to counteract the effects of the sedation, and resuscitation equipment should be immediately available.

> During this endoscopic procedure, perforation of the esophagus, stomach, or duodenum may occur. Any acute abdominal pain, drop in blood pressure, tachycardia,

or dyspnea should be considered possible indication of perforation requiring immediate medical and possibly surgical intervention.

Interfering Factors

➤ Uncooperative or combative client
➤ Barium from previous studies

Contraindications

➤ Allergy to contrast material without specific modifications
➤ Pregnancy, due to radiation exposure to fetus
➤ Gastrectomy clients with separation of the duodenum
➤ Esophageal diverticuli
➤ Pancreatitis
➤ Perforation of esophagus, stomach, or duodenum

Potential Complications

➤ Pancreatitis
➤ Sepsis
➤ Perforation of the esophagus, stomach, or duodenum resulting in sepsis, peritonitis, or hemorrhage
➤ Allergic reaction, including anaphylaxis
➤ Aspiration

NURSING CONSIDERATIONS

Prepare Your Client

➤ Explain that this test is used to look at parts of the digestive tract to make sure there are no blockages or other problems.
➤ Explain that the procedure usually takes about 1–1.5 hours to perform.
➤ Ensure that an informed consent is obtained, because of the possible complications associated with this procedure.
➤ Check to be sure the client has no allergy to contrast material or iodine.
➤ Withhold food and fluids for at least 8 hours before the test.

➤ Consult with the primary health care provider about intravenous antibiotics which may be administered 1 hour before the procedure to minimize or avoid pancreatitis as a potential complication of ERCP.
➤ Confirm that adults and older children have voided before the procedure.

Perform Procedure

Nurses do not perform this procedure, but should understand the process to prepare the client. Position the client on the x-ray table in a left lateral position with the left arm behind the back. IV sedation is administered according to the needs of the client and preference of the endoscopist. Local anesthetic is sprayed into the throat to minimize the gag reflex and the potential for aspiration. Endos-copy is performed, and once the duodenum is entered, medication (often glucagon) is given intravenously to paralyze the duodenum, facilitating the exam. The papilla of Vater is entered, and contrast material is administered to visualize ducts; detailed x-rays are taken. Stents may be placed as necessary. ERCP is rarely performed on children, usually only after repeated episodes of pancreatitis and under general anesthesia.

Care After Test

➤ Withhold food or fluids by mouth until client is fully awake and has regained protective reflexes.
➤ Monitor vital signs, especially observing for elevations in temperature and signs of respiratory depression from sedation.
➤ Report complaints of nausea, vomiting, and abdominal pain to primary health care provider—pancre-

atitis is a complication of ERCP.

➤ Encourage gargling or administer throat lozenges if ordered for symptomatic relief of sore throat due to endoscope.

➤ Observe for signs of allergic reaction to the contrast material, including urticaria, pruritus, fever, and dyspnea.

➤ Review related tests such as serum amylase, serum lipase, urine amylase, percutaneous transhepatic cholangiography, intravenous cholangiography, and oral cholecystography.

Educate Your Client and the Family

➤ Depending upon findings of the test, educate concerning further testing or therapeutic interventions which may be necessary.

➤ Alert client and family to the signs/symptoms of pancreatitis: fever, abdominal pain, nausea, and vomiting.

Epstein-Barr Virus Antibody

ep steen • bar • vie russ

(EBV, EBV Antibody Test, Infectious Mononucleosis Test, Heterophile Antibody Titer Test, Heterophile Agglutination Test, Monospot, Mono-Test, Monostican)

Normal Findings

<1:10 or negative titer
90% of individuals have antibodies to EBV by age 20
1:10–1:60 indicates exposure to EBV at some time
1:224 or greater indicates current infection or mononucleosis
Fourfold increase in titer in samples drawn 10–14 days apart indicates a current, active infection

What This Test Will Tell You

This blood test detects and measures antibody levels or titers to the Epstein-Barr virus, the organism most likely to cause infectious mononucleosis (mono).

The first line test to diagnose mononucleosis is the heterophile agglutination (monospot) test. Antibody titers are only necessary when the clinical picture resembles mononucleosis but the monospot is negative, typically occurring in immunosuppressed individuals and very young children.

EBV is implicated as the causative organism in chronic fatigue syndrome ("yuppie disease"), a persistent mononucleosis-like infection characterized by myalgia, fever, and malaise. The monospot is negative in this syndrome.

EBV can reactivate in transplant clients who receive immunosuppressant medication. Although most of these clients sustain a mononucleosis-like infection, some develop lymphoma as a result of reactivation following transplant. Antibodies are drawn to diagnose and track the course of the infection.

High titers of EBV antibody are found in nasopharyngeal cancer. Levels should be drawn on clients at risk and to monitor therapy. The antibody response to EBV is quite complex and involves the rise and fall of several different titers. No correlation exists between titer levels and severity of disease. Titers must be interpreted in light of the client's clinical picture. Most laboratories track the four antibodies listed in the table on page 285.

Abnormal Findings

▲ INCREASED TITERS may indicate infectious mononucleosis, Burkitt's lymphoma, nasopharyngeal carcinoma, chronic fatigue syndrome, sarcoidosis, systemic lupus erythematosus, lymphocytic leukemia, Hayden's disease, hepatitis A and B, or pancreatic carcinoma.

NURSING CONSIDERATIONS

Prepare Your Client

➤ Explain that this test looks for a virus called Epstein-Barr that may be causing symptoms.
➤ Explain that titers will be drawn in a series a few weeks apart.

Perform Procedure

➤ Collect 5–10 mL of venous blood in a red-top tube.
➤ Record the date of symptom onset on the lab slip.

Care After Test

➤ Assess for signs and symptoms of infection such as sore throat and lymphadenopathy, especially of the anterior and posterior cervical chains.
➤ Assess for splenomegaly, present in half of all cases, which can, though rarely, result in splenic rupture. Abdominal pain, postural hypoten-

sion, vertigo, or other signs of hemorrhage should be observed for and acted upon immediately.
➤ Administer antipyretics and analgesics to control fever and discomfort.
➤ Encourage fluids for febrile client. .
➤ Immunosuppressed client may be prescribed acyclovir. Carefully monitor renal function and hydration with this potentially nephrotoxic medication. .
➤ Isolation is not required.
➤ Evaluate related tests such as hematocrit, hemoglobin, white blood cell count with differential, white blood cell count, aspartate aminotransferase, alanine aminotransferase, and alkaline phosphatase.

Educate Your Client and the Family

➤ Explain that EBV is transmitted in the saliva, so toothbrushes, food, and drinking glasses should not be shared.
➤ Explain that EBV will probably not infect everyone in the household. Most people already have immunity to the virus, and only those people without immunity develop mononucleosis.
➤ Tell your client and family that most people recover completely in 4–6 weeks.
➤ Instruct your client and family that treatment is bed rest and fluids.
➤ Tell them to avoid contact sports or any activity that could cause the spleen to rupture. Splenomegaly (enlarged spleen) is a common occurrence in mononucleosis.
➤ Instruct client to inform the primary health care provider immediately if acute abdominal pain develops.

EPSTEIN-BARR ANTIBODY TITER COMPONENTS

- VCA (viral capsid antigen) IgM and IgG
- EAD (early antigen diffuse component) IgG
- EAR (early antigen restricted component) IgG
- EBNA (Epstein-Barr nuclear antigen)

E

RELATED DIAGNOSIS

Acute infectious mononucleosis

high VCA: IgM, IgG titers

negative EBNA titer

positive heterophile antibody test

Previous infection with EBV

negative VCA: IgM titer

positive VCA: IgG titer

positive EBNA titer

negative heterophile antibody test

Chronic fatigue syndrome

elevated serial titer peaks of VCA: IgG and EA: IgG

Erythrocyte Count
eh rith roe site • kownt
(Red Cell Count, Red Blood Cell Count, RBC)

Normal Findings
ADULT, ELDERLY, AND ADOLES-
CENT
Female: 4.2–5.4 million/mm^3(μL)
(SI units: 4.2–5.4 × 10^{12}/L)
Male: 4.5–6.2 million/mm^3(μL) (SI
units: 4.5–6.2 × 10^{12}/L)
PREGNANT
No differences in values due to preg-
nancy. However, reductions in RBC
count are common during normal
pregnancy.
NEWBORN
4.4–7.1 million/mm^3 (μL) (SI units:
4.4–7.1 × 10^{12}/L)
INFANT AND CHILD
2 months old: Drops to 3.0–3.8 mil-
lion/mm^3 (μL) (SI units: 3.0–3.8 ×

10^{12}/L), then rises slowly
Child: 4.6–5.5 million/mm^3 (μL) (SI
units: 4.4–7.1 × 10^{12}/L)

What This Test Will Tell You
This blood test evaluates anemia and
polycythemia, and calculates red
blood cell indices. Oxygen transport
to the cells throughout the body
depends upon sufficient numbers of
red cells with adequate amounts of
hemoglobin. The test is usually performed as part of a collection of
related tests called the complete
blood count (CBC).

Abnormal Findings
▼DECREASED LEVELS may indicate anemia, dietary deficiencies,

pregnancy, pernicious anemia, fluid overload, hemorrhage, renal failure, hemolysis, chronic illness, lupus erythematosus, Addison's disease, Hodgkin's disease, leukemia, multiple myeloma, antineoplastic chemotherapeutic medications, rheumatic disease, or subacute endocarditis.

▲INCREASED LEVELS may indicate living at high altitudes, polycythemia vera, dehydration, pulmonary fibrosis, cor pulmonale, or congenital heart disease.

███████ACTION ALERT!

➤ Marked elevations, above the normal limits for age and gender, may indicate polycythemia and increased viscosity of the blood and be associated with increased risk of thromboembolic events. Rehydration with oral and/or parenteral fluids or phlebotomy may be required emergently.

➤ Reductions of erythrocytes, below normal limits for age and gender, may indicate blood loss or anemia or diminished red cell production. Fluid resuscitation, blood transfusions, and oxygen therapy may be necessary as emergency interventions.

Interfering Factors

➤ Living at high altitudes causes physiologically normal increases in hematocrit (Hct) values.

➤ Hemolysis of blood cells due to rough handling of the specimen will invalidate test results.

➤ Collection of a sample above an existing intravenous (IV) fluid line may produce a diluted sample and falsely low value.

➤ If the tourniquet is left in place for longer than 1 or 2 minutes, hemoconcentration may occur within that extremity and increase the sample reading by 2%–5%.

➤ Failure to place the sample in a collection tube with the proper anticoagulant or failure to mix the sample sufficiently with the anticoagulant may affect the values.

➤ Medications that may produce elevated RBC counts include gentamicin, erythropoietin, and methyldopa.

➤ Medications that may produce reduced RBC counts include chloramphenicol, hydantoin, and quinidine.

➤ Lying in a recumbent position while blood is drawn will lower values.

➤ Excessive exercise raises values.

➤ Pregnancy and other conditions causing an increase in body fluids will decrease values.

NURSING CONSIDERATIONS

Prepare Your Client

➤ Explain that this test measures the number of red blood cells (erythrocytes) in the blood, and that high or low levels may be causing symptoms or problems.

Perform Procedure

➤ Collect 7 mL of venous blood in a lavender-top tube.

Care After Test

➤ Observe the client for signs and symptoms of anemia including pallor, dyspnea, chest pain, and fatigue.

➤Encourage rest periods for client experiencing fatigue related to anemia.

➤ Evaluate client's ability to perform activities of daily living.

➤ Refer to community health care services as needed if client is unable to meet basic daily needs.

➤ Obtain a dietary consult to assist the client and family in choosing a well-balanced diet, including foods high in iron and vitamin B_{12}.

> Review related tests such as hemo-globin, hematocrit, reticulocyte count, red blood cell indices, hemo-globin electrophoresis, ferritin level, total iron binding capacity (TIBC), bone marrow and liver biopsies, and iron absorption and excretion studies.

Educate Your Client and the Family

> If a low red cell count is part of the diagnosis of anemia, blood loss, or fluid overload, discuss with the client/family the significance of the findings.

> If a severe anemia is identified, explain how it may affect the client's activities. Severe anemia may pro-duce fatigue, shortness of breath with or without exertion, fainting, increases in heart rate, and even tis-sue damage, such as heart attack (myocardial infarction). Teach the client to pace activities and to main-tain regular patterns of sleep, rest, and activity to prevent fatigue.

> Discuss with your client and fam-ily the significance of red blood cell levels. For example, extreme in-creases may trigger a stroke (cere-brovascular accident) in some indi-viduals. Severe anemia can trigger heart pain (angina) or heart attack (myocardial infarction).

> If an anemia is identified, instruct the client in dietary sources of iron, such as red meat, organ meats, dark green vegetables, and fortified grains.

Erythrocyte Distribution, Fetal-Maternal

eh rith roe site • diss tri byu shun • fee tahl • mah tur nal
(Fetal Red Cells, Fetal-Maternal Bleed)

Normal Findings

Absence of fetal red blood cells in maternal whole blood

What This Test Will Tell You

This blood test detects and measures the amount of Rh+ fetal blood trans-ferred to the maternal circulatory system through transplacental bleeds or hemorrhage to determine the required dosage of Rh_o (D) immune globulin to prevent maternal isoim-munization. Rh is a genetically deter-mined factor on red blood cells or erythrocytes. When Rh(D)-positive red blood cells invade the circulatory system of an Rh(D)-negative individ-ual, antibodies are formed against the invading red cell antigens.

Rh_o (D) immune globulin is administered to unsensitized clients following abortion or delivery of an Rh(D)-positive baby and prophylac-tically at 28 weeks' gestation. At delivery or following abortion, when known fetal-maternal bleeds have occurred, an Rh(D)-negative mother is tested to determine the amount of Rh(D)-positive fetal red blood cells invading her system. As little as 0.5 mL of fetal blood can cause isoim-munization. If more than 30 mL of fetal blood enters the maternal circu-latory system, the dosage of Rh_o (D) immune globulin is increased to pre-vent maternal antibody formation.

Abnormal Findings

Presence of fetal blood cells in mater-nal whole blood indicates maternal isoimmunization.

Absence of fetal blood cells in maternal whole blood should not be interpreted as indicating that Rh_o (D) immune globulin is not required if the mother is known to be Rh– and the fetus is Rh+.

■■■■■■ ACTION ALERT

The Rh-negative (Rh–) client with evidence of fetal Rh-positive (Rh+) blood in her circulatory system will need an injection of Rh_o (D) immune globulin within 72 hours of delivery or abortion to prevent maternal isoimmunization.

Interfering Factors
➤ Blood specimen not stored at 2–8°C until tested
➤ Blood specimen not tested within 24 hours of collection
➤ Bacterial contamination of specimen
➤ Specimen drawn > 72 hours after delivery or abortion
➤ Hemolysis of red cells due to improper storage or handling

Contraindications
➤ Rh(D)-negative mother delivering an Rh(D)-negative fetus
➤ Isoimmunized client

NURSING CONSIDERATIONS
Prepare Your Client
➤ Explain to client that blood will be drawn to determine the amount of medicine needed to protect a developing baby from blood incompatibility in future pregnancies.
➤ Assess client's understanding of need for Rh_o (D) immune globulin; she should have received information during her pregnancy from her certified nurse-midwife, other advanced practice nurse, or physician. Clarify any misunderstanding and answer

any further questions she may have, or seek information for her.

Perform Procedure
➤ Perform venipuncture and collect a minimum of 1 mL of blood in a lavender-top tube.
➤ Notify lab of date of antepartum dose of Rh_o (D) immune globulin as there could still be detectable levels of passive anti-D in her serum.

Care After Test
➤ All Rh-negative mothers should be screened for Rh isoimmunization or irregular antibodies at their first visit for a pregnancy, and at 24, 28, 32, and 36 weeks gestation.
➤ All Rh-positive mothers with a history of the birth of a severely jaundiced infant, stillborn infant, maternal transfusions, cesarean delivery, or either spontaneous or elective abortions should also be screened for Rh isoimmunization and irregular antibodies.
➤ Collaborate with the primary health care provider about administering 1 vial of Rh_o (D) immune globulin if fetal packed RBCs are <15 mL, or 2 vials of Rh_o (D) immune globulin if fetal packed RBCs are >15 mL.
➤ Review related tests such as the maternal blood type.

Educate Your Client and the Family
➤ Explain that Rh_o (D) immune globulin should be given at any time she loses a baby during the first few months of pregnancy.
➤ Explain that Rh_o (D) immune globulin will be given during the next pregnancy as it was during this pregnancy if needed.
➤ Explain testing will take place when her next baby is born as was

done with this baby to determine whether Rh_o (D) immune globulin is needed.

Erythrocyte Indices

eh rith roe site · in dih sees

(Red Cell Indices, Mean Corpuscular Volume [MCV], Mean Corpuscular Hemoglobin [MCH], Mean Corpuscular Hemoglobin Concentration [MCHC])

E

Normal Findings

ADULT, PREGNANT, CHILD, ADOLESCENT, AND ELDERLY

MCV: 80–99 μm^3 (SI units: 80–99 fL)

MCH: 27–32 pg (SI units: 1.7–2.0 fmol)

MCHC: 30–36 g/dL (30%–36%) (SI units: 0.30–0.36 mmol/L)

INFANT

MCV: 96–108 μm^3 (SI units: 96–108 fL)

MCH: 32–34 pg (SI units: 2.0–2.1 fmol)

MCHC: 32–33 g/dL (32%–33%) (SI units: 0.32–0.33 mmol/L)

What This Test Will Tell You

This blood test compares red blood cell indices with other information, such as hemoglobin and hematocrit and erythrocyte count, providing valuable information in classifying types and causes of anemia. Red blood cell indices provide comparative information about the size, weight, and hemoglobin concentration of an average red cell. The MCV (Mean Corpuscular Volume) provides an indication of red cell size. MCV is stated as the ratio of the volume of packed cells to the red cell count (RBC). The MCH (Mean Corpuscular Hemoglobin) provides a measured weight of an average red cell. The measurement is stated in relation to the MCV, since larger red cells generally reflect a heavier weight. The MCHC (Mean Corpuscular Hemoglobin Concentration) is a measurement of the amount of hemoglobin in an average cell. The MCHC is stated as a ratio of the weight of hemoglobin to the volume of red cells.

Abnormal Findings

▼ LOW MCV (microcytic) may indicate iron deficiency anemia or thalassemia.

▲ HIGH MCV (macrocytic) may indicate liver disease, alcoholism, megaloblastic anemia, reticulocytosis, inherited disorders of DNA synthesis, pernicious anemia, folic acid deficiency, or antimetabolite therapy.

▼ LOW MCH may indicate microcytic anemia or hypochromic anemia.

▲ HIGH MCH may indicate macrocytic anemia.

▼ LOW MCHC may indicate iron deficiency anemia or thalassemia.

▲ HIGH MCHC may indicate spherocytosis.

Interfering Factors

➤ Hemolysis of blood cells due to rough handling of the specimen will invalidate test results.

➤ Failure to place the sample in a collection tube with the proper anticoagulant or failure to mix the sample sufficiently with the anticoagulant may affect the value.

➤ If the tourniquet is left in place for longer than 1 or 2 minutes, hemoconcentration may occur within that extremity and affect the sample values.

➤ Very high white blood cell counts may cause falsely elevated red cell counts in automated or semi-automated equipment and produce invalid MCV and MCH values.

➤ Conditions that cause red cells to stick together will produce falsely reduced red cell counts and invalid test results.

➤ Abnormal size of red blood cells will alter red cell indices.

NURSING CONSIDERATIONS

Prepare Your Client

➤ Explain that this test measures the amount, size, and iron content of red blood cells, and can help identify problems such as anemia or find the type of anemia.

Perform Procedure

➤ Collect 5–7 mL of venous blood in a lavender-top tube.

Care After Test

➤ Observe the client for signs and symptoms of anemia including pallor, dyspnea, chest pain, and fatigue.

➤ Encourage rest periods for client experiencing fatigue related to anemia.

➤ Evaluate client's ability to perform activities of daily living.

➤ Refer to community health care services as needed if client is unable to perform basic daily needs.

➤ Obtain a dietary consult to assist the client and family in choosing a well-balanced diet, including foods high in iron and vitamin B_{12}.

➤ Review related tests such as hemoglobin, hematocrit, reticulocyte count, hemoglobin electrophoresis, ferritin level, total iron binding capacity (TIBC), bone marrow and liver biopsies, and iron absorption and excretion studies.

Educate Your Client and the Family

➤ If low red cell indices indicate the possibility of blood loss or anemia, explain that further testing may be necessary to identify the cause of the condition, and to check the client's response to treatment.

➤ If a severe anemia is identified, explain how this may affect the client's activities. Severe anemia may produce fatigue, shortness of breath with or without exertion, fainting, increases in heart rate, and even tissue damage, such as heart attack (myocardial infarction). Teach the client to pace activities and to maintain regular patterns of sleep, rest, and activity to prevent fatigue.

➤ Discuss with your client or family the significance of the test values. Red cell indices may indicate a particular type of anemia. If the type of anemia indicates a dietary deficiency that can be remedied by change in diet, instruct the client and family in dietary sources and preparation to replace the vitamin or mineral that is lacking.

Erythrocyte Sedimentation Rate

eh rith roe site • sed ih men tay shun • rate
(ESR, Sed Rate)

Normal Findings

	Westergren	Wintrobe	Cutler	Smith
Adult male	0–15 mm/hr	0–9 mm/hr	0–8 mm/hr	0–10 mm/hr
Adult female	0–20 mm/hr	0–15 mm/hr	0–10 mm/hr	0–10 mm/hr
Child	0–10 mm/hr	0–13 mm/hr	4–13 mm/hr	
Newborn	0–2 mm/hr			

What This Test Will Tell You

This blood test evaluates the presence of an inflammatory process, including those caused by neoplasms, infections, autoimmune diseases, and necrosis. Because many factors can cause an increase in the rate that the red blood cells fall, the ESR is not diagnostic for any disease. It is useful as an indicator that something is wrong, but it does not reveal the site or cause. Some clinicians feel that the ESR has little value because it is so nonspecific, and because it is influenced by many factors. The ESR rises slowly and is often preceded by other objective signs such as fever and an increased white blood cell count. The C-reactive protein, also a nonspecific indicator of inflammation, rises and falls more quickly with the beginning and resolution of the inflammatory process. A negative ESR does not rule out serious disease.

This test has some value in detecting occult disease such as breast and colon cancer and lymphoma, all of which may have a very elevated ESR. The ESR is also useful in monitoring the therapeutic course of a client with known disease, especially rheumatic and collagen diseases. Finally, the sed rate is useful in helping make a differential diagnosis; for instance, it is elevated in rheumatic arthritis but not in osteoarthritis.

Abnormal Findings

▲ INCREASED LEVELS may indicate bacterial infections, pneumonia, rheumatoid arthritis, rheumatic fever, myocardial infarction, toxemia, venereal disease, pelvic inflammatory disease, nephritis, or cancer.

▼ DECREASED LEVELS may indicate congestive heart failure, infectious mononucleosis, angina pectoris, arthritis, polycythemia, sickle-cell anemia, or proteinemia.

Interfering Factors

➤ ESR is normal in 5% of clients with rheumatic arthritis and systemic lupus erythematosus.

➤ The ESR is elevated in pregnancy, early postpartum, menstruation, hypercholesterolemia, and normal elderly females.

➤ The ESR is decreased in hyperglycemia, polycythemia, congestive heart failure, and sickle-cell anemia.

➤ Medications that can increase the ESR include dextran, methyldopa, procainamide, theophylline, oral contraceptives, and vitamin A.

➤ Medications that can decrease the ESR include ethambutol, quinine, steroids, and salicylates (aspirin).

NURSING CONSIDERATIONS

Prepare Your Client
➤ Tell your client that this test is to help detect any active inflammation or infection.

Perform Procedure
➤ Collect 5–10 mL of venous blood in a lavender-top tube, or 4.5 mL in a black-top tube, or 4.5 mL in a blue-top tube, depending upon laboratory methods for determining the sed rate. Consult your institution's laboratory.
➤ Keep specimen at room temperature.
➤ Take to lab immediately; cells begin to settle in 2 hours.

Care After Test
➤ If the ESR is elevated, anticipate other laboratory work and diagnostic studies.
➤ Assess for signs and symptoms of inflammatory disease, infection, or neoplasms. Report any new symptoms immediately to the primary health care provider.
➤ If the ESR is elevated and the client has a known disease, expect a change or increase in medications or therapy.
➤ Review related tests such as C-reactive protein, complete blood count, and red cell indices.

Educate Your Client and the Family
➤ Explain to your client that if the ESR is elevated, additional studies will be needed to form an accurate diagnosis.
➤ Explain that the results of this test will improve as the inflammatory or infectious process resolves.

Erythrocyte Survival Time

eh rith roe site • sur vie val • time
(Red Blood Cell Survival Time, RBC Survival Time, CR-51 Red Cell Survival, ^{51}CR Red Blood Cell Survival)

Normal Findings
All ages: 25–35 days, half-life of red blood cells (RBC) (^{51}Cr)

What This Test Will Tell You
This blood test measures erythrocyte survival time to analyze unexplained anemia. The average life span of red blood cells is assessed by tagging a random sample of the client's red blood cells with radioactive chromium-51 sodium chromate (^{51}Cr). This tagged blood is allowed to circulate within the client's system and a series of blood samples are obtained over 3 to 4 weeks. Testing continues until 50% of the tagged cells disappear. Normal RBCs have a life span of 120 days, and therefore a half-life of 60 days, whereas the chromium-tagged red cells may have a shorter half-life of 25–35 days. In addition to a count of cells, the body (particularly the spleen, liver, and

pericardium) is scanned by a gamma camera for sites of radioactive concentration, indicating excessive sequestration and destruction of red cells. This scanning reports the ratio of radioactive sequestering in the spleen and pericardium. The splenic/pericardium ratio is normally <2:1. If a comparison is reported of sequestering in the spleen and liver, the normal ratio is 1:1.

Abnormal Findings

▼DECREASED *RBC survival time* may indicate hemolytic disease, megaloblastic anemia of pregnancy, sickle-cell anemia, pernicious anemia, chronic lymphocytic leukemia, congenital non-spherocytic hemolytic anemia, hemoglobin C disease, hereditary spherocytosis, splenomegaly, leukemia, uremia, or hemolysis.

▲INCREASED *RBC survival time* may indicate accelerated erythropoiesis or thalassemia minor.

Interfering Factors

➤ Dehydration, blood loss, or overhydration affects the circulating blood volume and will influence test results.
➤ Blood transfusions during the test period distort test results.
➤ Very high white cell counts (>25,000) reduce RBC survival time.
➤ Platelet counts greater than 500,000 will decrease RBC survival time.
➤ Splenomegaly can increase splenic/pericardium ratios.
➤ Splenic infarctions can decrease splenic/pericardium ratios.

Contraindications

➤ Pregnancy, because the potential for fetal damage from the radioactive

material is considered too great to warrant testing
➤ Significant active bleeding, because blood loss and transfusions may invalidate test results
➤ Need for repeated blood draws for other testing, which may interfere with test results

Complications

➤ Possible damage to fetus in pregnant women

NURSING CONSIDERATIONS

Prepare Your Client

➤ Explain to your client that this test measures if the body is destroying red blood cells too much and too early.
➤ Explain to the client that the small amounts of radioisotope will not cause any noticeable effect and will not expose the client or anyone nearby to large amounts of radiation.
➤ Assure the client that there is no sensation or pain associated with scanning.

Perform Procedure

➤ Collect 20–30 mL in green-top collection tubes for initial tagging. This sample will be mixed with 100 microcuries of ^{51}Cr and incubated.
➤ After preparation, the client's tagged blood will be readministered intravenously.
➤ When testing begins, perform venipuncture and collect 10 mL of blood into a green-top blood collection tube. This sample will be quantitated for counts of ^{51}Cr per minute.
➤ The client will undergo nuclear imaging of the spleen, liver and pericardium.
➤ Repeat testing of blood samples and nuclear imaging will be performed every 3 days for approxi-

mately 3 weeks.

Care After Test

➤ Observe the client for signs and symptoms of anemia including pallor, dyspnea, chest pain, and fatigue.

➤ Encourage rest periods for clients experiencing fatigue related to anemia.

➤ Evaluate client's ability to perform activities of daily living.

➤ Refer to community health care services as needed if client is unable to perform basic daily needs.

➤ Obtain a dietary consult to assist the client and family in choosing a well-balanced diet, including foods high in iron and vitamin B_{12}.

➤ Review related tests such as hemoglobin, hematocrit, reticulocyte count, red blood cell indices, hemoglobin electrophoresis, ferritin level, total iron binding capacity (TIBC), bone marrow and liver biopsies, and iron absorption and excretion studies.

Educate Your Client and the Family

➤ If testing indicates significant sequestering of red cells in the spleen, inform your client or family that a splenectomy may be necessary to reduce the speed of red cell destruction.

➤ If a hemolytic anemia or disorder is identified through testing, the client and family need to understand essential treatment related to the disorder. For example, teach the client with sickle-cell disease about behaviors that reduce the incidence of sickling events.

Esophageal Function Studies

ee sof ah jee al • funk shun • stud ees
(Esophageal Motility Studies, Esophageal Manometry, Esophageal Motility Study, Lower Esophageal Sphincter [LES] Pressure, LES Manometry, Swallowing Manometry, Acid Reflux Study, Acid Clearing, Bernstein Test, Acid Perfusion)

Normal Findings

LOWER ESOPHAGEAL SPHINCTER MANOMETRY

Resting lower esophageal sphincter (LES) pressure ≥10 mm Hg

Complete relaxation of the LES with swallowing

Mean LES pressure 15–30 mm Hg above the gastric pressure level

ACID REFLUX

pH 4.0 or greater

Absence of acid reflux

SWALLOWING MANOMETRY

Normal peristaltic waves with swallowing patterns

ACID CLEARING

Acid clearing in less than 10 swallows

ACID PERFUSION

Negative pain response to acid infusion in esophagus

What This Test Will Tell You

These tests are used primarily to diagnose esophageal reflux, abnormalities of peristalsis during swallowing, esophagitis, acid reflux, and heartburn, or to monitor the effectiveness of therapy for these conditions. Several tests make up the esophageal function studies series.

Measurement of lower esophageal sphincter pressures is used to detect abnormalities in the passage of food and liquids from the esophagus through the LES into the stomach. If LES pressures are low, the sphincter may be incompetent, allowing reflux to occur. If LES pressures are elevated, the sphincter may not adequately allow the passage of food from the esophagus into the stomach. Determination of acid reflux is an important element in the diagnosis of gastroesophageal reflux. Acid clearing is performed to evaluate the effectiveness of swallowing to propel the contents of the esophagus into the stomach. Finally, an acid perfusion test is also important in the evaluation of gastroesophageal reflux.

Abnormal Findings

➤ *LES pressure < 10 mm Hg* may indicate reflux esophagitis, gastroesophageal reflux, or chalasia.
➤ *LES pressure > 10 mm Hg* may indicate incomplete relaxation of LES, esophageal spasm, or achalasia.
➤ *pH less than 4* may indicate gastroesophageal reflux.
➤ *More than 10 swallows to clear acid infusion* may indicate gastroesophageal reflux as cause of heartburn symptoms.

ACTION ALERT!

Gastroesophageal intubation, especially in infants, carries significant risk for aspiration. Monitor closely for alterations in respiratory patterns including dyspnea, apnea, cyanosis, and labored breathing, which could indicate aspiration. Maintain a patent airway and support breathing as necessary while a definitive diagnosis and treatment are determined.

Interfering Factors

➤ Nitrates, calcium channel blockers, anticholinergics, promotility agents, and sedatives may invalidate results if taken in the 24 hours prior to esophageal function testing because these medications affect esophageal motor tone.
➤ Eating or drinking prior to the test may invalidate results.

Contraindications

➤ Cardiovascular instability.
➤ Recent gastric surgery.
➤ Severe esophageal ulcers.
➤ Uncooperative clients.
➤ Testing for acid reflux and/or acid clearance during esophageal function studies is contraindicated for clients with active or recent gastrointestinal bleeding, known active ulcer disease, and/or those who cannot tolerate intubation due to the risks of aspiration.

Potential Complications

➤ Aspiration

NURSING CONSIDERATIONS
Prepare Your Client

➤ Explain that the test is used to measure how well food moves through the esophagus (swallowing tube), through a sphincter (valve), and into the stomach.
➤ Restrict food and fluids for 8 hours prior to the test, or according to your institution's protocol.
➤ Explain that as the tube is inserted into the mouth or nose and guided into the stomach, a pressure sensation may be felt.
➤ Inform the cleint that although the test may be uncomfortable, it

should not be painful, and sedation is not required. Sedation may be used in certain pediatric clients, however.

Perform Procedure

Nurses do not perform this procedure, but should understand the process to prepare the client. Three to four small fluid-filled catheters are attached to a pressure transducer and hooked to a recorder. The catheters are inserted into the client directly through a tube placed through the mouth or nose and guided into the esophagus and stomach for pressure recording. Pressures are recorded over several respiratory cycles and during a sequence of swallowing efforts, and may also be recorded with the client in various positions. Lower esophageal sphincter (LES) pressure is recorded as a mean pressure taken from pressure values of the three or four recording catheters pulled slowly across the gastroesophageal junction.

Client being tested for acid reflux is asked to perform a series of respiratory maneuvers in different body positions, such as deep breathing, coughing, and the Valsalva maneuver in the supine, right side down and left side down positions and with the head down 20 degrees. A fall in the esophagus pH indicates the presence of reflux.

For client being tested for esophageal acid clearance, hydrochloric acid is infused and the client is asked to swallow. The number of swallows required to clear the acid from the esophagus is determined.

For acid perfusion testing, hydrochloric acid and saline are infused alternately to see which, if either, may cause symptoms of heartburn.

Care After Test

➤ Observe pediatric client for signs of reflux-related pulmonary complications.

➤ Feed infant with suspected reflux with the head elevated. Ensure the head of the infant is kept elevated after feeding as well to prevent dangerous reflux and aspiration.

➤ Assess for difficulty eating and swallowing. Take precautions to avoid aspiration by collaborating with a dietician and feeding specialist to select an appropriate diet for the client that facilitates effective passage of food and fluids and minimizes aspiration risks.

➤ Evaluate additional diagnostic tests used to assess gastroesophageal reflux such as esophagogastroduodenoscopy and biopsy, barium swallow, and/or gastroesophageal reflux scan.

Educate Your Client and the Family

➤ Teach client with gastroesophageal reflux to avoid lying on the right side or supine, as regurgitation is more likely to occur in these positions.

➤ Advise client with esophagitis to avoid hot and cold liquids, coffee, citrus juices, and alcoholic beverages, since these substances may worsen symptoms associated with gastroesophageal reflux.

➤ Encourage client with gastroesophageal reflux to avoid activities that require considerable bending or stooping, such as gardening, picking objects off the floor, tying shoes, or sitting slumped down in a chair. The bending and stooping associated with activities such as these can worsen the symptoms of gastroesophageal reflux.

➤ Inform the client that smaller, more frequent meals, rather than three large meals a day, can lessen the symptoms of gastroesophageal reflux.

➤ Teach the client to avoid foods with a high fat content, since they can worsen symptoms associated with gastroesophageal reflux.

➤ For infant with gastroesophageal reflux, stress the importance of feeding them in the upright position and maintaining them upright for 60 minutes after eating.

Esophagogastroduodenoscopy

eh **sof** ah goe **gass** troe doo **od** en **oss** koe pee

(EGD, Enteroscopy, Gastroscopy, Upper Gastrointestinal Endoscopy, UGI Endoscopy)

Normal Findings

Absence of bleeding, inflammation, hernias, mass lesions, strictures, and stenoses

What This Test Will Tell You

This endoscopic test evaluates and diagnoses clinical conditions of the upper gastrointestinal (GI) tract. Direct visualization of the upper GI tract using a long, flexible endoscope allows the endoscopist to assess mucosal vascular patterns for abnormalities such as bleeding sites or inflammation, and to obtain tissue samples or biopsies which can confirm or exclude small mass lesions such as cancerous tumors.

This procedure may also be used therapeutically, to treat disorders of the upper GI tract. Treatment of bleeding sites, balloon dilatation of strictures or stenoses, and removal of foreign bodies may all be performed during EGD.

Abnormal Findings

Gastrointestinal abnormalities may include reflux, polyps, hiatal hernia, esophagitis, varices, incompetency of the cardiac or pyloric sphincter, stric-tures, tumors, celiac disease, or arteriovenous malformations.

ACTION ALERT!

Conscious sedation or extreme vagal response to gastrointestinal intubation can result in cardiopulmonary arrest. Medications including atropine, drugs to reverse sedation, and other emergency pharmacologic agents should be immediately available with cardiopulmonary resuscitative equipment.

Severe, life-threatening hemorrhage can result from gastrointestinal intubation, especially in the presence of esophageal varices. Monitor for signs and symptoms of shock including diaphoresis, anxiety, hypotension, and tachycardia.

Interfering Factors

➤ Barium in the esophagus, stomach, and/or small intestine can prevent adequate visualization and tissue sampling of the upper GI tract.

➤ Lack of cooperation and severe anxiety can prevent gastrointestinal intubation or adequate visualization.

➤ Contents in the stomach may interfere with visualization.

➤ Gagging and emesis can prevent gastrointestinal intubation or adequate visualization.

Contraindications

➤ Recent myocardial infarction or pulmonary embolism, shock, and any conditions that result in unstable cardiovascular status increase the danger of cardiorespiratory compromise and arrest.

➤ Acute bleeding in the upper gastrointestinal tract.

➤ Recent gastrointestinal surgery where healing of suture lines cannot be assured.

➤ Esophageal varices, esophageal strictures, or other esophageal disease.

➤ Uncooperative clients or those who have depressed levels of consciousness.

➤ Suspected or actual perforated viscus, acute abdomen, acute oral or oropharyngeal inflammation, abnormal upper airway anatomy, seizures, and/or severe cervical arthritis.

➤ Significant coagulopathy.

Potential Complications

➤ Esophageal, stomach, or duodenal perforation

➤ Hemorrhage

➤ Cardiorespiratory depression, resulting from intravenous sedation given prior to the procedure

➤ Cardiac arrhythmias, resulting from intravenous medications to decrease duodenal spasms given during the procedure

➤ Vasovagal reactions

➤ Infection

NURSING CONSIDERATIONS

Prepare Your Client

➤ Explain that this test is used to look inside from the esophagus (where they begin swallowing) to the duodenum (just past the stomach) to see if any problems exist.

➤ Explain that the client will not be unconscious during the procedure, but that intravenous sedation will be given to promote comfort and relaxation, even light sleep. The procedure takes approximately 20–30 minutes.

➤ Advise the client that the procedure is uncomfortable, but should not be painful. As the endoscope is being inserted into the throat, a retching or gagging sensation may be felt, but there is usually no vomiting or severe pain. As the scope passes into the stomach and small intestine, pressure may be felt.

➤ Talk about how the client can notify the nurse if severe pain is felt.

➤ Make sure that an informed consent is obtained, because of the possible complications associated with this procedure.

➤ Restrict food and fluids for 8–12 hours before the procedure.

➤ Have the client urinate before the procedure.

➤ Administer sedation prior to the procedure as ordered. General anesthesia may be used in certain pediatric, uncooperative, or highly anxious clients.

Perform Procedure

Nurses do not perform this procedure, but should understand the process to prepare the client and to assist the endoscopist in obtaining the best results. A long, flexible endoscope is used to visualize the upper GI tract. The endoscope is equipped with suction to remove secretions and air controls that distend the mucosal lumen for safe passage through the abdominal structures. Water controls keep the fiber-optic tip of the instrument clean.

Assist the client into a left lateral decubitus position. Instruct the client to swallow as the endoscopist inserts the endoscope into the throat, and to breathe deeply as the scope passes into the stomach, in order to relax the abdominal muscles.

The endoscopist sprays the client's throat with a local anesthetic, inserts the instrument into the throat, and insufflates a small amount of air to help dilate the mucosal lumen. The endoscope is then passed through the esophagus, the stomach, and the duodenum. During the EGD, samples of tissue may be taken for evaluation, or bleeding sites may be treated by injecting sclerosing agents, electrocoagulation, or laser coagulation. Pictures may also be taken during this procedure.

During the procedure, assess the client's vital signs, oxygenation status, respiratory excursion, level of abdominal distention, level of consciousness, vagal response, and pain tolerance.

Care After Test

➤ Monitor vital signs every 15–30 minutes until the client is stable.

➤ Observe for signs of complications, such as bleeding, vomiting, change in vital signs, severe abdominal pain and/or distention, tachycardia, fever, dyspnea, subcutaneous emphysema in the neck, and abdominal rigidity.

➤ Keep the client in a semi-Fowler's position or turned to the side to help expectorate any fluids.

➤ Restrict food and fluids until the gag reflex has returned (approximately 2–4 hours).

➤ Observe the client carefully when fluids are first offered for signs of difficulty swallowing or aspiration.

➤ Saline gargles or throat lozenges may be used to decrease throat soreness and hoarseness.

➤ Evaluate related tests such as an upper gastrointestinal tract series, barium swallow, small bowel series, hypotonic duodenography, and barium enema.

Educate Your Client and the Family

➤ Inform the client that they will feel some abdominal discomfort and/or flatus following the procedure, due to the air inflated into the abdominal structures during the procedure. Getting up and walking around can help get rid of the air and minimize the discomfort.

➤ Advise client to avoid strenuous activities for 24 hours after the test.

➤ Inform client of the signs and symptoms of gastrointestinal bleeding including dark stools, tarry stools, abdominal or back pain, fever, pounding heart, and weakness. Tell the client to report these to the primary health care provider immediately.

➤ Teach the client and family a well-balanced diet, including the importance of adequate fluid and fiber intake.

Estriol Excretion

ess tree ole • eks kree shun
(Estrogen Fractions)

Normal Findings

Increasing estriol levels, demonstrating fetal growth and normally functioning fetal-placental unit

What This Test Will Tell You

This blood and 24-hour urine test assesses fetal growth and placenta function in high-risk pregnancies. Urine and serum estriol levels begin to increase in the 8th week of pregnancy and continue to rise until delivery. Both the placenta and the fetus make estriol. A continued increase in estriol levels indicates that the baby and placenta are functioning correctly. Decreasing levels indicate deterioration of the fetal-placenta unit, requiring the primary health care provider to evaluate whether to continue the pregnancy or deliver the baby early.

The daily, but more often weekly, studies usually begin around the 28th–30th week of the pregnancy. All the results are compared to the previous levels to demonstrate a steady increase (normal) or a fall in estriol levels (abnormal). For the urine test, a 24-hour collection is necessary to allow for circadian rhythms and differing levels throughout a day. Alternately, blood estriol levels can be assessed. This test is done less frequently now due to increased use of ultrasound and stress testing for fetal evaluation.

Abnormal Findings

▲ INCREASING LEVELS may indicate adrenal tumors, multiple pregnancy, glucosuria, ovarian tumors, urinary tract infections, or testicular cancer.

▼ DECREASING LEVELS may indicate an ill-functioning fetal-placental unit, pre-eclampsia, eclampsia, placental sulfatase deficiency, fetal death, anorexia nervosa, Rh isoimmunization, fetal adrenal insufficiency, congenital anomalies of fetus, maternal hypertension, anencephaly, Turner's syndrome, or maternal diabetes mellitus.

ACTION ALERT!

A 40% decrease in lab value from the average of the 2 previous days' studies or a 20% drop over 2 weeks requires immediate evaluation of fetal well-being.

Interfering Factors

➤ The test may not be useful for a multiple gestation as the urine estriol levels will simply be an average of the fetal-placental units' estriol contributions. One child may be doing very well while its twin may be starting to deteriorate.

➤ Uncontrolled gestational diabetes and urinary tract infections can increase estriol levels.

➤ Recent studies using radioisotopes can affect test results.

➤ Medications that may increase levels include steroids, estrogen, phenothiazines, and tetracyclines.

➤ Failure to collect all of the 24-hour urine.

➤ Failure to keep cold or transport immediately.

NURSING CONSIDERATIONS

Prepare Your Client

➤ Explain that this test is one way to see how well the baby and the womb (placenta) are growing.

➤ Tell client to drink fluids during the urine collection.

Perform Procedure

For 24-hour urine collection:

➤ Collect a 24-hour urine sample. Ensure container has a preservative.

➤ Keep urine iced or refrigerated.

For blood testing:

➤ Collect 5–7 mL of venous blood in a red-top tube.

Care After Test

➤ Evaluate fetal movements and heart rate.

➤ Ask the client if she is taking prenatal vitamins as ordered by her primary health care provider. Stress the importance of supplemental vitamins in providing good nutrition and normal growth and development of her baby.

➤ Assess the client's knowledge of prenatal care including diet, activity, rest, signs and symptoms of labor, and danger signs in pregnancy. Provide instruction as indicated.

➤ Assess the client's ability to provide adequate nutrition for the fetus. Refer to social services and Women, Infants, and Children program (WIC) if she needs assistance.

➤ Refer to a registered dietician if dietary deficiencies are suspected.

➤ Assess the client for use of cigarettes, tobacco products, alcohol, over-the-counter medications, and street drugs. Instruct the client as necessary to avoid these substances as they may cause intrauterine growth retardation.

➤ If the client reports decreased fetal movements, assess recent maternal history for maternal activity and relationship to fetal movement. Assess also her recent consumption of food or fluids and its relationship to fetal movement. Consult with the primary health care provider about instructing the client to eat, drink, and then rest. During rest, tell her to concentrate on fetal movements for 1 hour. Three fetal movements in 1 hour are reassuring.

➤ Review related tests such as fetal ultrasound.

Educate Your Client and the Family

➤ Explain that this is a screening test. If the estriol level begins to fall, further monitoring may be needed.

➤ Teach the client how to count fetal movements and to report decreased activity immediately. See *Daily Fetal Movement Count.*

➤ Instruct the client about normal signs of labor such as a gush of fluid, bloody show, and contractions that increase in frequency, intensity, and duration.

➤ Instruct the client about danger signs in pregnancy such as a gush of fluid, vaginal bleeding, abdominal pain, temperature elevation, dizziness, blurred vision, persistent vomiting, severe headache, edema, muscular irritability, difficult urination, or decreased/absent fetal movements.

➤ Tell the client to notify the primary health care provider if there are less than three movements in 1 hour. A nonstress test or biophysical profile may be ordered.

Estrogen and Progesterone Receptor Assay, Tissue

ess troe jen • and • proe jess tur one • ree sep tur • a say

Normal Findings

	Estrogen	Progesterone
Negative	<3 femtomoles (fmol)/mg of protein	<5 fmol/mg
Positive	>3 fmol/mg of protein	>5 fmol/mg

What This Test Will Tell You

This tissue analysis test identifies clients with breast cancer who are most likely to respond to ablative (removal of hormone-producing endocrine glands) or additive therapy (medication producing same hormone-suppressing effect as ablative therapy). Normal breast tissue contains estrogen-receptor sites; however, only about 33% of breast cancers are estrogen-receptor positive (ER+). Because tumor growth in ER+ clients depends on an estrogen supply, therapy is directed toward reducing estrogen. If the tumor is also progesterone-receptor positive (PR+), the client's prognosis improves with hormone-suppression therapy. Most tumors that are PR+ are also ER+. The rate of response to therapy for clients with ER+ tumors increases from 60% to 80% when the tumor is also PR+.

Abnormal Findings

Presence of ER+ and/or PR+ receptors may indicate tumors that will respond to hormone-suppression therapy.
Absence of ER+ and/or PR+ receptors may indicate tumors that are growing more rapidly and/or are less responsive to hormone-suppression therapy.

Interfering Factors

➤ Tissue specimen less than 200–500 mg
➤ Failure to trim fat from tissue, cut specimen into small pieces, place in vial, and freeze in liquid nitrogen within 30 minutes of surgical excision
➤ Failure to store frozen specimen at –70°C

Potential Complications

➤ Possible bleeding or hematoma formation at the surgical/biopsy site
➤ Possible numbness of the nipple after surgical excision of the mass; this should abate in 2 months, but may interfere with sexual arousal

---

NURSING CONSIDERATIONS

Prepare Your Client

➤ Explain to the client that this test is done following a breast biopsy to help determine the best therapy if breast cancer is found.
➤ Explain to client that if cancer is found, additional tests will be done on the tissue specimen to help determine the best treatment plan.
➤ See *Breast Biopsy.*

Perform Procedure

➤ See *Breast Biopsy.*
➤ Be sure tissue specimen for recep-

tor assay is placed in correct container (without formaldehyde), frozen correctly, and stored at appropriate temperature (see preceding Interfering Factors).

Care After Test

➤ See *Breast Biopsy*.

➤ Refer client to cancer support groups such as those offered by the American Cancer Society.

➤ Review related tests such as serum estrogen level, mammogram, computed tomography scan, and bone scan.

Educate Your Client and the Family

➤ Explain that hormone therapy is used to treat tumors that are dependent upon progesterone or estrogen for growth.

➤ Inform client that more than half of all primary and metastatic tumors that are receptor-positive respond to hormonal therapy.

E

Estrogen, Serum

ess troe jen • see rum

(Estrone [E_1], Estradiol [E_2], and Estriol [E_3])

Normal Findings

ADULT MALE
12–34 pg/mL (SI units: 40–120 pmol/L)

ADULT AND MENSTRUATING ADOLESCENT FEMALE
Proliferative phase (Days 1–10): 24–68 pg/ml (SI units: 90–250 pmol/L)
Midcycle (Days 11–20): 50–186 pg/ml (SI units: 180–690 pmol/L)
Luteal phase (Days 21–28): 73–149 pg/mL (SI units: 270–550 pmol/L)

PREGNANT
Levels increase throughout the pregnancy.

CHILD
1–6 years: 3–10 pg/mL (SI units: 10–40 pmol/L)
Levels gradually rise to adult levels with age.

ELDERLY
Levels are greatly decreased following menopause.

What This Test Will Tell You

This radioimmunoassay blood test identifies the serum levels of the only measurable estrogens, estrone (E_1), estradiol (E_2), and estriol (E_3). Estrogen is secreted by the ovaries, adrenal cortex, and testes. More than 30 estrogens have been identified, but estradiol is the principal estrogenic hormone produced by the ovary. The characteristics of the menstrual cycle, with the changing levels of estrogen, are in response to the release of pituitary gonadotropin. In the prepubescent female, pituitary gonadotropin release is suppressed by low levels of adrenal estrogen. At puberty, inhibition levels are reset.

Abnormal Findings

▲ INCREASED LEVELS may indicate menstrual irregularity and infertility, time of menstrual cycle, gynecomastia, precocious puberty in females, hepatic disease with decreased estrogen metabolism, testicular atrophy, estrogen-secreting ovarian tumors, testicular tumors, adrenal tumors, or congenital adrenal hyperplasia.

▼DECREASED LEVELS may indicate menopause, alteration in fetal well-being, fetal demise, ovarian dysfunction, delayed puberty in females, infertility, Turner's syndrome, amenorrhea due to hypopituitarism, anorexia nervosa, psychogenic stress, intense athletic activities, or testicular feminization syndrome in females.

Interfering Factors

➤ Medications that can increase levels include estrogens and oral contraceptives.
➤ Steroids and hormones of pituitary origin may alter results.
➤ Clomiphene can decrease levels.
➤ Pregnancy can increase levels.
➤ Hemolysis.

NURSING CONSIDERATIONS

Prepare Your Client

➤ Explain that this test will check the amount of the hormone estrogen that the body is producing.
➤ For the nonpregnant, premenopausal female, explain that the test may be repeated during the various phases of the menstrual cycle.
➤ Recognize that the client may have considerable anxiety about the outcome and implications of this test. These concerns will vary and include: (1) the pregnant client who is anxious about her baby; (2) male and female clients who are concerned about their physical well-being and their sexuality; (3) parents who are concerned about the sexual characteristics of their children.

Perform Procedure

➤ Perform venipuncture and collect 5–10 mL of blood in a red-top tube.
➤ Notify lab of time and date that steroid, estrogen, and pituitary-based hormone medications were last taken.
➤ Indicate on lab slip first day of last menstrual period for nonpregnant, premenopausal, postpubescent females.
➤ Indicate on lab slip if client is postmenopausal.

Care After Test

➤ Assess for feminization of males, masculinization of females, or signs of sexual maturation as indicated.
➤ Review related tests such as urine estrogen, follicle-stimulating-hormone levels, serum luteinizing-hormone levels, serum progesterone, serum testosterone, and serum estriol levels.

Educate Your Client and the Family

➤ Tell the client to make an appointment with the primary health care provider to discuss the results of the test.
➤ Tell the client that more tests may need to be done in order for the primary health care provider to make a diagnosis.
➤ Explain to the nonpregnant, premenopausal, postpubescent female client that the test will be repeated several times between her periods so that changes in estrogen levels can be measured.
➤ Explain to the pregnant client that the test may be repeated during her pregnancy to continue to check on the well-being of her baby.

Estrogen, Total Urine
ess troe jen • toe tal • yur in

Normal Findings

ADULT MALE
4–25 µg/24 hours (SI units: 10–80 nmol/24 hours)

ADULT PREMENOPAUSAL AND ADOLESCENT FEMALE
Preovulation: 5–25 µg/24 hours (SI units: 15–85 nmol/24 hours)
Follicular phase: 24–100 µg/24 hours (SI units: 80–350 nmol/24 hours)
Luteal phase: 12–80 µg/24 hours (SI units: 40–280 nmol/24 hours)

POSTMENOPAUSAL FEMALE
0–10 µg/24 hours (SI units: <40 nmol/24 hours)

PREGNANT
(See *Estriol Excretion*, which is the test of choice in pregnant women.)

CHILD, PREPUBESCENT
1 µg/24 hours

What This Test Will Tell You

This urine analysis identifies the total urine levels of the major measurable estrogens, estrone (E_1), estradiol (E_2), and estriol (E_3). Estrogen is secreted by the ovaries, adrenal cortex, testicles, and in pregnancy, by the placenta. In both sexes, estrogen metabolism occurs primarily in the liver. More than 30 estrogens have been identified, but estradiol is the principal estrogenic hormone and is produced by the ovaries. The characteristics of the menstrual cycle, with the changing levels of estrogen, are in response to the release of pituitary gonadotropin. In the prepubescent female, pituitary gonadotropin release is suppressed by low levels of adrenal estrogen. At puberty, inhibition levels are reset.

Abnormal Findings

▲ INCREASED LEVELS may indicate multiple pregnancy, ovarian tumors, testicular tumors, adrenocortical tumors, adrenocortical hyperplasia, glycosuria, hepatic disease with decreased estrogen metabolism, urinary tract infections, precocious puberty, corpus luteum cyst, or Stein-Leventhal syndrome.

▼ DECREASED LEVELS may indicate menopause, deterioration of fetoplacental unit, alteration in fetal well-being, fetal demise, ovarian dysfunction, ovarian agenesis, diabetes mellitus, Turner's syndrome, adrenogenital syndrome, hypopituitarism, adrenal hypofunction, or anorexia nervosa.

Interfering Factors

➤ Medications including adrenocorticosteroids, ampicillin, cascara sagrada, clomiphene, estrogen- and progesterone-containing drugs, steroids, thiazide diuretics, meprobamate, methenamine mandelate, hydrochloride, phenolphthalein, phenothiazines, senna, tetracyclines, and vitamins may interfere with accurate results.

➤ Glycosuria and urinary tract infections.

➤ Failure to refrigerate specimen or keep on ice.

➤ Failure to collect all urine in 24-hour period.

➤ Failure to place all urine in lab bottle with a preservative to maintain specimen at a pH of 3.0 to 5.0.

➤ Contamination of specimen with toilet paper, menses, or fecal material.

NURSING CONSIDERATIONS

Prepare Your Client

➤ Explain that this test will help to evaluate the amount of the hormone estrogen being produced by the body.

➤ Recognize that the client may have considerable anxiety about the outcome and implications of this test. These concerns will vary and include: (1) the pregnant client who is anxious about her baby; (2) male and female clients who are concerned about their physical well-being and their sexuality; (3) parents who are concerned about the sexual characteristics of their children.

Perform Procedure

➤ Collect 24-hour urine specimen.

➤ Where pertinent, indicate the first day of the last menstrual period on the laboratory slip.

➤ Transport refrigerated (cooled) specimen to lab before warming occurs.

Care After Test

➤ Assess for feminization of males, masculinization of females, or signs of sexual maturation as indicated.

➤ Review related tests such as cytologic examination of vaginal smear, urine pregnanediol, follicle-stimulating-hormone level, and progesterone level.

Educate Your Client and the Family

➤ Tell the postpubescent, premenopausal female client that this test may be repeated at different points in the menstrual cycle to evaluate changing estrogen levels.

➤ Explain to the pregnant client that the test may be repeated during her pregnancy to continue to check on the well-being of her baby.

Evoked Potential Studies

ee voekt • poe ten shul • stud ees

Normal Findings

Normal waveform latencies with no conduction delays

What This Test Will Tell You

This electrophysiologic test produces graphic recordings (traces) of the central nervous system response to sensory stimuli, which help in diagnosing both central and peripheral nervous system diseases. Electrical impulses causing nerve conduction of impulses are generated by electrodes placed on the client's skin and/or scalp. This information is analyzed by a computer, and a trac-ing of the activity is produced. This is a very sensitive test that detects lesions in the cortex, spinal cord, brain stem, and thalamus that other tests may not reveal. In addition to diagnosing disease, this procedure is performed to monitor neuro-electrical function during surgery, locate nerve damage, and predict outcome in brain-injured clients. A particular advantage of this test is the client does not have to be conscious, cooperative, or verbal in order for results to be obtained and analyzed.

Evoked potential tests consist of visual evoked potentials, brain stem auditory evoked potentials, and somatosensory evoked potentials.

Abnormal Findings

➤ *Visual evoked potentials* may reveal multiple sclerosis, optic neuritis, Parkinson's disease, optic nerve lesion, optic tract lesion, visual cortex lesion, and brain death.

➤ *Auditory evoked potentials* may reveal acoustic tumor, cerebrovascular accident, multiple sclerosis, lesions causing hearing disorders, central auditory pathway dysfunction, and brain death.

➤ *Somatosensory evoked potentials* may reveal peripheral nerve lesions, spinal cord lesion, cerebrovascular accident, multiple sclerosis, cervical myelopathy, tumors, or brain death. They are also used to monitor spinal cord function during surgery and during treatment for multiple sclerosis, and to evaluate extent and location of brain injury.

NURSING CONSIDERATIONS

Prepare Your Client

➤ Explain to your client and family that this test measures the ability of the brain to receive stimulation from the eyes, ears, or arms and legs.

➤ Tell them that small sensors will be placed on the scalp and/or skin to detect electrical activity. This test can be performed on clients that are confused, uncooperative, or even comatose.

➤ Assure client and family that the test is not painful.

➤ Wash the client's hair or affected body area before testing.

➤ Inform the client and family that a gel will be applied to the skin with each electrode.

➤ Tell the client there is no need to restrict food, fluids, or medications before the test. The tests are not affected by sedatives or anesthesia.

Perform Procedure

Nurses do not perform this procedure, but should understand the tests to explain to the client. Place the sensors on the scalp for the visual and brain stem auditory evoked potential studies. Place the sensors on specific areas of skin for somatosensory evoked potential study.

VISUAL EVOKED RESPONSES

During the visual evoked study the client is shown a flashing light or a rapidly changing geometric design such as a reversing checkerboard, or the retina is directly stimulated in other ways. One eye is tested at a time. Scalp electrodes measure the brain's response and a recording is made.

AUDITORY BRAIN STEM EVOKED RESPONSES

Earphones are placed on the client and sounds such as clicks or tones are transmitted into the earphones. Only one ear is tested at a time. Scalp electrodes measure the brain's response and a recording is made.

SOMATOSENSORY EVOKED RESPONSES

Somatosensory evoked potential testing measures the electrical activity of peripheral nerves. Electrodes are commonly placed on the medial nerve (over the wrists) and/or peroneal nerve (over the knees) to provide a mild electrical stimulation. This may cause mild discomfort or muscle twitches. Scalp electrodes measure the brain's response and a recording is made.

E

Care After Test

➤ Wash the gel from the body part tested.

➤ Assure that appropriate community health agency and occupational therapy referrals are made for client with compromised function.

➤ Evaluate related tests such as hearing screening, vision screening, electromyography, and other evaluations of brain stem function.

Educate Your Client and the Family

➤ Teach the client self-care strategies and the family ways to help the client meet basic needs (activities of daily living). Maintaining optimal independence despite compromised neurologic function is very important.

➤ Teach safety measures related to any alterations in sensory function.

Exercise Stress Test

ek sur size • stres • test
(Stress Test, Exercise Tolerance Test, Electrocardiogram Stress Test, Treadmill Test)

Normal Findings

All ages:
Normal exercise tolerance (85% of maximum heart rate predicted for age and sex)
No significant dysrhythmias, syncope, or myocardial ischemia
No significant complaints of symptoms such as lightheadedness, pain, fatigue

What This Test Will Tell You

This electrophysiologic test is used primarily to screen for and evaluate myocardial function as well as to monitor the client's response to therapies to improve function. The stress test is frequently used to diagnose the heart's ability to respond to and tolerate exercise. Abnormal heart rhythms, ischemic heart disease, coronary artery disease, and valvular abnormalities are some of the conditions that can affect normal exercise tolerance. This test is performed most commonly using a treadmill, but stair stepping or a stationary bicycle may also be used. Continuous electrocardiographic (ECG) monitoring is done throughout the test to identify abnormal rate responses and ischemia. The client's blood pressure is also monitored throughout the test.

The selected exercise is usually performed under continuous ECG monitoring until the target heart rate, 85% of the maximal heart rate for the age and sex of the client, is reached, or the client needs to quit because of abnormal symptoms or findings. With treadmill testing, stages are used to gradually increase the work of exercise by raising the speed and grade (elevation) of the treadmill at regular time intervals. Stationary bicycle testing is also done in stages with gradual increases in resistance to increase the work of exercise throughout the test. Oxygen consumption may also be monitored by using a special mouthpiece.

Abnormal Findings

This test may reveal coronary artery disease, failure of the blood pressure to rise to support increased activity, extreme rise in blood pressure in response to exercise, ST segment changes indicating myocardial ischemia, dysrhythmias, abnormal rate response (extreme tachycardia, bradycardia), ectopic rhythms or beats, or claudication.

ACTION ALERT!

Diagnostic indications of myocardial ischemia, myocardial infarction, second- or third-degree heart blocks, syncope, and ventricular dysrhythmias with accompanying symptoms all require immediate medical attention and intervention. These conditions may be associated with a high incidence of cardiopulmonary arrest.

Interfering Factors

➤ Improperly grounded recording equipment can distort electrical tracings.

➤ Improper placement of electrodes.

➤ Electrodes without adequate amounts of conduction gel.

➤ Dried conduction gel on electrodes.

➤ Medications such as calcium channel blockers, antidysrhythmics, beta blockers, other cardiac medications, and antihypertensives may impair exercise tolerance or identification of dysrhythmias.

➤ Heavy meals prior to testing can interfere with results.

➤ Tobacco can cause coronary artery spasms.

Contraindications

➤ Very young clients, generally under 5–8 years of age, because of their inability to safely use the exercise equipment

➤ Impaired mobility

➤ Unstable angina or severe aortic valvular disease

➤ Must be done with extreme caution in clients with pulmonary disease

Potential Complications

➤ Syncope
➤ Induction of serious dysrhythmias
➤ Cardiopulmonary arrest

E

NURSING CONSIDERATIONS

Prepare Your Client

➤ Explain that the test is to look at how the heart is working in response to exercise.

➤ Explain to the client or family that this test is performed by placing small discs or strips that stick to the skin on the chest, arms, and legs. Tell them they will be walking on a treadmill (or pedaling a stationary bike, or climbing stair steps) while the ECG machine is recording the heart's activity.

➤ Inform them that the test is usually done in a cardiac stress laboratory and takes about 30–45 minutes.

➤ Instruct client to inform the health professionals doing the stress test of any chest pain, dizziness, nausea, palpitations, extreme fatigue, and shortness of breath. Assure them that if they feel they cannot go on, the test will be terminated.

➤ Record baseline vital signs.

➤ Advise your client not to smoke for at least 4 hours before the test.

➤ Be sure your client hasn't skipped a meal before this type of strenuous test, but it should not be performed soon after eating a large meal.

➤ Inform client with heavy chest hair that small areas may need to be shaved or clipped to assure adequate electrode to skin contact.

➤ Note any medications the client is taking for hypertension or cardiac disease and inform the health care professional interpreting the ECG.

➤ Do not remove glasses, dentures, or hearing aids unless dictated by your hospital policy. The client may need these in order to communicate and cooperate during the procedure.

➤ Assist the client in selecting loose-fitting clothes that are not too warm and non-skid, well-fitting footwear such as sneakers.

Perform Procedure

Nurses do not usually perform this procedure but should understand the process to prepare the client and assist the primary health care provider. Electrodes are applied appropriately to continuously monitor the electrocardiogram throughout the test. The primary health care provider will select a protocol or adjust how fast and at how steep a grade the treadmill will be set. These adjustments are changed during stages of the test to achieve either a target heart rate without symptoms or until significant symptoms occur.

Ask the client to voice any complaints such as chest pain, dizziness, shortness of breath, or extreme fatigue. Record these subjective complaints.

Care After Test

➤ Evaluate the need for cardiac rehabilitation program for client with abnormal findings indicating cardiac disease.

➤ Monitor vital signs and assess for chest pain, dizziness, dysrhythmias, and other symptoms following the test.

➤ Evaluate other related tests such as an echocardiogram, cardiac enzymes, ECG, and cardiac catheterization.

Educate Your Client and the Family

➤ Teach client and family a heart-healthy diet, including no added salt, if there is evidence of atherosclerotic vessel disease.

➤ Encourage significant others to take cardiopulmonary resuscitation (CPR) courses.

➤ Teach client to pace activities if indicated by test results.

Febrile and Cold Agglutination Test

fee bril • and • kold • ah gloo tih nay shun
(Febrile and Cold Agglutinins, Widal's Test, O and H Antigen Test, Slide
Agglutination Test, Tube Dilution Test, Weils-Felix Reaction Test, Proteus
Antigen Test, Cold Agglutinins, Febrile Agglutinins)

Normal Findings

FEBRILE
≤ 1:80 titer is negative
COLD
≤ 1:16 titer is negative

What This Test Will Tell You

These blood tests diagnose specific
infectious diseases as well as reactions
to cold temperatures. Febrile agglutinins are antibodies that cause red
blood cells to aggregate or clump
together in the presence of high body
temperatures. Cold agglutinins cause
aggregation in the presence of lower
temperatures. Febrile agglutinin antibody titers are measured when
microorganisms are either extremely
difficult to culture or are so infectious
that they are hazardous to laboratory
personnel. Cold agglutinin testing is
indicated when an antibody screen or
panel suggests cold autoagglutina-
tion, in the workup for hemolytic
anemias, or as part of a workup of
painful extremities in cold weather
and other suspected cold reactions.

Abnormal Findings

➤ Febrile agglutinins: Fourfold
increase in serial titer confirms diagnosis. Elevated results may reveal
typhoid, paratyphoid, brucellosis,
tularemia, salmonella fever, or Rocky
Mountain spotted fever.
➤ Cold agglutinins: Positive findings
are titers > 1:40. Elevated results may
reveal *Mycoplasma pneumoniae*
infection, infectious mononucleosis,
cirrhosis, staphylococcemia, thymic

tumors, viral illnesses, multiple
myeloma, or scleroderma. See table
on page 312.

ACTION ALERT!

Isolation may be necessary for clients with
positive febrile agglutination titers and/or
fever of unknown origin (FUO) because of
the possibility of a highly contagious or carrier state in the client.

Interfering Factors

➤ Chronic exposure to infected animals may falsely elevate febrile titer
levels.
➤ Immunosuppressed clients may
be unable to mount an antibody
response and therefore have negative
results.
➤ Antibiotics taken early in the
course of the disease can depress
titers.
➤ Tularemia antibodies cross-react
with brucellosis antigen.
➤ Previous skin testing may elevate
titers (brucellosis).
➤ Hemolysis of specimen.
➤ Failure to collect the specimen in a
tube of the appropriate temperature.

NURSING CONSIDERATIONS

Prepare Your Client

➤ Explain as appropriate that the
test will help diagnose the cause of
the infection or if reactions to cold
may be causing symptoms.
➤ Tell your client that the test is done
at least twice, to measure rise and fall
in antibody levels.

Febrile and Cold Agglutinations in Common Infectious Diseases

Normal Antibody, Titer, Related Disease	Test Name	Titer Levels	Disease Transmission
Salmonella antibody <1:80 Detects typhoid or paratyphoid fever	Widal's test O and H antigen test	Antibodies appear in 1 week, rise in 3–6 weeks; O agglutinin falls in 6–12 months, H agglutinin can stay elevated for years.	Ingestion of contaminated food, milk, or water.
Brucellosis antibody <1:80 Detects brucellosis	Slide agglutination	Titers appear 2–3 weeks after infection, peak at 4–8 weeks.	Transmitted to humans from animals, especially goats, hogs, cattle, and dogs. Humans contract brucellosis from contact with infected animals or ingestion of infected meat or milk. Veterinarians, livestock workers, and dairy workers at greatest risk.
Tularemia antibody <1:40 Detects tularemia	Tube dilution test	Antibodies appear in 4 days; titers peak at 4–7 weeks, decline slowly over a year.	Spread to humans by infected rabbits, deer ticks, and fleas. Hunters, trappers, and agricultural workers at greatest risk.
Rickettsial antibody <1:40 Detects Rocky Mountain spotted fever, typhus	Weils-Felix reaction, Proteus antigen test	Antibodies appear 6–12 days after infection, peak in 1 month, decline in 5–6 months.	Spread by bite of infected tick or mite.

Perform Procedure

➤ The tube for febrile agglutination must be cooled to a specific temperature. Obtain properly cooled tube from the laboratory.

➤ The tube for cold agglutination testing must be warmed to a specific temperature. Obtain properly warmed tube from the laboratory.

➤ Collect 7 mL of venous blood into a properly prepared red-top tube.

➤ Document on lab slip any prior antibiotic therapy.

➤ Send specimen to laboratory immediately; any delay can alter results.

Care After Test

➤ Isolate the client with highly infectious disease processes if the results of the febrile agglutinin test are positive.

➤ Monitor febrile patterns. Medicate the client as ordered to reduce fever and symptoms.

➤ Evaluate the effectiveness of antibiotics administered by checking the resolution of titer levels.

➤ Monitor fluid and electrolytes. Febrile agglutinin–positive infections are associated with anorexia, weight loss, and dehydration.

➤ Obtain occupational and environmental history to determine exposure to infected animals (brucellosis, tularemia) if febrile agglutinins are present.

➤ For positive febrile agglutinins, check recent travel history to determine if client has been in areas where Rocky Mountain spotted fever, spread by tick bites, is endemic. Obtain diet history to determine if client has ingested contaminated food (typhoid, salmonella, paratyphoid). Inspect client's skin for rash characteristic of typhoid and Rocky Mountain spotted fever.

➤ Conduct a careful abdominal assessment for hepatomegaly, splenomegaly, and abdominal distention associated with infections causing elevated febrile agglutinin levels.

➤ Assess for pain or hemolytic anemia, which are often associated with positive cold agglutinin results.

➤ Review related tests including the complete blood count with differential, erythrocyte sedimentation rate, blood cultures, urine cultures, and chest x-ray.

Educate Your Client and the Family

➤ Stress importance of taking antibiotics as prescribed.

➤ Discuss importance of washing hands to avoid spreading infection to others.

➤ Teach client with occupational or environmental exposure (hunters, veterinarians, slaughterhouse workers, dairy farmers) to wear gloves when working with infected animals.

➤ Discuss signs and symptoms of infection with client and family: fever, weight loss, enlarged lymph nodes, distended abdomen.

➤ If client has splenomegaly or hepatomegaly, warn them to avoid contact sports or heavy lifting, which could damage the affected organ.

➤ If cold agglutinin titer is positive, warn client to avoid becoming cold and to protect themselves in cold weather.

➤ Instruct client with cold agglutinins and family to notify health care provider before any surgery where becoming cold is a possibility, such as heart surgery.

➤ Teach client with cold agglutinins and family to report any increase in extremity pain following exposure to cold.

Fecal Occult Blood

fee kal • oh kult • blud

(HemoQuant, Hemoccult, Hema-Chek)

Normal Findings

Absence of blood

What This Test Will Tell You

This stool test detects the presence of blood in the stool, and is most frequently used to screen for colon cancer. It is not useful in clients with frank gastrointestinal (GI) bleeding, actively bleeding hemorrhoids, or in women who are menstruating. Colon tumors, irritated by intestinal motion and content passage, bleed small amounts that are not detectable by naked eye inspection. Thus, occult (hidden) blood testing is a useful screening tool. However, other tests must be done to validate the presence of a tumor.

The most frequently used tests on the market (Hemoccult, Hema-Chek) utilize guaiac to detect the oxidation process in stool specimens. This process is catalyzed by hemoglobin, which turns the guaiac test blue if blood is present. Hemoglobin is degraded by pancreatic enzymes and becomes chemically altered as it passes through the GI tract; therefore, guaiac-based tests are less likely to detect occult upper GI bleeding than occult lower GI bleeding.

HemoQuant is less commonly used to test for fecal occult blood. The HemoQuant test is a quantitative assay that detects hemoglobin and hemoglobin breakdown products in stool specimens. Unlike guaiac-based tests, HemoQuant detects both upper and lower GI bleeding, and it does not cross-react with ascorbic acid, iron, or foodstuffs.

Abnormal Findings

Presence of blood may indicate colorectal carcinoma, colorectal adenomatous polyps, ulcers, hemorrhoids, varices, inflammatory gastrointestinal disorders, diverticular disease, gastrointestinal injury or trauma, esophagitis, or gastritis.

Interfering Factors

➤ Client noncompliance with dietary and/or medication restrictions can result in false positive results in guaiac-based tests.

➤ False negative results may be caused by vitamin C (ascorbic acid) or toilet bowl cleaners in guaiac-based tests.

➤ Recent ingestion of red meat, turnips, and horseradish.

➤ Nasopharyngeal or gingival bleeding will cause a positive result.

➤ Medications such as colchicine, rauwolfia, and iron may cause false positive results.

➤ False positive results may occur with oxidizing drugs such as iodine and bromides.

NURSING CONSIDERATIONS

Prepare Your Client

➤ Explain that this test is used to detect the presence of blood in the stool to help detect and diagnose problems early.

➤ Ensure adequacy of gastric preparation. In adults, this means that for 48–72 hours prior to the test, the client should adhere to a high-fiber diet with no red meat, avoid foods high in peroxidase, such as turnips, broccoli, or horseradish, and avoid iron preparations, bromides, iodides, and high doses of ascorbic acid.

➤ Advise the client to avoid salicylates and non-steroidal anti-inflammatory drugs (NSAIDs) for 1 week prior to the test.

➤ Teach the client that the stool specimen should be stored at room temperature.

➤ If samples are to be collected at home, teach client to keep urine, toilet paper, and water from the toilet out of the samples.

Perform Procedure

➤ Over a 3-day period, a small amount of stools are collected on a tongue blade and placed in a disposable container, after making sure that the specimens are not contaminated by urine, toilet tissue, or toilet bowl cleaners.

➤ Tap water or normal saline enemas may be used if needed to obtain a specimen.

➤ Laboratory testing of stool specimens must be performed within 4–5 days after collection, and the specimens should not be refrigerated.

➤ The Hemoccult test is most commonly used to detect occult fecal blood. This test consists of guaiac-impregnated paper slides or guaiac tape and a developing solution. A small piece of stool is placed on a slide or tape and rehydrated with developing solution, and a blue color appears within 30–60 seconds if blood is present.

➤ Follow manufacturer's directions for procedure.

Care After Test

➤ Correlate results of test with other signs and symptoms of GI disease, such as melena, abdominal cramping, weight loss, constipation, reduced stool caliber, hematochezia, and/or tenesmus.

➤ Evaluate other GI diagnostic and laboratory blood tests such as the sigmoidoscopy, colonoscopy, and hemoglobin/hematocrit.

Educate Your Client and the Family

➤ Encourage client and family to follow an anti-cancer diet, one which is low fat and includes high-fiber foods with plenty of fresh fruits and vegetables.

➤ Teach client the risk factors for colorectal cancer, which include a family history of colorectal cancer or polyps, a personal history of long-standing ulcerative colitis, adenomatous polyps, and/or endometrial, ovarian, or breast cancer.

➤ Encourage frequent health checkups for client with one or more risk factors for colon cancer.

➤ Tell the client to re-start medications that were put on hold prior to the test, but to avoid medications associated with blood loss in the GI tract, such as aspirin and other non-steroidal anti-inflammatory drugs (NSAIDs).

F

Ferritin, Serum
fair ih tin • see rum

Normal Findings
ADULT AND ELDERLY
Female: 10–150 ng/mL (SI units: 10–150 µg/L)
Male: 12–300 ng/mL (SI units: 12–300 µg/L)
PREGNANT
Slight to moderate decreases are common in pregnancy.
NEWBORNS
25–200 ng/mL (SI units: 25–200 µg/L)
INFANTS
1 month: 200–600 ng/mL (SI units: 200–600 µg/L)
2–5 months: 50–200 ng/mL (SI units: 50–200 µg/L)
CHILD
7–140 ng/mL (SI units: 7–140 µg/L)
ADOLESCENT
7–140 ng/mL up to age 15 (SI units: 7–140 µg/L)

What This Test Will Tell You
This blood test differentiates and classifies anemias and monitors their response to therapy. Serum ferritin levels measure the amount of ferritin, an important iron-storage protein.

Serum ferritin levels may vary throughout the lifespan for many reasons. They are lower in menstruating women than in postmenopausal women and may be reduced in elderly clients with poor dietary intake of iron. Levels do not begin to approximate adult normals until after age 15. Decreases in levels of serum ferritin are commonly seen during periods of rapid growth.

Abnormal Findings
▲INCREASED LEVELS may indicate chronic renal disease, acute or chronic hepatic disease, hemochromatosis, hemosiderosis, iron overload (may result from multiple transfusions), leukemia, breast cancer, Hodgkin's disease, acute or chronic infection, acute or chronic inflammation, chronic hemolytic anemias, sickle-cell anemia, or thalassemia.
▼DECREASED LEVELS may indicate chronic iron deficiency, malnutrition, or severe protein deficiency.

■ ACTION ALERT!
Women: <10 ng/mL
Men: <20 ng/mL
Newborn: <25 ng/mL
Child/adolescent: <7 ng/mL
These levels indicate significant potential for anemia, which may result in cardiac ischemia and dysrhythmias, respiratory distress, and organ system impairment.

Interfering Factors
➤ Hemolytic blood diseases may produce artificially high iron levels.
➤ Recent blood transfusions may cause elevated serum ferritin levels.
➤ Conditions such as acute inflammatory diseases, infections, and cancer may elevate serum ferritin levels.

NURSING CONSIDERATIONS
Prepare Your Client
➤ Explain that this test measures the amount of iron available in the body to produce healthy blood.

Perform Procedure
➤ Collect 5–7 mL of venous blood in a red-top tube.

Care After Test

➤ Observe the client for signs and symptoms of anemia including pallor, tachycardia, dyspnea, chest pain, and fatigue. Severe anemia may produce these symptoms because of tissue hypoxia.

➤ Encourage rest periods for clients experiencing fatigue related to anemia.

➤ Evaluate client's ability to perform activities of daily living.

➤ Refer to community health care services as needed if client is unable to perform basic daily needs.

➤ Obtain a dietary consult to assist the client and family in choosing a well-balanced diet, including foods high in iron and vitamin B_{12}.

➤ Review related tests such as hemoglobin, hematocrit, reticulocyte count, red blood cell indices, hemoglobin electrophoresis, total iron binding capacity (TIBC), bone marrow and liver biopsies, and iron absorption and excretion studies.

Educate Your Client and the Family

➤ If a severe anemia is identified through testing, explain how it may affect the client's activities. Severe anemia may produce fatigue, shortness of breath with or without exertion, fainting, increases in heart rate, and even tissue damage, such as heart attack (myocardial infarction). Teach the client to pace activities and to maintain regular patterns of sleep, rest, and activity to prevent fatigue.

➤ If an anemia is identified, instruct the client in dietary sources of iron, such as red meat, organ meats, dark green vegetables, and fortified grains.

➤ If your client is placed on oral iron replacement therapy for iron deficiency, explain that oral iron supplements are often better tolerated when taken with food and that iron supplements will cause darkened stools.

Fetal Scalp Blood pH
fee tahl • skalp • blud • pee aych
(Continuous Fetal pH Monitoring, Intermittent Fetal pH Monitoring)

Normal Findings
Fetus: Normal pH: 7.25–7.35

What This Test Will Tell You

This test is performed when suspicious or inconclusive fetal heart rate (FHR) patterns are observed and additional information regarding fetal status is needed to determine whether to expedite delivery. This fetal blood test is the most useful measure of fetal status, helping diagnose and evaluate fetal hypoxia and acid-base imbalances that occur when the fetus is deprived of oxygen and in distress. Mild, transient decreases in fetal blood pH are normally associated with contractions.

Continuous fetal tissue pH monitoring is now being conducted on an experimental basis, using a pH monitoring electrode attached to the presenting part with a probe just below the skin surface.

Abnormal Findings

▼DECREASED *fetal pH* may indicate fetal distress or fetal hypoxia.

███████ ACTION ALERT!
Borderline pH: 7.20–7.25
Acidotic pH: 7.20 or less on two consecutive measurements
With a borderline pH, a second sample should be reanalyzed in 15–30 minutes to monitor for a downward trend. A pH below 7.20 is pathological and prompts evaluation for immediate forceps delivery or cesarean section. Low Apgar scores are associated with a pH of 7.15 or below and fetal demise is common with a 6.8 pH.

Interfering Factors

➤ Cervix less than 2–3 cm dilated
➤ Intact amnion; will need to be ruptured
➤ Station of presenting part above −2
➤ Mixing maternal blood with fetal blood specimen
➤ Mixing air with sample, causing cellular respiration

Contraindications

➤ Known obstetrical emergencies such as prolapsed cord, placenta previa, abruptio placenta, definitive ominous FHR patterns, and amniotic fluid embolus which require immediate delivery of the fetus. Taking time to perform this test or awaiting results can lead to further deterioration of the fetus.
➤ Premature rupture of the membranes.
➤ Client with active cervical infections including gonorrhea and chlamydia.

Potential Complications

➤ Continued fetal bleeding from puncture site
➤ Ecchymosis
➤ Hematoma
➤ Infection at puncture site

NURSING CONSIDERATIONS

Prepare Your Client

➤ Explain to the client that the fetal scalp blood sampling is important when there is any question about how well the baby is doing, or if the baby is having trouble during labor.
➤ Be sure that the client understands that immediate delivery of her baby will be indicated if the test reveals that the baby is not getting enough oxygen. The delivery will be by forceps or cesarean section depending on such factors as labor status and the fetal-maternal cephalo-pelvic relationship.
➤ Ensure that an informed consent is obtained, because of the possible complications associated with this procedure.
➤ Explain that the procedure takes 10–20 minutes.
➤ Explain that this is a sterile procedure and that she must keep her hands above her waist so as not to touch anything.
➤ Warn the client that she may be uncomfortable while the procedure is being done, especially during contractions. However, if the client has had an epidural block during labor, she may not experience any discomfort.
➤ Advise the client that it may be necessary to repeat the test, depending upon the results.

Perform Procedure

Nurses do not perform this procedure, but need to understand it to explain it to clients, to ready the proper equipment, and to assist in the procedure. Help the client into the lithotomy position. Cleanse the perineal and vaginal area with an antiseptic solution, usually povidone-iodine (betadine) unless the client has an allergy to iodine or shellfish.

An amnioscope is inserted into the vagina and through the cervical canal to view the fetus's head (or buttocks if breech). The scalp of the fetus is cleansed with an antiseptic solution such as betadine, and dried. A silicone gel is applied to scalp to facilitate beading, or the formation of a bubble of blood. The fetal scalp is pierced with a microscalpel and blood is collected in long, heparinized, capillary tubes.

Seal the tubes with wax and store on ice to prevent cellular respiration, which can alter pH. Firm pressure is applied to the puncture site throughout 1–2 contractions to promote hemostasis. Observe the site during the next contraction to verify absence of bleeding. Labeled, iced specimen is taken to lab for immediate analysis; results are critical in determining labor management.

Care After Test

➤ Assess for other possible signs of distress such as meconium-stained amniotic fluid.

➤ Promote maternal-fetal well-being by providing oxygen to client and discontinuing any oxytocin infusion with evidence of fetal distress.

➤ Alternate maternal position from side to side to relieve fetal cord, maternal aorta, and maternal vena caval compression.

➤ Observe for any change in bloody show indicating bleeding from fetal scalp puncture site.

➤ Assist with preparation for immediate delivery, if indicated.

➤ Provide support to client/couple/family in the event of emergency delivery.

➤ After delivery, assess newborn, identifying and documenting puncture site(s); cleanse site(s) with antiseptic solution such as betadine and apply an antibiotic ointment, if prescribed.

➤ Review related tests such as maternal serum pH and fetal heart rate and trends.

Educate Your Client and the Family

➤ Inform the client and family that changes can occur during labor that keep the baby from getting as much oxygen as needed.

➤ Tell the mother that oxygen given to her will help her baby.

➤ Explain to the client that lying on her back causes pressure on her large blood vessels from the weight of the baby. This can slow down her circulation and may result in less oxygen being delivered to her baby.

➤ Tell the client and family that if the baby is showing signs of not getting enough oxygen, the baby will be taken (delivered) immediately.

➤ Warn client that the baby will have a small cut on the scalp (or buttocks, if breech) and the site may be bruised.

Fetoscopy
fee toss koe pee

Normal Findings

Fetus: No abnormalities

What This Test Will Tell You

This endoscopic and microscopic examination diagnoses fetal abnormalities not detectable by amniocentesis. An endoscope inserted through the abdominal wall allows for direct visualization of the fetus. The examination is performed at about 18 weeks' gestation; at this time, placental surface vessels are of adequate size and fetal parts are easy to identify. Therapeutic abortion, if elected, would be less hazardous at this time than later in pregnancy. Fetoscopy is also used for fetal therapy, such as ventricular shunts for hydrocephalus, bladder shunts for obstruction, and blood transfusions for the severely anemic fetus due to Rh sensitization. A fetal blood sample can be collected to diagnose congenital blood disorders such as hemophilia, sickle cell, or fetal distress indicated by blood gas measurements.

Abnormal Findings

External body defects may be detected and indicate neural tube defects, limb or finger defects, or facial clefts. *Blood analysis–detected disorders* may indicate thalassemia, hemophilia, sickle-cell anemia, muscular dystrophy, or chronic granulomatous diseases. *Skin biopsy–detected disorders* may indicate ichthyosiform erythroderma or epidermolysis bullosa. (See *Amniotic Fluid Analysis* for additional implications.)

Interfering Factors

➤ Morbid obesity
➤ Improper handling of specimens

Contraindications

➤ Client with anteriorly placed placenta that prohibits access without placental disruption
➤ Client with a history of spontaneous abortions and premature labor
➤ Client with an incompetent cervix

Potential Complications

➤ There is an increased risk of spontaneous abortion (5%–10%) and of preterm delivery (10%) associated with this procedure. It should be offered only to those women who have a significant risk of producing a child with a birth defect that can only be diagnosed by fetoscopy.
➤ Trauma to the fetus, umbilical cord, or placenta.
➤ Infection.
➤ Amniotic fluid leakage.
➤ Rh sensitization from fetal bleeding into maternal circulation.
➤ Fetal demise.
➤ Amniotic fluid embolism.
➤ Accidental puncture of maternal bladder or intestines.
➤ Amnionitis.

NURSING CONSIDERATIONS

Prepare Your Client

➤ Explain to the client that this procedure allows the primary health care provider to look directly at the baby for any possible problems that would be found by simply being able to see the baby or sampling blood or skin.

➤ Ensure that an informed consent is obtained, because of the possible complications associated with this procedure.

➤ Advise the client to eat light, mild foods that will not cause digestive problems or nausea.

➤ Tell the client the procedure will take 1–2 hours.

➤ Ask the client if she is allergic to iodine, as a povidone-iodine (beta-dine) skin preparation may be done prior to the test.

➤ Ask the client if she has any drug allergies, especially noting the medications ordered for the procedure. Sedation may be ordered prior to the test to sedate both the mother and fetus and decrease fetal movement.

➤ Take baseline vital signs and fetal heart rate (FHR) before the procedure.

Perform Procedure

Nurses do not perform this procedure, but need to understand it to explain it to clients. Position the client on her back during the procedure and ask her to place her hands behind her head or across her chest to avoid touching the sterile field. Ultrasound will be used prior to and during the test to guide the physician. Generally, sedation is administered intravenously. The abdomen is cleansed with a disinfecting solution at the site selected for cannula and fetoscope entry, and a local anesthetic is injected.

A small abdominal incision (0.5 cm through abdomen to peritoneum) is made and the fetoscopy equipment is inserted under ultrasound guidance. A cannula containing a trocar is inserted through incision into uterus and amniotic cavity. The trocar is withdrawn, amniotic fluid is obtained for analysis (see *Amniocentesis*), and the needlescope is inserted. The fetus, umbilical cord, and placenta are visually inspected, and then blood samples and tissue specimens are obtained using special attachments.

The amnioscope is removed, and the abdomen cleansed to remove disinfecting solution. Apply a sterile bandage to incision.

Care After Test

➤ Assess and record maternal vital signs and FHR; report deviations from normal to primary care provider.

➤ Assess the client for rupture of membranes and uterine contractions after the procedure by looking for a leak or gush of fluid from the vagina and rhythmical tightening of the uterine muscles resulting in effacement (taking up) and dilatation (opening) of the cervix.

➤ Assess fetal activity.

➤ Assess client for bleeding or drainage from the vagina or puncture site.

➤ Administer Rh immune globulin to Rh-negative client within 72 hours of procedure to prevent Rh isoimmunization unless fetal blood is found to be Rh-negative.

➤ Arrange for a repeat ultrasound to be performed the day after the test to confirm fetal viability and an adequate amount of amniotic fluid.

➤ Administer prophylactic antibiotic to prevent amnionitis and/or a tocolytic drug to inhibit uterine contractions, if prescribed.

➤ Review related tests such as amniotic fluid studies and genetic cytology.

Educate Your Client and the Family

➤ Instruct client to avoid strenuous activity for 1–2 weeks following test.

➤ Instruct client that after the procedure she should notify her primary maternity care provider if she has a gush of fluid, vaginal bleeding, abdominal pain, temperature elevation, dizziness, blurred vision, persistent vomiting, severe headache, edema, muscular irritability, difficult urination, or decreased/absent fetal movements.

➤ Advise the client to lie down on her side and notify the primary health care provider if preterm labor is suspected.

Fibrin Degradation Products

fie brin • deg rah day shun • prod ucts
(Fibrin Split Products, FSP, Fibrin Breakdown Products)

Normal Findings

ALL AGES
Screening assay: <10µg/mL (SI units: <10 mg/L)
Quantitative assay: <3 µg/mL (SI units: <3 mg/L)

What This Test Will Tell You

This blood test screens for disseminated intravascular coagulation (DIC). Elevations of fibrin degradation products occur with excessive breakdown of clots (fibrinolysis). Fibrin molecules are broken down by the enzyme plasmin, resulting in the release of fibrin degradation products. Elevations also occur in a variety of conditions that stimulate fibrinolytic activity.

Abnormal Findings

▲INCREASED *fibrin degradation products* (>10 µg/mL) may indicate disseminated intravascular coagulation (DIC), primary fibrinolysis, alcoholic cirrhosis, liver disease, preeclampsia, abruptio placentae, intrauterine death, burns, heatstroke, pulmonary embolus, renal disease, septicemia, massive blood transfusions, transplant rejection states, leukemia, congenital heart disease, deep-vein thrombosis (transient increase), or myocardial infarction (after 24–48 hours), and also occur following cardiopulmonary pump surgery.

ACTION ALERT!

Fibrin split products in excess of 40 µg/mL may indicate disseminated intravascular coagulation or other bleeding/coagulation disorders. Observe closely for bleeding and signs of shock.

Interfering Factors

➤ Heparin administration prior to testing will produce false positive results.

➤ Fibrinolytic medications, such as urokinase or streptokinase, or large doses of barbiturates produce increased levels of fibrin degradation products.

➤ Incorrect collection or handling of the blood sample will interfere with test results.

NURSING CONSIDERATIONS

Prepare Your Client

➤ Explain that this test helps to evaluate how well the system that breaks down blood clots is working.

➤ Review other clotting studies whenever available *before* venipuncture is performed to ascertain if excessive bleeding from the site can be anticipated.

Perform Procedure

➤ Collect 2 mL of venous blood in a blue-top tube.

Care After Test

➤ Assess client for unusual bruising or prolonged bleeding from venipuncture site. Delayed clotting is a complication of many conditions for which this test is ordered.

➤ Avoid intramuscular (IM) injections, if possible. If it is not possible to avoid injections, use the smallest possible needle for the injection. Rotation of the injection sites allows healing time for these sites. Pressure rather than massage after injection may reduce the potential for the development of a hematoma at the injection site.

➤ Test all body secretions including stool, gastrointestinal aspirate, and tracheal aspirate for occult blood. Closely inspect mucous membranes for bleeding.

➤ Review related tests such as prothrombin time, partial thromboplastin time, bleeding time, and activated clotting time.

Educate Your Client and the Family

➤ Clients with impaired clotting have prolonged bleeding times. Instruct the client and family on safety measures such as electric razors, non-skid shoes, and soft toothbrushes.

➤ Instruct the client or family to report prolonged or unusual bleeding or bruising.

➤ Significant elevations, which indicate a bleeding tendency, require that the client be protected from trauma. Injuries may result in uncontrolled bleeding, which is difficult to manage. Teach family and client how to evaluate the home environment and increase safety.

➤ Instruct the client or family in diet, activity, and/or medication regimens to prevent constipation. Hard stools may be traumatic to anal and rectal mucosa.

➤ Instruct the client with a bleeding tendency to avoid taking medications that prolong bleeding time, such as aspirin or products containing aspirin. Instruct client to avoid large quantities of alcohol and its regular use. A written list of products to avoid will provide the client or family with a reference when shopping or selecting home remedies for minor ailments.

F

Fibrinogen
fie brin oe jen
(Plasma Fibrinogen, Factor I, Quantitative Fibrinogen)

Normal Findings
ALL AGES
200–400 mg/dL
PREGNANT
Elevations greater than baseline fibrinogen level may occur during the third trimester of pregnancy. Elevations may exceed 400 mg/mL.

What This Test Will Tell You
This blood test evaluates bleeding disorders by assessing the levels of fibrinogen, a critical element in the normal clotting cascade.

Fibrinogen is a plasma protein synthesized in the liver and converted by thrombin to fibrin during normal functioning of the clotting cascade. If fibrinogen is not produced in adequate amounts by a diseased liver, clotting is prolonged or severely impaired because fibrin is not available to form stable clots. If, however, fibrinogen is produced in normal amounts, but excessive bleeding and clotting in the body require more than the liver can produce, a *consumptive coagulopathy* occurs.

Abnormal Findings
▼DECREASED LEVELS *of fibrinogen* (<200 mg/100 mL) may indicate disseminated intravascular coagulation (DIC), neoplasms (carcinoma of the prostate or lung, pancreatic cancer), bone marrow disorders (leukemia, multiple myeloma, hemolytic anemia), severe hepatic disease or hepatic failure, afibrinogenemia, hypofibrinogenemia, dysfibrinogenemia, fibrinolysis, thrombocytopenia, or hemolytic transfusion reaction.

▲INCREASED LEVELS *of fibrinogen* (>400 mg/100 mL) may indicate cancer of breast, stomach, or kidney; hepatitis; multiple myeloma; uremia; menstruation; postsurgery; systemic inflammatory disorders; nephrosis; burns; recovering or compensated DIC; or pregnancy (third trimester).

ACTION ALERT!
Levels less than 100 mg/100 mL are significantly low and are indicative of a serious coagulation disorder. They also affect the reliability of all coagulation tests that have a fibrin clot as an end point. Observe the client closely for signs of occult as well as overt blood loss, shock, and signs of microthrombi in the circulation.

Interfering Factors
➤ Heparin therapy requires use of a non-heparin reagent for testing.
➤ Hemolysis.
➤ Medications including oral contraceptives, estrogen therapy, asparaginase, phenobarbital, urokinase, streptokinase, and heparin may increase fibrinogen levels.
➤ Recent blood transfusions may change *effective fibrinogen levels* since the fibrinogen in stored blood undergoes spontaneous deterioration.
➤ High concentrations of plasmin will interfere with the reliability of the test.

Contraindications
➤ Individuals who have received blood transfusions, particularly multiple units of blood products, in

recent days or weeks will display unreliable fibrinogen levels.

➤ Some authorities discourage assessment of fibrinogen levels in clients with active bleeding or with acute infectious process.

NURSING CONSIDERATIONS

Prepare Your Client

➤ Tell your client that this test helps to evaluate how well the blood can clot.

Perform Procedure

➤ Collect 4.5 mL of venous blood in a blue-top tube.

➤ Transport the sample to the laboratory immediately. Some laboratories request the sample be placed on ice for transport.

Care After Test

➤ Assess client for unusual bruising or prolonged bleeding from venipuncture site. Delayed clotting is a complication of many conditions for which this test is ordered.

➤ Avoid intramuscular injections, if possible. If it is not possible to avoid injections, use the smallest possible needle for the injection. Rotation of the injection sites allows healing time for these sites. Pressure rather than massage after injection may reduce the potential for the development of a hematoma at the injection site.

➤ Test all body secretions including stool, gastrointestinal aspirate, and tracheal aspirate for occult blood. Closely inspect mucous membranes for bleeding.

➤ Review related tests such as prothrombin time, thrombin time, partial thromboplastin time, bleeding time, and activated clotting time.

Educate Your Client and the Family

➤ Clients with impaired clotting have prolonged bleeding times. Instruct the client and family on safety measures such as electric razors, non-skid shoes, and soft toothbrushes.

➤ Instruct the client or family to report prolonged or unusual bleeding or bruising.

➤ Significant elevations, which indicate a bleeding tendency, require that the client be protected from trauma. Injuries may result in uncontrolled bleeding, which is difficult to manage. Teach family and client how to evaluate the home environment and increase safety.

➤ Instruct the client and family in diet, activity, and/or medication regimens to prevent constipation. Hard stools may be traumatic to anal and rectal mucosa.

➤ Instruct the client with a bleeding tendency to avoid taking medications that prolong bleeding time, such as aspirin or products containing aspirin. Instruct client to avoid large quantities of alcohol and its regular use. A written list of products to avoid will provide the client or family with a reference when shopping or selecting home remedies for minor ailments.

Follicle-Stimulating Hormone, Serum

fahl lik ahl • stim yu lay ting • hor mone • see rum
(FSH)

Normal Findings

ADULT MALE
5–20 mIU/mL (SI units: 5–20 U/L)
ADULT PREMENOPAUSAL AND
ADOLESCENT FEMALE
Follicular phase: 5–20 mIU/mL (SI units: 5–20 U/L)
Midcycle peak: 15–30 mIU/mL (SI units: 15–30 U/L)
Luteal phase: 5–15 mIU/mL (SI units: 5–15 U/L)
POSTMENOPAUSAL FEMALE
50–100 mIU/mL (SI units: 50–100 U/L)
CHILD
5–10 mIU/mL (SI units: 5–10 U/L)

What This Test Will Tell You

This blood test is most commonly used to assist in diagnosing the cause of infertility. The test evaluates the proper release of follicle-stimulating hormone (FSH) by the anterior pituitary. In women, the rise and fall of FSH coincides with the phases of the menstrual cycle.

Abnormal Findings

▲ INCREASED LEVELS may indicate ovarian inadequacy, precocious puberty, menopause, orchitis, testicular failure in males, seminoma, Turner's syndrome, congenital hypogonadism, absence of gonads, or early acromegaly.

▼ DECREASED LEVELS may indicate infertility, pituitary insufficiency, hypothalamic disorders, pituitary tumors, ovarian tumors, or anorexia nervosa. Ovarian failure is associated with levels > 40 mIU/mL.

Interfering Factors

➤ Use of oral contraceptives, estrogen, progesterone, phenothiazines, and androgens may alter results.
➤ Radioactive scans within 1 week of blood sampling may interfere with obtaining accurate results because this test is done by radioimmunoassay.
➤ Levels may fluctuate throughout a 24-hour period.
➤ Hemolysis.

NURSING CONSIDERATIONS

Prepare Your Client

➤ Explain that this test is done to evaluate a certain sex hormone, especially to help find out if there is a problem in being able to become pregnant.
➤ Assure that the client has been lying down for at least 30 minutes prior to obtaining the venous sample.

Perform Procedure

➤ Collect 7 mL of blood into a red-top tube, preferably between 6 A.M. and 8 A.M.
➤ Mark on the lab slip if the woman is postmenopausal, or note the date of the last menstrual period.
➤ Handle and transport the specimen carefully to avoid hemolysis of sample.

Care After Test

➤ If infertility is diagnosed, assure that a referral is made to a fertility specialist if necessary.

> If indicated, help the couple identify adoptive agencies and/or infertility support groups.

> Review related tests such as luteinizing hormone, serum estrogen, urine FSH, and progesterone levels.

Educate Your Client and the Family

> If a client is undergoing an infertility workup, explain that the test may need to be repeated on several occasions.

> Tell client that frequently there are multiple causes of infertility, requiring tests for both partners.

F

Fragile X Chromosome Study

fra jil • X • kroe mah zome • stuh dee
(Fra X)

Normal Findings

Negative for fragile X chromosome. Although those testing negative are unlikely to have fra X syndrome, the sensitivity of this test is not 100%.

What This Test Will Tell You

This blood test diagnoses a newly identified chromosomal disorder, fragile X (fra X) syndrome, and detects female carriers. Fra X may be transmitted by a carrier female who is not affected, by a heterozygous female with signs of active mutant X in her cells, and by a normal male with little clinical demonstration of the problem who transmits fra X to his daughter. Fra X syndrome occurs in about 1 in 2000 births with females usually being less severely affected. Fra X syndrome is second only to Down syndrome as a cause of mental retardation.

Abnormal Findings

Presence of >4% fragile X chromosomes in sample may indicate fragile X syndrome or carrier of fragile X syndrome.

Interfering Factors

> Ingestion of folic acid or vitamins with folic acid during the month preceding the study interferes with identification of fra X chromosome in the culture.

> Failure to specify suspected diagnosis when ordering chromosome studies may result in an inadequate number of examined cells. Fra X abnormality cannot be detected in all cells even though the fra X chromosome will be present as an inherited disorder; 50–100 cells need to be examined in males, and 100–200 in females.

> Age of client, due to a decreased proportion of fra X positive cells in older clients.

> Failure of carrier females to demonstrate fra X chromosomes.

> Hemolysis of specimen by inappropriate handling and agitation of specimen.

> Failure to maintain specimen at ambient temperature after collecting.

> Delay of more than 24 hours in preparing blood specimen for analysis.

➤ Failure to use sodium heparin as the anticoagulant in the specimen tube. Other anticoagulants can alter cell viability.

NURSING CONSIDERATIONS

Prepare Your Client

➤ Explain that this test is used to help diagnose a genetic problem called fragile X. As appropriate, explain that the test is being done either to discover if a female is a carrier of this syndrome or if the client has this syndrome.

➤ Instruct the client not to take folic acid or vitamins containing folic acid for at least 1 month prior to the test.

Perform Procedure

➤ Collect 7–10 mL of blood in a green-top tube.

➤ Label specimen noting suspected fra X diagnosis, maintain at ambient temperature, and send to cytogenic laboratory immediately.

Care After Test

➤ If a positive diagnosis is made, refer the client and/or family for genetic counseling.

➤ If the fragile X syndrome is diagnosed in the client, refer for developmental testing and early interventional programs.

➤ Assess the client for other signs and symptoms of fragile X syndrome including mental retardation, large ears, large testes in males, and loose connective tissue.

➤ Review related tests such as developmental testing and cytologic genetics.

Educate Your Client and the Family

➤ Instruct client to make an appointment to discuss the test results with the clinical geneticist or physician who prescribed the test and who should be familiar with the fra X syndrome.

➤ Explain that if the test is positive for fra X syndrome, testing of other members of the client's family may be prescribed.

➤ Explain that the test may be repeated if the results are negative because many factors can interfere with the study and cause an error in testing.

➤ Encourage and assist the client and/or family to arrange an appointment for counseling.

➤ Explain the importance of testing other family members for the syndrome or as carriers of the syndrome. Assist these family members also in obtaining referral appointments.

➤ If folic acid supplements are prescribed for an affected child, explain to the family the importance of having the child take the vitamin as directed; explain that some affected children have shown improvement in behavior when taking this supplement. This treatment has shown no benefit in adults.

Free Fatty Acids
free • fat tee • ass ids
(FFA, Nonesterified Fatty Acids, NEFA)

Normal Findings
All ages: 8–20 mg/dL (SI units: 0.2–0.7 mmol/L)

What This Test Will Tell You
This blood test measures one of the types of lipids carried in the bloodstream to diagnose or evaluate the control of diabetes, detect malnutrition, or detect hyperlipoproteinemia. Free fatty acids (FFAs) are important components of lipoproteins and triglycerides. When lipoproteins or triglycerides are broken down, FFAs accumulate in fatty tissues until needed during times of stress such as physical exercise, fasting, malnutrition, or stress. Free fatty acids are most commonly regulated by neurohormones such as norepinephrine, epinephrine, and ACTH, as well as glucagon, cortisol, thyroxine, and growth hormone. FFAs are converted in the liver to very low density lipoproteins, and an accompanying rise of triglycerides also normally occurs.

Abnormal Findings
▲INCREASED LEVELS may indicate uncontrolled diabetes mellitus, secondary hyperlipoproteinemia, hyperthyroidism, prolonged starvation, chronic hepatitis, acute renal failure, pheochromocytoma, or acute alcohol intoxication.

Interfering Factors
➤ Fever, vigorous exercise, and recent weight loss may increase levels.
➤ Medications including heparin, adrenocorticotropic hormone, epinephrine, amphetamines, cortisone, growth hormone, thyroid-stimulating hormone, thyroxine, nicotine, caffeine, isoproterenol, tollutamide, reserpine, and oral contraceptives may increase levels.
➤ Aspirin, glucose, insulin, and neomycin may decrease FFAs.

NURSING CONSIDERATIONS
Prepare Your Client
➤ Explain, as indicated, that this test is used to help diagnose or evaluate the control of diabetes, evaluate nutritional status, or detect problems with breaking down fat and starches.
➤ Withhold food and all fluids other than water for 12 hours before sampling.
➤ Restrict alcohol consumption for 24 hours before sampling.
➤ Assure the client is relaxed and has not experienced recent stress or physical activity.

Perform Procedure
➤ Collect 10–15 mL of venous blood in a red-top tube.
➤ Take to lab immediately as the sample will need to be spun down at once.

Care After Test
➤ Arrange for new diabetic instruction or reevaluate instruction if indicated.
➤ Consult a registered dietician if abnormal levels are detected.
➤ Assess for signs and symptoms of malnutrition such as dry skin, body weight less than fifth percentile,

recent weight loss, hair loss, and amenorrhea.

➤ Evaluate related tests such as serum cholesterol, triglyceride levels, alanine aminotransferase (ALT), aspartate aminotransferase (AST), blood urea nitrogen (BUN), and serum creatinine.

Educate Your Client and the Family

➤ Reinforce the diet prescribed by a registered dietician.

➤ Assist the client in learning how to select a well-balanced diet.

Free Thyroxine T$_4$

free • thie **rok** sin • tee • 4

(FT$_4$ Index, FT$_4$, Free Thyroxine Index, FTI)

Normal Findings

ADULT, PREGNANT, AND ELDERLY

Free thyroxine index: 0.8–2.4 ng/dL (SI units: 10–31 pmol/L)

For clients on levothyroxine sodium: Up to 5.0 ng/dL

Free thyroxine level: 1–3 ng/dL (SI units: 13–39 pmol/L)

NEWBORN

Values will be increased.

ADOLESCENT

Values will be decreased.

What This Test Will Tell You

This blood test rules out hypothyroidism and hyperthyroidism, and evaluates thyroid replacement therapy. Because free thyroxine (FT$_4$) is not dependent upon thyroxine-binding globulin (TBG), it is more useful in providing an accurate picture of thyroid function when TBG levels are abnormal.

Abnormal Findings

▲ INCREASED LEVELS may indicate hyperthyroidism, Graves' disease, thyrotoxicosis due to T$_4$, or cirrhosis of the liver (slight elevation).

▼ DECREASED LEVELS may indicate hypothyroidism, early thyroiditis, or thyrotoxicosis due to T$_3$.

Interfering Factors

➤ Heparin will cause falsely elevated levels.

➤ Radionuclear scan tests within 1 week may affect results.

NURSING CONSIDERATIONS

Prepare Your Client

➤ Explain that this is a blood test to help find any problems there may be in a gland in the neck called the thyroid gland.

➤ For the free thyroxine index, first or simultaneously obtain the value of the T$_3$ uptake ratio.

Perform Procedure

➤ Collect 5 mL of venous blood in a red-top tube.

➤ 0.5 cc is sufficient for pediatric testing.

➤ For neonates, perform a heelstick.

➤ To calculate the free thyroxine index, use the following formula:

T$_4$ × T$_3$ uptake ratio = free thyroxine index

Care After Test

➤ Assess for signs of hypothyroidism including hypothermia, bradycardia, weight gain, thick and dry skin, thin hair, hypotension, cold extremities, masklike expression, fatigue, slowed mental processes, myalgia, weakness, and constipation.

➤ Assess for signs of hyperthyroidism including nervousness, apprehension, tachycardia, diaphoresis, flushed skin, tremor in hands, constipation, diarrhea, weight loss, weakness, amenorrhea, and cardiac dysrhythmias.

➤ Institute safety measures if weakness is noted.

➤ Review related tests such as levels of serum thyroxine, radioactive iodine uptake (RAI), protein-bound iodine, thyrotropin-releasing hormone, thyroid-stimulating hormone, and triiodothyronine suppression test.

Educate Your Client and the Family

➤ Teach client that thyroid hormone replacement must be taken for life if hypofunction is found or if the thyroid is removed surgically.

➤ Teach client how to meet rest and nutritional needs required by a hyperfunctioning thyroid. This includes frequent rest periods and a high-calorie, high-protein diet.

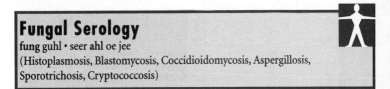

Fungal Serology
fung guhl • seer ahl oe jee
(Histoplasmosis, Blastomycosis, Coccidioidomycosis, Aspergillosis, Sporotrichosis, Cryptococcosis)

Normal Findings
Negative
Complement fixation titer < 1:8
Immunodiffusion method—Negative results
For sporotrichosis, agglutination titer < 1:40

What This Test Will Tell You
This blood test helps diagnose fungal infections (mycoses) by detecting and measuring the presence of antibodies in the serum.

The diagnosis of deep fungal disease is best made by tissue, body fluid, or sputum cultures. There are many different types of antibody tests for the various fungal infections. Most have a secondary role in diagnosis because of the high percentage of false positives.

Blastomycosis has no occupational predisposition and occurs in the non-immune-compromised host. Antibody titers are positive in less than 50% of infections. The geographical range is the southeast and midwest United States.

Coccidioidomycosis-antibody testing is extremely useful for diagnosis with specificity as high as 90%. Coccidioidomycosis in the U.S. is found mainly in the southwest. This fungal infection may often cause meningitis.

Histoplasmosis-antibody tests have false positives in 10% of cases. It is the most common fungal infection and is found east of the Mississippi. It grows on moist surfaces, and is commonly found in bird and bat droppings.

Abnormal Findings

Presence of fungal antibodies may indicate systemic fungal disease, pulmonary fungal disease, or coccidioidomycosis meningitis.

Interfering Factors

➤ Fungal antibodies may be found in normal people.

➤ Histoplasmosis has high level of false positives in people with tuberculosis or other fungal diseases.

➤ Blastomycosis testing may cross-react with histoplasmosis.

➤ Recent skin testing for fungal infections.

➤ Immunosuppression may result in low or negative titers despite infection.

➤ Failure to fast may alter results.

NURSING CONSIDERATIONS

Prepare Your Client

➤ Explain that this test will detect any evidence that fungus or mold is growing in the lungs or other organs and causing symptoms.

➤ Explain that fungal disease can be quite serious and that all diagnostic efforts including antibody testing need to be done.

➤ Restrict food and fluids for 8–12 hours before venous sampling.

Perform Procedure

➤ Obtain antibody tests 3–4 weeks after exposure whenever possible.

➤ Collect 7 mL of venous blood in a red-top tube.

Care After Test

➤ Obtain client's occupation and travel history to help discover which fungi may be causing symptoms.

➤ Monitor the client's fever patterns. Fungal infections cause fever in spite of antibiotics.

➤ Assess client for respiratory difficulty, cough, dyspnea, chest pain, hemoptysis, and hypoxia.

➤ If amphotericin B is used, monitor renal function due to its potential nephrotoxicity.

➤ Obtain an order to premedicate with acetaminophen, diphenhydramine, and corticosteroids before starting infusion of amphotericin.

➤ Isolation is not necessary since fungal infections are not contagious.

➤ Review related tests such as complete blood count with differential and culture results.

Educate Your Client and the Family

➤ Tell client and family that fungal infections cannot be transmitted person to person.

➤ Tell client to use a mask when cleaning bird cages or chicken coops.

➤ Warn client about the side effects of amphotericin B including fever, chills, headache, appetite loss, nausea, and vomiting.

➤ Reassure client that most of the side effects can be controlled with premedication.

Galactose-1-phosphate Uridyl Transferase

gah lak tose • wun(1) • foss fate • yur ih dill • trans fur ase
(GALT, Galactokinase, Gal-1-PUT, Galactosemia Screen)

Normal Findings
All ages: 18.5–28.5 U/g hemoglobin

What This Test Will Tell You
This blood test detects an inborn error of carbohydrate metabolism called galactosemia caused by the hereditary absence of the enzyme galactose-1-phosphate uridyl transferase. Commonly performed on newborns, this test may also be performed on adults to assess their status as carriers of this metabolic disorder. This enzyme is normally present on all red blood cells. Its absence indicates galactosemia, an inability to metabolize galactose, which is found most commonly in milk, and convert it to glucose.

Abnormal Findings
Galactosemia

 ACTION ALERT!

Galactosemia must be detected in the first weeks of life to prevent serious and life-threatening complications. Galactosemia may be caused by other enzyme deficiencies, so if there are strong reasons to suspect galactosemia, such as symptoms or a family history, other tests must be performed to assure accurate diagnosis.

Interfering Factors
➤ If the person is a carrier of the disease, but does not actually have the disease, the result may show a "normal" finding.
➤ Hemolysis of sample.

NURSING CONSIDERATIONS G

Prepare Your Client
➤ Explain that this test is being done to see if the baby has a serious problem with digesting a sugar found in milk.

Perform Procedure
➤ A micro-stick (heelstick) is used on infants to collect blood in heparinized capillary tubes.
➤ Collect 5 mL of venous blood in a green- or purple-top tube for adults who are undergoing screening as carriers.

Care After Test
➤ Evaluate family history for galactosemia.
➤ If galactosemia is diagnosed, recommend that siblings be tested for the disease and for status as carriers. Parents also should be tested for carrier status.
➤ Arrange genetic counseling referral if galactosemia is diagnosed.
➤ Assess for signs and symptoms of galactosemia including hepatomegaly, renal function, visual acuity, developmental delay, and other organ disease.
➤ Arrange for a consultation with a registered dietician.
➤ Review related tests such as the Beutler fluorometric test, Paigen assay, visual acuity, liver and renal function tests, and developmental status.

Educate Your Client and the Family

➤ Inform parents that all future children and grandchildren should also be screened for galactosemia at birth.

➤ Reinforce importance of dietary restrictions and assist family in making dietary selections appropriate for these infants and children by removing galactose from the diet. Primary source is milk and dairy products. Children need another source of calcium.

➤ Ensure that the parents understand the serious consequences to the child's health if dietary restrictions are not observed.

Gallbladder Scan

gahl bla dur • skan

(Hepatobiliary Scintigraphy, HIDA Scan, Cholescintigraphy, DISIDA Scanning, Iminodiacetic Acid Analogue Gallbladder Scanning, IDA Gallbladder Scanning, Hepatobiliary Imaging, Biliary Tract Radionuclide Scan)

Normal Findings

Patent biliary tract including cystic and common bile ducts

Visualization of normal structures within 1 hour of injection of radionuclide material

Ejection fraction greater than 35%

What This Test Will Tell You

This nuclear scanning test detects obstruction of the cystic and common bile duct, acute cholecystitis, and other defects of the gallbladder. Intravenous injection of a radionuclide material results in normal filling of the gallbladder and biliary tree, or helps reveal delays, obstructions, and abnormalities.

Abnormal Findings

Abnormalities may indicate acute cholecystitis, chronic cholecystitis, or obstruction of bile duct due to gallstone, tumor, or stricture.

ACTION ALERT!

Perforation and peritonitis may occur with acute cholecystitis. Monitor carefully for increase in abdominal pain, fever, tachycardia, hypotension, and signs or symptoms of shock. Notify the primary health care provider immediately if these symptoms occur.

Interfering Factors

➤ Fasting for the past 24 hours will interfere with normal filling of the gallbladder.

Contraindications

➤ Pregnancy, due to radiation exposure of the fetus

Potential Complications

➤ Allergic reaction to the radionuclide, though this is uncommon

---

NURSING CONSIDERATIONS

Prepare Your Client

➤ Explain that the test is to make sure that a part of the body called the gallbladder and tiny tubes called the bile ducts are working properly.

➤ Ensure your client has eaten within the past 24 hours, but has fasted for the past 2 hours.

➤ Explain to the client they will need an intravenous fluid infusion in order to administer the radionuclide. Explain the venipuncture process clearly.

➤ Provide a fatty meal or cholecystokinin if gallbladder function is also to be determined, to evaluate emptying of the gallbladder.

➤ Tell your client or family the test will last approximately 1–2 hours, but may take as long as 4 hours to complete.

➤ Assure your client and family that there is a minimal exposure to radioactivity and it is not dangerous.

Perform Procedure

Nurses do not perform this procedure, but should understand the process to prepare the client. The client is taken to the nuclear medicine department, and a radionuclide labeled with technetium-99m (Tc-99m) is administered intravenously. The client lies supine while serial images are obtained over 1 hour. Subsequent images may be taken at intervals of 15–30 minutes as indicated, until the gallbladder, common bile duct, and duodenum are visualized. If function is to be evaluated, the gallbladder is continually scanned to measure the percentage of isotope ejected. An ejection fraction below 35% indicates primary gallbladder disease.

Care After Test

➤ Reassure client and family that only tracer doses of the radioisotope were used, so no precautions need to be taken by others against exposure to radioactivity.

➤ Assess for right upper quadrant pain, nausea, and vomiting, which are often associated with cholecystitis. Especially monitor for signs and symptoms of perforation, which include nausea, vomiting, Murphy's sign, and a leukocyte count greater than 20,000 cells/mm^3.

➤ Carefully assess fluid and electrolyte balance. Collaborate with the primary health care provider regarding the need for intravenous fluid therapy and withholding oral fluid and nutrition.

➤ Consult with a registered dietician to assist the family and client in meeting special dietary needs.

➤ Administer medications as ordered to decrease the size of existing stones or even dissolve small ones. Monitor for side effects such as diarrhea, cramps, and liver enzyme elevations.

Educate Your Client and the Family

➤ Educate your client and family about any additional testing that may be required.

➤ Teach the client and family about changes in diet that may be required. Most commonly a low-fat diet is indicated.

Gallium Scan
gal lee um • skan

Normal Findings
No evidence of abnormal increased uptake of gallium within the body
No evidence of abscesses, tumors, inflammation, or other areas of abnormal uptake

What This Test Will Tell You
This nuclear scan detects benign, malignant, and recurrent tumors and their response to therapy, and it detects infectious or inflammatory lesions such as abscesses. Gallium is a radionuclide that concentrates in pathologic areas, but is not specific enough to distinguish between tumors and infectious lesions. However, this test is more useful than other diagnostic imaging tests in detecting metastatic tumors, especially lymphomas and bronchogenic carcinomas, and in clarifying focal hepatic defects. Bronchogenic carcinoma and non-Hodgkin's lymphoma are often staged using gallium scanning. In clients with fever of unknown origin, a gallium scan may detect sources of infection.

Abnormal Findings
Abnormal uptake areas may indicate bronchogenic carcinoma, Hodgkin's disease, lymphomas, abscesses, inflammatory lesions, non-Hodgkin's lymphomas, brain tumors, hypernephromas, carcinoma, vaginal melanomas, pneumonia, sarcoidosis, tuberculosis, chronic osteomyelitis, adenocarcinomas, hepatoma, sarcomas, testicular tumors, Wilms tumor, peritonitis, or recurrent tumors of most types.

ACTION ALERT!
Assess client carefully for allergic reaction to contrast material including dyspnea, itching, urticaria, flushing, hypotension, and shock. Life-threatening anaphylactic reactions can occur and need to be recognized and treated immediately.

Interfering Factors
➤ Some organs (liver, spleen, bone, and colon) normally retain gallium, but in less concentration.
➤ Not all types of tumors will concentrate gallium.
➤ If client moves during the scanning procedure, the scan may be inaccurate.
➤ A negative study does not rule out the presence of disease as there are approximately 40% false negatives.
➤ Degeneration or necrosis of tumor and antineoplastic drugs given immediately before scan can result in false negative results.
➤ Single solitary nodules are difficult to detect.
➤ Abnormal concentration of gallium in bowel or fecal matter as gallium is excreted in feces can interfere with visualization.
➤ Barium studies done within 7 days of scan interfere with gallium activity in the bowel.
➤ Normal uptake of gallium in liver and spleen may obscure the detection of abnormal lymph nodes causing false negative test results.
➤ In the presence of leukopenia, false positive results may be obtained.

Contraindications

➤ This test is contraindicated in pregnancy, due to radiation exposure to the fetus.

➤ This test is usually not recommended for women who are breast-feeding, due to exposure to radiation. If benefits greatly outweigh risk, then breast-feeding should be discontinued for at least 4 weeks following testing.

➤ This test is usually not recommended for young children due to exposure to radiation unless the benefits greatly outweigh risk.

Potential Complications

➤ Allergic reaction to radionuclide-gallium

NURSING CONSIDERATIONS

Prepare Your Client

➤ Explain that this test helps find abnormal or inflamed tissues. If appropriate, explain that the test shows if cancer has spread or shows the response to cancer therapy.

➤ An intravenous (IV) injection of gallium, a radionuclide, is administered 4–24 hours before the first scan.

➤ Inform client that the dose of radioactive material is small and not harmful.

➤ Warn client that the IV injection will cause a very transient discomfort from the needle puncture.

➤ Explain the need to increase oral fluid intake beginning 24 hours prior to the scan to assure the body is well hydrated.

➤ Administer a laxative and/or cleaning enema as ordered to empty the gastrointestinal tract when the abdomen is to be scanned.

➤ Inform client the total body scan will take 30–90 minutes.

➤ Tell client that delayed image scans may be scheduled at 24-hour intervals up to 72 hours to help determine normal from abnormal concentrations.

➤ Ensure that an informed consent is obtained, because of the possible complications associated with this procedure.

➤ Administer sedation as ordered if client is unable to lie still during procedure.

➤ Confirm that client has voided before the scanning procedure.

Perform Procedure

Nurses do not perform this procedure but should understand the process to prepare the client and assist the physician. The client is positioned on the x-ray table and repositioned for various images throughout the procedure. Prepare client by explaining there may be a sound made by the scanning machine, and that they will need to lie motionless during the scan. Explain the scanner detects rays emitted from the radioactive material that was injected and converts the information into video screen images.

Care After Test

➤ Inform client if other scans will be done and at what intervals.

➤ Explain the need for oral laxatives and enemas prior to repeating scans.

➤ Assess for occult gastrointestinal bleeding with routine stool guaiac testing. Clients with cancer often have coagulopathies.

➤ Evaluate related laboratory tests such as alpha fetoprotein (AFP), carcinoembryonic antigen (CEA), tumor markers, and coagulopathy studies, and imaging results including those from ultrasounds, magnetic resonance imaging, computed tomography scan, and x-rays.

Educate Your Client and the Family

➤ Urge client to eat a diet high in bulk and to drink lots of fluids to encourage normal urinary and bowel elimination, as gallium is excreted by the kidney and colon.

➤ Client with cancer may have prolonged bleeding times. Instruct the client and family on safety measures such as electric razors, non-skid shoes, and soft toothbrushes if indicated.

➤ Explain that results may take up to a few days to be reported.

Gamma-Glutamyl Transferase

gam mah • gloo tah mil • tranz fur ase

(GGT, Y-Glutamyltransferase, Glutamyl Transpeptidase, Y-GTP, GGTP)

Normal Findings

ADULT, PREGNANT, CHILD, AND ADOLESCENT

Males 18–50 years: 10–39 U/L
Females < 45 years: 6–29 U/L
Males > 50 years: 10–48 U/L
Females > 45 years: 8–38 U/L

NEWBORN

Values up to 5 times greater than adult (if premature baby, results can be 10 times greater than adult).

What This Test Will Tell You

This blood test detects liver cell damage by measuring blood levels of the enzyme gamma-glutamyl transferase (GGT), which is involved in the transfer of amino acids and peptides across cell membranes. This enzyme is found primarily in liver and kidney tissue and to a lesser degree in the spleen, prostate gland, and heart. This test is sometimes used in alcoholic rehabilitation programs to detect alcohol ingestion because high levels of GGT are present 12–24 hours after consuming a large amount of alcohol. GGT is a more sensitive indicator of cholestatic liver disease than is alkaline phosphatase, especially in children.

Abnormal Findings

▲ INCREASED LEVELS indicate obstructive liver disease; cirrhosis; acute or chronic hepatitis; cancer of the liver, pancreas, prostate gland, breast, kidney, lung, or brain; alcoholism; alcohol ingestion; infectious mononucleosis; hepatic ischemia or necrosis; congestive heart failure with hepatomegaly; myocardial infarction; hepotoxic drugs; cholestasis; or hemochromatosis.

Interfering Factors

➤ Medications that can increase GGT levels include large amounts of acetaminophen, alcohol, barbiturates, phenytoin, and streptokinase.

➤ Decreased levels of GGT can be caused by oral contraceptives.

➤ Moderate to heavy intake of alcohol can cause elevated levels for up to 2–3 weeks.

➤ GGT levels are elevated 4–10 days after an acute myocardial infarction, most likely due to hepatic insult.

NURSING CONSIDERATIONS

Prepare Your Client

➤ Explain that this test will help determine if the liver has damage or, if appropriate, assure they haven't had any alcohol to drink if they are in an alcohol rehabilitation program.

➤ Consult with the primary health care provider about the need to withhold medications known to alter the results.

Perform Procedure

➤ Collect a 7–10 mL sample of venous blood in a red-top tube. (For small infants, draw blood from a heelstick.)

➤ Observe the venipuncture site closely for hematoma formation or bleeding. Coagulopathies are common in liver disease. Apply a pressure dressing to the venipuncture site.

Care After Test

➤ Assess client for unusual bruising or prolonged bleeding from venipuncture site. Delayed clotting is a complication of severely impaired liver function.

➤ Assess skin, sclera of eyes for jaundice and note findings.

➤ Consult with a registered dietician to design a high-calorie, well-balanced diet. Clients with advanced liver disease have poor absorption of nutrients due to decreased bile flow into the intestines. As appropriate, reduce sodium or protein in the diet if edema and ascites, or increased ammonia levels are present.

➤ Evaluate other liver function tests such as aspartate aminotransferase (AST), alanine aminotransferase (ALT), direct and indirect bilirubin levels, alkaline phosphatase, serum ammonia, and prothrombin time.

Educate Your Client and the Family

➤ Instruct the client and family to report any jaundice—yellow discoloration of skin or whites of eyes.

➤ As appropriate, instruct client and family on a high-calorie, well-balanced diet. If sodium restrictions or protein restrictions are indicated, assist client and family to make dietary selections with these limitations.

➤ Clients with impaired liver function have prolonged bleeding times. Instruct the client and family on safety care measures such as electric razors, non-skid shoes, and soft toothbrushes.

➤ Instruct the client and family to report prolonged or unusual bleeding or bruising. Also report very dark colored or tarry stools; esophageal varices are a complication of liver disease.

Gastric Analysis

gas trik • ah **nal** ah sis

(Gastric Aspirate Analysis, Tube Gastric Analysis, Tubeless Gastric Analysis)

Normal Findings

TUBE

(Measured in milliequivalents [mEq] of hydrochloric acid per hour)

See data at bottom of page.

TUBELESS

Dye detectable in urine

What This Test Will Tell You

This test measures the acidity and volume of the gastric contents to diagnose gastric hypersecretory and hyposecretory diseases such as pernicious anemia and atrophic gastritis. The test also evaluates clients with symptoms of peptic ulcer disease and the effectiveness of treatment. Clients with peptic ulcer disease, however, may have gastric secretions that are normal in amount and composition. Gastric acid is secreted by the parietal cells of the stomach. The amount secreted and its pH is altered by many disorders and diseases.

Two tests are performed in the gastric analysis: the basal acid output and the gastric acid stimulation test. Basal acid output measures the amount of hydrochloric acid (HCl) secreted by the stomach in an unstimulated state, expressed as milliequivalents of HCl per hour. Maximal acid output is measured in the gastric acid stimulation test. It is the total acid output during the hour following pentagastrin (a gastric secretory stimulant) subcutaneous injection.

The recent development of a test to measure serum gastrin levels has largely replaced the use of gastric analysis in determining Zollinger-Ellison syndrome.

Abnormal Findings

▲ INCREASED LEVELS of acid may indicate peptic ulcer disease, Zollinger-Ellison syndrome, hypersecretory disease, or gastroesophageal reflux disease.

▼ DECREASED LEVELS of acid may indicate atrophic gastritis or pernicious anemia.

Interfering Factors

➤ Smoking or chewing gum prior to the procedure will increase gastric acid secretion and increase levels measured.

➤ Histamine receptor antagonists, anticholinergics, tricyclic antidepressants, sucralfate, beta blockers, alcohol, antacids, and adrenocorticosteroids can decrease levels.

Contraindications

FOR TUBE TEST

➤ Gastric outlet obstruction, recent upper gastrointestinal bleeding, inability to freely pass a nasogastric tube, or when food particles or fresh blood are present in the gastric aspirate

➤ Aortic aneurysm, congestive heart failure, esophageal varices, coagu-

Basal acid output (BAO)	Maximal acid output (MAO)
Male: 2–5 mEq/hour	*Male*: 5–26 mEq/hour
Female: 1–4 mEq/hour	*Female*: 7–15 mEq/hour

lopathies, esophageal malignancy, esophageal stenosis, and pregnancy

Potential Complications

➤ Nosebleeds
➤ Tube misplacement
➤ Mild adverse reaction to the gastric stimulant pentagastrin, which may include transitory dizziness, faintness, flushing, tachycardia, and numbness of the extremities
➤ Bronchial, uterine, or intestinal spasms resulting from histamine

---

NURSING CONSIDERATIONS

Prepare Your Client

➤ Explain that this test is used to measure the amount of the stomach juices and examine their components to see if any problems exist, or to evaluate the effectiveness of treatment.
➤ Explain that the procedure will take place with the client awake; intravenous sedation is not usually required.
➤ Inform the client that although the procedure may be uncomfortable, it should not be painful.
➤ Obtain an informed consent, because of the possible complications associated with this procedure.
➤ Ensure adequacy of gastric preparation. In adults, this means that the client should fast for 12 hours before gastric analysis, and that all histamine receptor antagonists, anticholinergics, tricyclic antidepressants, sucralfate, beta blockers, alcohol, caffeine, smoking, chewing gum, adrenocorticosteroids, and antacids should be withheld for 48 hours before testing.
➤ Advise the client that swallowing during tube placement will help the physician guide it to the proper location in the stomach.

➤ Tell the client that while the tube is in place, they should spit rather than swallow. Provide a container.

Perform Procedure

TUBE GASTRIC ANALYSIS

Nurses do not perform this procedure, but should understand the process to prepare the client and to assist the gastroenterologist in obtaining the best results from the procedure.

Position the client lying on their left side. The nares are anesthetized and a radiopaque polyethylene tube passed through the nares into the stomach so the tube tip lies along the stomach's greater curvature. Tube placement is verified by x-ray and aspiration of stomach contents. The stomach contents are removed as completely as possible by manual aspiration through the nasogastric tube.

Next, with the client still lying on the left side, four 15-minute basal acid output samples of gastric secretions are obtained separately, via the tube. The sum of the acid outputs for the four samples is measured in milliequivalents per hour, and is referred to as the basal acid output.

Pentagastrin, a gastric secretory stimulant, is given in a dose of 6 µg/kg by intramuscular or subcutaneous injection, and four 15-minute maximal acid output samples of gastric secretions are again collected. The milliequivalents of acid secreted in the hour following pentagastrin injection are referred to as the maximal acid output.

All acid samples are labeled with the amount and time of collection, and are analyzed for volume, pH, color, consistency, and presence of occult blood.

G

TUBELESS GASTRIC ANALYSIS

After ingesting a gastric stimulant such as a tablet of caffeine, a resin dye is also ingested. The presence of hydrochloric acid (HCl) in the stomach will create a blue color, which is absorbed in the intestinal tract and eliminated by the renal system within about 2 hours. The urine is noted to be blue if HCl is present normally in the stomach, and not to be blue if HCl is absent.

Care After Test

➤ Monitor vital signs closely until stable.

➤ Look for signs of an adverse reaction to pentagastrin, such as nausea, abdominal pain, tachycardia, or excessive sweating.

➤ Observe for signs of electrolyte imbalance, since removal of gastric secretion also removes fluid rich in electrolytes such as sodium and potassium.

➤ Evaluate other gastric secretory function tests such as the serum gastrin.

Educate Your Client and the Family

➤ Teach client or family to keep client well hydrated after the test, so that fluid and electrolytes are replaced.

➤ Instruct the client to re-start medications put on hold prior to the test.

➤ Advise client with peptic ulcer disease and/or other gastric hypersecretory diseases to avoid cigarette smoking, foods and products that contain alcohol and caffeine, and aspirin because they stimulate gastric secretion.

Gastric Cytology and Culture

gass trik • sie tahl oe jee • and • kuhl chur

Normal Findings

Absence of inflammation, infection, malignant cells, and/or mass lesions

What This Test Will Tell You

This endoscopic test and microscopic evaluation evaluate and diagnose a number of clinical conditions of the upper gastrointestinal (GI) tract involving pathogenic organisms. The presence of infection, bleeding, and cancerous tumors can be verified by inspecting mucosal vascular patterns for abnormalities such as bleeding sites or inflammation, obtaining tissue samples for cytology, culture, or biopsies, and examining cells and organisms in the GI tract. Simple nasogastric intubation may be done without endoscopic examination to obtain gastric washings for cytologic analysis and culture.

Abnormal Findings

Abnormalities may indicate gastrointestinal abnormalities, gastric cancer, gastritis, or tuberculosis.

ACTION ALERT!

➤ Conscious sedation or extreme vagal response to gastrointestinal intubation can result in cardiopulmonary arrest. Medications including atropine, drugs to reverse sedation, and other emergency pharmacologic agents should be immediately available with cardiopulmonary resuscitative equipment.

➤ Severe, life-threatening hemorrhage can result from gastrointestinal intubation, especially in the presence of esophageal varices.

➤ Tube placement into the trachea results in respiratory distress and requires immediate removal of tube.

Interfering Factors

➤ Barium or food in the esophagus, stomach, and/or small intestine can prevent adequate visualization, tissue sampling, and examination of cells in the upper GI tract.

➤ Lack of cooperation and severe anxiety can prevent gastrointestinal intubation or adequate visualization.

➤ Gagging and emesis can prevent gastrointestinal intubation or adequate visualization.

Contraindications

➤ Recent myocardial infarction or pulmonary embolism, shock, and any other conditions that result in unstable cardiovascular status. There is a danger of cardiorespiratory compromise and arrest associated with gastrointestinal intubation and a vagal response.

➤ Esophageal varices, esophageal strictures, or other esophageal disease.

➤ Uncooperative client or client with depressed level of consciousness.

➤ Suspected or actual perforated viscus, acute abdomen, acute oral or oropharyngeal inflammation, abnormal upper airway anatomy, seizures, and/or severe cervical arthritis.

➤ Significant derangements in coagulation, as measured by partial thromboplastin time, bleeding time, and other tests of the coagulation system.

➤ Cardiorespiratory depression re-

sulting from intravenous sedation given prior to the procedure.

➤ Cardiac arrhythmias, resulting from intravenous medications to decrease duodenal spasms given during the procedure.

➤ Vasovagal reactions.

➤ Infection.

➤ Pulmonary aspiration of blood, secretions, or regurgitated gastric contents.

G

NURSING CONSIDERATIONS

Prepare Your Client
FOR ENDOSCOPY

➤ If samples are taken during endoscopy, explain that this test is used to look at the throat where swallowing occurs, the stomach, and the beginning of the intestinal tract in order to see problem areas and to take small samples of the stomach contents.

➤ Inform the client or family that the client will not be unconscious during the procedure, but that intravenous sedation will be given to promote comfort and relaxation, even light sleep.

➤ Advise the client that the procedure is uncomfortable, but should not be painful. As the endoscope is being inserted into the throat, a retching or gagging sensation may be felt, but there is usually no vomiting or severe pain. As the scope passes into the stomach and small intestine, a pressure sensation may be felt.

➤ Teach the client to notify the nurse if severe pain is felt.

➤ Make sure that an informed consent is obtained, because of the possible complications associated with this procedure.

➤ Restrict food and fluids for 8–12 hours before the procedure.

➤ Give the client preoperative sedation. General anesthesia may be used in certain pediatric, uncooperative, or highly anxious clients.

(Done by placing a nasogastric tube and aspirating stomach contents)
➤ Explain that this test is done to look at and evaluate the contents of the stomach for any problems.
➤ Advise the client that the procedure is uncomfortable, but should not be painful. As the tube is being inserted into the throat, a retching or gagging sensation may be felt, but there is usually no vomiting or severe pain. As the tube passes into the stomach, a pressure sensation may be felt.
➤ Discuss how the client will notify the nurse if severe pain is felt.
➤ Restrict food and fluids for 8–12 hours before the procedure.

Perform Procedure
ENDOSCOPY
Nurses do not perform this procedure, but should understand the process to prepare the client and to assist the endoscopist in obtaining the best results from the procedure.

Assist the client into a left lateral decubitus position. A long flexible endoscope is used to visualize the upper GI tract. The endoscope is equipped with suction to remove secretions. It also has air controls that distend the mucosal lumen for safe passage through the abdominal structures, and water controls that keep the fiber-optic tip of the instrument clean. The endoscopist sprays the client's throat with a local anesthetic, inserts the instrument into the throat, and insufflates a small amount of air to help dilate the mucosal lumen. The endoscope is then passed through the esophagus, the stomach, and the duodenum.

Instruct the client to swallow as the endoscopist inserts the endoscope into the throat, and to breathe deeply as the scope passes into the stomach, in order to relax the abdominal muscles. Once the endoscope is satisfactorily placed in the target tissue, a small sheathed cytology brush is passed through the scope's biopsy channel. The endoscopist then extends the brush beyond its plastic sheath, rubbing it across the mucosa. After cells are obtained in this manner, the head of the brush is withdrawn into the outer sheath and then removed from the endoscope. Multiple specimens may be taken from the target area, to improve the accuracy of histopathologic interpretation. After the cytology brush is removed from the endoscope, it is gently rotated in one direction across several clean microscope slides, resulting in thin smears of cells.

Cell specimen slides should be placed in a slide holder or alcohol solution, labeled, and sent to the laboratory for examination or to microbiology for culture and sensitivity.

Assess the client's vital signs, oxygenation status, level of abdominal distention, level of consciousness, vagal response, and pain tolerance during the procedure. Administer atropine or glucagon as needed to decrease bowel spasms and/or motility. Monitor for the cardiovascular side effects of these drugs.

NASOGASTRIC INTUBATION
➤ This procedure is commonly performed by nurses.

➤ Insert a nasogastric tube into the stomach. Verify placement by aspiration of stomach contents.

➤ If samples are for cytology, instill approximately 100 cc of normal saline into the stomach after proper placement has been verified.

➤ The client is moved in several different positions to help the saline "wash" the stomach walls completely.

➤ If samples are for culture, particularly for tuberculosis, do not instill saline, but simply aspirate stomach contents.

➤ Aspirate the fluid and send to the laboratory for analysis in sealed containers.

➤ Remove the nasogastric tube unless otherwise indicated.

Care After Test

FOLLOWING ENDOSCOPY

➤ Monitor vital signs every 15–30 minutes until the patient is stable.

➤ Observe for signs of complications, such as bleeding, vomiting, change in vital signs, severe abdominal pain and/or distention, tachycardia, fever, dyspnea, subcutaneous emphysema in the neck, and abdominal rigidity.

➤ Keep the client in a semi-Fowler's position or turned to the side to help expectorate any fluids.

➤ Restrict food and fluids until the gag reflex has returned.

➤ Observe the client carefully when fluids are first offered for signs of difficulty swallowing or aspiration.

➤ Saline gargles or throat lozenges may be used to decrease throat soreness and hoarseness.

➤ Evaluate related tests such as an upper gastrointestinal tract series, barium swallow, small bowel series, hypotonic duodenography, and barium enema.

FOLLOWING NASOGASTRIC INTUBATION

➤ Observe the nares, sputum, and oral cavity for bleeding.

➤ Evaluate related tests such as upper gastrointestinal tract series, barium swallow, small bowel series, abdominal ultrasound, computed tomography, and barium enema.

Educate Your Client and the Family

REGARDING ENDOSCOPIC PROCEDURE

➤ Inform client that they will feel some abdominal discomfort and/or flatus following the procedure, because air is put into the abdominal structures during the procedure. Getting up and walking around can help get rid of the air and minimize the discomfort.

➤ Advise clients to avoid strenuous activities for 24 hours after the test.

➤ Inform clients of the signs and symptoms of gastrointestinal bleeding including dark stools, tarry stools, abdominal or back pain, fever, pounding heart, and weakness.

➤ Teach client and the family a well-balanced diet, including the importance of adequate fluid and fiber intake.

REGARDING NASOGASTRIC INTUBATION

➤ Instruct client not to forcefully blow their nose for 6 hours to avoid bleeding.

Gastric Emptying Scan
gas trik • emp tee ing • skan

Normal Findings
Normal gastric emptying time for all ages: 70–125 minutes. The average time is 90 minutes.
FEMALES
Solids: 92 minutes ±7.5 minutes
Liquids: 53.8 ±4.9 minutes
MALES
Solids: 59.8 minutes ±3.7 minutes
Liquids: 30.3 minutes ±2.3 minutes

What This Test Will Tell You
This nuclear radiographic test measures the rates of solid and/or liquid emptying of the stomach in order to help diagnose tumors, obstructions, or nervous system problems that affect emptying. This test may also be ordered if recent gastrointestinal surgery has been performed, and a leakage at a suture or anastomosis site is suspected. This study involves scanning the stomach after ingesting a solid or liquid test meal containing a radionuclide. In the individual with normal structure and function of the stomach, gastric emptying should be complete within 2–6 hours of a typical meal.

Abnormal Findings
▲ INCREASED *gastric emptying* may indicate dumping syndrome following ulcer surgery.
▼ DECREASED *gastric emptying* may indicate diabetic gastroparesis, peptic ulcer disease, gastric malignancy, or nonfunctional gastrointestinal anastomosis.

Interfering Factors
➤ Medications such as opiates, anticholinergics, antidepressants, lev-odopa, beta-adrenergic agonists, progesterone, aluminum hydroxide antacids, alcohol, and cigarettes can delay gastric emptying.
➤ Medications such as beta-adrenergic antagonists, metoclopramide, domperidone, and cisapride can increase gastric emptying.
➤ Positioning the scintigraphic camera close to the stomach may be difficult in obese clients, which may limit the information available from the test.
➤ Lying in a fixed supine position for a period of time, as required by the test, may be difficult for some disabled or hospitalized elderly clients.
➤ Malignant cachexia and/or effects of chemotherapy or radiation therapy may make test interpretation difficult in clients with metastatic malignancy.

Contraindications
➤ Unstable metabolic states such as sepsis, hyperglycemia, electrolyte imbalance, acidosis, parenteral nutrition, hyperosmolarity, and the immediate postsurgical period
➤ Pregnancy and lactation, due to the possible exposure of the fetus/infant to the radionuclide material

Potential Complications
➤ Fetal abnormalities due to radiation exposure if test is performed inadvertently during pregnancy

NURSING CONSIDERATIONS
Prepare Your Client
➤ Explain to the client that the test is

used to measure the stomach's ability to empty liquids and solids and takes approximately 90 minutes.

➤ Inform the client that the radiation hazard from radionuclide testing is very slight since the doses used are very small and the length of time the radionuclide material is in their body is very short.

➤ Vegetarians can be given an isotope-labeled egg salad sandwich instead of chicken liver.

➤ Withhold any medications that influence motility at least 12 hours before a gastric emptying test.

➤ Ensure that gastric emptying studies in premenopausal women are performed during the first 14 days of the menstrual cycle, since gastrointestinal transit is prolonged during the progesterone-influenced luteal phase.

➤ Tell the client to notify the nurse if nausea occurs. Anti-emetic drugs may be given before or during the gastric emptying scan, since in single doses they do not alter gastric emptying, and they will minimize central nervous system–induced nausea.

Perform Procedure

Nurses do not perform this procedure, but should understand the process to prepare the client and to assist the gastroenterologist in obtaining the best results from the procedure.

In the solid-emptying study, a test meal of cooked egg white or chicken liver containing technetium-99m (Tc-99m) is eaten. In the liquid-emptying study, the client drinks orange juice which contains Tc-99m. Sequential images from the gamma camera are then recorded every 2 minutes for 60–90 minutes, until less than 50% of solid food material remains in the stomach. Instruct the client to consume the test meal in less than 5 minutes. The client should alternate ingestion of solids and liquids for adequate food mixing during meal consumption. If emptying is prolonged, metoclopramide may be given to assess its efficacy in improving gastric motility.

Care After Test

➤ Resume medications that were withheld for testing purposes.

➤ If client is symptomatic and having difficulty taking in an adequate nutritional diet, obtain a dietary consult with a registered dietician.

➤ Evaluate additional tests used to evaluate gastric motility such as endoscopy with antral biopsy, gastric analysis, and esophageal function tests.

Educate Your Client and the Family

➤ Advise the client with dumping syndrome that lying down immediately after a meal can slow gastric emptying and reduce symptoms associated with the dumping syndrome.

➤ Instruct the client with gastroparesis that maintaining an upright posture after a meal can increase the rate of gastric emptying and reduce the symptoms of gastric fullness, bloating, and nausea associated with gastroparesis.

➤ Inform the client with delayed gastric emptying that mild to moderate exercise can prove beneficial in increasing the rate of gastric emptying and reducing symptoms of gastric fullness, bloating, and nausea associated with reduced gastric emptying states.

Gastrin

gas trin
(Gastrin Stimulation Test)

Normal Findings

ADULT, 16–60 YEARS
Male: <200 pg/mL (ng/L, SI units)
Female: <75 pg/mL (ng/L, SI units)
NEONATE, 0–4 DAYS
120–183 pg/mL (ng/L, SI units)
Cord: 20–290 pg/mL (ng/L, SI units)
CHILD
<10–125 pg/mL (ng/L, SI units)
ELDERLY, OVER 60 YEARS OLD
>100 pg/mL (ng/L, SI units)

What This Test Will Tell You

This blood test differentiates Zollinger-Ellison syndrome (ZES) and G-cell hyperplasia from peptic ulcer disease as the cause of gastrointestinal disorders. Peptic ulcer disease is more common and is associated with normal gastrin levels, whereas ZES and G-cell hyperplasia generally have markedly increased levels. In instances where there is not a significant increase in serum gastrin, a gastrin stimulation test is performed. Calcium or secretin is infused for this test, with exaggerated serum gastrin levels noted in ZES or G-cell hyperplasia.

Gastrin is normally produced by the G-cells of the distal stomach, and stimulates gastric secretion and gastric emptying in response to the pH of the stomach. Gastrin is secreted when the pH is elevated (alkaline), such as when food or antacids are ingested. Once the pH is reduced (acidic), a negative feedback system suppresses secretion of gastrin.

Abnormal Findings

▲ INCREASED LEVELS may indicate Zollinger-Ellison syndrome, retained antrum, gastric outlet obstruction, antral G-cell hyperplasia, post-vagotomy, pernicious anemia, atrophic gastritis, renal failure, or short gut syndrome.

Interfering Factors

➤ Smoking, alcohol consumption, or chewing gum prior to the procedure will increase gastric secretion and may cause decreased levels.
➤ Histamine receptor antagonists and anticholinergic medications may increase levels.
➤ Previous ulcer surgery may be associated with elevated results.
➤ Hemolysis of the specimen will invalidate the results.
➤ Insulin-induced hypoglycemia will result in elevated findings.
➤ A nonfasting specimen will show high levels.

NURSING CONSIDERATIONS

Prepare Your Client

➤ Explain that this test is to measure the amount of a hormone called gastrin in the blood to see if any problems exist, or to evaluate the effects of treatment for peptic ulcer disease.
➤ Instruct the client to fast for 12 hours prior to the test. Water is permitted, but gum chewing is prohibited.
➤ Withhold histamine receptor antagonists and anticholinergic medications for 24 hours prior to the test.
➤ Instruct the client to abstain from alcohol and tobacco for 24 hours prior to the test.

Perform Procedure

SERUM GASTRIN

➤ Collect 1–5 mL of venous blood in a 10–15 mL red-top tube.

GASTRIN STIMULATION TEST

➤ If a gastrin stimulation test is ordered, a pre-infusion level is obtained and compared to timed post-infusion levels.

➤ For the calcium infusion test, calcium gluconate is given intravenously over 3 hours and a specimen is drawn every 30 minutes for 4 hours.

➤ For the secretin test, secretin is injected intravenously and gastrin levels are taken every 15 minutes for 1 hour.

Care After Test

➤ Evaluate the nutritional status of the client. Seek the assistance of a registered dietician in evaluating and planning an effective dietary plan when indicated.

➤ Evaluate other gastric secretory function tests such as the gastric analysis.

Educate Your Client and the Family

➤ Instruct client with ulcerative conditions to avoid gastric secretion stimulants such as cigarette smoking, alcohol, caffeine, and aspirin.

Gastroesophageal Reflux Scan

gas troe ee sof ah jee al • ree fluks • skan
(GE Reflux Scan, Aspiration Scan)

Normal Findings

Absence of gastroesophageal reflux

What This Test Will Tell You

This radiographic test detects reflux of gastroduodenal contents across the gastroesophageal (GE) junction to diagnose disorders of the esophagus and evaluate the efficacy of anti-reflux medications. This test may be used with children to identify gastroesophageal reflux as a cause of recurrent pneumonia, recurrent vomiting, sleep apnea, and/or failure to thrive.

Abnormal Findings

Gastroesophageal reflux

Interfering Factors

➤ Movement during testing may impair imaging quality.

Contraindications

➤ Pregnancy, due to possible exposure of the fetus to radionuclide material

➤ Unstable metabolic states such as sepsis, hyperglycemia, electrolyte imbalance, acidosis

➤ The immediate postoperative period

NURSING CONSIDERATIONS

Prepare Your Client

➤ Explain that this test is used to look at swallowing and the stomach, in order to tell if any backward flow is occurring.

➤ Explain that during the scan a soft, irregular clicking noise is heard as the special camera moves across the body. There is no pain associated with this test.

➤ Collaborate with the primary health care provider about the need to restrict food and fluids for 4–6 hours (2 hours for infants) prior to the test. Alternatively, a large meal may be ordered just prior to testing.

Perform Procedure

Nurses do not perform this procedure, but should understand the process to prepare the client. After ingesting an oral mixture containing technetium-99m, the client is positioned supine with an abdominal binder in place. As the binder is inflated, the scintigraphic camera takes pictures of the gastroesophageal area for 30–60 minutes. The client's position may be changed frequently to determine the effect position has on reflux. The camera records the distribution and amount of radioactivity within the gastroesophageal junction.

Care After Test

➤ Encourage the client to drink extra fluids to help excrete the contrast material.

➤ Observe client for signs of reflux-related pulmonary complications such as tachypnea, dyspnea, cyanosis, apnea, and choking.

➤ Observe client closely while they are eating or drinking if reflux is con-firmed or suspected.

➤ Review related tests including esophagogastroduodenoscopy and biopsy, barium swallow, and/or esophageal function tests.

Educate Your Client and the Family

➤ Teach client with gastroesophageal reflux to avoid hot and cold liquids, coffee, citrus juices, and alcoholic beverages. These substances may worsen symptoms associated with GE reflux.

➤ Encourage the client to avoid activities that require considerable bending or stooping such as gardening, picking objects off the floor, tying shoes, and sitting slumped down in a chair. These activities can exacerbate the symptoms of GE reflux.

➤ Instruct the client that smaller, more frequent meals, rather than 2–3 large meals per day, can lessen the symptoms of GE reflux.

➤ Inform the client that foods with high fat content can also worsen symptoms of GE reflux.

➤ For infant with gastroesophageal reflux, instruct the family on the importance of feeding the infant in the upright position and maintaining them upright for 60 minutes after feeding.

Gastrointestinal Bleeding Scan

gass troe in tes ti nal • bleed ing • skan

(Gastrointestinal [GI] Scintigraphy, Gastrointestinal Scintigram, Abdominal
Scintigraphy, Abdominal Scintigram, Abdominal Bleeding Scan)

Normal Findings

Absence of bleeding

What This Test Will Tell You

This radiographic test locates sites of active gastrointestinal or abdominal bleeding. A scanner or gamma camera records the distribution and amount of radioactivity within the abdomen after the client's red blood cells are tagged with an intravenous injection of the radionuclide technetium-99m (Tc-99m). Alternatively, injection of sulfur colloid labeled Tc-99m may be administered intravenously. By registering the pooling of this tagged blood, sites of active gastrointestinal bleeding can be identified. This test is superior to endoscopy and arteriography for locating hemorrhaging when the bleeding is in the small intestines, excessive, or intermittent. Scintigraphy is not, however, able to locate bleeding to an exact area, but only to an abdominal quadrant.

Abnormal Findings

➤ *Upper gastrointestinal bleeding* is associated with peptic ulcer, gastritis, esophagitis, duodenitis, Mallory-Weiss tears, and esophageal varices.
➤ *Lower gastrointestinal bleeding* is associated with colitis, polyps, cancer, diverticulosis, and hemorrhoids.
➤ *Other sources of abdominal bleeding* are associated with angiodysplasia and trauma.

Interfering Factors

➤ Obesity may make positioning the scintigraphic camera close to the

stomach difficult and limit imaging.
➤ Musculoskeletal disorders or changes in mentation that make lying in a fixed supine position for a long period difficult may interfere.
➤ Areas of the intestinal tract posterior to the liver, spleen, and bladder may not be imaged well.
➤ Barium in the intestinal tract from previous studies can interfere with visualization.

Contraindications

➤ Unstable metabolic states such as sepsis, hyperglycemia, electrolyte imbalance, acidosis, and the immediate postoperative period
➤ Pregnancy, due to the risks to the fetus

NURSING CONSIDERATIONS

Prepare Your Client

➤ Explain that the test is used to look inside the stomach and intestines, as well as the abdomen in general, to find out if any bleeding is occurring.
➤ Ensure that an informed consent is obtained.
➤ Collaborate with the primary health care provider to determine if foods and fluids should be withheld prior to the test. Although foods and fluids are not routinely withheld for this test, it may be important if surgery or other invasive procedures are anticipated as a result of the test.

Perform Procedure

Nurses do not perform this procedure, but should understand the process to prepare the client. Red blood cells or sulfur colloid are tagged with Tc-99m and then injected intravenously. The client is positioned supinely, and the scintigraphic camera takes pictures of the abdominal area over 30–60 minutes. A soft, irregular clicking noise will be heard as the scanner moves across the abdomen. Multiple images are recorded.

Care After Test

➤ Encourage the client to drink extra fluids to help the body excrete the Tc-99m.

➤ Monitor gastric drainage for bright red blood or material resembling coffee grounds.

➤ Observe for the presence of black, tarry stools (melena).

➤ Take frequent vital signs, watching for signs of hypovolemia (increased heart rate, lowered blood pressure) due to bleeding.

➤ In client with peptic ulcer, monitor for signs of perforation, such as acute upper abdominal pain and guarding, rebound tenderness, and absent bowel sounds.

➤ Evaluate additional laboratory and diagnostic tests used to assess gastrointestinal bleeding such as esophagogastroduodenoscopy, clotting factors, upper gastrointestinal studies, and the complete blood count.

Educate Your Client and the Family

➤ Advise client to avoid medications and substances that can cause and/or worsen gastrointestinal bleeding, such as aspirin, non-steroidal anti-inflammatory drugs (NSAIDs), nicotine, and alcohol.

➤ Teach client to monitor for gastrointestinal bleeding by noting and reporting to their primary health care provider black, tarry stools, weakness, nausea, abdominal distention, and cramping.

Gastrointestinal Tract Biopsy

gass troe in tess tin ahl • trakt • bie op see

Normal Findings

Absence of inflammation, infection, and/or mass lesions

What This Test Will Tell You

This test evaluates and diagnoses a number of upper gastrointestinal (GI) tract problems, including gastritis, duodenitis, peptic ulcer, esophagitis, gastric ulcer, and gastric or esophageal cancer. Direct visualization of the upper GI tract using a long flexible endoscope allows the endoscopist to assess mucosal vascular patterns for abnormalities such as bleeding sites or inflammation, and to obtain tissue samples or biopsies which can confirm or exclude small mass lesions such as cancerous tumors.

Abnormal Findings

Abnormalities may indicate gastritis, esophagitis, gastric ulcers, polyps, Crohn's disease, chronic ulcerative colitis, gastric cancer, esophageal cancer, lymphoma, or Barrett's esophagus.

➤ Conscious sedation or extreme vagal response to gastrointestinal intubation can result in cardiopulmonary arrest. Medications including atropine, drugs to reverse sedation, and other emergency pharmacologic agents should be immediately available with cardiopulmonary resuscitative equipment.

➤ Severe, life-threatening hemorrhage can result from gastrointestinal intubation, especially in the presence of esophageal varices.

Interfering Factors

➤ Barium in the esophagus, stomach, and/or small intestine can prevent adequate visualization and tissue sampling of the upper GI tract.

➤ Lack of cooperation and severe anxiety can prevent gastrointestinal intubation or adequate visualization.

➤ Gagging and emesis can prevent gastrointestinal intubation or adequate visualization.

➤ Contents in the stomach may interfere with visualization.

Contraindications

➤ Recent myocardial infarction or pulmonary embolism, shock, and any conditions that result in unstable cardiovascular status. There is a danger of cardiorespiratory compromise and arrest associated with gastrointestinal intubation and a vagal response.

➤ Esophageal varices, esophageal strictures, or other esophageal disease.

➤ Uncooperative client or client with depressed level of consciousness.

➤ Suspected or actual perforated viscus, acute abdomen, acute oral or oropharyngeal inflammation, abnormal upper airway anatomy, seizures, and/or severe cervical arthritis.

➤ Significant derangements in coagulation, as measured by partial thromboplastin time, bleeding time, and other tests of the coagulation system.

➤ Recent gastrointestinal surgery where healing of suture lines cannot be assured.

Potential Complications

➤ Esophageal, stomach, or duodenal perforation

➤ Hemorrhage

➤ Cardiorespiratory depression, resulting from intravenous sedation given prior to the procedure

➤ Cardiac arrhythmias, resulting from intravenous medications to decrease duodenal spasms given during the procedure

➤ Vasovagal reactions

➤ Infection

➤ Pulmonary aspiration of blood, secretions, or regurgitated gastric contents

---

NURSING CONSIDERATIONS

Prepare Your Client

➤ Explain that this test is used to look at the throat where swallowing occurs, the stomach, and the beginning of the intestinal tract in order to see problem areas or to take small samples of tissue.

➤ Inform the client or family that the client will not be unconscious during the procedure, but that intravenous sedation will be given to promote comfort and relaxation, even light sleep.

➤ Advise the client that the procedure is uncomfortable, but should not be painful. As the endoscope is being inserted into the throat, a retching or gagging sensation may be felt, but there is usually no vomiting or severe pain. As the scope passes into the stomach and small intestine, a pressure sensation may be felt.

➤ Teach the client to notify the nurse if severe pain is felt.

➤ Make sure that all risks are understood by the client.

➤ Make sure that an informed consent is obtained, because of the possible complications associated with this procedure.

➤ Restrict food and fluids for 8–12 hours before the procedure.

➤ Have the client urinate before the procedure.

➤ Give the client preoperative sedation. General anesthesia may be used in certain pediatric, uncooperative, or highly anxious clients.

Perform Procedure

Nurses do not perform this procedure, but should understand the process to prepare the client and to assist the endoscopist in obtaining the best results from the procedure.

Assist the client into a left lateral decubitus position. A long flexible endoscope is used to visualize the upper GI tract. The endoscope is equipped with suction to remove secretions and air controls that distend the mucosal lumen for safe passage through the abdominal structures. Water controls keep the fiber-optic tip of the instrument clean. The endoscopist sprays the client's throat with a local anesthetic, inserts the instrument into the throat, and insufflates a small amount of air to help dilate the mucosal lumen. The endoscope is then passed through the esophagus, the stomach, and the duodenum.

Instruct the client to swallow as the endoscopist inserts the endoscope into the throat, and to breathe deeply as the scope passes into the stomach, in order to relax the abdominal muscles.

Once the endoscope is satisfactorily placed in the target tissue, biopsy forceps are passed down the biopsy channel. With the forceps in place, the nurse opens and closes the forceps in response to the endoscopist's request. Closing the forceps and pulling on the tissues tears off a specimen of the target tissues. Multiple specimens are taken from the target area, to improve the accuracy of histopathologic interpretation. Photographs may also be taken through the scope. When tissue sampling is complete, the biopsy forceps are withdrawn through the channel of the endoscope, and secretions should be wiped clean from the endoscope shaft.

Specimen containers are labeled with client information and the site of the biopsy. Assess the client's vital signs, oxygenation status, respiratory excursion, level of abdominal distention, level of consciousness, vagal response, and pain tolerance during the procedure.

Care After Test

➤ Monitor vital signs every 15–30 minutes until the client is stable.

➤ Observe for signs of complications, such as bleeding, vomiting, change in vital signs, severe abdominal pain and/or distention, tachycardia, fever, dyspnea, subcutaneous emphysema in the neck, and abdominal rigidity.

➤ Keep the client in a semi-Fowler's position or turned to the side to help expectorate any fluids.

➤ Restrict food and fluids until the gag reflex has returned.

➤ Observe the client carefully when fluids are first offered for signs of difficulty swallowing or aspiration.

➤ Saline gargles or throat lozenges

may be used to decrease throat soreness.

➤ Evaluate related tests such as an upper gastrointestinal tract series, barium swallow, small bowel series, hypotonic duodenography, and barium enema.

Educate Your Client and the Family

➤ Inform client that they will feel some abdominal discomfort and/or flatus following the procedure, due to the air forced into the abdominal structures during the procedure.

Getting up and walking around can help get rid of the air and minimize the discomfort.

➤ Advise client to avoid strenuous activities for 24 hours after the test.

➤ Inform clients of the signs and symptoms of gastrointestinal bleeding including dark stools, tarry stools, abdominal or back pain, fever, pounding heart, and weakness.

➤ Teach client and family a well-balanced diet, including the importance of adequate fluid and fiber intake.

G

Glomerular Basement Membrane Antibody, Serum

gloe **mehr** yu lur • **base** ment • **mem** brane • **an** ti bod ee • see rum
(Antiglomerular Basement Membrane Antibodies in Serum, Anti–GBM Antibody, AGBM)

Normal Findings
Negative: <10 units

What This Test Will Tell You
This blood test detects circulating glomerular basement membrane antibodies that are associated with anti–glomerular basement membrane (anti-GBM) glomerulonephritis and Goodpasture's syndrome. Less than 5% of clients with glomerulonephritis demonstrate glomerular basement membrane antibodies as the causative factor. Generally the antibody is implicated in crescent-forming histologic types of glomerular injury, pulmonary hemorrhage, and respiratory failure.

Abnormal Findings
Weakly positive: 10–19 units
Positive: ≥20 units

Positive results may reveal anti-GBM glomerulonephritis, Goodpasture's syndrome, or pulmonary hemosiderosis.

NURSING CONSIDERATIONS

Prepare Your Client
➤ Explain that this test is important to see if the immune system is making antibodies that may be causing kidney or lung problems.

Perform Procedure
➤ Collect 5–10 mL of venous blood into a red-top tube.
➤ Label the specimen container and send it to the lab. The test should be run immediately.

Care After Test
➤ Maintain an intake and output record to monitor renal function.

➤ Assess for signs and symptoms of glomerulonephritis. They may include occult to gross hematuria, proteinuria, elevated temperature, edema, decreased urine output, elevated blood pressure, fatigue, and anxiety.

➤ Assess for signs and symptoms of Goodpasture's syndrome, which may include hemoptysis, pulmonary insufficiency, rales, rhonchi, hematuria, weakness, pallor, and anemia.

➤ Evaluate other laboratory and diagnostic tests such as blood urea nitrogen, serum creatinine, serum albumin, complete blood count, urinalysis, renal biopsy, and sputum analysis.

Educate Your Client and the Family

➤ Encourage rest to allow the kidney to heal.

➤ Explain fluid and dietary restrictions. A renal diet consists of low sodium, low protein, and low fluid intake.

Glucagon, Serum
gloo kah gon • see rum

Normal Findings
All ages: 50–200 pg/mL (SI units: 50–200 ng/L)

What This Test Will Tell You
This blood test detects alterations in glucose metabolism, most often when the pancreas is affected. There are two hormones needed for glucose metabolism: insulin and glucagon. Insulin allows glucose into the cells, thereby lowering blood glucose. Glucagon, a polypeptide hormone secreted by the pancreas, promotes the breakdown of glycogen in the liver, causing the blood sugar to increase.

Abnormal Findings
▲ INCREASED LEVELS may indicate pancreatitis, diabetes mellitus, glucagonoma (an alpha-cell tumor of the pancreas), uremia, or pheochromocytoma.

▼ DECREASED LEVELS may indicate pancreatic inflammation, pancreatic cancer, or surgical removal of pancreas.

Interfering Factors
Increased levels can result from the following:

➤ Hemolysis of cells

➤ Transporting sample at room temperature

➤ Vigorous exercise, stress, trauma, prolonged fasting, and use of insulin prior to sampling

---

NURSING CONSIDERATIONS

Prepare Your Client

➤ Explain that this test is used to measure a hormone or chemical in the body that helps control blood sugar.

➤ Ensure the client has had nothing to eat for 10–12 hours before sampling unless this test is performed simultaneously with a glucose tolerance test.

➤ Keep the client lying down and

quiet for at least 30 minutes prior to obtaining the blood sample to decrease effects of exercise and stress.
➤ Consult with the primary health care provider to withhold insulin or catecholamines during the fasting period. If they must be given, note these on the laboratory slip.

Perform Procedure
➤ Collect 10 mL of venous blood into a *chilled* lavender-top tube.
➤ Transport the blood sample on ice immediately.

Care After Test
➤ Observe the client for signs and symptoms of disruptions in glucose metabolism. Hypoglycemia may be indicated by change in level of consciousness, diaphoresis, and tachycardia. Hyperglycemic signs include fatigue, decreased level of consciousness, sweet or fruity breath odor, excessive thirst, and increased urinary output.
➤ Observe for signs and symptoms of pancreatitis which include severe abdominal pain, nausea, vomiting, low-grade fever, diarrhea, weight loss, dark brown or frothy urine, Grey Turner's sign, or Cullen's sign.
➤ If pancreatitis is suspected, assess for a history of alcohol abuse.
➤ Review related tests such as serum glucose level, serum somatostatin levels, and amylase levels.

Educate Your Client and the Family
➤ For client with diabetes mellitus, review dietary intake and instruct on diabetic diet as needed to assist the client in achieving better control.

G

Glucose, Fasting
gloo kose • fast ing
(FBS, Fasting Blood Sugar)

Normal Findings
ADULT
Serum: 70–110 mg/dL (SI units: 3.89–6.11 mmol/L)
Whole blood: 60–100 mg/dL (SI units: 3.33–5.53 mmol/L)
PREGNANT
Serum: 80–150 mg/dL (SI units: 4.4–8.25 mmol/L)
NEWBORN
Serum: 30–70 mg/dL (SI units: 1.65–3.85 mmol/L)
Cord blood in newborn, serum: 45–96 mg/dL (SI units: 2.47–5.28 mmol/L)
CHILD
<24 months old, serum: 60–100 mg/dL (SI units: 3.30–5.50 mmol/L)

24 months through adolescence, serum: 60–105 mg/dL (SI units: 3.30–5.78 mmol/L)
ADOLESCENT
Serum: 70–105 mg/dL (SI units: 3.85–5.78 mmol/L)
ELDERLY
Serum: 80–140 mg/dL (SI units: 4.40–7.70 mmol/L)

ACTION ALERT!
Serum values:
Adult male: <50 or >400 mg/dL
Adult female: <40 or >400 mg/dL
Infant: <40 mg/dL
Newborn: <30 or >300 mg/dL
These values signify either severe hypo-

glycemia or hyperglycemia requiring immediate interventions, which include oral or intravenous glucose administration, glucagon, or insulin administration. Prolonged hypoglycemia, especially in the neonate, can result in permanent and irreversible brain damage. If symptoms of hypoglycemia are present, but no glucose monitoring is immediately available, give glucose, as fruit juice if possible. Hypoglycemia presents a more immediate emergency than hyperglycemia.

What This Test Will Tell You

This blood test detects alterations in glucose metabolism, most often to diagnose diabetes mellitus or help evaluate the control of this disease. Two hormones are needed for glucose metabolism: insulin and glucagon. Insulin allows glucose into the cells, thereby lowering blood glucose. Glucagon encourages the breakdown of glycogen in the liver, causing the blood glucose to increase. The blood glucose will fluctuate depending upon the client's activity level and length of time from the last meal. A fasting blood glucose is used as a baseline measurement, as it is not influenced by dietary intake as a variable factor.

Abnormal Findings

▲ INCREASED LEVELS may indicate diabetes mellitus, stress, Cushing's disease, steroid use, pancreatitis, pituitary adenoma, pancreatic adenoma, chronic liver disease, hypokalemia, crushing injuries, brain trauma, acromegaly, congestive heart failure, or pheochromocytoma.

▼ DECREASED LEVELS may indicate insulin overdose, cachexia, hypothyroidism, Addison's disease, islet cell carcinoma of the pancreas, bacterial sepsis, glycogen storage disease, cancer, erythroblastosis fetalis, increased

exercise, or liver disease.

Interfering Factors

➤ Levels may be increased by intravenous infusions of a dextrose-containing solution, steroids, anesthesia, stress, infection, caffeine/nicotine, beta blockers, adrenal gland infection, total parenteral nutrition, diuretics, estrogen, and phenytoin.

➤ Levels may be decreased by insulin, alcohol, anabolic steroids, and oral antidiabetic agents.

NURSING CONSIDERATIONS

Prepare Your Client

➤ Explain that this test is used to determine blood levels of sugar.

➤ Ensure that the client fasts from food for 8–12 hours before the test. They may drink water.

➤ Do not give their insulin/antidiabetic agents until the blood is drawn. Confer with the primary care provider if symptoms of hyperglycemia develop during the period that insulin is withheld.

Perform Procedure

➤ Collect 5 mL of venous blood into red (for plasma level) or green-top (for whole blood) tube.

➤ Although this test is usually done using venous blood, it may also be performed on capillary blood using a glucometer and reagent strips. If so, follow specific directions for the particular brand of machine and reagent strips.

Care After Test

➤ Administer medications previously withheld for testing purposes.

➤ Ensure the client receives food promptly in accordance with the ordered diet.

➤ Observe for signs and symptoms of hypoglycemia such as diaphoresis, palpitations, tachycardia, and change in level of consciousness.

➤ Observe for signs and symptoms of hyperglycemia such as thirst, increased urination, hunger, mental status changes, and fruity or acetone breath.

➤ Obtain a dietary consult with a registered dietician for client with abnormal glucose levels related to diabetes mellitus.

➤ Monitor fluid and electrolyte status. Hyperglycemia leads to dehydration and hypokalemia, and intravenous insulin administration may lead to hypokalemia.

➤ Review related tests such as serum glucagon, random glucose level, and urine glucose level.

Educate Your Client and the Family

➤ Teach client or family to self-monitor their blood sugar if appropriate. Many insurance companies will provide the monitors and test strips.

➤ Inform client or family about diabetic support groups and offer referrals.

➤ Teach signs/symptoms of hypoglycemia including nausea, lightheadedness, hunger, and shakes.

➤ Teach client and family to administer orange juice, hard candy, or another suitable source of quick sugar for these symptoms if the client's level of consciousness is unimpaired. If the level of consciousness is questionable, then oral glucose gels may be more suitable. Instruct them to seek medical attention immediately.

Glucose, Postprandial

gloo kose • poest pran dee uhl

(PPG, Plasma Postprandial Glucose 2-hour PPG, 2-hour Postprandial Blood Sugar, PPBS, 2-hour PPBS, 2-hour Glucose)

Normal Findings

ADULTS < 50 YEARS OF AGE AND CHILDREN

70–140 mg/dL (SI units: <7.8 mmol/L)

PREGNANT

Normally there is a slight elevation of glucose during pregnancy.

OLDER ADULTS

50–60 years of age: 70–150 mg/dL (SI units: <8.3 mmol/L)

60 years of age and older: 70–160 mg/dL (SI units: <8.8 mmol/L)

What This Test Will Tell You

This blood glucose test screens for diabetes and monitors insulin therapy. The blood glucose is measured 2 hours after a test meal (postprandial). The glucose concentration in a postprandial specimen is rarely elevated in normal persons, but is significantly elevated in diabetics. In clients with normal glucose metabolism, the pancreas is able to secrete adequate amounts of insulin in response to a glucose load produced by eating a meal. With normal insulin production, the serum glucose level should return to normal within 2 hours after eating. For clients with impaired pancreatic function, insulin is not released in response to a high carbohydrate load, causing blood glucose levels to remain elevated 2 hours following the meal.

Abnormal Findings

▲ INCREASED LEVELS may indicate diabetes mellitus, Cushing's syndrome, hyperthyroidism, acromegaly, cirrhosis, pheochromocytoma, some malignancies, or infection.

▼ DECREASED LEVELS may indicate Addison's disease, anterior pituitary insufficiency, hypothyroidism, islet cell adenoma, or steatorrhea.

ACTION ALERT!

Glucose values less than 50 mg/dL or greater than 400 mg/dL can signify critical glucose imbalances resulting in coma or death. Both hypoglycemia and hyperglycemia require prompt medical attention.

Interfering Factors

➤ Coffee, smoking, excessive stress, pregnancy, infection, and current illness can cause elevations in blood glucose levels.
➤ Strenuous exercise may decrease levels.
➤ Failure to consume a high-carbohydrate meal prior to test causes decreased levels.
➤ Medications that may increase levels include thiazide diuretics, oral contraceptives, phenytoin, corticosteroids, chlorthalidone, furosemide, ethacrynic acid, and glucose infusions.
➤ Medications that may decrease glucose levels include beta-adrenergic blockers, amphetamines, insulin,

oral hypoglycemics, alcohol, monoamine oxidase inhibitors, and amphetamines.

NURSING CONSIDERATIONS

Prepare Your Client

➤ Explain that this test is used to help diagnose "sugar" diabetes or, if appropriate, to see how insulin treatment is working.
➤ Instruct the client to fast for 12 hours prior to breakfast the day of the test. The breakfast should contain at least 75 grams of carbohydrates by including such content as fruit juice, cereal with sugar, toast, and milk.
➤ If client is a known diabetic, check with the primary health care provider about withholding regularly scheduled insulin dosages.
➤ For a known diabetic, ask the last time they took insulin. Record the time, amount, and type of insulin.
➤ Ensure the client does not smoke, eat, or drink fluids other than water after the meal is consumed and before the blood sample is drawn.

Perform Procedure

➤ Collect 7 mL of venous blood in a red-top or gray-top tube exactly 2 hours after the client finishes breakfast.

Care After Test

➤ Assess for signs and symptoms of hyperglycemia including thirst, hunger, dehydration, and increased urination.
➤ Assess for complications of diabetes such as impairment of integumentary, digestive, circulatory, and sensory functions.
➤ Monitor results of other endocrine function tests such as the glucose tolerance test, glycosylated hemoglobin level, blood glucose, and

urine glucose and ketones.

Educate Your Client and the Family

➤ If diagnosis of diabetes is established, begin individualized diabetic education.

➤ Review client's knowledge of and compliance with diet and insulin administration before adjustments are made in treatment, if this test reveals poor glucose control in an established diabetic.

➤ Teach client signs and symptoms of hypoglycemia and hyperglycemia, especially if postprandial hypoglycemia seems to be a particular problem.

➤ Teach client to keep a source of glucose available, such as raisins or juice. When experiencing hypoglycemia, $1/2$ cup of milk or other protein should be consumed to keep glucose stable until mealtime.

G

Glucose-6-Phosphate Dehydrogenase
gloo kose • siks • fos fate • dee hie drah jeh nase
(G-6-PD Screen)

Normal Findings

Screening: Negative
Quantitative: 8.0–8.86 U/g hemoglobin
Findings may simply be reported as normal.

What This Test Will Tell You

This blood test identifies a hereditary enzyme-deficient hemolytic anemia. G-6-PD deficiency is a sex-linked, recessive genetic disorder found mostly in males that results in hemolysis of red blood cells, producing anemia. Women are usually asymptomatic carriers of the affected X chromosome. This condition is seen primarily in Sephardic Jews (Mediterranean) and in the African-American population (Type A).

Abnormal Findings

▲INCREASED LEVELS may indicate pernicious anemia, idiopathic thrombocytopenic purpura, hepatic coma, hyperthyroidism, myocardial infarction, chronic blood loss, and other megaloblastic anemias.

ACTION ALERT!

Do not administer sulfonamides or antipyretics to clients with known G-6-PD deficiency, as acute hemolytic episodes may result.

Interfering Factors

➤ Medications that cause increased levels of G-6-PD include ascorbic acid, aspirin, phenacetin, primaquine, quinidine, sulfonamides, nitrofurantoin, vitamin K, antipyretics, and tolbutamide.

NURSING CONSIDERATIONS

Prepare Your Client

➤ Explain that this test is to find a problem in the red blood cells, which carry oxygen throughout the body.

Perform Procedure

➤ Collect 3–5 mL of venous blood in a lavender-top tube containing ethylenediaminetetraacetic acid (EDTA) or a blue-top tube containing acid citrate dextrose or a green-top tube containing heparin.

Care After Test

➤ Assess client history for factors that may precipitate a hemolytic episode including diabetic acidosis, fava bean ingestion, infection (viral, bacterial), and septicemia.

➤ Collaborate with the primary health care provider to ensure that medications that may cause an acute hemolytic episode are not ordered or administered. These medications include acetanilid, nalidixic acid, naphthalene, acetylphenylthydrazine, aspirin, chloramphenicol, nitrofurantoin, nitrofuran, pentaquine, probenecid, antipyrine, ascorbic acid, quinacrine, quinidine, quinine, sulfonamides, and vitamin K.

➤ Assess the client for signs and symptoms for hemolytic anemia including pallor, dyspnea, chest pain, and fatigue.

➤ Encourage rest periods for client experiencing fatigue related to anemia.

➤ Evaluate client's ability to perform activities of daily living and refer to community health care services as needed if client is unable to perform basic daily needs.

➤ Obtain a dietary consult to assist the client and family in choosing a well-balanced diet, including foods high in iron and vitamin B_{12}.

➤ Refer client and family for genetic counseling.

➤ Review related tests such as hemoglobin, hematocrit, reticulocyte count, red blood cell indices, hemoglobin electrophoresis, ferritin level, total iron-binding capacity (TIBC), bone marrow and liver biopsies, and iron absorption and excretion studies.

Educate Your Client and the Family

➤ If a severe anemia is identified through testing, the client needs to understand the impact this may have upon activities. Severe anemia may produce increased fatigue, dyspnea with or without exertion, syncope, increases in heart rate, and even tissue damage such as myocardial infarction.

➤ If an anemia is identified, instruct the client in dietary sources of iron, such as red meat, organ meats, dark green vegetables, and fortified grains.

➤ If hemoconcentration is identified from dehydration, instruct the client and family in how to increase fluids in dietary intake. Interventions vary greatly depending upon the cause of the dehydration.

➤ If low hemoglobin level is from blood loss, blood transfusion may be necessary. Explain to your client or family that blood products undergo sophisticated testing for human immunodeficiency virus (HIV) and hepatitis, as well as compatibility with the client's blood. Discuss with your client or family the options available to them in their particular circumstance. Blood product transfusion may be possible through a general donor pool, family donors, or even self-donated (autologous) blood (either blood taken from the client if surgery is expected or a cell-saving device in surgery to recycle the client's own blood). Explain the transfusion process to the client or family and describe the anticipated experience so that they will understand what to expect.

Glucose Tolerance
gloo kose • tahl ur ens
(GTT, Oral Glucose Tolerance Test, OGTT, Intravenous Glucose Tolerance Test, IGTT)

Normal Findings
ADULT
Fasting: 70–115 mg/dL (SI units: <6.4 mmol/L)
30 minutes: <200 mg/dL (SI units: <11.1 mmol/L)
1 hour: <200 mg/dL (SI units: <11.1 mmol/L)
2 hours: <140 mg/dL (SI units: <7.8 mmol/L)
3 hours: 70–115 mg/dL (SI units: <6.4 mmol/L)
4 hours: 70–115 mg/dL (SI units: <6.4 mmol/L)
PREGNANT
Fasting: <105 mg/dL (SI units: <5.8 mmol/L)
1 hour: <190 mg/dL (SI units: <10.5 mmol/L)
2 hours: <165 mg/dL (SI units: <9.1 mmol/L)
3 hours: <145 mg/dL (SI units: <8.0 mmol/L)
ELDERLY
Same as adult except 2-hour level is <160 mg/dL (SI units: <8.8 mmol/L)
CHILD
Diagnosis of diabetes mellitus in children requires either (1) a random serum glucose level greater than 200 mg/dL (SI units: >11.1 mmol/L) *and* symptoms, OR (2) fasting glucose levels >140 mg/dL (SI units: >7.8 mmol/L) on at least two different samplings and elevated levels of glucose on at least two OGT tests.

What This Test Will Tell You
This screening blood test helps diagnose conditions of impaired glucose metabolism. The fasting client consumes a set amount of carbohydrate and the blood sugar is monitored at $1/2$ hour, 1 hour, and 2 hours, sometimes continuing to 3 and 4 hours. While a client with normal glucose metabolism will demonstrate a rise and then a fall in the glucose level, the diabetic client will demonstrate a continued rise in the blood sugar level throughout the testing period. Urine testing may also be used during this test. Urine testing is less accurate than serum determinations. There is normally no glucose found in the urine.

Abnormal Findings
Abnormal levels may indicate diabetes mellitus, hypoglycemia, gestational diabetes, Cushing's syndrome, or pancreatic tumor.

ACTION ALERT!
If the blood sugar is <60 mg/dL or >400 mg/dL, the test may need to be stopped to prevent serious illness, even cardiopulmonary arrest. Monitor for signs/symptoms of hypoglycemia/hyperglycemia throughout the test and be prepared to administer glucose or insulin as ordered.

Interfering Factors
➤ If the client is unable to drink the entire glucose load or vomits it, the test will not be accurate. The test should be modified to give an intravenous glucose load for clients unable to tolerate the oral load (for example, because of short bowel syndrome, malabsorption, gastrectomy).
➤ Glucose levels are elevated with smoking, stress, coffee, and tea.
➤ Exercise lowers glucose levels.

➤ Medications that may increase glucose levels and indicate an intolerance include aspirin, beta blockers, furosemide, oral contraceptives, many antipsychotic medications, steroids, thiazide diuretics, antihypertensive medications, and anti-inflammatory agents.

Contraindications

➤ Seriously ill clients with infection, fever, or endocrine diseases, since elevated blood sugar would not be diagnostic.

➤ If the fasting blood sugar is >300 mg/dL, the test is usually not done.

➤ Clients with a surgical history of gastrectomy or a medical history of either short bowel or malabsorption cannot tolerate oral glucose loads. These clients should receive intravenous glucose loads.

➤ This test is not performed on a known diabetic, due to risk of hyperglycemic reactions.

Potential Complications

Vertigo, tachycardia, sweating, syncope, anxiety, and tremor. If any of these symptoms are noted, draw a blood sugar sample immediately and consult with the primary health care provider about the need to administer insulin and stop the test.

NURSING CONSIDERATIONS

Prepare Your Client

➤ Explain that this test is done to see how well the body can use sugar for energy.

➤ Provide written and verbal instructions regarding pretest diet.

➤ Verify that the client has consumed a moderate carbohydrate diet for the previous 3 days, and has fasted for 12 hours prior to the test.

➤ Ask the client about nausea prior to the test to minimize vomiting potential.

➤ Collaborate with the primary health care provider regarding restrictions of prescribed medications which may affect test results.

➤ Do not give A.M. insulin or oral hypoglycemics until the test is completed.

➤ Weigh the client to assist in calculation of the glucose dose.

Perform Procedure

➤ Collect 3–5 mL of venous blood in a red-top tube.

➤ Obtain urine specimen if required.

➤ Have client drink the entire glucose load.

➤ Instruct client not to eat or drink anything during the test except water.

➤ Instruct the client not to smoke or exercise during or prior to the test.

➤ Collect 3–5 mL of blood into a red-top tube after 30 minutes, 1 hour, 2 hours, and possibly 3 and 4 hours as ordered.

➤ Monitor for nausea, dizziness, rapid heart rate, sweating, tremors, anxiety, and syncope throughout the testing period. If any of these occur, obtain a blood sample immediately and be prepared to stop the testing and administer insulin or glucose.

Care After Test

➤ Resume previous diet.

➤ Administer insulin or oral hypoglycemics if they were withheld for the test.

➤ Assess for signs or symptoms of hypoglycemia or hyperglycemia.

➤ If client is a newly diagnosed diabetic, arrange for a consultation with a registered dietician and diabetic teaching.

➤ Review related tests such as fasting blood glucose level and glycosylated hemoglobin values.

Educate Your Client and the Family

➤ Discuss signs and symptoms of hypoglycemia including dizziness, tremor, hunger, and sweating. Teach client to have emergency sources of glucose readily available and to eat a protein such as milk as soon as possible.

➤ Discuss signs and symptoms of hyperglycemia including headache, thirst, and hunger.

Gonorrhea Culture
gon oe ree ah • kul chur

Normal Findings
Negative culture

What This Test Will Tell You
This culture and microscopic examination identifies the presence or absence of *Neisseria gonorrhoeae*, the causative gram-negative organism in gonorrhea. A gonorrhea culture is a part of the prenatal laboratory workup. If a prenatal culture is positive, treatment during pregnancy is necessary to prevent fetal and maternal complications. Gonorrhea is also associated with cervicitis, chlamydia, conjunctivitis, prostatitis, epididymitis, salpingitis, trichomonas, and vaginitis.

A Papanicolaou smear (Pap smear) is done with a gonorrhea culture. Many primary health care providers do a chlamydia test with a gonorrhea culture because the organisms often coexist.

ACTION ALERT!

➤ Gonorrhea is a sexually transmitted disease that must be reported to the local health department.
➤ Observe men closely for nausea, vertigo, diaphoresis, bradycardia, hypotension, and pallor, which may occur when urethral cultures are obtained. Take precautions to prevent injury, such as placing the client in a supine position during culturing.

Interfering Factors
➤ Menstrual flow.
➤ Lubricants and feminine hygiene products.
➤ Female douching within 24 hours of a cervical culture leaves fewer organisms to culture.
➤ Fecal material may contaminate a rectal culture.
➤ Male voiding within 1 hour of a urethral culture washes secretions from the urethra.

NURSING CONSIDERATIONS

Prepare Your Client
➤ Explain that this test will help determine if the client has an infection called gonorrhea.
➤ Explain that a culture will be taken from the vagina, urethra, rectum, and/or the throat according to the location of symptoms.
➤ Explain that the throat and rectum should be cultured in people who engage in oral or anal sex.
➤ Instruct the female client not to douche or tub bathe before a cervical culture.

➤ Instruct male client that cultures must be taken at least 1 hour after voiding.

Perform Procedure

Nurses do not usually perform this procedure, but should understand the process to prepare the client and assist the primary health care provider. Avoid touching your face—gonorrhea can be spread to the eyes of the examiner with contaminated fingers.

A throat culture is obtained from males and females who engage in oral intercourse. The posterior pharynx and area around the tonsils are swabbed with a cotton-tipped applicator.

For female cervical cultures, no lubricants are used because they may inhibit bacterial growth. The vaginal speculum is moistened only with warm water. A sterile cotton swab is moved from side to side in the cervix. At least 30 seconds are allowed for the organisms to be absorbed by the swab.

Rectal cultures are obtained after a cervical culture in females. The cotton-tipped swab is inserted 1 inch into the anal canal and moved from side to side. At least 30 seconds are allowed for the organisms to be absorbed by the swab.

For male urethral cultures, again no lubricants are used because they may inhibit bacterial growth. A sterile bacteriologic wire loop or a sterile urethral swab is used. The specimen is obtained from the anterior urethra by inserting the wire loop or swab no more than 2 inches and scraping the mucosa.

Newborns of mothers with gonorrhea have rectal and orogastric cultures taken.

Care After Test

➤ Assess newborns of mothers with gonorrhea for pneumonia and eye involvement.

➤ Perform follow-up cultures 3–7 days after treatment because treatment is not always 100% effective.

➤ Interview the client for sexual contacts. Instruct the client to have all sexual contacts tested.

➤ Assess for signs and symptoms of infection including greenish-yellow discharge from the cervix, vagina, or urethra in males as well as painful urination in males. Females are, however, often asymptomatic.

➤ Administer antibiotic therapy as ordered.

➤ Review related tests such as cultures for syphilis and chlamydia as well as human immunodeficiency virus (HIV).

Educate Your Client and the Family

➤ Explain the importance of testing for other sexually transmitted diseases because these diseases often coexist.

➤ Instruct the client that after treatment is received, follow-up cultures are important to be sure the infection has disappeared.

➤ Instruct the client to avoid any sexual contact until finished with treatment and partner(s) complete treatment as well.

➤ Teach the client the importance of completing all of the prescribed antibiotic.

➤ Instruct client on use of condoms to prevent reinfection or infection with another sexually transmitted disease.

Group B Streptococcus Test of the Vagina

grupe • Bee • strep toe kok uss • of • the • vah jie nah

(Group B Strep, GBS, B Strep)

Normal Findings

Absence of group B streptococcus

What This Test Will Tell You

This test screens for the presence of group B streptococcus (GBS) in the vagina in women with suspected infections to prevent transmission to and resultant sepsis in neonates. Group B strep is normally found in the gastrointestinal tract and may be transmitted to the genital tract by sexual transmission of an infected partner or stool contamination of the vagina. Most carriers harbor GBS intermittently. GBS may be transmitted from mother to newborn at delivery.

Abnormal Findings

Group B streptococcus

ACTION ALERT!

Group B strep transmitted to the fetus/newborn may result in sepsis at birth, in 48 hours, or after 1 week. GBS may lead to meningitis or death of a newborn.

NURSING CONSIDERATIONS

Prepare Your Client

➤ Explain that this is a test to look for a specific germ or bacteria in the vagina.

Treatment of GBS is controversial. Some health care professionals culture clients at risk for GBS at 26–28 weeks and treat. Others treat during pregnancy and/or labor, and treat the newborn after birth as needed. Clients with a positive culture of GBS who are going to give birth because of premature rupture of membranes or other reasons will probably be given intravenous antibiotics such as ampicillin for treatment.

Perform Procedure

➤ A cotton-tipped swab is inserted into the vagina and moved around the vaginal mucosa. The swab is transferred to the culture media provided by the laboratory.

Care After Test

➤ Assess the newborn for signs of sepsis such as respiratory distress, temperature regulation problems, and signs of shock.

➤ Assess for allergy to any antibiotics that may be ordered if culture is positive. Penicillin, ampicillin, and erythromycin are frequently used.

➤ Review related tests such as the biophysical profile, nonstress test, and blood cultures.

Educate Your Client and the Family

➤ Instruct the client who has GBS how to properly take antibiotics if ordered prior to delivery. Instruct the client to take the antibiotics until they are finished.

➤ Reinforce explanations to the client with GBS in labor that IV antibiotics are given and may be given to the baby after delivery.

➤ Instruct the pregnant client with GBS about danger signs in pregnancy such as a gush of fluid, vaginal bleeding, abdominal pain, temperature elevation, dizziness, blurred vision, persistent vomiting, severe headache, edema, muscular irritability, difficult urination, or absence of fetal movement.

➤ Instruct the pregnant client with GBS about daily fetal movement count (DFMC).

➤ Instruct the pregnant client with GBS to come to the hospital or birthing center when her membranes rupture (water breaks).

➤ Instruct the client about the signs of preterm labor (20th–37th week) such as uterine contractions every 10 minutes or less, menstrual-like cramps in the lower abdomen, low dull backache, pelvic pressure, and an increase or change in vaginal discharge. If any of these occur, client should lie down on left side and notify the primary health care provider.

➤ Teach client to wash hands thoroughly and always wipe from the front to the back after toileting.

Gynecology Ultrasound

gie neh kol oe jee • ul tra sownd
(Gynecologic Sonogram, Transabdominal Ultrasound, Transvaginal Ultrasound, Transvaginal Scan)

Normal Findings

No cysts, foreign bodies, tumors, or stones

Normal shape, size, and position of uterus, bladder, fallopian tubes, and ovaries

What This Test Will Tell You

This ultrasound test helps detect problems with the bladder, ovaries, uterus, fallopian tubes, or vagina. The procedure can be performed transabdominally (across the abdomen) or transvaginally (in the vagina). Sound waves are transmitted to a screen in the form of echoes from the area being tested.

Transvaginal ultrasound is most useful for providing information about individual organs and detecting ectopic pregnancies and endometrial problems. It is also useful for evaluating cysts and fibroids.

Abnormal Findings

Abnormalities may indicate pelvic cysts; pelvic abscesses; ectopic pregnancy; foreign body (IUD); endometrial abnormality; hydatidiform mole; neoplasms of uterus, bladder, ovaries, or fallopian tubes; pelvic tumor; or abnormal cervical or uterine vasculature.

Interfering Factors

➤ Barium or gas in the intestines prevents correct transmission of sound waves in the pelvis.

➤ Abdominal fat in large amounts decreases sound wave transmission and clarity.

➤ Large masses are difficult to visualize completely with the transvaginal technique.

➤ Dehydration decreases clarity of the picture between organs and body fluids.

NURSING CONSIDERATIONS

Prepare Your Client

➤ Explain that this test is to detect any problems with the womb (uterus), tubes, ovaries, or bladder.

➤ Schedule this examination before a barium enema or upper gastrointestinal (GI) series if those tests are needed. Barium in the colon may prevent a clear picture.

➤ Instruct the client who is going to have a transabdominal scan to drink 1 quart (four 8-ounce glasses) of water 1 hour before the exam and not void until after the procedure is completed. Drinking the water enhances sound wave transmission and produces better images. Assure the client that the only discomfort with the transabdominal procedure is a full bladder.

➤ Instruct client who is going to have a transvaginal scan to fast from fluids for 4 hours prior to the test and void before the test is started.

➤ A female should be present to reassure the client and serve as a witness to the examination when a transvaginal ultrasound is performed.

Perform Procedure

TRANSABDOMINAL SCAN

➤ Position client on the procedure table.

➤ The pelvic area is covered with the conductive gel.

➤ The transducer is moved over the lower abdomen at different angles.

➤ The client is turned slightly to the right or left to visualize the ovaries and adnexal area.

➤ Photographs are obtained by taking pictures of the oscilloscope images for both methods.

TRANSVAGINAL SCAN

➤ Place the client in lithotomy position or place a pillow under the buttocks to raise the pelvis.

➤ The vaginal transducer is covered with a sheath containing conduction gel. The transducer is lubricated with a sterile lubricant and inserted into the mid-vagina. Either the client or examiner may insert the transducer.

➤ The transducer is rotated 90 degrees to obtain different scans of the uterus, tubes, and ovaries.

Care After Test

TRANSABDOMINAL SCAN

➤ Remove the conductive gel from the client's skin with a warm, moist washcloth and towel.

➤ Allow the client to void.

➤ Disinfect the transducer.

TRANSVAGINAL SCAN

➤ Remove the transducer.

➤ Provide the client with a towel and washcloth to remove any lubricant.

➤ Disinfect the transducer.

➤ Review related tests such as the bimanual pelvic examination, computed tomography of the pelvis and abdomen, and x-rays.

Educate Your Client and the Family

➤ Evaluate your client's knowledge of early detection such as yearly Papanicolaou (Pap) smears, mammograms, and self-exams of breasts.

➤ If an infertility problem is diagnosed, offer emotional support and clarify any instructions for further testing and/or medications.

➤ Refer to social services to explore alternatives such as adoption if appropriate.

➤ Ensure client has been referred to a fertility expert if indicated.

➤ If the client has an ectopic pregnancy, offer emotional support to the client and family and prepare the client for surgery.

➤ If the client has a mass, offer emotional support to the client and family. Explain any further testing that is ordered.

Haptoglobin

hap toe gloe bin

(Heptoglobin, Serum; Hp)

Normal Findings

ADULT, PREGNANT, CHILD, ADOLESCENT, AND ELDERLY

38–270 mg/dL (SI units: 380–2700 µmol/L)

Haptoglobin is absent in approximately 1% of the total population as a genetically transmitted trait. The majority of individuals who have ahaptoglobinemia are African American and do not demonstrate evidence of disease or dysfunction.

INFANT AND NEWBORN

Newborn: 0–10 mg/dL (SI units: 0–1.6 µmol/L)

Infant: 0–30 mg/dL (SI units: 0–4.8 µmol/L)

Not present in 90% of newborns. By 4 months of age, haptoglobin levels and hemoglobin-binding capacity have risen to normal adult levels.

What This Test Will Tell You

This blood test identifies and analyzes hemolysis of red blood cells. Produced by the liver, haptoglobin is a protein that binds with hemoglobin released in the destruction of red blood cells. The bound hemoglobin is eliminated by the liver. If haptoglobin is absent or insufficient, free hemoglobin is excreted in the urine.

In hemolytic anemia (diseases or conditions that result in rapid destruction of red blood cells), haptoglobin is quickly bound with the excessive available hemoglobin and serum levels of haptoglobin decrease.

Abnormal Findings

▲INCREASED LEVELS may indicate pyogenic infections, trauma, rheumatoid arthritis, obstructive biliary disease, nephritis, pyelonephritis, ulcerative colitis, peptic ulcer, myocardial infarction, infectious mononucleosis, rheumatic fever, amyloidosis, nephrotic syndrome, adrenal steroid therapy, or some cancers (such as Hodgkin's disease and lymphosarcoma).

▼DECREASED LEVELS may indicate untreated pernicious anemia, acute or chronic hemolytic anemia, hemolytic transfusion reaction, prosthetic heart valves, systemic lupus erythematosus, erythroblastosis fetalis, malaria, paroxysmal nocturnal hemoglobinuria, uremia, hypertension, thrombotic thrombocytopenic purpura, sickle-cell disease, hereditary spherocytosis, thalassemia, Hp O-O disorder, hepatocellular disease, or hemorrhage.

ACTION ALERT!

Values less than 40 mg/dL haptoglobin in blood may indicate an acute hemolytic process, especially if clinical symptoms are present (chills, fever, back pain, tachycardia, tachypnea, distended neck veins, and hypotension). Individuals with symptoms of acute febrile illness, shock, and low haptoglobin levels will require immediate intervention and supportive care, including sepsis workup and circulatory support.

Interfering Factors

➤ Steroids and androgens may produce high haptoglobin levels. These substances may also mask a hemolytic process.

➤ Hemolysis of the sample causes decreased results.

➤ A current or chronic infection

may produce transient elevations in haptoglobin levels.

➤ Low haptoglobin levels may result from use of medications such as oral contraceptives, chlorpromazine, diphenhydramine, indomethacin, quinidine, streptomycin, isoniazid (INH), and nitrofurantoin.

Contraindications

➤ Since the majority of newborns (90%) do not demonstrate any level of haptoglobin, testing is not indicated for neonates.

NURSING CONSIDERATIONS

Prepare Your Client

➤ Explain that the test helps to evaluate if red blood cells are being destroyed too quickly, and how well the liver is able to help clear the waste products.

Perform Procedure

➤ Collect 2–7 mL of venous blood in a red-top tube.
➤ Avoid rough handling during collection, which might cause hemolysis of the sample.

Care After Test

➤ If severe hemolysis is occurring and the client is demonstrating signs of shock, prepare to draw blood cultures, begin intravenous (IV) antibiotics, initiate IV fluid replacement and maintenance, administer acetaminophen for fever > 101°F, administer supplemental oxygen administration if indicated, and frequently assess vital signs for hypotension.
➤ If blood product administration preceded a transfusion reaction, follow transfusion reaction protocol: stop blood product administration but maintain IV access with normal saline; obtain urine specimen for lab-oratory analysis for potential red blood cells (RBCs) in urine; obtain blood specimen for repeat typing, and repeat cross-matching procedures and identification of antibodies. In some instances, the client may receive an injection of diphenhydramine.

➤ Review related tests such as hemoglobin, hematocrit, red blood cell count, red blood cell indices, prothrombin time, partial thromboplastin time, white blood cell count with differential, agglutinins, and erythrocyte sedimentation rate.

Educate Your Client and the Family

➤ If low haptoglobin levels identify an acute hemolytic process, such as a hemolytic blood transfusion reaction, hemolytic anemia, or an acute exacerbation of an inflammatory disorder, explain that this test may be used again to assess changes in condition or response to treatment.
➤ If the client has a prosthetic heart valve that contributes to increased hemolysis of erythrocytes (and thus lowered haptoglobin levels), explain the need to assess the effect of the prosthetic valve on the blood and prevent any further complications.
➤ If increased levels of haptoglobin are due to acute infection, instruct your client that treatment (to lower fever, replace fluids, kill disease organisms) is designed to keep the infection from getting worse. Haptoglobin levels and breakdown of red blood cells will return to normal when the infection is gone.
➤ If hemolytic anemia is diagnosed, teach the client and family to conserve energy, reduce oxygen demand, and prevent compromise of the circulation, including keeping well hydrated to prevent clotting.

Hematocrit

hee mat oe krit
(Hct, Packed Cell Volume, PCV)

Normal Findings

ADULT AND ADOLESCENT
Female: 37%–47%
Male: 42%–54%
PREGNANT
>33%
NEWBORN
42%–64%
INFANT
30%–40%
CHILD
31%–43%
ELDERLY
Normal values may be slightly decreased from adult values.

What This Test Will Tell You

This blood test evaluates blood loss, anemia, blood replacement therapy, and fluid balance, and screens red blood cell status. The hematocrit (Hct) is a measure of the concentration of red blood cells within the blood volume and is expressed as a percentage. Normal values depend on the ratio of two components, the number of red cells present and the plasma volume, so the hematocrit is also a useful tool in evaluating dehydration and hypervolemia.

Abnormal Findings

▼DECREASED LEVELS may indicate anemia, blood loss, dietary deficiency, malnutrition, bone marrow failure, leukemia, hemolytic reaction, rheumatoid arthritis, cirrhosis, hyperthyroidism, Hodgkin's disease, fluid volume overload, or multiple myeloma.

▲INCREASED LEVELS may indicate polycythemia vera, severe dehy-

dration, burns, trauma, surgery, eclampsia, congenital heart disease, or erythrocytosis.

H

ACTION ALERT!

A hematocrit below 20% may signal severe anemia or blood loss and may result in cardiac ischemia and dysrhythmias, respiratory distress, and organ system impairment. Fluid resuscitation, blood transfusions, and oxygen therapy may be necessary as emergency interventions. A hematocrit above 55% (except in the newborn) may signal polycythemia or hemoconcentration from fluid loss and be associated with increased risk of thromboembolic events. Rehydration with oral and/or parenteral fluids or phlebotomy may be required emergently.

Interfering Factors

➤ Living at high altitudes causes physiologically normal increases in Hct values.

➤ Hemolysis of blood cells due to rough handling of the specimen will invalidate test results.

➤ Collection of a sample above an existing intravenous (IV) fluid line may produce a diluted sample and falsely low value.

➤ If the tourniquet is left in place for longer than 1 or 2 minutes, hemoconcentration may occur within that extremity and increase the sample reading by 2%–5%.

➤ Failure to place the sample in a collection tube with the proper anticoagulant or failure to mix the sample sufficiently with the anticoagulant may affect the values.

➤ Chloramphenicol and penicillin may decrease levels.

➤ High-dose diuretics may increase levels.

➤ Fluid overload decreases hematocrit by hemodilution.

➤ Dehydration increases hematocrit by hemoconcentration.

➤ Very high white blood cell counts may increase the hematocrit value.

➤ Hemodilution associated with pregnancy causes lower levels.

➤ Abnormalities in red blood cell size may increase or decrease the hematocrit.

NURSING CONSIDERATIONS

Prepare Your Client

➤ Explain that this test helps evaluate if there are enough red blood cells in the blood, or if there is too much or too little water in the body.

Perform Procedure

➤ Collect 7 mL of venous blood in a lavender-top tube.

➤ Alternately, collect the sample in a heparinized capillary tube (red-banded tube) and seal one or both ends after collection.

Care After Test

➤ Observe the client for signs and symptoms of anemia including pallor, tachycardia, dyspnea, chest pain, and fatigue. Severe anemia may produce these symptoms from tissue hypoxia.

➤ Encourage rest periods for client experiencing fatigue related to anemia.

➤ Evaluate client's ability to perform activities of daily living.

➤ Refer to community health care services as needed if client is unable to perform basic daily needs.

➤ Obtain a dietary consult to assist the client and family in choosing a well-balanced diet, including foods high in iron and vitamin B_{12}.

➤ Review related tests such as hemoglobin, hematocrit, reticulocyte count, red blood cell indices, hemoglobin electrophoresis, ferritin level, total iron binding capacity (TIBC), bone marrow and liver biopsies, and iron absorption and excretion studies.

Educate Your Client and the Family

➤ If a low hematocrit level indicates the possibility of blood loss or anemia, explain that further testing will be necessary to identify the cause of the condition, and to check the client's response to treatment.

➤ If a severe anemia is identified, explain how this may affect the client's activities. Severe anemia may produce fatigue, shortness of breath with or without exertion, fainting, increases in heart rate, and even tissue damage, such as heart attack (myocardial infarction). Teach the client to pace activities and to maintain regular patterns of sleep, rest, and activity to prevent fatigue.

➤ Discuss with your client or family the significance of the hematocrit levels. For example, extreme increases in red blood cells may trigger a stroke (cerebrovascular accident) in some individuals. Acute dehydration can start a sickling crisis.

➤ If an anemia is identified, instruct the client in dietary sources of iron, such as red meat, organ meats, dark green vegetables and fortified grains.

➤ If hemoconcentration is identified from dehydration, instruct the client/family in measures to supply increased fluids in dietary intake. Interventions vary greatly depending upon the cause of the dehydration.

Hemoglobin
hee mo gloe bin
(Hb, Hgb)

Normal Findings
ADULT AND ADOLESCENT
Female: 12–16 g/dL (SI units: 7.4–9.9 mmol/L)
Male: 14–18 g/dL (SI units: 8.7–11.2 mmol/L
PREGNANT
12–16 g/dL, but slight decreases in hemoglobin levels are common in pregnancy
NEWBORN
11–22 g/dL (SI units: 6.7–13.5 mmol/L)
CHILD
11–16 g/dL (SI units: 6.7–9.9 mmol/L)
ELDERLY
Female: 11.7–13.8 g/dL (SI units: 7.2–8.6 mmol/L)
Male: 12.4–14.9 g/dL (SI units: 7.6–9.2 mmol/L)

What This Test Will Tell You
This test evaluates blood loss, erythropoietic ability, anemia, and response to therapy. Hemoglobin is an important component of red blood cells that carries oxygen and carbon dioxide to and from tissues. Normally performed as a part of the complete blood count (CBC), this test can be performed individually. The hemoglobin level is directly related to the red blood cell count (RBC).

Abnormal Findings
▲INCREASED LEVELS may indicate polycythemia vera, congenital heart disease, congestive heart failure, hemoconcentration of the blood, dehydration, chronic obstruc-

tive pulmonary disease, severe burns, or polycythemia secondary to high altitudes.

▼DECREASED LEVELS may indicate anemia from blood loss, dietary deficiency, malnutrition, sickle-cell anemia; hemolysis from splenomegaly; kidney diseases; systemic lupus erythematosus; malignancies; hemoglobinopathies; or sarcoidosis.

ACTION ALERT!
<5 g/dL. Clinical manifestations of low hemoglobin levels are related, to a degree, to the length of time over which the abnormal value developed. Rapid drops in hemoglobin are more poorly tolerated and clients are more symptomatic than if the change was gradual over time. These levels may cause heart failure. These clients should be monitored closely and their activity limited.

Interfering Factors
➤ Living at high altitudes produces a physiologically normal increase in hemoglobin levels.
➤ Hemolysis of blood cells due to rough handling of the specimen will alter test results.
➤ Failure to place the sample in a collection tube with the proper anticoagulant or failure to mix the sample sufficiently with the anticoagulant may affect the values.
➤ Increased levels may occur if the client is taking medications such as gentamicin or methyldopa.
➤ Reduced levels may occur if the client is taking medications such as antibiotics, antineoplastic drugs, aspirin, indomethacin, rifampin, or sulfonamide.

H

➤ Conditions that may produce falsely elevated levels include lipemia, very high white cell counts, or red cells that are resistant to lysis.

➤ Because the hemoglobin is calculated based on the amount contained in a deciliter of blood, the value can be influenced by fluid losses or gains.

NURSING CONSIDERATIONS

Prepare Your Client

➤ Explain that this test measures a part of the blood that carries oxygen.

Perform Procedure

➤ Collect 5–7 mL of venous blood in a lavender-top tube.

➤ Alternately, a fingerstick or heelstick method may be used to collect venous blood in a heparinized capillary tube.

Care After Test

➤ Observe the client for signs and symptoms of anemia including pallor, dyspnea, chest pain, and fatigue.

➤ Encourage rest periods for client experiencing fatigue related to anemia.

➤ Evaluate client's ability to perform activities of daily living.

➤ Refer to community health care services as needed if client is unable to perform basic daily needs.

➤ Obtain a dietary consult to assist the client and family in choosing a well-balanced diet, including foods high in iron and vitamin B_{12}.

➤ Review related tests such as hemoglobin, hematocrit, reticulocyte count, red blood cell indices, hemoglobin electrophoresis, ferritin level, total iron binding capacity (TIBC), bone marrow and liver biopsies, and iron absorption and excretion studies.

Educate Your Client and the Family

➤ If a low hemoglobin level indicates the possibility of blood loss or anemia, instruct the client or family that further testing will be necessary to identify the cause of the condition, as well as the client's response to treatment.

➤ If a severe anemia is identified, explain how this may affect the client's activities. Severe anemia may produce fatigue, shortness of breath with or without exertion, fainting, increases in heart rate, and even tissue damage, such as heart attack (myocardial infarction). Teach the client to pace activities and to maintain regular patterns of sleep, rest, and activity to prevent fatigue.

➤ If an anemia is identified, instruct the client in dietary sources of iron, such as red meat, organ meats, dark green vegetables and fortified grains.

➤ If hemoconcentration is identified from dehydration, instruct the client or family in measures to supply increased fluids in dietary intake. Interventions vary greatly depending upon the cause of the dehydration.

➤ If low hemoglobin level is from blood loss, blood transfusion may be necessary. Explain to your client or family that blood products undergo sophisticated testing for HIV and hepatitis, as well as compatibility with the client's blood. Discuss with your client or family the options available to them in their particular circumstance. Blood product transfusion may be possible through a general donor pool, family donors, or even self-donated (autologous) blood (unless a surgical procedure is anticipated and donations made in advance, this may be limited to a cell-saving device in surgery to recycle the client's own blood). Explain the transfusion process to the client or family and describe the anticipated experience so that they will understand what to expect.

Hemoglobin Electrophoresis
hee mo gloe bin • ee lek troe for ee sis
(Hemoglobinopathy Test, Hgb A$_1$, Hgb A$_2$, Hgb F, Hgb S, Hgb C)

Normal Findings

ADULT, CHILD, ADOLESCENT, AND PREGNANT
Hgb A$_1$ 95%–98%
Hgb A$_2$ 2%–3%
Hgb F < 2%
Hgb S 0%
Hgb C 0%

NEWBORN
Hgb F 50%–80%; adult levels are reached at about 6 months
Hgb A$_1$ 48%
Hgb A$_2$ 2%
Hgb S 0%
Hgb C 0%

What This Test Will Tell You

This blood test screens and diagnoses hemolytic disorders when abnormal hemoglobins are detected. Hemoglobin electrophoresis measures the amounts of normal and abnormal hemoglobin molecules by using a cathode (negative charge) and anode (positive charge) in a medium to which red cells are added. The hemoglobins of various types are attracted to different degrees to either the positive or negative pole. This produces a leveling or "banding" of differing hemoglobins, which can be quantified.

Abnormal Findings

Elevations of hemoglobin A$_2$	4%–5.8%	thalassemia minor
Elevations of hemoglobin F	1%–3%	thalassemia minor
	10%–90%	thalassemia major
	5%–35%	heterozygous hereditary persistence of fetal hemoglobin (HPFH)
	100%	homozygous HPFH
	15%	sickle-cell disease
Elevations of hemoglobin S	70%–98%	sickle-cell disease
Elevations of homozygous Hgb C	90%–96%	Hgb C disease
Elevations of heterozygous Hgb C	24%–44%	hemoglobin C trait
Low hemoglobin A$_1$	0%	sickle-cell disease
	0%	hemoglobin C disease
	5%–20%	thalassemia major

Low hemoglobin A₁, continued

50%–85%	thalassemia minor
60%–80%	sickle-cell trait
65%–90%	hemoglobin H disease

ACTION ALERT!

Presence of hemoglobin S or C, or elevations in hemoglobin F in individuals other than newborns, may indicate hemolytic disease.

Interfering Factors

➤ A blood transfusion from a donor within the preceding 3–4 months may obscure test results.

➤ Hemolysis of the blood sample through rough handling of the sample during venipuncture or handling after collection may obscure test results.

➤ Failure to fill the blood collection tube completely may affect test results.

➤ The correct anticoagulant must be used in the blood collection tube to ensure accurate test results.

NURSING CONSIDERATIONS

Prepare Your Client

➤ Explain that this test looks at red blood cells and the part that carries oxygen called hemoglobin to discover any unusual problems.

Perform Procedure

➤ Collect 7 mL of venous blood in a lavender-top tube.

Care After Test

➤ Observe the client for signs and symptoms of unstable hemoglobins including pallor, jaundice, splenomegaly, cyanosis, and hemoglobinuria.

➤ Encourage rest periods for client experiencing fatigue related to anemia.

➤ Evaluate client's ability to perform activities of daily living.

➤ Refer to community health care services as needed if client is unable to perform basic daily needs.

➤ Obtain genetic referral if appropriate.

➤ Review related tests such as hemoglobin, hematocrit, reticulocyte count, red blood cell indices, globin chain analysis, hemoglobin electrophoresis, peripheral blood smear for Heinz bodies, serum bilirubin, urine bilirubin, and Schilling test.

Educate Your Client and the Family

If sickle-cell disease is diagnosed:

➤ Initiate a pain management regimen—usually with little or no use of narcotics. Explore pain relief methods such as imagery and ice packs.

➤ Teach client to continue light physical activity if experiencing fatigue, but to rest when needed and not to plan too strenuous or prolonged activities.

➤ Inform clients that maintaining regular patterns of sleep, rest, and activity are important to prevent fatigue.

➤ Stress the importance of a well-balanced diet to provide optimal energy stores, and of preventing dehydration.

➤ Teach client to avoid acute infections, which may precipitate a sickling crisis, by getting immunizations, avoiding obvious exposures to individuals with respiratory infections, employing stress-reduction activities, and maintaining healthy daily living habits such as a nutritious diet and adequate rest.

➤ Tell client to avoid exposure to temperature extremes and high altitudes, which may worsen the disease or precipitate a sickling event.
➤ Inform client that moderate exercise is probably acceptable, but vigorous and very strenuous exercise may precipitate a sickling event.

If β-thalassemia major is diagnosed:
➤ Teach client about anticipated treatments for the disease: blood transfusions at fairly regular intervals, and administration of an iron chelating medication to reduce the deposit of iron in the muscle tissue.

H

Hemoglobin, Glycosylated

hee mo gloe bin • glie koe sih lay ted
(Hemoglobin A_{1C}, Hgb A_{1c})

Normal Findings

ADULT, INFANT, ADOLESCENT, AND ELDERLY

Hgb A_{1c}: 2.2%–5%. Although Hgb A_{1c} is usually measured, Hgb A_1 may be measured to give more specific information. See chart below.

PREGNANT

Slight reductions in glycosylated hemoglobin may occur during pregnancy.

CHILD

Hgb A_{1c}: 1.8%–4%

What This Test Will Tell You

This blood test monitors blood glucose control over a period of weeks, rather than during a single period of time. A portion of the hemoglobin in the red blood cell combines with blood glucose as it circulates. This forms glycohemoglobin, which is permanently bound to that portion of the hemoglobin during the life span of the red cell. Because old red cells are continuously being destroyed and new ones formed, the process of binding of glucose with part of the hemoglobin is ongoing. The fluctuations in blood glucose over the preceding 100–120 days are averaged, producing a reflection of the stability or instability of the blood glucose over that time. This provides a broader perspective of client compliance and response to therapy in diabetic management. The advantage of glycosylated hemoglobin (or hemoglobin A_{1c}) is that the test is not affected by food intake just before the test. Additionally, the glucose level found within the red cells is more stable and reliable than that within the plasma.

	Hemoglobin A_{1c}	Glycosylated hemoglobin (A_{1a}, A_{1b}, A_{1c})
Good diabetic control	2.5%–6.0∞	<7.5%
Fair diabetic control	6.1%–8.0%	7.6%–9.0%
Poor diabetic control	>8.0%	>9.0%

This measurement is very useful for diabetic children, those with brittle diabetes who may have wide changes in daily blood glucose levels, clients who may alter their behavior to come into diabetic compliance just before their health care appointment, and for individualizing and evaluating control treatment plans.

Abnormal Findings

▼DECREASED LEVELS of *glycosylated hemoglobin* may indicate adequate control in diabetes, pregnancy, chronic renal failure, or sickle-cell anemia.

▲INCREASED LEVELS of *glycosylated hemoglobin* levels may indicate:
2.5%–6%: Good diabetic control
6.1%–8%: Fair diabetic control
>8%: Poor diabetic control
Increased levels may also indicate newly diagnosed diabetes or thalassemia.

■■■■ ACTION ALERT!

Levels above 8% Hgb A$_{1c}$ represent poor glucose control. Extremely high levels require immediate workup for hyperglycemia and ketoacidosis.

Interfering Factors

➤ Failure to place the sample in a collection tube with the proper anticoagulant or failure to mix the sample sufficiently with the anticoagulant may affect the values.

➤ Conditions that produce deceptively low values include sickle-cell anemia, chronic renal failure, and pregnancy.

➤ Conditions such as thalassemia that have a prolonged RBC life span may produce a falsely high value.

NURSING CONSIDERATIONS

Prepare Your Client

➤ Explain that this test measures the average glucose levels over 3–4 months and provides excellent information about how well their blood sugar has been controlled during this time.

Perform Procedure

➤ Collect 7 mL of venous blood in a lavender-top blood collection tube (note: some laboratories use a gray-top tube).

Care After Test

➤ Review diabetic diet with client and family depending upon results.
➤ Observe for signs and symptoms of hypoglycemia such as diaphoresis, tachycardia, and change in level of consciousness.
➤ Observe for signs and symptoms of hyperglycemia such as thirst, increased urinary output, hunger, and fruity breath.
➤ Obtain a dietary consult with a registered dietician for client demonstrating abnormal glucose levels related to diabetes mellitus.
➤ Review related tests such as serum glucagon, random glucose level, urine glucose level, fasting blood sugar, glucose tolerance test, 2-hour postprandial glucose test, and urine acetones.
➤ Refer for or initiate diabetic teaching.

Educate Your Client and the Family

➤ Explain the test results to your client or the family as good, fair, or poor control.

> If the results are within the "good–fair" range for a diabetic, encourage them to continue the plan.

> If the results are in the "poor" range, discuss areas that may be modified such as diet and amount of exercise.

> If the client is an established diabetic, review with the client the dietary, activity, and insulin parameters. Explore any areas of difficulty experienced with facets of diabetes management.

> If the test reveals a newly diagnosed diabetic client, contract with the client and family for a schedule of instruction and learning sessions about diabetes management. For best results, instruction in home management of diabetes requires multiple teaching methods. Because of the extensive and complex nature of diabetes and its management, instruction is best done in multiple segments, with sufficient time for the client and family to absorb and reflect on the content.

> Explore with the client and family options for responses to medical crises. Family and significant others need to be aware of signs and symptoms of fluctuations in blood glucose that signal potentially dangerous conditions. Client's judgments may be impaired by blood glucose extremes and therefore they may be unable to intervene on their own behalf. If family, friends, or co-workers are educated about behaviors that may signal high or low blood glucose levels, discuss potential responses to these behaviors.

> Instruct the client and family on the importance of wearing medical alert identification.

Hemoglobin S

hee mo **gloe** bin • ess

(Sickle-Cell Test, Sickledex [trade name], Sickle Prep, Sickle-Cell Preparation, Hgb S)

Normal Findings

All ages: Negative or 0%

What This Test Will Tell You

This screening blood test identifies sickle-cell disease and sickle-cell trait. For definitive diagnosis, hemoglobin electrophoresis is necessary. Sickle-cell disease is transmitted genetically by a recessive gene. When two such genes are present, sickle-cell anemia results. Sickle-cell disease exhibits itself as a disorder of the hemoglobin. Acidemia, hypoxia, dehydration, environmental temperature changes, infection, trauma, strenuous activity, fatigue, or pyrexia can cause the hemoglobin to change shape, resulting in deformed, sickle-shaped red blood cells. Once these conditions are reversed, the red cells resume their normal shapes. However, repeated sickling leads to permanent red blood cell deformity.

Abnormal Findings

Positive results may indicate sickle-cell trait or sickle-cell disease.

Interfering Factors

➤ False negative results may occur with hemoglobin concentrations under 10%, in infants less than 3–6 months of age, or in cases of blood transfusions within the past 3 months, phenothiazine drug therapy, concurrent iron deficiency, insufficient sample size (<7 mL of blood), polycythemia, or thalassemia.

➤ False positives occur with polycythemia vera, hemoglobin abnormalities, systemic lupus erythematosus, multiple myeloma, or improper sampling size.

➤ Hemolysis or clotting of the specimen invalidates the results.

NURSING CONSIDERATIONS

Prepare Your Client

➤ Explain that the purpose of the test is to check the blood for sickle cells.

➤ Ask whether the client has received a blood transfusion within the prior 3 months. If there is a history of blood transfusion, consult with the primary health care provider about performing this test.

Perform Procedure

➤ Collect 7 mL of venous blood in a lavender-top tube.

Care After Test

➤ Observe the client for signs and symptoms of sickle-cell disease including fatigue, dyspnea, bone pain, joint swelling, and chest pain.

➤ Assess for signs and symptoms of infection, because individuals with sickle-cell disease are susceptible to infection.

➤ Assess the client carefully for acute or chronic pain, which is common in sickle-cell disease. Consult with a pain management team experienced with clients who have sickle-cell disease.

➤ As indicated, administer oxygen therapy and restrict activity during acute exacerbations of disease.

➤ Evaluate related tests such as hemoglobin electrophoresis (used to distinguish between homozygous and heterozygous forms of the disease), serum osmolarity, arterial blood gases, hematocrit, hemoglobin, red blood cell indices, and complete blood cell count.

Educate Your Client and the Family

➤ Support the client emotionally while awaiting test results. A diagnosis of sickle-cell disease can have far-reaching impact on the client and offspring.

➤ Explain that genetic counseling is essential for sickle-cell carriers.

➤ Teach family and client the common precipitating factors of sickle-cell crises. Loss of appetite, weakness, fatigue, and pale coloring may indicate the onset of a crisis.

➤ Tell client with sickle-cell disease to avoid traveling to high-altitude regions, traveling in an unpressurized aircraft, performing very strenuous exercise, and being in extreme cold. These activities can result in hypoxia, which can exacerbate a sickling crisis.

➤ Instruct the client to inform hospital personnel of a sickle-cell condition. Surgical and maternity clients with sickle-cell disease require very close observation.

➤ Instruct the client that a medical alert card or jewelry with the sickle-cell diagnosis is crucial in identifying that problem in an emergency situation.

➤ Children with sickle-cell disease must have all their childhood immunizations, meticulous wound care, regular dental checkups along with good oral care, and a well-balanced diet.

➤ Teach client with sickle-cell disease to seek prompt attention for infections and to avoid becoming dehydrated.

Hemoglobins, Unstable
hee mo gloe bins • un stay bul

Normal Findings
All ages:
Negative (less than 5%) with the heat labile test
Stable (no precipitation at 40 minutes) with the isopropanol precipitation test

What This Test Will Tell You
This blood test is used in the differential diagnosis of hemolytic anemias. Its purpose is to detect unstable hemoglobins that weaken the structure of the hemoglobin molecule. This congenital defect in hemoglobin structure may produce no signs or symptoms, or may produce a mild, moderate, or severe hemolytic anemia.

Unstable hemoglobin is normally absent from the blood and it precipitates faster than normal hemoglobin. After precipitation, these unstable hemoglobins form Heinz bodies, small inclusions that attach to the red blood cell membranes and increase the fragility of the cell, leading to hemolysis.

More than 60 varieties of unstable hemoglobins exist, each named after the city in which they were discovered. The effects vary according to their number, severity of instability, the condition of the spleen, and the oxygen-carrying abilities of the abnormal hemoglobins.

Abnormal Findings
Positive findings may indicate unstable hemoglobins and Heinz body anemia.

Interfering Factors
➤ False positive results may occur from medications such as antimalarial agents, antipyretics, analgesics, furazolidone (in infants), nitrofurans, phenacetin, phenazopyridine, procarbazine, sulfonamides, tolbutamide, and vitamin K, which cause Heinz bodies to be formed.
➤ High levels of hemoglobin F (fetal hemoglobin) may cause a false positive with the isopropanol test.
➤ Hemolysis or hemoconcentration due to prolonged tourniquet constriction may result in false positive findings.

NURSING CONSIDERATIONS

Prepare Your Client

➤ Explain that this test is done to look for problems in the red blood cells, especially the part that contains iron.

Perform Procedure

➤ Collect 7 mL of venous blood in a lavender-top tube.

Care After Test

➤ Observe the client for signs and symptoms of unstable hemoglobins including pallor, jaundice, spleno-megaly, cyanosis, and hemoglobin-uria.

➤ Encourage rest periods for client who experiences fatigue related to anemia.

➤ Evaluate client's ability to perform activities of daily living.

➤ Refer to community health care services as needed if client is unable to perform basic daily needs.

➤ Review related tests such as hemoglobin, hematocrit, reticulocyte count, red blood cell indices, globin chain analysis, hemoglobin electrophoresis, peripheral blood smear for Heinz bodies, serum bilirubin, urine bilirubin, and Schilling test.

Educate Your Client and the Family

➤ Teach client to continue light physical activity if experiencing fatigue, but to rest when needed and not to plan too strenuous or prolonged activities.

➤ Inform client that maintaining regular patterns of sleep, rest, and activity are important to prevent fatigue.

➤ Stress the importance of a well-balanced diet to provide optimal energy stores.

Hemoglobin, Urine

hee mo gloe bin • yur in
(Hgb Urine Screening)

Normal Findings

All ages: Negative

What This Test Will Tell You

This urine test identifies the presence of free hemoglobin in the urine, which can result from extensive hemolysis of red blood cells. When red blood cell destruction occurs in the circulation, rather than normally in the reticuloendothelial system, free hemoglobin enters the plasma and binds with haptoglobin. If the plasma level of hemoglobin becomes higher than the level of haptoglobin,

the excess of unbound hemoglobin is eliminated through the urine. Free hemoglobin can often be found by this test when red blood cells cannot because red blood cells lyse in strongly alkaline or dilute urine.

Abnormal Findings

Presence of hemoglobin may indicate extensive burns or crushing injuries, transfusion reactions to incompatible blood, pyrexia, chemical or drug reactions, malaria, irrigation of operated prostate bed with water, congenital or acquired hemolytic anemias, paroxysmal hemoglobinuria, carbon monoxide poisoning, severe electric shock, barbiturate overdose, urethritis, cystitis, or ureteral calculus.

Interfering Factors
➤ False positive results can occur in the presence of hematuria, with either abnormal conditions or menstrual flow.
➤ Large doses of vitamin C or of drugs that contain vitamin C as a preservative (as with antibiotics) can produce false negative results.
➤ Antifungal, antibacterial, and antineoplastic agents, gold salts, nephrotoxic medications, and anticoagulants may result in positive results.

NURSING CONSIDERATIONS
Prepare Your Client
➤ Explain that this test looks for a part of red blood in the urine.
➤ If the female client is menstruating, reschedule the test, since contamination of the specimen with blood will alter test results.

Perform Procedure
➤ Fresh random urine (minimum of 50 cc) is collected from the first voiding of the morning.

Care After Test
➤ Observe the client for signs and symptoms of hemoglobinuria including pallor, jaundice, abdominal pain, anemia, and splenomegaly.
➤ Encourage rest periods for client who experiences fatigue related to anemia.
➤ Evaluate client's ability to perform activities of daily living.
➤ Refer to community health care services as needed if client is unable to perform basic daily needs.
➤ Review related tests such as hemoglobin, hematocrit, reticulocyte count, red blood cell indices, hemoglobin electrophoresis, peripheral blood smear for Heinz bodies, serum bilirubin, urine bilirubin, and Schilling test.

Educate Your Client and the Family
➤ Teach client to continue light physical activity if experiencing fatigue, but to rest when needed and not to plan too strenuous or prolonged activities.
➤ Inform client that maintaining regular patterns of sleep, rest, and activity are important to prevent fatigue.
➤ Stress the importance of a well-balanced diet to provide optimal energy stores.
➤ Teach client diagnosed with paroxysmal hemoglobinuria to avoid crowds and other sources of infection, which can stimulate hemolysis.

Hemosiderin, Urine

hee moe sid eh rin • yur in

(Hemosiderin Stain, Hemosiderin, Iron Stain, Siderocyte Stain)

Normal Findings

All ages: Negative

What This Test Will Tell You

This urine test aids in the diagnosis of iron-storage disorders. Hemosiderin is one form of an iron oxide that the body uses to store iron. When intake is excessive, or in congenital iron tissue storage disorders, iron may abnormally accumulate in different tissues and cause severe damage. When tissue damage occurs due to abnormal deposition of iron, a condition called hemochromatosis occurs. When damage does not occur with abnormal iron deposition, the condition is called hemosiderosis. The tissues and organs most susceptible to damage from iron storage disorders are the liver, heart, pancreas, kidneys, bone marrow, and skin.

Abnormal Findings

▲ INCREASED LEVELS may indicate hemochromatosis, hemosiderosis, hemolytic anemias associated with intravascular hemolysis, mechanical trauma to erythrocytes (as with heart valve hemolysis), hemolysis due to body burns, hemolysis associated with oxidant drugs, thalassemia major, sickle-cell anemia, severe megaloblastic anemia, malarial infection, multiple transfusions, pancreatitis, pernicious anemia, excessive iron injections, or excessive dietary intake of iron.

Interfering Factors

➤ Hemosiderin is not detected in alkaline urine.

➤ Delay in sending the specimen to the laboratory may result in inaccurate findings.

NURSING CONSIDERATIONS

Prepare Your Client

➤ Explain that this test helps determine how well the body is storing iron.

Perform Procedure

➤ Collect a minimum of 15 cc of freshly voided urine with the first voiding of the morning.

➤ Send the specimen to the laboratory within 2 hours after the voiding.

Care After Test

➤ Observe the client for signs and symptoms of anemia including pallor, fatigue, shortness of breath, and activity intolerance.

➤ Encourage rest periods for client who experiences fatigue related to anemia.

➤ Evaluate client's ability to perform activities of daily living.

➤ Refer to community health care services as needed if client is unable to perform basic daily needs.

➤ Assess the client's intake of iron supplements. Carefully analyze any vitamins taken regularly. This condition may result from excessive oral iron intake. Clues to excessive iron intake may include constipation, diarrhea, nausea, and vomiting.

➤ Review health history for conditions requiring multiple blood transfusions, which can also lead to abnormal iron storage.

> Evaluate renal and hepatic function to assess if end organ damage is occurring.

> Review related tests such as hemoglobin, hematocrit, reticulocyte count, red blood cell indices, globin chain analysis, hemoglobin electrophoresis, peripheral blood smear for Heinz bodies, serum bilirubin, urine bilirubin, Schilling test, bone marrow biopsy, liver biopsy, urinalysis, serum iron, total iron binding capacity, and ferritin levels.

Educate Your Client and the Family

> Teach client to continue light physical activity if experiencing fatigue, but to rest when needed and not to plan too strenuous or prolonged activities.

> Inform client that maintaining regular patterns of sleep, rest, and activity are important to prevent fatigue.

> Stress the importance of a well-balanced diet to provide optimal energy stores.

> If client is taking oral iron excessively, explain the adverse effects and assist the patient in terminating or taking appropriate oral iron supplement doses.

H

Hepatitis Viral Studies, Serum

hep ah tie tis • vie rahl • stud ees • see rum

Normal Findings

Normal results are negative for hepatitis B surface antigen (HBsAg), hepatitis B surface antibody (HBsAb), hepatitis B e antigen (HBeAg), hepatitis B e antibody (anti-HBe, HBeAb), hepatitis B virus deoxyribonucleic acid (HBV-DNA), hepatitis B core antibody (anti-HBc IgM, HBcAb), Dane particle, Delta hepatitis, and/or Australian antigen.

What This Test Will Tell You

This blood test detects an acute or convalescent viral hepatitis infection. Tests are available to detect hepatitis A, B, and non-A/non-B, also known as hepatitis C.

Hepatitis B, also known as serum or transfusion hepatitis (HAB), has a relatively long incubation period of 1–6 months. This form of hepatitis is transmitted largely by blood transfusion, intravenous drug abuse with contaminated needles, and sexual activity. Both the virus and the antibodies against it can be detected in the blood by laboratory testing.

Hepatitis A, also known as infectious hepatitis, has a much shorter incubation period of only 2–6 weeks. In hepatitis A, intravenous transmission is rare; the most common method for transmission is the oral-fecal route. The virus itself cannot be detected by laboratory testing, but the antibody formed against HAV can be detected in the serum.

Hepatitis C, also known as non-A/non-B hepatitis (HAC), also has a relatively short incubation period of 2–12 weeks. This form of hepatitis is most commonly transmitted through blood transfusions. Laboratory determination of the presence of antibodies for HAC is available.

Abnormal Findings

➤ *Positive hepatitis B surface antigen* may indicate early, active HBV infection or carrier state.

➤ *Positive hepatitis B surface antibody* may indicate later stage of infection, successful immunity following immunization or infection, or presence of antibody following passive immunization with gamma globulin.

➤ *Positive hepatitis B core antibody* may indicate chronic hepatitis or active infection.

➤ *Positive hepatitis B e antigen* indicates early hepatitis, active hepatitis, and highly infectious hepatitis.

➤ *Positive hepatitis B e antibody* indicates later stages of infection and reduction of infectious state.

➤ *Hepatitis A antibody* (HAV AB, anti-HAV) is positive about 5 weeks after infection.

➤ *HAV-IgM* indicates an acute infection.

➤ *HAV-IgG* indicates a past exposure.

➤ *Hepatitis C antibody* (anti-HCV) is positive for both acute and chronic hepatitis C infections.

NURSING CONSIDERATIONS

Prepare Your Client

➤ Explain that this test is used to look for an infection in the liver called viral hepatitis.

Perform Procedure

➤ Collect 5–7 mL of venous blood into a red-top tube.

Care After Test

➤ Assess client for signs and symptoms of acute infection such as lethargy, anorexia, nausea and vomiting, jaundice, and fever.

➤ Assess client for unusual bruising or prolonged bleeding from venipuncture site. Delayed clotting is a complication of severely impaired liver function.

➤ Assess skin, sclera of eyes for jaundice and note findings.

➤ Consult with a registered dietician to design a high-calorie, well-balanced diet. People with advanced liver disease have poor absorption of nutrients due to decreased bile flow into the intestines. As appropriate, reduce sodium or protein in the diet if edema and ascites, or increased ammonia levels are present.

➤ Evaluate history for risk factors such as intravenous drug use, prostitution, homosexuality, treatment by hemodialysis, organ or tissue transplantation, and blood transfusion.

➤ Administer immunoglobulin as indicated to individuals exposed to hepatitis B virus.

➤ Evaluate other liver function tests such as aspartate aminotransferase (AST), alanine aminotransferase (ALT), direct and indirect bilirubin levels, alkaline phosphatase, serum ammonia, and prothrombin time.

Educate Your Client and the Family

➤ Instruct client who tests positive for hepatitis and their family on the client's need for a well-balanced diet and increased rest and fluids.

➤ Instruct other close family members to be tested for infection, and administer hepatitis B immunoglobulin as appropriate. Encourage immunization with hepatitis B vaccine.

➤ Educate client and family to

obtain proper immunization for newborns. Approximately 90% of infants born to mothers positive for HBsAg and HBcAb develop HBV infections.

➤ Educate client and family on measures to prevent the spread to other close contacts including not sharing toothbrushes, not breast-feeding infants, using male or female condoms during sexual activity, not reusing or sharing needles, and preventing contact with blood.

➤ Instruct the client and family to report signs/symptoms or additional complaints to primary health care provider. These would include jaundice (yellow skin or eyes), lethargy, loss of appetite, nausea, vomiting, and fever.

➤ Educate the client who is at high risk of hepatitis exposure (such as health care personnel) of the importance of the hepatitis B vaccine.

H

Herpes Simplex Antibodies, Serum

hur pees • sim pleks • an ti bod ees • see rum
(Herpes Simplex Virus Antibody, IISV-1, HSV-2, Herpes 1-2 Antibody Titer)

Normal Findings

Titer < 1:10 is considered negative for antibodies

What This Test Will Tell You

This blood test determines the presence and level of the herpes simplex virus antibody in blood. Herpes simplex virus type 1 (HSV-1) is generally associated with infection of the eyes, face, mouth, upper respiratory tract, and central nervous system. It is transmitted through contact with contaminated saliva, lesions, and mucous membranes. Herpes virus type 2 (HSV-2) is associated with infection of the urogenital tract and perineum. It is transmitted by sexual contact, transplacentally, and during delivery of the neonate.

Abnormal Findings

➤ 1:10–1:100, first week of infection
➤ 1:100–1:500, current late primary infection

➤ Greater than 1:500, established latent infection

➤ An antibody titer increase of fourfold or greater between acute and convalescent specimens is needed to determine infection.

➤ An increase in titers may be associated with skin lesions, HSV-1 encephalitis, HSV-2 meningitis, pharyngitis, stomatitis, upper respiratory infection, pneumonia, bronchitis, intestinal herpes ulcerations, neonatal congenital herpes (eye infection, central nervous system disorders, infection of liver, heart, adrenals), or cervical neoplasia.

Interfering Factors

➤ Hemolysis of sample.
➤ Bacterial contamination of sample.
➤ Lipemia.
➤ Fats naturally occurring in foods and fluids may interfere with test results.

NURSING CONSIDERATIONS

Prepare Your Client

➤ Explain that this test is to help diagnose a specific virus in the body called herpes.

➤ Tell the client that one blood sample is taken at the onset of symptoms, and another is taken 2–3 weeks later to see if there is an increase in antibodies.

➤ Restrict food and fluids for 8 hours prior to the test.

Perform Procedure

➤ Collect 5 mL of venous blood in a red-top tube.

➤ Draw the specimen before antiviral medications are administered; they may cause falsely low titer results.

Care After Test

➤ Evaluate other tests such as cerebrospinal fluid culture for herpes simplex, herpes simplex viral cultures, and levels of aspartate aminotransferase (AST), alanine aminotransferase (ALT), bilirubin, and serum ammonia.

Educate Your Client and the Family

➤ Inform client that the sores (lesions) go away with time. Treatment is usually aimed at the symptoms or problems the client has.

Antibiotics do not work on a virus.

➤ Client with HSV-2 should keep the genital area clean and dry. Encourage client to wear loose-fitting cotton undergarments. Sitz baths may soothe affected areas and reduce inflammation.

➤ Inform client that herpes is spread through direct contact with herpes lesions. Encourage client to avoid activity that would expose other people to the herpes virus. Sexual contact should be avoided while lesions are present.

➤ Inform client that herpes is a recurrent disease. Some people are able to predict a recurrence by noting symptoms such as tingling, burning, and itching at the site of recurring lesions. Successive outbreaks of herpes tend to be less severe and lesions heal within 10–12 days.

➤ If client is receiving acyclovir to treat herpes symptoms, make sure they know how to use it. If acyclovir ointment is used, instruct client to cover all lesions with the ointment. Oral acyclovir may be prescribed for recurrent outbreaks.

➤ Suggest to a female client with genital herpes that she have yearly Papanicolaou (Pap) smears. Some references cite an increased risk of cervical cancer in women after positive cervical HSV-2 cultures.

Herpes Simplex Virus Culture

hur pees • sim pleks • vie rus • kul chur

(HSV Viral Culture, Herpes Culture)

Normal Findings

Negative

What This Test Will Tell You

This microbiological test isolates and cultures the herpes simplex virus to aid in diagnosis of herpes simplex infection. Herpes simplex virus (HSV) culture is not necessarily diagnostic of HSV infection. HSV-1 has been cultured from healthy controls. The diagnosis is strengthened by a rise in antibody titer and a positive viral culture.

Abnormal Findings

Positive cultures may be associated with skin lesions, HSV-1 encephalitis, HSV-2 meningitis, pharyngitis, stomatitis, upper respiratory infection, pneumonia, bronchitis, intestinal herpes ulcerations, neonatal congenital herpes (eye infection, central nervous system disorders, infection of liver, heart, adrenals), or cervical neoplasia.

Interfering Factors

➤ Contamination of the specimen.

➤ Delays in delivering the specimen to the lab promptly. The specimen may be refrigerated if necessary, but do not freeze it.

NURSING CONSIDERATIONS

Prepare Your Client

➤ Explain that this test is used to help diagnose a specific virus that might be causing sores.

➤ Explain the procedure for culture collection to your client. Culture specimens may be collected from sites such as the lesion, cerebrospinal fluid, cervical mucosa, or blood. Prepare your client for the procedure necessary for specimen collection.

➤ Instruct female clients not to douche or take a tub bath prior to a cervical culture.

➤ Inform your client another viral culture will be collected approximately 2 weeks after the onset of symptoms.

Perform Procedure

➤ Collect the specimen from a lesion by rolling a sterile swab over the area.

➤ Collect 7 mL of venous blood in a red-top tube for testing of blood. Cervical mucosa specimens are collected during an internal gynecological examination. Cerebrospinal fluid is tested by obtaining a specimen from a spinal tap.

➤ The specimen should be placed in a viral transport media for transport to the lab because the specimen can dry out very quickly and yield false negative results.

Care After Test

➤ Implement symptomatic treatments for the HSV client. These may include cold soaks onto open sores and giving oral acyclovir or topical lidocaine if prescribed.

➤ Evaluate related tests such as cerebrospinal fluid HSV titer, herpes simplex antibody titer, and levels of aspartate aminotransferase (AST), alanine aminotransferase (ALT), bilirubin, and serum ammonia.

Educate Your Client and the Family

➤ Inform your client that the sores (lesions) go away with time. Treatment is usually aimed at the symptoms or problems the client has. Antibiotics do not work on a virus.

➤ Your client with HSV-2 should keep the genital area clean and dry. Encourage your client to wear loose-fitting cotton undergarments. Sitz baths may soothe affected areas and reduce inflammation.

➤ Inform your client that herpes is spread through direct contact with herpes lesions. Encourage your client to avoid activity that would expose other people to the herpes virus. Sexual contact should be avoided while lesions are present.

➤ Inform your client that herpes is a recurrent disease. Some people are able to predict a recurrence by noting symptoms such as tingling, burning, and itching at the site of recurring lesions. Successive outbreaks of herpes tend to be less severe and lesions heal within 10–12 days.

➤ If your client is receiving acyclovir to treat herpes symptoms, make sure they know how to use it. If acyclovir ointment is used, instruct your client to cover all lesions with the ointment. Oral acyclovir may be prescribed for recurrent outbreaks.

➤ Suggest to a female client with genital herpes that she have yearly Papanicolaou (Pap) smears. Some references cite an increased risk of cervical cancer in women after positive cervical HSV-2 cultures.

Heterophile Agglutination Test

het ur ah fil • ah gloo tih nay shun
(Infectious Mononucleosis Screening Test)

Normal Findings

All ages: Negative

What This Test Will Tell You

This blood test diagnoses infectious mononucleosis. Heterophile antibody is produced in infectious mononucleosis and is found in the serum of 80% of patients with this disorder. Elevated levels are also found in other conditions. This test assesses the reaction of agglutinins (indicated by clumping) to the red blood cells of horses or sheep.

With infectious mononucleosis, the titer of antibodies gradually increases to about 1:224 during weeks 3–4 after infection, followed by a gradual decrease during weeks 4–8. It is this pattern of titer increase and decrease that is most diagnostic of infectious mononucleosis.

Abnormal Findings

▲INCREASED LEVELS may indicate infectious mononucleosis, Epstein-Barr virus infection, serum sickness, systemic lupus erythematosus, syphilis, or cryoglobulinemia.

Interfering Factors

➤ If treatment has already begun for infectious mononucleosis before the development of heterophile antibodies, the titer is usually negative.

➤ Addiction to narcotics, leukemia,

hepatitis, and pancreatic cancer may result in false positive titers.

➤ Hemolysis of the sample can interfere with the interpretation of the results.

NURSING CONSIDERATIONS

Prepare Your Client

➤ Explain that this test helps detect a viral illness called "mono" (infectious mononucleosis).

Perform Procedure

➤ Collect 7 mL of venous blood in a red-top tube.

Care After Test

➤ Assess for signs and symptoms of infection such as sore throat and lymphadenopathy, especially of the anterior and posterior cervical chains.

➤ Assess for splenomegaly, present in half of all cases, which can, though rarely, result in splenic rupture. Abdominal pain, postural hypotension, vertigo, or other signs of hemorrhage should be observed for and acted upon immediately.

➤ Administer antipyretics and analgesics to control fever and discomfort.

➤ Encourage fluids for febrile clients.

➤ Immunosuppressed clients may be prescribed acyclovir. Carefully monitor renal function and hydration with this potentially nephrotoxic medication.

➤ Evaluate related tests such as hematocrit, hemoglobin, white blood cell count with differential, aspartate aminotransferase, alanine aminotransferase, and alkaline phosphatase.

Educate Your Client and the Family

➤ Explain that the virus causing mononucleosis can be transmitted in the saliva, so toothbrushes, food, and drinking glasses should not be shared.

➤ Inform client and family that the virus will probably not infect everyone in the household. Most people already have immunity to the virus, and only those people without immunity develop mononucleosis.

➤ Tell client and family that most people recover completely in 4–6 weeks.

➤ Instruct your client and family that treatment is bed rest, fluids, and painkillers such as aspirin or acetaminophen.

➤ Teach client to avoid contact sports or any activity that could cause the spleen to rupture. Splenomegaly (enlarged spleen) is a common occurrence in mononucleosis.

➤ Instruct client to inform the primary health care provider immediately if acute abdominal pain develops.

➤ If the titer is positive and infectious mononucleosis is confirmed, instruct the client in the treatment plan.

➤ If the titer is positive but infectious mononucleosis is not confirmed or if the titer is negative, explain to the client that additional testing may be necessary in a few days or weeks.

H

Hexosaminidase A and B

hek sah sa min ih dase • A • and • B

Normal Findings

ALL AGES

Total hexosaminidase—type A and type B: 5–12.9 U/L (SI units: 10.4–23.8)

Type A: 56%–80% of total.

PREGNANT

The total values are increased during pregnancy.

What This Test Will Tell You

This blood test screens for Tay-Sachs disease or its carrier state, as well as Sondhoff's disease, a more severe and rapidly progressive form. This test may be performed during pregnancy on amniotic fluid.

Abnormal Findings

➤ *Deficiency of the A component* may indicate Tay-Sachs disease.

➤ *Deficiency of the A and B components* may indicate Sondhoff's disease.

Interfering Factors

➤ Hemolysis of the blood sample invalidates the results.

➤ Pregnancy or oral contraceptives may make determinations of the mother's results invalid.

NURSING CONSIDERATIONS

Prepare Your Client

➤ Explain that this is a screening test for Tay-Sachs disease, a disease that affects the brain.

➤ Explain to adult client that this test is used to determine if they are carriers of this rare disease.

➤ If this test is being performed on the fetus of a pregnant woman, explain that an amniocentesis is required, and review the procedure for amniocentesis.

Perform Procedure

➤ Collect 7 mL of venous or cord blood in a red-top tube. A heelstick may be used to sample blood from infants.

Care After Test

➤ Assess for evidence of Tay-Sachs disease in infants, including signs and symptoms of impaired neuromuscular development and function.

➤ If the results come back positive, the client and family should be referred to a genetic counseling center.

➤ Review related tests including electroencephalogram, and computed tomography and magnetic resonance imaging of the central nervous system.

Educate Your Client and the Family

➤ Explain that being the "carrier" of genetic disease means that the client has the genetic makeup to pass the disease on to offspring. However, explain that for this disease, both parents must be carriers for the offspring to be affected.

➤ Educate the family of a child diagnosed with Tay-Sachs disease about care related to muscle weakness, excessive mucus production, blindness, and seizures.

➤ Instruct family of a child with Tay-Sachs disease of the need to contact support groups and other people to assist in dealing with physical and emotional stressors involved in caring for a child whose life expectancy is less than 4 years.

HLA-B27 Antigen

H · L · A · B · 27 · an ti jen

(HLA Testing, HLA Typing, Human Leukocyte Antigen Serum)

Normal Findings

Histocompatibility match or non-match

What This Test Will Tell You

This blood test determines whether a client has HLA-B27 antigens associated with susceptibility to specific diseases. Human leukocyte antigen (HLA) is located on the cell membrane of all nucleated cells and platelets as well as on many tissue cells. There are five series in the HLA system: A, B, C, D, and DR (D-related). HLA typing is used for organ tissue matching, paternity testing, and disease associations, but HLA-B27 antigen testing is used primarily in disease susceptibility recognition.

Abnormal Findings

Abnormalities may reveal ankylosing spondylitis, Reiter's syndrome, psoriatic arthritis, juvenile rheumatoid arthritis, sacroiliitis, salmonella arthritis, acute anterior uveitis, or chronic juvenile uveitis.

Interfering Factors

➤ Hemolysis of the blood sample
➤ Blood transfusion within 3 days of test

NURSING CONSIDERATIONS

Prepare Your Client

➤ Explain that this test will determine if your client has markers called HLA-B27 antigens that may be found with certain diseases.

➤ Ensure there have been no blood transfusions within the last 3 days.

Perform Procedure

➤ Collect 10 mL of venous blood in a green-top or yellow-top tube. The sample should be tested as soon as possible.

Care After Test

➤ Treat HLA-associated rheumatic disease symptoms. Pain may be controlled with anti-inflammatory medications. Assist your client to maintain as much independence as possible by encouraging them to remain active. Exercises may assist in maintaining range of motion and flexibility.
➤ Obtain physical and occupational therapy consults if needed to promote independence in daily activities.
➤ Evaluate other lab values and diagnostic studies such as rheumatoid arthritis (RA) factor, erythrocyte sedimentation rate, synovial fluid analysis, and radiographic changes in bone structure.

Educate Your Client and the Family

➤ Educate your client regarding medications and side effects of prescribed medications.
➤ Teach your client range-of-motion exercises.
➤ Instruct client and family to establish a routine for completing daily tasks and meeting self-care needs within the physical limits of the client.

Holter Monitoring

hole tur • mon ih tur ing

(Ambulator Electrocardiography, Ambulatory ECG Monitoring)

Normal Findings

All ages: Normal sinus rhythm, normal conduction patterns, absence of areas of infarct or ischemia

What This Test Will Tell You

This electrophysiologic test is used to assess and document cardiac rhythm disturbances, and to monitor the effectiveness of antidysrhythmic and pacemaker therapy. The Holter monitoring test is a continuous ambulatory electrocardiogram (ECG) that can document abnormal heart rhythms and cardiac causes of dizziness, chest pain, and syncope. By having the client or family keep a careful journal of symptoms and activities while the recording is taking place, any rhythm disturbances can be documented. Many Holter monitors also have an event recording button that can be activated to mark the ECG tape if symptoms such as palpitations, pain, or skipped beats are felt. The effectiveness of pacemaker or pharmacologic management of dysrhythmias can also be evaluated by documenting the absence or improvement of rhythm disturbances during activities of daily living. See *Electrocardiogram* for further information.

Abnormal Findings

The test may reveal dysrhythmias, myocardial infarction, myocardial ischemia, ventricular hypertrophy, conduction defects, heart block, or Wolff-Parkinson-White syndrome.

ACTION ALERT!

Diagnostic indications of myocardial ischemia, myocardial infarction, ventricular dysrhythmias, and second- or third-degree heart blocks with accompanying symptoms all require immediate medical attention and intervention. These conditions may be associated with a high incidence of cardiopulmonary arrest.

Interfering Factors

➤ Improperly placed or loose electrodes
➤ Failure of the client or family to keep an accurate diary
➤ Tampering with the monitor by the client or family
➤ Early removal of the electrodes and monitoring device by the client or family

NURSING CONSIDERATIONS

Prepare Your Client

➤ Explain to client and family that this test records heart rhythms using small discs or strips that stick to the skin on the chest and a recording box the client wears. Tell them they will need to leave these in place throughout the recording period.
➤ Assure the client there is no pain with this test.
➤ Tell client with heavy chest hair that small areas may need to be shaved or clipped to assure adequate electrode-to-skin contact.
➤ Instruct the client to avoid or minimize the use of electrical devices that may interfere with the recording such as electric shavers, toothbrushes, and blankets; microwave

ovens; remote controls for appliances; citizen band (CB) radios; high voltage areas; magnets; and metal detectors.

➤ Instruct the client not to shower or tub bathe, only sponge bathe.

➤ Reinforce instructions to note any symptoms they may feel by pushing a button located on the outside of the recorder.

➤ Teach client to record symptoms such as shortness of breath, dizziness, angina, indigestion, headache, weakness, and palpitations in the diary or journal for the test. Activities such as sleep, exercise, eating, bowel movements, smoking, sexual activity, and emotional stress should be recorded as well.

➤ Inform the client and family of the recording period (usually 24–48 hours).

➤ Teach clients and family a heart-healthy diet, including no added salt, if there is evidence of atherosclerotic vessel disease.

➤ Note any medications the client is taking for hypertension or cardiac disease and inform the professional interpreting the ambulatory ECG.

➤ Instruct the client and family to keep the electrodes and monitor intact for the duration of the monitoring period.

➤ Do not put the electrodes on arms, legs, or shoulders as skeletal movement can make interpretation of the tracings difficult.

Perform Procedure

Nurses do not often perform this procedure but should understand the process to prepare the client. Electrodes are placed on the chest wall and attached to a recording box, which is usually worn around the neck or waist.

Care After Test

➤ Gently remove the electrodes and wipe the conduction gel from the skin.

➤ Review the need for or results of exercise tolerance and cardiac rehabilitation program for client with abnormal findings indicating cardiac disease.

➤ Reassess the client's pharmacologic therapy and administration of medications if rhythm disturbances are being medically managed. Return of abnormal rhythms might be related to noncompliance with or self-management of antidysrhythmic medications.

➤ Evaluate related tests such as an electrocardiogram, echocardiogram, cardiac enzymes, cardiac stress test, and cardiac catheterization.

Educate Your Client and the Family

➤ Show client or family how to replace electrodes that may come loose.

➤ Explain carefully that although the test checks how the body's own natural electrical system in the heart is working, the recording box and wires cannot carry electricity to the body. By looking at the heart's own natural flow of current, the primary health care provider can get information on how well the heart is pumping and receiving blood.

➤ Encourage family members to learn cardiopulmonary resuscitation.

➤ Teach client to seek medical assistance immediately if rest or prescribed medications do not relieve chest pain or symptomatic dysrhythmias.

Homovanillic Acid, Urine

hoe moe va nil ik • ass id • yur in

(HVA)

Normal Findings

ADULT

1–7 µg/mg creatinine in urine

CHILD

10–15 years: .25–12 µg/mg creatinine

5–10 years: .5–9 µg/mg creatinine

2–5 years: .5–13.5 µg/mg creatinine

1–2 years: 4–23 µg/mg creatinine

INFANT

6–12 months: 3–30 µg/mg creatinine

1–6 months: 3–40 µg/mg creatinine

1 week: 5–50 µg/mg creatinine

NEWBORN

5–20 µg/mg creatinine

PREMATURE NEWBORN

3 days: 10–50 µg/mg creatinine

1–2 days: 5–20 µg/mg creatinine

What This Test Will Tell You

This urine test measures the level of the terminal metabolite of dopamine, homovanillic acid (HVA), in order to diagnose specific brain tumors in infants and children (neuroblastomas or ganglioneuromas) and to rule out pheochromocytoma. Dopamine is a major catecholamine produced by the brain and is broken down into other chemicals by the liver. One of these metabolites is HVA and is excreted in the urine. Abnormally high levels of HVA in the urine may signify increased secretion of catecholamine substances by tumors. Urine HVA is frequently analyzed in conjunction with another catecholamine metabolite test, vanillylmandelic acid, to increase the accuracy of tumor diagnosis.

Abnormal Findings

▲ INCREASED LEVELS may indicate neuroblastoma, ganglioneuroma, ganglioblastoma, malignant pheochromocytoma, or polycystic ovary syndrome.

Interfering Factors

➤ Monoamine oxidase (MAO) inhibitors decrease HVA levels.

➤ Aspirin, methocarbamol, and levodopa alter HVA results, causing levels to be either increased or decreased.

➤ Failure to collect all urine during the 24-hour period.

➤ Failure to store the urine specimen in preservative or to keep it cool.

➤ Increased emotional stress or physical exercise during the urine collection period may cause elevated levels.

➤ Excessive physical activity or stress may increase results and interfere with interpretation.

NURSING CONSIDERATIONS

Prepare Your Client

➤ Instruct the client and family on 24-hour urine collection.

➤ Ensure the client refrains from excessive physical activity during the collection period.

➤ Inform the client that increased emotional stress may alter the test results. If the client becomes excessively stressed during the testing period, the primary health care provider should be informed in order to appropriately evaluate results.

Perform Procedure

➤ Collect all urine for 24 hours and place in a container with boric acid or hydrochloric acid.

➤ Keep the urine on ice or refrigerated during the collection period.

Care After Test

➤ Evaluate neurological function and ensure that there are no deficiencies that are a threat to safety, such as difficulty walking.

➤ Evaluate other urinary levels of catecholamines such as vanillylmandelic acid, norepinephrine, normetanephrine, and dopamine.

Educate Your Client and the Family

➤ Instruct parents involved in mass pediatric neuroblastoma screening projects to keep scheduled appointments. Early detection improves prognosis.

➤ Teach client and family ways to promote safety such as use of hand rails and keeping walkways free of clutter.

Human Chorionic Gonadotropin

hyoo man • kor ee on ik • goe nad ah troe pin
(HCG, HCG-beta Subunit, Pregnancy Test)

Normal Findings

ADULT

Serum:

Negative or 3 IU/L (mIU/mL) or less in males

Negative or 3 IU/L (mIU/mL) or less in nonpregnant females

Urine:

Negative in males and nonpregnant females

PREGNANT

Serum:

Rising 0–14 weeks gestation

100 mU/mL 10–14 weeks gestation

20 mU/mL 15 weeks to term

Urine:

First trimester: up to 500,000 IU

Second trimester: 10,000–25,000 IU

Third trimester: 5,000–15,000 IU

What This Test Will Tell You

This blood or urine test diagnoses pregnancy, hydatidiform mole, and some forms of cancer. Human chorionic gonadotropin (HCG) is a glyco-protein hormone that is secreted by the placenta and many germ cell tumors. It is one of the earliest hormones secreted during pregnancy by the chorionic tissue, which is the origin of the placenta. HCG production begins 8–10 days after conception, peaks at about 10 weeks of gestation, and should be undetectable within 3–4 days after delivery. The beta subunit is used to monitor tumor response to surgery and/or chemotherapy. The alpha subunit may give a false positive pregnancy test if not tested with the beta subunit.

Abnormal Findings

▲ INCREASED LEVELS may indicate pregnancy; hydatidiform mole; choriocarcinoma; ovarian and testicular teratomas; multiple pregnancy; seminoma; neoplasms of colon, liver, pancreas, stomach, lung, or breast; gynecomastia; ectopic pregnancy; or erythroblastosis fetalis.

▼ DECREASED LEVELS may indicate ectopic pregnancy, threatened abortion, abortion, or fetal death.

Interfering Factors

➤ Hemolysis, lipemia, and icterus may result in inaccurate blood test findings.

➤ Excessive production of luteinizing hormone (LH) may cause false positive results.

➤ HCG-producing tumors may cause false positive results in a test conducted to determine pregnancy.

➤ Absence of gonadal hormones in menopausal women may cause false positive results.

➤ Medications that may cause false positive results include anticonvulsants, antiparkinsonians, hypnotics, and tranquilizers.

➤ Heparin and phenothiazines may decrease blood HCG levels.

➤ If performed too early after conception, in ectopic pregnancy or with threatened abortion, false negative results may be obtained.

➤ If the blood test is done using radioimmunoassay, a radionuclide scan within 1 week of testing may falsely elevate the levels.

➤ Proteinuria and hematuria may cause false positive urine test results.

➤ Diuretics and promethazine may cause false negative urine test results.

NURSING CONSIDERATIONS

Prepare Your Client

➤ Explain that this is a test to check a hormone level and, as appropriate, to diagnose pregnancy or to help detect tumors or other problems.

Perform Procedure

➤ Blood test: Collect 7–10 mL of venous blood in a red-top tube.

➤ Urine test: Collect the first urine voided in the morning.

➤ Write the date of the last menstrual period on the lab slip.

Care After Test

➤ If the client is pregnant, assess knowledge of prenatal care including diet, activity, rest, signs and symptoms of labor, and danger signs in pregnancy. Provide instruction as indicated.

➤ Assess pregnant woman's readiness to meet parental role functions by reviewing infant care knowledge, methods of infant feeding, and ability to obtain needed supplies. Provide instruction and/or community health service referrals as indicated.

➤ Assess the client for use of cigarettes, tobacco products, alcohol, over-the-counter medications, and street drugs. Instruct the client as necessary to avoid these substances as they may cause intrauterine growth retardation.

➤ Review related tests such as amniocentesis, nonstress test, nipple stimulation test, and biophysical profile.

Educate Your Client and the Family

➤ Instruct the client about the importance of prenatal care if pregnant.

➤ Explain to the client that abnormal levels will need to be followed up by a primary health care provider, who may want to repeat the test to rule out any errors.

➤ Explain that follow-up testing is necessary even though they may feel fine.

➤ Instruct the client about danger signs in pregnancy such as a gush of fluid, vaginal bleeding, abdominal pain, temperature elevation, dizziness, blurred vision, persistent vomiting, severe headache, edema, muscular irritability, difficult urination, or decreased/absent fetal movements.

➤ Teach the client the signs of preterm labor such as abdominal cramping with or without diarrhea, uterine contractions every 10 minutes or more frequently, menstrual-like cramps in the lower abdomen, low backache, increase or change in vaginal discharge, or pelvic pressure.

➤ Explain to the client who has had trophoblastic disease or tumors that birth control is necessary if remission is to be ascertained, because HCG levels go up normally in pregnancy.

H

Human Placental Lactogen, Serum

hyoo man • plah sen tal • lak toe jen • see rum
(HPL, hPL, HCS, Human Chorionic Somatomammotropin)

Normal Findings

NONPREGNANT FEMALES AND MALES
<0.5 µg/mL
PREGNANT
5–27 weeks' gestation: 4.6 µg/mL
28–31 weeks: 2.4–6.1 µg/mL
32–35 weeks: 3.7–7.7 µg/mL
36 weeks to term: 5–8.6 µg/mL
At term, diabetic: 9–11 µg/mL
Values should progressively increase during pregnancy.

What This Test Will Tell You

This blood test evaluates placental function and diagnoses choriocarcinoma or hydatidiform mole. Human chorionic somatomammotropin is a hormone produced by the placenta that is critical to lactation, maternal protein synthesis and breakdown of fats, and fetal nutrition and growth. Levels tend to rise with the size or number of placentas, as evidenced by higher levels as pregnancy progresses and with multiple fetuses. Serial results over time produce more meaningful and reliable information than single values alone.

Abnormal Findings

▲ INCREASED LEVELS may indicate diabetes mellitus, multiple pregnancy, Rh isoimmunization, maternal liver disease, maternal sickle-cell disease, or cancers such as bronchogenic carcinoma, lymphoma, hepatoma, or pheochromocytoma.

▼ DECREASED LEVELS may indicate postmaturity, intrauterine growth retardation, fetal distress, threatened abortion, hydatidiform mole, choriocarcinoma, or pregnancy-induced hypertension (PIH).

ACTION ALERT!

A level of less than 3.5 µg/mL after 30 weeks' gestation may indicate placental dysfunction. Further evaluation of fetal well-being must be initiated immediately.

Interfering Factors

➤ Radioactive scans within 7–10 days will make accurate determinations by this radioimmunoassay impossible.

NURSING CONSIDERATIONS

Prepare Your Client

➤ Explain that this test measures hormone levels produced by the placenta, the part of the womb responsible for getting adequate oxygen and nutrition to the baby.

Perform Procedure

➤ Collect 7–10 mL of venous blood in a red-top tube.

Care After Test

➤ If the client reports decreased fetal movements, assess recent maternal history for maternal activity and relationship to fetal movement. Also assess the mother's recent consumption of food or fluids and its relationship to fetal movement. Consult with the primary health care provider about instructing the client to eat, drink, and then rest. During rest, tell her to concentrate on fetal movements for 1 hour. Three fetal movements in 1 hour are reassuring.

➤ Review related tests such as amniocentesis, nonstress test, nipple stimulation test, biophysical profile, estriol levels, and prolactin levels.

Educate Your Client and the Family

➤ Instruct the client with decreased levels that further evaluation with amniocentesis and nonstress testing should be done.

➤ Tell the client to notify the primary health care provider if they have less than 3 movements in 1 hour. A nonstress test or biophysical profile may be ordered.

➤ Instruct the client about normal signs of labor such as a gush of fluid, bloody show, and contractions that increase in frequency, intensity, and duration.

➤ Instruct the client about danger signs in pregnancy such as a gush of fluid, vaginal bleeding, abdominal pain, temperature elevation, dizziness, blurred vision, persistent vomiting, severe headache, edema, muscular irritability, difficult urination, or decreased/absent fetal movements.

➤ Teach the client the signs of preterm labor such as abdominal cramping with or without diarrhea, uterine contractions every 10 minutes or more frequently, menstrual-like cramps in the lower abdomen, low backache, increase or change in vaginal discharge, or pelvic pressure.

➤ Advise the client to lie down on her side and notify the primary health care provider if preterm labor is suspected.

17-Hydroxycorticosteroids

17 • hie **drok** see **kor** ti koe **stair** oids
(17-OH, 17-OCHS)

Normal Findings

ADULT AND ADOLESCENT
Male: 4.5–12.0 mg/24 hours (SI units: 12–23 μmol/24 hours)
Female: 2.5–10.0 mg/24 hours (SI units: 7–27 μmol/24 hours)
PREGNANT
Levels increase slightly during first trimester.
CHILD
8–12 years old: <4.5 mg/24 hours (SI units: <12 μmol/24 hours)
<8 years old: <1.5 mg/24 hours (SI units: <4 μmol/24 hours)
ELDERLY
Values may be lower than adult levels.

What This Test Will Tell You

This 24-hour urine test assesses adrenal cortex function and helps diagnose Cushing's syndrome. 17-hydroxycorticosteroids (17-OH) are the end products of the corticosteroids as they break down during the regulation of glyconeogenesis. Cortisol accounts for the majority of adrenocortical steroids measured by this test. A 24-hour test is used because the amount of 17-OH excreted varies throughout a full day.

This test is only an indirect method of determining adrenal sufficiency. Both the urine free cortisol measurement and the serum cortisol measurements are more frequently ordered because they are more specific tests.

Abnormal Findings

▲ INCREASED LEVELS may indicate stress, hypertension, Cushing's syndrome, adrenal cancer, adrenocorticotropic hormone–producing tumor, eclampsia, hyperpituitarism, hyperthyroidism, pituitary tumor, virilism, adrenal hyperplasia, acute pancreatitis, or pre-eclampsia.

▼ DECREASED LEVELS may indicate Addison's disease, hypopituitarism, hypothyroidism, adrenal infarct, adrenogenital syndrome, hemorrhage, or congenital enzyme deficiency.

Interfering Factors

➤ Drugs that increase levels of 17-OH include erythromycin, anabolic steroids, chlorpromazine, meprobamate, phenothiazines, spironolactone, penicillin G, ascorbic acid, chloral hydrate, chlordiazepoxide, erythromycin, acetazolamide, inorganic iodines, quinidine, quinine, paraldehyde, colchicine, and methenamine.

➤ Drugs that decrease levels of 17-OH include phenytoin, estrogen, oral contraceptives, thiazide diuretics, calcium gluconate, corticosteroids, phenothiazine, and reserpine.

➤ Clients who are obese or very muscular may have increased levels.

➤ Emotional and physical stress increase levels.

➤ Licorice in the diet increases levels.

NURSING CONSIDERATIONS

Prepare Your Client

➤ Explain that the test is to see if there is a problem with two specific glands called the adrenal glands, and the hormones they put out.

➤ Encourage client to consume adequate fluids.

➤ Ensure the client avoids physical exercise and excessive stress prior to and during the collection period.

➤ Explain procedure for collecting a 24-hour urine specimen and the importance of not contaminating the specimen with feces, menses, or toilet paper.

Perform Procedure

➤ Collect a 24-hour urine specimen. Use a preservative.

➤ Keep specimen on ice.

Care After Test

➤ Institute special skin care precautions if Cushing's syndrome is diagnosed. Skin is often thin and fragile in this condition.

➤ Assess mental status and mobility. Institute safety precautions for client with slowed mental functioning or impaired musculoskeletal function.

➤ Review related tests such as plasma cortisol levels, urine free cortisol, adrenocorticotropic hormone stimulation test, adrenocorticotropic hormone suppression test, and urine 17-ketosteroids.

Educate Your Client and the Family

➤ Teach client and family to inspect the skin often for red or broken-down areas because the skin tends to be fragile.

➤ Instruct the family to assess the home environment for possible safety threats, evaluating stairs, throw rugs, furniture placement, and other conditions that could compromise a safe environment.

➤ Instruct family to seek health care immediately at any sign of infection as Cushing's syndrome makes one more prone to infection.

➤ Teach client that hormone replacement is lifelong and doses will need to be increased during times of physical or emotional stress.

➤ Alert the client that abruptly discontinuing the medications on their own may be life-threatening.

➤ Educate the client on the need of wearing medical alert identification to inform health care providers of the condition if they cannot do so themselves.

5-Hydroxyindoleacetic Acid

5 • hie **drok** see in dole ah **see** tik • **ass** id
(5-HIAA)

Normal Findings

All ages: 1–9 mg/24 hours (SI units: <30 μmol/24 hours)
Female: slightly lower than male

What This Test Will Tell You

This urine test measures 5-hydroxyindoleacetic acid (5-HIAA), the metabolite of serotonin, to determine if carcinoid tumors of the appendix or intestine are present. Serotonin is produced by cells of the gastrointestinal tract. Normally, the intestinal mucosa contains 95% serotonin; 5% is converted to 5-HIAA and excreted in very low concentrations in the urine. Carcinoid tumors in the appendix and/or intestine produce elevated amounts of serotonin, resulting in abnormally high levels of 5-HIAA in the urine.

Abnormal Findings

▲ INCREASED LEVELS (200–600 mg/24 hours or more) may indicate carcinoid tumors of the appendix and/or intestine, endocarditis, ganglioneuroblastoma, or sprue.

Interfering Factors

➤ Falsely elevated 5-HIAA levels may occur with certain foods and medications, such as avocados, bananas, eggplants, pineapples, plums, walnuts, acetanilid, glycerol guaiacolate, melphalan, fluorouracil, mephenesin, pindolol, naproxen, diazepam, atenolol, methocarbamol, phenacetin, and reserpine.

➤ Falsely decreased 5-HIAA levels may occur with certain medications, such as chlorpromazine (large doses), imipramine, phenylalanine, prochlorperazine, promethazine, promazine (large doses), methyldopa, monoamine oxidase (MAO) inhibitors, adrenocorticotropic hormone (ACTH), heparin, ethanol, and isoniazid (INH).

➤ Phenothiazines, salicylates, acetaminophen, methenamine, guaifenesin, mephenesin, and methocarbamol may either raise or lower levels.

➤ Diarrhea or gastroenteritis may invalidate results.

NURSING CONSIDERATIONS

Prepare Your Client

➤ Explain that this test is important to screen for cancer in the appendix and/or intestine.

➤ Tell clients to avoid eating bananas, pineapples, avocados, plums, tomatoes, walnuts, and eggplant for at least 4 days prior to testing.

➤ Instruct the client to collect all urine for 1 day. Explain the 24-hour urine collection process clearly, emphasizing the importance of not contaminating the urine specimen with stool, toilet paper, or menstrual blood flow.

Perform Procedure

➤ Collect a 24-hour urine sample in a large container with preservative.

➤ Refrigerate or keep the urine on ice during the collection period.

Care After Test

➤ Observe for signs and symptoms of carcinoid tumors including alterations in patterns of bowel elimination, cramping, and abdominal pain.

➤ Consult with a registered dietician to assist the family and client in meeting special dietary needs.

➤ Review related tests such as colonoscopy, stool for occult blood, tissue biopsies, and lower gastrointestinal studies.

Educate Your Client and the Family

➤ Encourage client with a family history of carcinoid tumors to get regular medical checkups because of their increased risk of developing cancer.

➤ Teach client and family how to choose foods that will promote more normal patterns of bowel elimination, taking into account personal patterns and disease state.

5-Hydroxyindoleacetic Acid, Urine

5 • hie drok see in dole ee a see tik • ass id
(5-HIAA)

Normal Findings

All ages: <6 mg/24 hours (SI units: <30 μmol/24 hours)

Female levels may be slightly lower than male.

What This Test Will Tell You

This urine test detects or monitors carcinoid tumors. Carcinoid tumor cells release an excess of serotonin, a powerful vasopressor produced primarily in the intestinal mucosa that regulates smooth muscle contraction and peristalsis. The test measures the amount of 5-HIAA, a metabolite of serotonin, that is excreted in the urine as the result of the excessive serotonin. Generally, a random urine sample is obtained to detect the presence of 5-HIAA. If that is positive, a 24-hour urine collection and serial testing may be ordered to further diagnose the presence of 5-HIAA, as well as to indicate progression of the tumor or of therapeutic response.

Abnormal Findings

▲ INCREASED LEVELS may indicate carcinoid tumors. Levels over 100 mg/24 hours are indicative of large carcinoid tumor.

▼ DECREASED LEVELS may indicate positive response to treatment.

Interfering Factors

➤ Bananas, pineapple, plums, walnuts, eggplant, tomatoes, and avocados may result in false positives as these foods are rich in serotonin.

➤ Medications that may increase values include phenacetin, guaifenesin (often in cough syrups), reserpine, meprobamate, phenothiazine, spironolactone, ascorbic acid, penicillin G, hydroxyzine, methenamine, quinidine, chloral hydrate, and quinine.

➤ Levels may be decreased by adrenocorticotropic hormone (ACTH), heparin, isoniazid, monoamine oxidase (MAO) inhibitors, methyldopa, phenothiazines, promethazine, acetaminophen, ethanol, fluorouracil, and tricyclic antidepressants.

➤ A 24-hour urine sample that has not been refrigerated and/or does not have a preservative may interfere with accurate results.

➤ Diarrhea may interfere with accurate results.

NURSING CONSIDERATIONS

Prepare Your Client

➤ Explain that this test is important to help detect special tumors called carcinoid tumors.

➤ Explain that a 24-hour urine test usually follows if the random urine test is positive for 5-HIAA.

➤ Explain to the client that the test often needs to be repeated for accuracy.

➤ Tell the client not to eat bananas, pineapple, avocados, plums, eggplant, tomatoes, or walnuts for 4 days before the test.

➤ Assess any drugs the client may be taking that could cause a false positive or false negative result, and collaborate with the primary health care provider regarding restrictions of prescribed medications which may affect test results.

Perform Procedure

➤ Collect a random urine sample for the qualitative random test used to initially detect a tumor.

➤ Collect a 24-hour urine sample for the quantitative test used to monitor a tumor.

Care After Test

➤ Assess carefully for chronic and acute pain. Obtain pain management consultation if indicated.

➤ Assess for signs and symptoms of metastatic cancer including bone pain, fatigue, and recurring symptoms of the tumor.

➤ Assess for the psychosocial needs of the client and family including values, beliefs, resources, and coping ability.

➤ Assess the client for signs and symptoms such as bleeding from injection sites, petechia, ecchymosis, occult blood, and decreasing platelet count related to increased risk for bleeding.

➤ Assess oral mucous membranes for signs and symptoms of stomatitis. Routinely give oral hygiene care.

➤ Assess for the client's ability to cope with changes in body image such as weight loss or gain, loss of hair, changes in body functions, and decreased sexual function, and with role changes.

➤ Provide the client opportunities to have control over care issues such as times for treatment, settings for care, and presence of significant others.

➤ Refer client and family to a cancer support group if appropriate.

➤ Refer to social services to assist with the financial and economic impact of cancer.

➤ Clients with impaired bone marrow function may have prolonged bleeding times. Institute safety measures such as electric razors, nonskid shoes, no intramuscular injections, no rectal temperatures, and soft toothbrushes.

➤ Encourage verbalization of fears related to cancer, prognosis, treatment, and death.

➤ Review related tests such as plasma and platelet serotonin tests, complete white blood cell count with differential, and tissue biopsies.

Educate Your Client and the Family

➤ Explain that carcinoid tumors are usually of low-grade malignancy and that early removal provides a high cure rate.

➤ If the test is positive, teach client to avoid foods rich in serotonin including bananas, pineapple, plums, walnuts, eggplant, tomatoes, and avocados.

➤ Develop and constantly update a teaching plan for the learning needs of client and family related to diagnosis, testing, therapy, and home care.

Hydroxyproline, Urine

hie drok see proe lin • yur in

Normal Findings

ADULT

Total hydroxyproline:

14–45 mg/24 hours in males and females (SI units: 110–350 µmol/24 hours)

0.4–5 mg/2 hours in males (SI units: 3–40 µmol/2 hours)

0.4–2.9 mg/2 hours in females (SI units: 3–20 µmol/2 hours)

Free hydroxyproline less than 10% of total.

Most of the amino acid is protein bound.

PREGNANT

Elevations expected during third trimester due to rapid fetal growth.

NEWBORN

Elevated levels are expected in infants due to rapid growth. Hydroxyproline is measured through blood serum in newborns.

CHILD AND ADOLESCENT

Ages 1–5: 20–65 mg/24 hours (SI units: 150–510 µmol/24 hours)

Ages 6–10: 35–99 mg/24 hours (SI units: 270–770 µmol/24 hours)

Ages 11–18: 63–180 mg/24 hours (SI units: 480–1400 µmol/24 hours)

Elevated levels expected during periods of rapid skeletal growth. Peak levels occur between 11 and 18 years of age.

ELDERLY

Elevated levels may be related to mild osteoporosis.

What This Test Will Tell You

This urine test provides information regarding bone resorption (destruction) as well as the client's response to treatment. Hydroxyproline is an amino acid found primarily in colla-gen, which is an insoluble protein found in connective tissue such as bone, skin, teeth, ligaments, and cartilage. This amino acid is produced when collagen is broken down through disease, injury, or digestion of foods.

Abnormal Findings

▲ INCREASED FREE LEVELS may indicate hydroxyprolinemia and familial iminoglycinuria.

▲ INCREASED TOTAL LEVELS may indicate osteoporosis, hyperparathy-roidism, bone tumor, Paget's disease, multiple myeloma, Marfan's syn-drome, Klinefelter's syndrome, acromegaly, osteomyelitis, Albright's syndrome, or rickets.

▼ DECREASED TOTAL LEVELS may indicate response to drug therapy for bone resorption conditions (slow decrease), hypoparathyroidism, hypopituitarism, hypothyroidism, malnutrition, or muscular dystrophy.

ACTION ALERT!

This test is performed on clients who may be at high risk for pathological fractures. Maintain proper body alignment and do not apply pulling or pressure forces.

Interfering Factors

➤ Dietary collagen will cause increased levels, especially of free hydroxyproline.

➤ Drugs that can cause decreased levels include ascorbic acid, vitamin D, aspirin, glucocorticoids, calci-tonin, and mithramycin.

➤ Psoriasis and burns can increase the levels due to collagen turnover.

➤ Failure to collect all the urine or store the specimen properly.

NURSING CONSIDERATIONS

Prepare Your Client

➤ Explain that this test detects problems that cause damage to the bones, skin, and other tissues in the body, or to see how well treatment is working.

➤ Assure the client has had a diet free of collagen-rich foods for at least 24 hours prior to beginning the test and throughout the urine collection period. Foods to be avoided include meat, poultry, fish, jelly, and any food containing gelatin.

➤ Explain to the client the importance of collecting all urine during the collection period for accurate results.

Perform Procedure

➤ Obtain from the laboratory a large container with a preservative to prevent breakdown of the hydroxyproline.

➤ Follow procedures for continuous urine collection (24-hour or 2-hour collection).

➤ Refrigerate specimen or keep it in an ice bucket during the collection period.

Care After Test

➤ Maintain proper body alignment and apply no pulling or pressure forces to bones to avoid pathological fractures when tests indicate bone destruction.

➤ Obtain a dietary consult to evaluate dietary intake of calcium and make recommendations in diet.

➤ Collaborate with the primary health care provider to evaluate the need for oral calcium supplemental therapy.

➤ Institute safety precautions in the environment to prevent accidental injury.

➤ Evaluate related tests such as alkaline phosphatase, bone x-rays, bone scans, serum calcium, serum phosphorus, and serum magnesium levels.

Educate Your Client and the Family

➤ Teach client and family proper body mechanics and positioning to support bones that may not be able to tolerate stress.

➤ Inform client and family how to prevent falls, which may lead to serious fractures. This includes providing adequate lighting, handrails on stairs and in bathrooms, and removal of scatter rugs and clutter.

➤ Instruct client and family on sources of dietary and supplemental calcium if indicated.

Hysterosalpingography

his teh roe **sal** ping **gah** grah fee
(Uterotubography, Uterosalpingography, Hysterogram, Hysterosalpingogram)

Normal Findings

No defects in the uterine cavity and normal, patent fallopian tubes.

What This Test Will Tell You

This x-ray test with contrast media detects abnormalities of the uterus and fallopian tubes, especially when a woman has not been able to conceive. Malformations of the uterus and fallopian tubes or blockage can be visualized when contrast material is injected into the fallopian tubes through the cervix and the material's passage is followed. This test may be especially useful for clients with a history of pelvic inflammatory disease (PID), which can kink the tubes, immobilize the uterus and tubes, and isolate the ovaries by scarring the tubes. The passage of dye may clear obstructions. This test is also used to document the effectiveness of a tubal ligation.

Abnormal Findings

Abnormalities may include tubal obstruction, uterine tumors, internal scarring, fallopian tube occlusion, extrauterine pregnancy, adhesions, uterine fistulas, or developmental anomalies.

ACTION ALERT!

Assess clients carefully for allergic reaction to contrast material, including dyspnea, itching, urticaria, flushing, hypotension, and shock. Life-threatening anaphylactic reactions can occur and need to be recognized and treated immediately.

Interfering Factors

➤ Gas or feces may prevent visualization.
➤ Tubal spasm may give a false appearance to normal fallopian tubes.

Contraindications

➤ Suspected pregnancy, since contrast medium may induce abortion
➤ Uterine bleeding, since contrast medium may enter the body via open blood vessels
➤ Infections of the fallopian tubes, cervix or vagina, because the test may promote extension of the infection
➤ Purulent vaginal drainage
➤ Fever
➤ Menstruation

➤ Recent curettage
➤ Serious cardiac and/or systemic disease

Potential Complications

➤ Allergic reaction to the contrast material
➤ Infection of the fallopian tubes or endometrium
➤ Uterine or tubal perforation
➤ Spontaneous abortion

NURSING CONSIDERATIONS

Prepare Your Client

➤ Explain, as appropriate, that this test is to detect problems of the uterus and fallopian tubes, especially to find possible reasons why it may have been difficult to become pregnant, or to see if tubal ligation is successful.
➤ Determine the date of the last menstrual period. Schedule 2–5 days after menstruation to avoid flushing a potential fertilized ovum out through a tube.
➤ Assess for allergy to iodine or shellfish. Allergic reactions are rare.
➤ Inform the client that the procedure may be uncomfortable or cause menstrual-type cramping, but should not be painful.
➤ Administer laxatives, suppositories, or enemas prior to the test as ordered.
➤ Administer antispasmodic or sedative if ordered.
➤ Withhold food and fluids for up to 4–8 hours prior to the test if ordered. Some primary health care providers do not require fasting.
➤ Have the client void before the procedure.
➤ Ensure that an informed consent form is signed if required by the institution.

Perform Procedure

Nurses do not perform this procedure but should understand the process to prepare the client and assist the physician. An x-ray of the abdomen is taken to check for gas or feces. The client is placed in a lithotomy position on the fluoroscopy table. A vaginal speculum is inserted and the cervix is cleansed.

X-ray contrast medium is injected to fully fill the uterus and fallopian tubes. Films are taken.

Assist the client to relax during the procedure. Observe the client throughout the procedure and monitor for possible allergic reaction.

Care After Test

➤ Assess for signs of perforation including abdominal pain, fever, or shock. Report to the primary health care provider immediately.

➤ Assess for signs and symptoms of infection including fever, odorous discharge, pain, and malaise.

➤ Inspect vaginal discharge, which may normally include small amounts of blood for a few days following the test.

➤ Assess for late signs of allergic reaction, which are very rare in this procedure. Prepare to treat with antihistamines or steroids as ordered.

➤ Assess for referred shoulder pain caused by dye in the peritoneal cavity and provide pharmacologic as well as nonpharmacological pain management interventions.

➤ Review related tests including laparoscopy, pregnancy test, and abdominal x-ray.

Educate Your Client and the Family

➤ Instruct the client that she may have menstrual-like cramps and/or shoulder pain caused by the dye leaking into the peritoneal cavity and irritating tissue including the diaphragm, which causes referred pain in the shoulder. Dizziness may occur.

➤ Explain that vaginal discharge may occur for 1–2 days after the procedure. The discharge may be bloody or contain dye. A sanitary pad rather than a tampon should be worn to control discharge without increasing the risk of infection.

➤ Instruct the client to report signs and symptoms of infection such as fever, increased pulse, and pain to the primary health care provider.

➤ Inform the client of available support groups for infertile women and men.

Immunoglobulin Electrophoresis

ih **myoo** noe **glob** yu lin • ee **lek** troe foe **ree** sis
(Gamma Globulin Electrophoresis, Immunoelectrophoresis, IEP,
Immunoglobulins, Ig, Protein Electrophoresis)

Normal Findings

ADULT

IgG: 650–1600 mg/dL
IgA: 50–400 mg/dL
IgM: 40–375 mg/dL
IgD: 0.5–8 mg/dL
IgE: 0.1–0.4 mg/dL

PREGNANT

IgE may decrease during pregnancy.

NEWBORN

IgG: 640–1450 mg/dL
IgA: 0–12 mg/dL
IgM: 5–30 mg/dL

CHILD

2–8 months:
IgG: 140–1190 mg/dL
IgA: 5–90 mg/dL
IgM: 14–167 mg/dL

15 months–3 years:
IgG: 300–1620 mg/dL
IgA: 2–192 mg/dL
IgM: 40–240 mg/dL

5–6 years:
IgG: 550–1530 mg/dL
IgA: 44–334 mg/dL
IgM: 38–248 mg/dL

7–10 years:
IgG: 620–1660 mg/dL
IgA: 42–435 mg/dL
IgM: 24–348 mg/dL

ADOLESCENT

Adult values are reached by late teens.

ELDERLY

The immune response tends to be less active in the elderly, resulting in lower-than-average adult levels.

What This Test Will Tell You

This blood test screens for a variety of immune system diseases related to immunoglobulin abnormalities. There are five major immunoglobulin groups found in gamma globulin: IgG, IgA, IgM, IgD, and IgE. These immunoglobulins are proteins produced by B lymphocytes (B cells) in response to antigen stimuli.

Each type of immunoglobulin (antibody) has specific clinical significance. IgG has a relative serum concentration of 75%–80% and is located in plasma and interstitial fluid. It is the only immunoglobulin that crosses the placental barrier and thus provides passive immunity to the newborn until the infant begins sufficient production at 6 months to 1 year. IgG is responsible for antibody production against viruses, bacteria, and toxins.

IgA comprises approximately 15% of the immunoglobulins. It is responsible for protecting the respiratory, gastrointestinal, and urinary tracts from viruses and bacteria. IgA is found in blood, saliva, tears, breast milk, and colostrum.

IgM has a relative serum concentration of 8% and is located in intravascular serum. Its levels increase within 24–72 hours after an antibody enters the body, indicating a primary immune response to an active infection. IgM is produced in response to rheumatoid factors, gram-negative organisms, Rh antibodies, heterophile antibodies, and ABO blood group isoantibodies.

IgD is present in small quantities and its role in the immune response is not known.

IgE is also found in small amounts in the body. Its production is increased during allergic reactions, anaphylaxis, and parasite infestation.

Abnormal Findings

▲INCREASED LEVELS *of IgG* may reveal infections, severe malnutrition, sarcoidosis, chronic granulomatous infection, liver disease, rheumatic fever, rheumatoid arthritis, hyperimmunization, infectious hepatitis, lupus erythematosus, or IgG multiple myeloma.

▼DECREASED LEVELS *of IgG* may reveal combined immunodeficiency, agammaglobulinemia, X-linked hypogammaglobulinemia, common variable immunodeficiency, protein-losing gastroenteropathies, acute thermal burns, nephrotic syndrome, lymphoid hyperplasia, pre-eclampsia, lymphocytic leukemia, or amyloidosis.

▲INCREASED LEVELS *of IgA* may reveal autoimmune disorders, tuberculosis, Laënnec's cirrhosis, rheumatoid arthritis, rheumatic fever, chronic infections, liver disease, inflammatory bowel disease, alcoholism, or carcinoma of the gastrointestinal or hepatobiliary tract.

▼DECREASED LEVELS *of IgA* may reveal agammaglobulinemia, X-linked hypogammaglobulinemia, protein-losing gastroenteropathies, acute thermal burns, nephrotic syndrome, chronic lymphocytic leukemia, or a malignancy.

▲INCREASED LEVELS *of IgM* may reveal infectious mononucleosis, subacute bacterial endocarditis, rheumatoid arthritis, lupus erythematosus, rubella virus in newborns, lymphosarcoma, brucellosis, malaria, or fungal infection.

▼DECREASED LEVELS *of IgM* may

reveal agammaglobulinemia, lymphoid hyperplasia, lymphocytic leukemia, or amyloidosis.

▲INCREASED LEVELS *of IgE* may reveal allergy such as hay fever, asthma, or anaphylaxis; skin sensitivity; or drugs recently given such as tetanus toxoid, tetanus antitoxin, or gamma globulin.

▼DECREASED LEVELS *of IgE* may reveal agammaglobulinemia.

Interfering Factors

➤ Blood transfusions and blood component therapy (including gamma globulin) within 6 weeks affect results.

➤ Immunizations within prior 6 months.

➤ Toxoids within prior 6 months.

➤ Drugs that may increase immunoglobulin levels include hydralazine, isoniazid, phenytoin, and procainamide.

➤ Use of immunosuppressive drugs may decrease IgA.

NURSING CONSIDERATIONS

Prepare Your Client

➤ Explain that this test is to see how well the body is able to fight infections and take care of itself by making antibodies. The levels of specific antibodies are useful in screening for certain diseases.

➤ Ask your client about recent blood transfusions, blood product therapy, immunizations, and current medications. Some of these factors may affect the test results.

Perform Procedure

➤ Collect 5–15 mL of blood in a red-top tube.

➤ Indicate on the lab slip if your client has received blood, blood product therapy, or immunizations within the last 6 months.

➤ Indicate on the lab slip any medications your client is taking that may affect lab results.

➤ Label the sample and send to the lab immediately.

Care After Test

➤ Assess your client for signs and symptoms of the specific disease process being evaluated.

➤ Institute protective measures for immunosupressed client such as strict hand washing, use of gowns and masks, and other measures to reduce exposure to infection.

➤ Evaluate other tests such as urine immunoelectrophoresis, bone marrow studies, protein electrophoresis, rheumatoid factor, erythrocyte sedimentation rate, bacterial cultures, and viral cultures.

Educate Your Client and the Family

➤ Instruct your client and family about medications to treat the disease.

➤ If a chronic disease process is diagnosed, assist your client and family to obtain information about local support groups.

➤ Instruct immonosupressed client to avoid crowds, small children, and individuals with respiratory infections.

Insulin, Serum
in suh lin • see rum
(Insulin Assay)

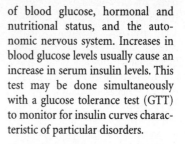

Normal Findings
ADULT, PREGNANT, AND ELDERLY
0–25 μU/mL (SI units: 0–145 pmol/L)
NEWBORN
0–20 μU/mL (SI units: 0–116 pmol/L)
CHILD AND ADOLESCENT
0–24 μU/mL (SI units: 0–139 pmol/L)

What This Test Will Tell You
This radioimmunoassay blood test diagnoses glucose imbalances from a variety of causes as well as disorders of lipid, carbohydrate, and insulin metabolism. Insulin is important in the regulation and metabolism of carbohydrates, lipids, and amino acids. Normally, the rate of insulin secretion is determined by the level of blood glucose, hormonal and nutritional status, and the autonomic nervous system. Increases in blood glucose levels usually cause an increase in serum insulin levels. This test may be done simultaneously with a glucose tolerance test (GTT) to monitor for insulin curves characteristic of particular disorders.

Abnormal Findings
▲INCREASED LEVELS may indicate insulinoma, acromegaly, insulin-resistant diabetes, or Cushing's syndrome.
▼DECREASED LEVELS may indicate diabetes mellitus.

ACTION ALERT!
Severe hypoglycemia may occur in clients with insulinoma during this test. Evaluate the client closely for signs of hypoglycemia

including tachycardia, diaphoresis, mental status changes, and hypotension. Be prepared to administer 50% glucose solution intravenously if ordered.

Interfering Factors

➤ Levels are increased with obesity, use of oral contraceptives, steroids, insulin administration, oral hypoglycemic agents, epinephrine, levodopa, and thyroid hormones.

➤ Recent radioisotope testing makes determining insulin levels by radioimmunoassay inaccurate.

➤ Failure to observe dietary restrictions prior to sampling.

➤ Exercise prior to sampling.

➤ Hemolysis.

➤ Failure to keep the sample on ice.

NURSING CONSIDERATIONS

Prepare Your Client

➤ Explain that this test measures the body's level of insulin, which is an important chemical to control blood sugar.

➤ Ensure the client is lying down and resting for 30 minutes prior to blood sampling to reduce the influence of physical activity or stress.

➤ Restrict food and fluids (except water) for 10–12 hours prior to the test.

Perform Procedure

➤ Collect 7 mL of venous blood in a red-top tube and another 7 mL of venous blood in a gray-top tube.

➤ Send the samples packed in ice to the laboratory immediately.

➤ When the test is being performed with the GTT, collect pairs of samples prior to ingestion of the glucose load and at designated intervals throughout the test.

Care After Test

➤ Resume previous diet.

➤ Administer insulin or oral hypoglycemics if they were held for the test.

➤ Assess for signs or symptoms of hypoglycemia or hyperglycemia.

➤ If client is a newly diagnosed diabetic, arrange for a dietary consult with a registered dietician and diabetic teaching.

➤ Review related tests such as fasting blood glucose level, anti-insulin receptor antibodies, oral glucose tolerance test, and glycosylated hemoglobin values.

Educate Your Client and the Family

➤ Discuss signs and symptoms of hypoglycemia including dizziness, tremor, hunger, and sweating. Teach client to have emergency sources of glucose readily available.

➤ Discuss signs and symptoms of hyperglycemia including headache, thirst, and hunger.

➤ Instruct the client about the lifetime need to maintain blood sugar control through diet, exercise, and medication.

➤ Teach the client of the need to wear medical alert identification to communicate their disorder to health care personnel in case they are unable to do so themselves.

Intravenous Pyelography

in trah vee nus • pie eh log rah fee

(IVP, Excretory Urography, EUG, Intravenous Urography, IUG, IVG
Intravenous Pyelogram)

Normal Findings

ALL AGES

Kidneys, ureters, and bladder are of normal size, shape, and position. Structures are free from obstruction and masses.

Within 5 minutes contrast material will outline kidney and calyces. The renal pelvis is visualized within 7 minutes. The ureters and bladder are then visualized as the contrast material flows through the lower urinary tract.

PREGNANT

Slight to moderate hydroureter and hydronephrosis; right kidney larger than left kidney.

CHILD

Bladder size differs widely among individual children and is generally greater in girls than boys.

ELDERLY

Defects in the ureters are related to the vesicoureteral junction and the possible reflux of urine into the ureter or subsequent renal pelvis. Bladder capacity is reduced. Bladder muscles weaken, causing incomplete emptying. Bladder outlet changes may cause obstruction in the male (benign prostatic hypertrophy) or incontinence in the female. Progressive loss of the whole nephrons and renal mass (mainly cortex) occurs in the kidney, resulting in smaller size.

What This Test Will Tell You

This radiographic procedure evaluates the structure and function of the urinary tract, assesses trauma to the kidneys, identifies congenital anomalies, and evaluates the ability to maintain normal urine flow. The test determines shape, size, and location of the kidneys, the ureters, and the bladder as well as the arterial and venous vascularity of the kidneys. This test is the cornerstone of a urologic examination. The ability to maintain normal flow is determined by the amount of time required for the contrast dye to fill and leave each structure. Disorders such as renal disease, ureteral or bladder stones, and tumors may inhibit the flow of the dye and thus be detected by this procedure.

Abnormal Findings

➤ *Renal abnormalities* may indicate renal calculi, abnormal size, abnormal shape, renal hematomas, abnormal structure, pyelonephritis, space-occupying lesion, polycystic kidney, congenital anomalies, renovascular hypertension, hydronephrosis, renal tuberculosis, supernumary kidney, absent kidney, renal hypertrophy, or redundant kidney pelvis.

➤ *Ureteral abnormalities* may indicate ureteral calculi, abnormal size, abnormal shape, abnormal structure, compression from external structures, redundant ureter, prostate hypertrophy, or space-occupying lesion.

➤ *Bladder abnormalities* may indicate bladder calculi, abnormal size, abnormal shape, abnormal structure, or space-occupying lesion.

Assess clients carefully for allergic reaction to contrast material, including dyspnea, itching, urticaria, flushing, hypotension, and shock. Life-threatening anaphylactic reactions can occur and need to be recognized and treated immediately.

Interfering Factors

➤ Views of the urinary tract may be obscured by feces or gas in the intestinal tract.

➤ Barium retention can obscure views of the urinary tract.

➤ End-stage renal disease may impair film quality.

➤ Insufficient injection of contrast medium may cause inaccurate interpretation of the film.

Contraindications

➤ Oliguria and/or blood urea nitrogen level exceeding 40 mg/dL, because of the inability to excrete contrast material

➤ Allergy to contrast material without modification

➤ Pregnancy, due to radiation exposure to the unborn fetus

➤ Combined hepatic and renal failure, because of client's inability to excrete the contrast material

Potential Complications

➤ Allergic reactions including anaphylaxis

➤ Dehydration

➤ Weakness

➤ Hematoma at the injection site

➤ Dysuria

➤ Renal failure

NURSING CONSIDERATIONS

Prepare Your Client

➤ Explain that this test is used to examine the shape, size, location, and the working ability of the kidneys, ureters, and bladder to make sure that they are working properly.

➤ Explain to client and family that a dye will be injected through their vein, causing a temporary burning sensation and metallic taste. They should report any other unusual sensations.

➤ Evaluate blood urea nitrogen and serum creatinine studies. If elevated, collaborate with the primary health care provider about the need to cancel the test because of the potential adverse effect of contrast material on renal function.

➤ Assess the chart for history of allergic reaction to iodine, shellfish, or radiographic dye.

➤ Make sure that an informed consent is obtained, because of the possible complications associated with this procedure.

➤ Record baseline vital signs.

➤ Assist the client to disrobe below the waist.

➤ Administer a laxative, if ordered, the night before the procedure to increase visualization on the x-ray film.

➤ Be sure the client is sufficiently hydrated, then instruct them to fast for 8 hours preceding the test. Some institutions do, however, allow a clear liquid breakfast. Pediatric client will have a shorter fasting period.

➤ Do not remove glasses, dentures, or hearing aids unless dictated by your hospital policy. The client may need to communicate and cooperate during the test.

➤ Schedule barium studies after intravenous pyelogram, if one has been ordered.

➤ Collaborate with the primary health care provider to determine if the intravenous fluid rate needs to be decreased to avoid dilution of intravenous contrast.

Perform Procedure

Nurses do not perform this procedure, but should understand the process to prepare the client. Assist the client to a supine position on the x-ray table. Observe client for possible reaction to the contrast dye (flushing, nausea, hives, dyspnea). The first x-ray is obtained to view the renal parenchyma 1 minute following intravenous contrast injection. Repeated x-rays are taken 5, 10, and 15 or 20 minutes following dye injection.

Ureteral compression is performed following exposure of the 5-minute film. In some individuals, two small inflated rubber bladders are placed on the abdomen on both sides of the midline and secured with a fastener around the torso of the client. This occludes the ureters (without client discomfort) and retains contrast medium in the upper urinary tract. The rubber bladders are released following exposure of the 10-minute film.

An x-ray film is obtained after the contrast medium reaches the lower ureters and as it reaches the bladder. The client is asked to void and a final film is obtained to assess for residual urine.

Care After Test

➤ Monitor vital signs closely until stable; usually every 15 minutes for the first hour, every 30 minutes for the next hour, and then every 4 hours for 24 hours.

➤ Monitor fluid intake and urine output for at least 24 hours. Notify the health care provider if the client is unable to void for 4 hours.

➤ Observe urine for hematuria. Report hematuria that persists after third voiding.

➤ Encourage drinking fluids, if not contraindicated, due to diuretic effect of contrast material.

➤ Observe for delayed reaction to contrast material (hives, skin rash, nausea), which could occur up to 6 hours after the test. Notify primary health care provider and administer antihistamines if ordered.

➤ Encourage bed rest for up to 8 hours for elderly or debilitated client. Maintain a safe environment because client may be weak from fasting and cathartic administration.

➤ Observe injection site for leakage of contrast material at site. Extravasation of the iodine in the material may cause tissue sloughing, requiring the administration of hyaluronidase to reabsorb the iodine.

➤ Evaluate related tests such as renal ultrasound, kidney-ureter-bladder x-rays, and renal tomograms.

Educate Your Client and the Family

➤ Teach client and family the importance of adequate fluid intake unless oliguria is present.

➤ Instruct client to request assistance when getting up for at least the first 8 hours following this test.

Intrinsic Factor Blocking and Binding Antibody, Serum

in trin sik • fak tor • blok ing • and • bine ding • an ti bod ee • see rum
(Intrinsic Factor Antibody, Blood; IF Antibody)

Normal Findings

All ages: Negative

What This Test Will Tell You

This blood test helps diagnose pernicious anemia by detecting the presence of antibodies to intrinsic factor (IF) in the blood. The intrinsic factor is produced by the gastric mucosa and joins with vitamin B_{12} in the gastrointestinal tract. If there is a lack of intrinsic factor, pernicious anemia results. In most clients with pernicious anemia, the serum shows antibodies to the intrinsic factor. There are two types of antibodies to the intrinsic factor: type I, the blocking antibody, and type II, the binding antibody.

Abnormal Findings

Presence of IF blocking or binding antibodies may indicate pernicious anemia.

ACTION ALERT!

If the test is positive, it is highly indicative of pernicious anemia, which can result in serious neurologic, gastric, and intestinal abnormalities. If left untreated, it may lead to permanent neurologic disability or death.

Interfering Factors

➤ Do not collect the sample if the client was injected with or has ingested vitamin B_{12} within 48 hours prior to the test.
➤ If the client has received a radioisotope or treatment with methotrexate or any other folic acid agonist within 7 days prior to the

test, the test results may be altered.
➤ Only about 50% of people with pernicious anemia have a positive result. A negative result does not rule out a diagnosis of pernicious anemia.

NURSING CONSIDERATIONS

Prepare Your Client

➤ Explain that the test is important to help diagnose a type of anemia, or lack of red blood, called pernicious anemia.
➤ Question the client about recent ingestion or injection of vitamin B_{12}.
➤ Check the client's history for recent exposure to a radioisotope or treatment with methotrexate or any other folic acid antagonist.

Perform Procedure

➤ Collect 5 mL of venous blood in a red-top tube.
➤ Let the tube stand undisturbed for 1 hour to form a clot. Send to the laboratory immediately to be frozen.

Care After Test

➤ Encourage rest periods for client experiencing fatigue related to anemia.
➤ Evaluate client's ability to perform activities of daily living.
➤ Refer to community health care services as needed if client is unable to perform basic daily needs.
➤ Consult with a registered dietician to assist the family and client in meeting special dietary needs.
➤ Review related tests such as hemoglobin, hematocrit, reticulocyte

count, red blood cell indices, globin chain analysis, hemoglobin electrophoresis, peripheral blood smear for Heinz bodies, serum bilirubin, urine bilirubin, and Schilling test.

Educate Your Client and the Family

➤ Teach client to continue light physical activity if experiencing fatigue, but to rest when needed and not to plan too strenuous or prolonged activities.

➤ Inform client that maintaining regular patterns of sleep, rest, and activity are important to prevent fatigue.

➤ Stress the importance of a well-balanced diet to provide optimal energy stores.

➤ If the test results indicate pernicious anemia, instruct the client that they will require vitamin B_{12} injections on a routine schedule (weekly at first, then monthly for maintenance). Teach self-injection or teach family how to inject.

➤ Instruct the client to contact the primary health care provider immediately with any signs of infection, which may quickly progress to a serious illness with pernicious anemia.

Iron Level, Serum

ie yurn • lev el • see rum
(Iron, Fe)

Normal Findings

ADULT, ADOLESCENT, AND ELDERLY
Male: 70–150 μg/dL (SI units: 12–27 μmol/L)
Female: 80–150 μg/dL (SI units: 14–27 μmol/L)
Pregnant: Values are slightly decreased from the female adult values if the client is not receiving iron supplements.
NEWBORN
100–250 mg/dL (SI units: 17–43 μmol/L)
CHILD
50–120 μg/dL (SI units: 9–21 μmol/L)

What This Test Will Tell You

This blood test estimates the total iron storage in the body, aids in the diagnosis of hemochromatosis, differentiates anemias, and evaluates nutritional status. Iron is a mineral found predominantly in hemoglobin and it acts as a carrier of oxygen from the lungs to the tissues. It indirectly aids in the return of carbon dioxide to the lungs. Iron is absorbed in the small intestine and transported, bound to a protein called transferrin, to the bone marrow for incorporation into hemoglobin.

Abnormal Findings

▲INCREASED LEVELS may indicate pernicious anemia, aplastic anemia, hemolytic anemia, hemochromatosis, acute leukemia, lead poisoning, acute hepatitis, thalassemia, excessive iron therapy, repeated blood transfusions, acute iron poisoning in children, or nephritis.

▼DECREASED LEVELS may indicate iron deficiency anemia, malnutrition, acute or chronic infection, carcinoma, nephrosis, hypothyroidism, postoperative state, kwashiorkor, gastrointestinal bleeding, dysmenorrhea, chronic diseases such as systemic lupus erythematosus or rheumatoid arthritis, third trimester of pregnancy, myocardial infarction, blood loss, burns, gastrectomy, malabsorption syndrome, chronic schizophrenia, or uremia.

ACTION ALERT!

Excessive ingestion of oral iron supplements is a serious, life-threatening poisoning emergency. Chelating agents need to be administered immediately in the event of toxic ingestions.

Interfering Factors

➤ Chloramphenicol, cisplatin, estrogens, ethanol, iron, dextran, methotrexate, and oral contraceptives may result in increased levels.

➤ Recent blood transfusions and hemolytic anemias can interfere with accurate findings.

➤ Adrenocorticotropic hormone (ACTH), colchicine, methicillin, testosterone, and chloramphenicol may result in decreased levels.

➤ Sleep deprivation or stress can lower iron levels.

➤ Ingestion of iron supplement tablets can result in serum iron concentrations of 300–500 µg/dL.

➤ Recent consumption of a meal high in iron can elevate serum levels of iron.

➤ Vitamin B_{12} that has been taken in the previous 48 hours can also increase results.

➤ Hemolysis of blood sample can result in elevated findings.

NURSING CONSIDERATIONS

Prepare Your Client

➤ Explain that this test helps to detect the body's levels of iron, which the red blood cells must have for transporting oxygen.

➤ The client should not receive iron supplements for at least 24 hours prior to the test.

➤ Evaluate recent (24–48-hour) dietary history for signs of ingestion of foods high in iron content.

Perform Procedure

➤ Collect 7–10 mL of venous blood in a red-top tube.

Care After Test

➤ Observe the client for signs and symptoms of anemia including pallor, dyspnea, chest pain, and fatigue.

➤ Encourage rest periods for client who experiences fatigue related to anemia.

➤ Evaluate client's ability to perform activities of daily living.

➤ Refer to community health care services as needed if client is unable to perform basic daily needs.

➤ Obtain a dietary consult to assist the client and family in choosing a well-balanced diet, including foods high in iron and vitamin B_{12}.

➤ Observe for signs and symptoms of acute iron poisoning in children, which include convulsions, shock, acidosis, blood loss, and electrolyte disturbances. Administer the chelating agent deferoxamine by subcutaneous, intramuscular, or slow intravenous infusion with normal saline solution as ordered. Watch for adverse effects of rapid intravenous infusion such as flushing, urticaria, hypotension, or shock. Explain that deferoxamine may give urine a reddish tint.

➤ Review related tests such as hemoglobin, hematocrit, reticulocyte count, red blood cell indices, hemoglobin electrophoresis, ferritin level, total iron binding capacity (TIBC), bone marrow and liver biopsies, and iron absorption and excretion studies.

Educate Your Client and the Family

➤ Teach client to continue light physical activity if experiencing fatigue, but to rest when needed and not to plan too strenuous or prolonged activities.

➤ Inform client that maintaining regular patterns of sleep, rest, and activity are important to prevent fatigue.

➤ Stress the importance of a well-balanced diet to provide optimal energy stores.

➤ Investigate whether the client or a caregiver plans and cooks the meals and include that person in teaching.

➤ Instruct your client in the foods that are rich in iron such as liver, egg yolks, lean beef, and prune juice.

➤ Instruct your client in the foods that are rich in vitamin C, which is a promoter of iron absorption. Foods rich in vitamin C include oranges, grapefruit, cabbage, and potatoes.

➤ Teach family with small children the dangers of oral ingestion of iron supplements, including children's vitamins with iron. Instruct on poison prevention in the home.

➤ Teach client with high levels of iron or client initiating iron therapy to include plenty of fluids and foods rich in fiber, as iron may cause constipation.

K

Normal Findings

ADULT
Male: 8–20 mg/24 hours (SI units: 28–87 µmol/24 hours)
Female: 6–15 mg/24 hours (SI units: 17–53 µmol/24 hours)
PREGNANT
Expect increased levels in the third trimester.
NEWBORN
<1 mg/24 hours. Expect increased levels in premature infants.
CHILD
≤10 years old: 0.1–5.0 mg/24 hours
ADOLESCENT
11–15 years old: 2–12 mg/24 hours
ELDERLY
Production of 17-ketosteroids can be expected to decline with age in both sexes.

What This Test Will Tell You

This 24-hour urine test measures adrenal and gonadal function. 17-ketosteroids (17-KS) are metabolites of adrenocortical and reproductive hormones that are secreted by the adrenal glands, testes, and minimally, the ovaries. The adrenal cortex is responsible for most of the 17-KS measured in urine, but in men, the testes also account for the production of about one-third of the level. Women's and children's levels are lower than men's levels because ovaries contribute minimally to 17-KS levels, and prepubescent children have little gonadal contribution to the level. Overall, these hormones have androgenic or masculinizing effects.

Abnormal Findings

▲INCREASED LEVELS may indicate adrenal hyperplasia, adrenal carcinoma, adrenal adenoma, hyperpituitarism, Cushing's syndrome, testicular interstitial cell tumors, luteal cell ovarian tumors, nonmalignant virilizing adrenal tumors, polycystic ovaries, androgenic arrhenoblastoma, severe stress, chronic illness, adrenocorticotropic hormone (ACTH) administration, or pregnancy (third trimester).

▼DECREASED LEVELS may indicate Addison's disease, panhypopituitarism, myxedema, nephrosis, gout, chronic illness, thyrotoxicosis, hypogonadism, or castration.

Interfering Factors

➤ Severe stress and obesity will cause increased levels.
➤ Levels are often increased during the third trimester of pregnancy.
➤ Medications that may increase levels include ACTH, antibiotics, secobarbital, dexamethasone, spironolactone, phenothiazines, nalidixic acid, quinidine, chlorpromazine, chloramphenicol, meprobamate, oleandomycin, and testosterone.
➤ Estrogens, oral contraceptives, penicillin, phenytoin, ethacrynic acid, probenecid, salicylates, promazine, reserpine, and thiazide diuretics can cause decreased levels.

NURSING CONSIDERATIONS
Prepare Your Client

➤ Explain that this test helps determine any problems with hormones in the body called the 17-keto-steroids.

➤ Explain the method for 24-hour collection of urine.

➤ Confer with the primary health care provider to see if medications need to be withheld.

➤ Assess for signs of stress.

Perform Procedure

➤ Collect urine in a 24-hour urine container with preservative.

➤ Refrigerate the specimen or keep on ice throughout the collection period.

➤ Encourage liberal drinking of fluids unless contraindicated.

Care After Test

➤ Observe for signs and symptoms of androgenic effects including hirsutism, ambiguous genitalia, and increase in clitoral or phallic size.

➤ Monitor results of other endocrine function tests such as 17-ketogenic steroid levels and plasma testosterone levels.

➤ Assess the effects on self-concept and provide emotional support.

Educate Your Client and the Family

➤ Explain to the client and family that problems in the adrenal glands as well as other organs or tissues can cause changes in sexual organs. Give specific information for the problem diagnosed.

➤ Teach family and client to report any new symptoms to the primary health care provider including new or increased growth of hair, changes in sexual function, or other new or unusual symptoms.

Kidney Sonogram

kid nee • son oe gram

(Kidney Ultrasonography, Kidney Ultrasound, Renal Sonogram, Renal Ultrasonography, Renal Ultrasound)

Normal Findings

Bilateral kidneys are present, with normal size and shape. Kidney contours are smooth, capsules sharply outlined. Kidneys are positioned between iliac crests and diaphragm. Renal veins can be seen. There should be no cysts, tumors, or calculi.

What This Test Will Tell You

This ultrasound test is usually done in conjunction with other urinary diagnostic tests to clarify or verify the presence of an abnormality in the genitourinary tract. The test is not limited to kidney ultrasound but

may also include ultrasound of the ureters, bladder, and gonads. Because renal function is not required, this test may be a substitute for excretory urography. This test may be used as a guide to locate the kidney in order to perform a kidney biopsy.

Abnormal Findings

Abnormalities may indicate hydronephrosis, cysts, tumors, renal abscesses, perirenal abscesses, horseshoe kidney, ectopic kidney, duplicated kidney, obstruction, calculi, polycystic kidney, end-stage glomerulonephritis, end-stage pyelonephritis, perirenal hematoma, nonfunctional kidney, adrenal gland abnormalities, tumors, cysts, or renal dysfunction.

Interfering Factors

➤ Retained barium from a previous test. The kidney sonogram should precede any barium procedure.

➤ Excessive trunk or perirenal fat impairs transmission of ultrasonic waves.

➤ Dehydration impairs contrast between organs and surrounding fluids.

➤ Flatus.

Contraindications

➤ Open flank wounds or dressings

NURSING CONSIDERATIONS

Prepare Your Client

➤ Explain that this test evaluates the size, shape, and position of the kidney and any obvious problems of these organs.

➤ Tell the client that this test is safe, painless, and will take about 30 minutes.

Perform Procedure

➤ Nurses do not usually perform this procedure, but should understand the process to prepare the client. Assist the client to a prone position on the x-ray table. A very young child may be positioned on the side. Expose the area to be scanned. Ultrasound lubricant is applied to the flank area. Transverse scans of the upper and lower renal poles are scanned to locate the longitudinal axis of the kidney. These areas are marked on the skin as points of reference. The transducer is moved longitudinally and transversely to obtain sectional images. Ask the client to breathe deeply several times to determine kidney movement during respiration.

Care After Test

➤ Remove the lubricant from the client's skin.

➤ Observe for signs of renal impairment including decreased urine output, edema, and electrolyte imbalances.

➤ Evaluate additional tests that may be performed such as the kidney-ureter-bladder (KUB) x-ray, excretory urography, intravenous pyelogram (IVP), serum creatinine, blood urea nitrogen, and creatinine clearance.

Educate Your Client and the Family

➤ Teach your client and family about additional tests requiring the use of contrast medium, such as the excretory urogram or the intravenous pyelogram.

➤ Encourage adequate fluid intake unless otherwise contraindicated.

➤ Educate client as indicated concerning dietary modifications required by renal calculi or renal function impairment.

Kidney, Ureter, and Bladder X-Ray Study

(Flat Plate X-Ray of Abdomen, KUB, Scout Film, Abdominal Plain Film, Three-Way Film)

Normal Findings

Both kidneys should appear approximately the same size, with the left kidney slightly higher than the right. The superior portion of the kidneys should tilt slightly toward the vertebral column. The ureters should normally not be visible. The bladder visualization is dependent upon the bladder's muscular wall density and the amount of urine present at the time of the x-ray. There should be no ascites or excessive gas in the abdomen, and no evidence of calculi.

What This Test Will Tell You

This radiographic test examines the abdomen to determine the size, structure, and position of the kidneys, ureters, and bladder, and to reveal gross, nonspecific urinary abnormalities. This test is often the first in a series evaluating the urinary tract. The plain x-ray film, without contrast medium, assesses the organs from three views: supine, left lateral, and upright. This test does not require nor does it confirm normal renal function. Because symptoms associated with urinary and gastrointestinal disorders are often similar to each other in the client's clinical presentation, a KUB may precede a series of gastrointestinal tests. The size, shape, and position of the liver and spleen, and abnormal collection of gas or ascites may be noted by this test. This test has limitations in its diagnostic information; therefore, other tests such as intravenous pyelography and barium studies may indicated.

Abnormal Findings

Abnormalities may indicate bilateral renal enlargement, unilateral enlargement, abnormally small kidney(s), renal displacement, absence of one kidney, abnormal kidney location, horseshoe kidney, lobulated kidney, renal calculi, renal calcification, ascites, foreign bodies, ureteral calculi, excessive gas, intestinal obstruction, or bladder fusion anomalies.

Interfering Factors

➤ Barium will obscure visualization of abdominal structures.

➤ Obesity, excessive air, feces, ascites, foreign bodies, or contrast media in the gastrointestinal tract may obscure viewing of the abdominal organs.

➤ The kidneys, ureters, and bladder may not be seen if calcified uterine fibromas or ovarian lesions are present.

Contraindications

➤ Pregnancy, due to radiation exposure to the fetus

NURSING CONSIDERATIONS

Prepare Your Client

➤ Explain that this test evaluates the size, structure, and position of the kidneys, ureters, and bladder and any glaring problems of these organs.

➤ Review diagnostic tests which have or might be ordered. Make sure that this test precedes any barium studies because barium can interfere with imaging.

➤ Tell the client that no discomfort is involved, and the test lasts only a few minutes.

Perform Procedure

Nurses do not perform this procedure, but should understand the process to prepare the client. One to three x-ray images are taken of the abdomen. A supine, left lateral, and standing x-ray may be done. If the client is unable to lie flat, they are assisted to a left lateral position with the right arm over head. Shielding is provided for male client over the penis and testicles to prevent radiation exposure. Female ovaries cannot be protected because of their proximity to the kidneys. The client is asked to breathe out and hold a breath as the x-ray is taken. The x-ray is repeated in a standing or sitting position if required. The supine film is done on an x-ray table or in bed, if portable. It requires the client to position their arms over head.

Care After Test

➤ Observe for signs and symptoms of renal or urinary tract dysfunction such as oliguria, edema, and abnormalities in electrolytes, serum creatinine, or blood urea nitrogen.
➤ Evaluate patterns of urinary elimination for any abnormalities.
➤ Review related tests that may follow the KUB, such as excretory urography and intravenous pyelogram.

Educate Your Client and the Family

➤ Encourage the client to increase fluid intake, unless contraindicated, if urinary tract infection or calculi are suspected.
➤ If urinary tract infection is suspected, teach client to report signs to the primary health care provider: burning, chills, fever, and/or hesitancy. Teach treatment including dietary modifications and drug therapy, if appropriate.
➤ Teach the client primary prevention of calculi formation if indicated. These include avoiding immobility and fluid-depleted states.
➤ Educate the client about measures taken to prevent recurrences of stone formation, including taking medications to combat infection and alter the pH of the urine, testing the pH of the urine with reagent strips daily, modifying the diet based on the type of stone-forming process (avoiding calcium-containing and other foods known to promote calculus formation), eating a well-balanced diet, and maintaining a liberal fluid intake.
➤ Instruct the client about the importance of recognizing any signs of recurrence.

K

Lactic Acid, Serum

lak tik • ass id • see rum

(Lactate, Blood Lactate)

Normal Findings

ALL AGES

Arterial blood: 0.5–1.8 mEq/L

Venous blood: 0.5–2.2 mEq/L

What This Test Will Tell You

This blood test measures the amount of lactic acid in the blood and assesses acid-base balance. Lactic acid accumulates in conditions such as severe hypoxia, diabetes, shock, hypermetabolism, and liver disease, resulting in an acid-base imbalance in the body. When cells are forced to catabolize glucose without adequate oxygen (anaerobic metabolism), glucose is incompletely catabolized to lactic acid. Lactic acid leaves the cell and enters the extracellular fluid where it readily donates a hydrogen ion (H^+) and causes acidemia.

This condition occurs when the metabolic rate increases to the point where the normal amount of intracellular oxygen is not adequate, as occurs with strenuous exercise, fever, or seizure activity. Lactic acidosis also may occur when the metabolic rate is normal but the amount of oxygen available to the tissues is low, as in any condition producing hypoxia, such as cardiac arrest, shock, respiratory failure, congestive heart failure, arterial insufficiency, or trauma. Lactic acidosis may also happen in hepatic failure because the liver is unable to properly metabolize lactate, even when it may be present in normal levels. Finally, lactic acidosis occurs in diabetic acidosis because of abnormal glucose metabolism.

Because it is essential to determine the cause of acidemia, other tests such as arterial blood gases, serum electrolytes, liver function, and renal function tests should be evaluated.

Abnormal Findings

▲INCREASED LEVELS may indicate hypoxia, shock, cardiac arrest, hemorrhage, diabetes, trauma, liver disease, heavy skeletal muscle exercise, seizure activity, fever, ingestion of acids such as ethanol or methanol intoxication, salicylate intoxication, renal failure, malignancy, or peritonitis.

▼DECREASED LEVELS may indicate hypothermia.

ACTION ALERT!

High levels of lactic acid can lead to a dangerous drop in blood pH, metabolic acidosis, and death.

Interfering Factors

➤ Strenuous exercise prior to blood sampling causes a rise in lactic acid because blood flow and oxygenation cannot keep pace with increased needs of exercising muscle.

➤ Clenching the fist prior to venipuncture may cause an elevated level due to release of lactic acid from the muscle of the clenched hand.

➤ Prolonged tourniquet application prior to venipuncture may cause an elevated lactic acid level due to insufficient oxygenated blood supply to the tissues.

➤ Failure to ice an arterial sample could cause an elevated level.

NURSING CONSIDERATIONS

Prepare Your Client

➤ Explain that the test is to determine if there are too many acids in the blood.

➤ Check with your laboratory to see if fasting for 8 hours prior to sampling is required.

➤ Ensure the client has not engaged in activity for at least 60 minutes prior to blood sampling.

➤ Explain that you will need to draw blood from the vein or artery as indicated. Describe the venipuncture process or procedure for the arterial puncture clearly.

➤ Instruct the client not to clench the fist prior to venipuncture as this could affect results.

Perform Procedure

➤ Avoid use of a tourniquet if possible.

➤ Perform a venipuncture to collect 5–7 mL of venous blood in a gray-top or green-top tube, depending on laboratory method.

➤ If an arterial sample is ordered, perform an arterial puncture to obtain 2–3 mL of blood in a heparinized syringe.

➤ Label the tube as arterial or venous and transport to the laboratory immediately. Arterial samples should be placed on ice.

Care After Test

➤ Assess clients with suspected elevated lactic acid levels for symptoms of acidemia, such as decreased level of consciousness, weakness, cardiac arrhythmias, deep and rapid breathing, or warm flushed skin.

➤ Review the client's history for factors that may contribute to acidosis, such as diabetes, liver disease, hypoxia, renal failure, heart disease, pulmonary disease, or hypotensive episodes.

➤ Evaluate related tests, such as arterial blood gases, electrolytes, liver function, and renal function.

Educate Your Client and the Family

➤ Inform client with elevated lactic acid levels that repeated blood samples may need to be drawn to monitor the response to treatment.

➤ Describe the treatment for acidemia, depending on the cause of the disorder.

➤ Educate client on the importance of following prescribed treatment and activity restrictions associated with their condition.

➤ Teach client and family the signs of acidemia: decreased level of consciousness, weakness, irregular heartbeat, warm flushed skin, and deep, rapid breathing.

Lactic Dehydrogenase

lak tik • dee hie **droj** en ase

(LD, LDH, Lactic Acid Dehydronase, Isoenzymes)

Normal Findings

Normal values vary with laboratory methods. Check with your laboratory for normal values.

ADULT AND ADOLESCENT
45–90 U/L, or 115–225 IU/L (SI units: 0.4–0.9 μmol/L)

PREGNANT
Slightly increased levels

NEWBORN
160–450 U/L, or 400–1125 IU/L (SI units: 1.4–4.1 μmol/L)

INFANT
100–250 U/L, or 250–625 IU/L (SI units: 2.2–5.6 μmol/L)

CHILD
60–170 U/L, or 150–425 IU/L (SI units: 0.5–1.5 μmol/L)

ELDERLY
50–102 U/L, or 125–255 IU/L (SI units: 0.4–0.9 μmol/L)

ALL AGES
Distribution of isoenzymes:
LDH_1: Cardiac fraction 17%–33%
LDH_2: Cardiac fraction 27%–48%
LDH_3: Pulmonary fraction 16%–30%
LDH_4: Hepatic fraction 2%–17%
LDH_5: Hepatic fraction 0%–13%
Note that reference ranges are method dependent.

What This Test Will Tell You

This blood test is used to diagnose myocardial infarction, pulmonary infarction, and liver disease, and less commonly in disorders of the bones, kidneys, brain, and red blood cells. Lactic dehydrogenase (LDH) is an intracellular enzyme present in almost all metabolizing cells. Cellular damage caused by hypoxia causes an elevation of serum LDH level, but because it is present in numerous tissues, its usefulness is limited by this factor. By using electrophoresis or heat inactivation of the specimen, five tissue-specific isoenzymes can be identified for more specific tissue evaluation: LDH_1 and LDH_2 are found primarily in the heart, red blood cells, and kidneys, LDH_3 primarily in the lungs, LDH_4 and LDH_5 primarily in the liver and skeletal muscles.

Abnormal Findings

▲INCREASED LEVELS may indicate an acute myocardial infarction, cerobrovascular accident, cancer, liver disease, renal infarction, hemolytic anemia, intestinal infarction, pancreatitis, muscular dystrophy, acute pulmonary infarction, mononucleosis, anemias, acute hepatitis, or shock.

▼DECREASED LEVELS may indicate positive responses to cancer treatment.

███████ ACTION ALERT!

An LDH_1 level that is greater than an LDH_2 level or greater than 40% is strongly indicative of a myocardial infarction.

Interfering Factors

➤ Hemolysis of sample may elevate serum LDH levels. This is due to high LDH activity in erythrocytes.
➤ Use of general anesthetic agents, narcotic analgesics, alcohol, anabolic steroids, aspirin, clofibrate, procainamide, mithramycin, and intramuscular injections can elevate LDH levels.

➤ Recent surgery, labor contractions, pregnancy, strenuous exercise, and prosthetic heart valves may also increase LDH levels.

NURSING CONSIDERATIONS
Prepare Your Client
➤ Explain to client and family that this test helps diagnose a variety of problems including a heart attack, blood clot to the lungs, and problems of the blood, kidneys, or liver.
➤ Inform the client and family that levels will most likely be drawn more than once to see if they are rising or falling.

Perform Procedure
➤ Collect 3–7 mL of venous blood into a red-top tube.
➤ Note any intramuscular injections within the past 8 hours.
➤ If test is being performed as part of a workup for myocardial infarction (MI), be sure to draw samples as scheduled to avoid missing a peak level. Serial levels will be performed.

Care After Test
➤ Evaluate the client's history for coronary and vascular disease if the test is being done to help diagnose an MI.
➤ Assess and collaborate with the primary health care provider to relieve the client's chest pain.
➤ Carefully evaluate vital signs and cardiovascular function if the client is being evaluated for heart disease. Vital signs are important in many of these disorders.

➤ In client with a potential MI, assess color for paleness, mucous membranes for moisture and color, and note any complaints of dyspnea, nausea, and chest or arm pain.
➤ In client with liver disease, assess skin and sclera of eyes for jaundice and note findings. Also note unusual bruising or prolonged bleeding from venipuncture site. Delayed clotting is a complication of severely impaired liver function.
➤ Review related tests including isoenzymes of creatinine phosphokinase (CPK), alanine aminotransferase (ALT), and aspartate aminotransferase (SGOT or AST).

Educate Your Client and the Family
➤ Instruct client with suspected heart disease to notify the nurse or primary health care provider immediately if chest pain or feelings of indigestion should occur or worsen.
➤ Instruct client with liver disease to report any jaundice, excessive or easy bruising, or fullness of the abdomen (ascites) to primary health care provider.
➤ If a myocardial infarction is diagnosed, teach the client and family behaviors associated with a heart-healthy lifestyle such as eating a low-salt, low-fat diet and engaging in a regular exercise program that has been reviewed by the primary health care provider.
➤ Discuss with the family the importance of learning cardiopulmonary resuscitation (CPR) and provide information about available courses.

Lactose Tolerance
lak tose • tol ur ans
(Oral Lactose Tolerance)

Normal Findings

ALL AGES

Blood sample: >20 mg/dL rise in plasma glucose over fasting levels with no abdominal symptoms such as diarrhea or pain. (SI units: >1.1 mmol/L)

Stool sample: pH 7–8 with low glucose content

What This Test Will Tell You

This blood and stool test identifies lactose intolerance. Lactose, a disaccharide found in dairy products, is normally broken down by lactase (an enzyme in the small intestines) to form glucose and galactose, which can be absorbed by the intestinal epithelium. In the absence of lactase there is no breakdown of lactose, and the undigested lactose is excreted. As the undigested lactose moves through the bowel it creates a cathartic effect and the client may experience abdominal cramps, diarrhea, nausea, flatulence, and bloating. Lactase levels decrease throughout the life span and many clients develop a lactose intolerance as a result.

Abnormal Findings

20% of individuals will have either a false positive or false negative test result.

▼DECREASED LEVELS (flat curve of less than 20 mg/dL rise over the fasting glucose blood level, or stool pH < 5.5) may indicate lactose intolerance or enterogenous diarrhea.

Interfering Factors

➤ Enterogenous steatorrhea (fatty stools) may interfere with the test results.

➤ Strenuous exercise may affect the blood glucose level.

➤ Failure to follow dietary restrictions may alter the test results.

➤ Delayed emptying of stomach contents, as seen with gastroparesis or diabetes mellitus, may decrease the glucose levels.

➤ Drugs such as insulin, thiazide diuretics, oral contraceptives, propranolol, benzodiazepines, glucagon, or oral hypoglycemics may alter the test results.

➤ Smoking may increase glucose levels.

➤ Glycolysis, often associated with excessive exercise, may cause false negative results.

Contraindications

➤ Previous documentation of a lactose intolerance, because the test itself may result in unpleasant symptoms.

Potential Complications

➤ Abdominal cramping
➤ Diarrhea
➤ Nausea
➤ Flatulence
➤ Abdominal bloating

NURSING CONSIDERATIONS

Prepare Your Client

➤ Explain that the test is to see if the body makes enough of a particular chemical (enzyme) needed to help digest milk and milk products.

➤ Restrict food and fluids for at least 8 hours before the test.

➤ Instruct the client to omit strenuous exercise for at least 8 hours prior to the test as it will alter the test results.

Perform Procedure

➤ Collect 7 mL of venous blood in a gray-top tube.

➤ Administer the test load of lactose (50–100 g of lactose) diluted in 200–400 mL of water. For a child, the dose is based on the child's size (50 g per square meter of body surface area).

➤ Instruct the client to drink the loading dose of lactose within 5–10 minutes and document the time when the loading dose is completed.

➤ Draw blood samples at 15, 30, 60, and 120 minutes from the time the loading dose was ingested. These are also 7-mL venous blood samples in gray-top tubes.

➤ If the stool specimen is required, collect it 5 hours after the loading dose.

Care After Test

➤ After the loading dose, monitor the client for the symptoms of lactose intolerance (abdominal cramps, nausea, bloating, flatulence, diarrhea).

➤ Advise client that this is a screening test and further testing for final diagnosis may be required.

➤ If the results are positive, arrange for a consult with a registered dietician.

➤ Evaluate other diagnostic tests such as D-xylose absorption test, glucose tolerance test, lactose/hydrogen breath test, small bowel mucosal biopsy, or urinary galactose excretion.

Educate Your Client and the Family

➤ If the test is positive for a lactose intolerance, instruct the client about lactose-free milk, which can be purchased at most grocery stores, and commercially available lactase preparations.

Laparoscopy

lap ah ross koe pee
(Peritoneoscopy, Pelvic Endoscopy, Gynecologic Laparoscopy, Abdominal Laparoscopy)

Normal Findings

Gynecologic examination: Normal size and shape of the uterus, fallopian tubes, and ovaries. The fallopian tubes are free of adhesions and mobile. There are no ovarian cysts or endometriosis present.

Medical examination: Normal liver, gallbladder, spleen, and greater curvature of the stomach.

What This Test Will Tell You

This endoscopic test detects cysts, adhesions, fibroids, or infection of the uterus, fallopian tubes, and/or ovaries. Laparoscopy is also used as a diagnostic examination of the liver, gallbladder, pancreas, and lymph nodes. In this procedure, direct visualization of internal abdominal and reproductive organs is performed to detect abnormalities or disease. Surgical procedures such as removal of tissue for biopsy, ligation of fallopian tubes, lysis of adhesions, and removal of diseased tissues or organs may also accompany the endoscopy. The laparoscopy is beneficial in that it requires only a small incision, takes little time, causes little physiologic stress, may be performed under local or general anesthetics, shortens healing time, and poses a reduced risk of postoperative adhesion formation.

Abnormal Findings

Abnormalities may indicate endometriosis, infertility, enlarged fallopian tubes, ectopic pregnancy, ovarian cysts, pelvic inflammatory disease, pelvic abscess, fibroids, cirrhosis, ascites, gallbladder disease, jaundice, lymphoma or other malignancy (which may be staged using laparoscopy), pelvic adhesions, salpingitis, fibroids, pancreatic disease, or engorged vessels in the peritoneum indicating portal hypertension.

ACTION ALERT!

Monitor the client carefully after the procedure for severe abdominal pain, a rigid boardlike abdomen, and/or rapidly increasing temperature, which could indicate peritonitis and/or perforation of the internal organs.

Interfering Factors

➤ Adhesions or extreme obesity may impair direct visualization.
➤ Blood may obstruct the field of vision.

Contraindications

➤ Advanced abdominal wall cancer
➤ Severe respiratory or cardiovascular disease
➤ Palpable abdominal mass
➤ Large abdominal hernia

➤ Chronic tuberculosis
➤ Peritonitis
➤ Intra-abdominal hemorrhage, because visualization through the scope would be obscured by the blood
➤ Multiple abdominal surgeries, due to possible adhesions

Potential Complications

➤ Perforation of an internal organ could result in spilling of the organ's contents (for example, stool, urine, or bile) into the peritoneal cavity and peritonitis.
➤ Hemorrhage from injury to the underlying structures.
➤ Acidosis from the carbon dioxide inflation of the abdominal cavity.
➤ Nausea.
➤ Subcutaneous emphysema.
➤ Infection at the incision site.
➤ Untoward reactions to the drugs used during the procedure such as topical anesthetics, narcotics, tranquilizers, or sedatives. The primary side effects of the above drugs are respiratory depression or hypotension.
➤ Seeding of cancer cells.

NURSING CONSIDERATIONS

Prepare Your Client

➤ Explain that this test is used to look directly at the organs inside the abdomen or stomach wall. If appropriate, explain that abnormal tissues may be removed.
➤ Explain that a local anesthetic at the insertion site will produce a brief burning sensation before the area becomes numb.
➤ Restrict food and fluids for 8–12 hours prior to the test.
➤ Ensure that an informed consent is obtained, because of the possible

complications associated with this procedure.

➤ Check the client's coagulation results prior to the test and be sure that the results are posted on the client's chart. Report abnormal coagulation results to the primary health care provider prior to the procedure.

➤ Have the client empty their bladder immediately before the procedure or insert a Foley catheter if ordered by the primary health care provider.

Perform Procedure

Nurses do not perform this procedure, but should understand the process to prepare the client. The client is placed in a Trendelenburg or modified lithotomy position to move organs from the pelvic cavity into the abdominal cavity, where they are more visually accessible. A fiberoptic scope is inserted through the abdominal wall into the peritoneum through an incision in or near the umbilicus. Up to 4 L of carbon dioxide are introduced into the peritoneal cavity to improve visualization of the organs by causing the omentum to rise from the organs. After the inspection or procedure is completed, carbon dioxide is allowed to escape passively. Following the procedure, the incision for the endoscope is closed with two or three stitches or steri-strips and covered with an adhesive bandage.

Care After Test

➤ Monitor vital signs closely until stable, usually every 15 minutes for the first hour, every 30 minutes for the next hour, and then every 4 hours for 24 hours.

➤ Observe the client closely for bleeding, increasing temperature, purulent drainage from the incision site, severe abdominal pain, or rigidity of the abdomen, as these symptoms could indicate infection, hemorrhage, organ perforation, or peritonitis.

➤ Advise the client that shoulder discomfort may be present for 1–2 days as the carbon dioxide gas may remain in the abdominal cavity and irritate the diaphragm, which causes referred pain in the shoulder area.

➤ Provide analgesics as needed for abdominal or shoulder discomfort.

➤ Monitor the urine output to ensure that there is no injury to the bladder following the test.

➤ Instruct the client to restrict activity for 2–7 days or as ordered by the primary health care provider.

➤ Evaluate related tests such as abdominal ultrasounds, abdominal computed tomography (CT) scans, abdominal magnetic resonance imaging (MRI) scans, hemoglobin, hematocrit, serum electrolytes, and/or abdominal flat plate x-rays.

Educate Your Client and the Family

➤ Instruct the client or family to notify the primary health care provider if the client's temperature becomes elevated, the incision becomes red or has a pus-like discharge, bleeding occurs from the incision site, or if there is increased severe abdominal pain following the procedure. These signs could indicate infection, hemorrhage, or peritonitis.

➤ Inform client about infertility support groups when indicated.

Lead, Serum

led • see rum

Normal Findings

All ages: <20 mg/dL (SI units: <1.0 µmol/L)

What This Test Will Tell You

This blood test determines exposure to dangerous levels of lead. Lead is a metal that interferes with synthesis of heme. Symptoms of lead toxicity are related to the type and amount of exposure from low chronic to high acute exposures. The most common exposure is frequent small doses over a period of time. Lead is normally excreted in the urine. Excessive levels are deposited in bone and soft tissues such as the brain.

Abnormal Findings

ADULT
>30 mg/dL are elevated (SI units: >1.5 µmol/L)
>60–80 mg/dL are toxic (SI units: >3–4 µmol/L)
INFANT AND CHILD
>25 mg/dL are toxic (SI units: >1.25 µmol/L)
>60–80 mg/dL indicate lead encephalopathy (SI units: >3–4 µmol/L)

ACTION ALERT!

Lead levels greater than 25 mg/dL in children are elevated and need to be aggressively investigated and treated with chelation therapy to promote renal excretion of lead and prevent serious sequelae such as mental retardation.

Interfering Factors

➤ Contamination of specimen with a lead-containing container.
➤ High-calcium diet prior to specimen collection may result in a false negative result because calcium facil-

itates lead being deposited in bone.

NURSING CONSIDERATIONS

Prepare Your Client

➤ Explain that this test looks for the amount of lead in the blood.
➤ Tell your client to limit calcium intake for at least 3 days prior to the test to allow movement of lead stores out of bones. Foods high in calcium include milk, cheese, some antacids, and multivitamins with minerals.

Perform Procedure

➤ Collect 5–10 mL of venous blood in a lavender-, black-, or green-top tube. Some laboratories prefer venous collection from specially treated lead-free brown-top tubes.
➤ Check with your laboratory to see if a 24-hour urine collection in a lead-free container is required. The specimen is stable at room temperature.

Care After Test

➤ Obtain history concerning potential lead exposure. Include occupation, ceramic pottery use, well water, and age of home as common sources of lead exposure.
➤ Monitor your client's urine output. Lead poisoning can decrease renal function.
➤ Assess for neurological changes such as aggression, lethargy, tremors, irritability, apathy, headaches, peripheral neuropathy, confusion, and seizures.
➤ Assess for gastrointestinal symptoms including anorexia, abdominal pain, vomiting, constipation, and encephalopathy.

➤ Assess for other signs and symptoms of lead poisoning including anemia, muscle pain, bluish-black line at gingival margin, and mental retardation.

➤ Assure client with toxic levels receives chelation therapy using edetate calcium disodium to promote excretion of lead.

➤ Encourage fluids to prevent hemoconcentration of lead.

➤ Evaluate other lab results such as porphyrins and urine delta-aminolevulinic acid (ALA).

Educate Your Client and the Family

➤ If your client has industrial or occupational lead exposure, explain the importance of having frequent blood tests to monitor the amount of lead in the blood.

➤ Inform your client that any adult with occupationally elevated levels (greater than 30 mg/dL) cannot return to the work site until levels fall below 30 mg/dL. This is a standard set by the Occupational Safety and Health Administration, which requires the worker to be compensated while unable to work.

➤ Teach parents that children may not have symptoms of lead poisoning but still receive damage to their brain. Reinforce the importance of having blood levels regularly monitored.

➤ If the level is elevated, tell your client to drink plenty of fluid to help eliminate lead through the urine.

➤ Assist parents in contacting the public health department to help them investigate environmental sources of lead.

➤ Tell parents how to limit their children's lead exposure. Suggestions include giving the child something to chew on that does not contain lead paint, providing drinking water that does not come from lead pipes, and keeping children away from chipping paint or dust that may contain lead.

➤ Explain that food must be stored in lead-free containers and that glazed pottery should not be used for food unless known to be lead-free.

Legionella Pneumophilia, Culture
lee jun el ah • **noo** moe fil ya • kul chur
(*Legionella* Culture, Legionnaires' Disease)

Normal Findings
Negative culture

What This Test Will Tell You
This culture diagnoses Legionnaires' disease by testing for the gram-negative bacillus *Legionella pneumophilia,* which causes acute respiratory infection and pneumonia. It is not transmitted from person to person. The bacteria, which is in soil, lakes, reservoirs, and streams, enters plumbing and air conditioning systems. The aerosolized bacteria is transmitted to humans through such devices as showers, whirlpools, air conditioners, or air-cooling towers. The bacteria has been isolated in blood, sputum, pleural fluid, bronchial washings, and lung tissue.

Abnormal Findings

A positive culture may reveal Legionnaires' disease.

Interfering Factors

➤ Anesthetic agents and saline used when obtaining bronchial washings may dilute the organism, causing difficulties in culturing the organism.

NURSING CONSIDERATIONS

Prepare Your Client

➤ Explain that this test is to help diagnose a specific infection of the lungs called Legionnaires' disease.

➤ Obtain a history from your client including possible environments where the bacillus may have been contracted, such as hotels or institutional showers.

➤ Teach the client how to collect a sputum for culture. The best time to obtain a sputum culture is early morning. Instruct your client to brush teeth and rinse mouth before obtaining the specimen to decrease the amount of contaminating flora.

➤ Instruct your client to inform you as soon as a specimen is collected so you can transport it to the lab.

Perform Procedure

➤ Collect the sputum culture. Transport the specimen to the lab as soon as possible after collection to prevent overgrowth of oral flora.

Care After Test

➤ Assess your client's respiratory status. Clinical manifestations of Legionnaires' disease include myalgia, headache, fever, chills, nonproductive cough, and pleuritic chest pain. Respiratory failure is a major complication.

➤ Assess your client's ability to care for self. Instruct your client to take adequate rest periods between activities.

➤ Administer oxygen therapy as ordered for respiratory distress.

➤ Evaluate other tests such as pulmonary function tests, blood cultures, chest x-rays, and arterial blood gases.

Educate Your Client and the Family

➤ Instruct your client to take the prescribed antibiotic therapy until it is gone. Treatment usually includes erythromycin and rifampin. Observe for side effects associated with antibiotic therapy.

➤ Teach your client coughing and deep breathing exercises.

➤ Inform your client about the importance of keeping follow-up appointments.

Leucine Aminopeptidase

loo seen • am in noe pep tie dase
(LAP, Arylamidase, Amino Acid Arylamidase)

Normal Findings

ADULT, CHILD, AND ELDERLY
Male: 80–200 U/mL
Female: 75–185 U/mL

Pregnant: Values may be normally increased. However, values are very elevated in pre-eclamptic pregnancies.

NEWBORN

Values over 500 U/L in an infant may suggest biliary atresia.

What This Test Will Tell You

This blood test evaluates the source of liver dysfunction. Leucine aminopeptidase (LAP) is a proteolytic enzyme that is produced in the liver and found mainly in the small intestine, pancreas, and liver. It is often used to make a differential diagnosis in cases of elevated alkaline phosphatase (ALP). The levels of this enzyme tend to parallel serum alkaline phosphatase, with the exception that LAP levels remain normal in bone disease. It is best used as an indicator for biliary obstruction. This test is not frequently ordered.

Abnormal Findings

▲ INCREASED LEVELS may indicate obstructive hepatobiliary disease including tumors and cholestasis, severe pre-eclamptic pregnancy, hepatitis, hepatic ischemia, hepatic necrosis, cirrhosis, metastatic carcinoma involving liver or pancreas, biliary atresia, or pancreatitis.

Interfering Factors

➤ Oral contraceptives (estrogens, progesterones), chlorpromazine, estrogens, and morphine may increase results.

➤ Hemolysis of specimen may interfere with results.

NURSING CONSIDERATIONS

Prepare Your Client

➤ Explain that this test is used with other tests to check how well the liver is working.

Perform Procedure

➤ Collect 5–10 mL of venous blood in a red-top tube.

➤ Observe the venipuncture site closely for hematoma formation or bleeding. Coagulopathies are common in liver disease. Apply a pressure dressing to the venipuncture site.

Care After Test

➤ Assess client for unusual bruising or prolonged bleeding from venipuncture site. Delayed clotting is a complication of severely impaired liver function.

➤ Assess skin, sclera of eyes for jaundice and note findings.

➤ Consult with a registered dietician to design a high-calorie, well-balanced diet. People with advanced liver disease have poor absorption of nutrients due to decreased bile flow into the intestines. As appropriate, reduce sodium or protein in the diet if edema and ascites, or increased ammonia levels are present.

➤ Evaluate other liver function tests such as aspartate aminotransferase (AST), alanine aminotransferase (ALT), direct and indirect bilirubin levels, alkaline phosphatase, serum ammonia, and prothrombin time.

Educate Your Client and the Family

➤ Instruct the client and family to report any jaundice—yellow discoloration of skin or whites of eyes.

➤ As appropriate, instruct client and family on a high-calorie, well-balanced diet. If sodium restrictions or protein restrictions are indicated, assist client and family to choose dietary selections with these limitations.

➤ Clients with impaired liver function have prolonged bleeding times. Instruct the client and family on safety measures such as electric razors, non-skid shoes, and soft toothbrushes.

> Instruct the client and family to report prolonged or unusual bleeding or bruising. They should report very dark colored or tarry stools; esophageal varices are a complication of liver disease.

Leukoagglutinin
loo koe ah gloo tih nin
(White Cell Antibodies)

Normal Findings
All ages: Negative

What This Test Will Tell You
This blood test detects antibodies that react with white blood cells. These reactions are responsible for some of the febrile, non-hemolytic responses that can occur with blood transfusions. With the detection of these antibodies, the primary health care provider then knows to transfuse only with leukocyte-poor blood.

This study is performed after a reaction occurs when compatible blood has been given, when blood containing leukoagglutinins is infused, or when the donor's plasma contains an antibody that reacts with recipient's white blood cells. This reaction results in a clinical syndrome of fever, dyspnea, cough, pulmonary infiltrates, and occasionally cyanosis and hypertension. This type of reaction must be differentiated from hemolytic reactions before further transfusions can be safely administered.

Abnormal Findings
▲ INCREASED LEVELS may indicate the presence of leukoagglutinins and the potential for blood transfusion reactions.

■ ACTION ALERT!
Severe blood transfusion reactions can occur if the client's or donor's blood possesses leukoagglutinins. If a transfusion reaction occurs, stop the transfusion immediately and infuse a minimal rate of normal saline to maintain vascular access while notifying the primary health care provider and preparing for emergency medical and nursing intervention if required.

Interfering Factors
> Dextran infusion
> Intravenous contrast material administration

NURSING CONSIDERATIONS
Prepare Your Client
> Explain that this test is to check the blood for proteins that can react badly with white blood cells found in blood transfusions.
> Obtain a thorough health history including prior blood transfusions and any adverse reactions. Clients who have had previous pregnancies as well as tissue or organ transplants are also at increased risk for forming leukoagglutinins.

Perform Procedure
> Collect 10 mL of venous blood in a red-top tube.
> Include on the laboratory slip any

suggestive health history including the number of pregnancies, organ or tissue transplants, and prior blood transfusions.

Care After Test

➤ Support the client emotionally whose life may depend on blood transfusions.

➤ Observe carefully for signs and symptoms of blood transfusion reactions including fever, chills, headache, nausea, vomiting, nonproductive cough, hypotension, hypertension, chest pain, dyspnea, skin rash, back pain, flushing, hematuria, tachycardia, or cyanosis. If these symptoms occur, stop the transfusion immediately and keep the vein accessible by infusing normal saline slowly. Notify the primary health care provider and the blood bank.

Monitor vital signs closely and prepare to administer emergency life support in severe reactions.

➤ Review related tests such as type and crossmatch.

Educate Your Client and the Family

➤ Teach your client that fever reactions can be decreased by treating all blood transfusions to remove the white blood cells. This is accomplished by using special blood filters and/or by irradiating the blood prior to transfusion.

➤ Teach the client that they must notify health care personnel about a positive leukoagglutinin test prior to any blood or blood product transfusion. A medical alert card or jewelry is recommended.

Leukocyte Alkaline Phosphatase Stain

loo koe site • al kah lin • foss fah tase • stane
(LAP)

Normal Findings

All ages: 30–130 units of precipitated dye/neutrophils; each laboratory will set specific norms.

Pregnant: The values will be elevated, especially in third trimester, because alkaline phosphatase is present in the placental tissue.

What This Test Will Tell You

This blood test differentiates chronic granulocytic leukemia from leukemoid or myeloid reaction resulting from infection, pregnancy, or estrogen therapy. A leukemoid or myeloid reaction is an elevation in white blood cell count (leukocytosis) that can resemble leukemia. This test

measures the presence of the enzyme alkaline phosphatase in the cytoplasm of neutrophilic granulocytes. Low to negative concentrations of the enzyme will be found in the leukemic leukocytes and a high concentration will be found in normal white blood cells. This test is used to support a diagnosis rather than being a definitive diagnostic test.

Abnormal Findings

▲ INCREASED LEVELS may indicate polycythemia vera, myelofibrosis, neutrophilic leukemoid reaction, infection, chronic inflammation, Hodgkin's disease, thrombocytopenia, or pregnancy.

▼ DECREASED LEVELS may indicate chronic myelogenous leukemia, acute or chronic granulocytic leukemia, paroxysmal nocturnal hemoglobinuria, aplastic anemia, infectious mononucleosis, idiopathic thrombocytopenia purpura, sarcoidosis, or granulocytopenia.

Interfering Factors
➤ Pregnancy

NURSING CONSIDERATIONS

Prepare Your Client
➤ Explain that this test is to determine the reason there are too many white blood cells in the blood.

Perform Procedure
➤ Collect 7 mL in a green-top tube, or perform a finger stick.
➤ Some laboratories may only require a peripheral finger stick to obtain a smear.
➤ Observe the venipuncture site closely for hematoma formation or bleeding. Coagulopathies may occur in leukemias. Apply a pressure dressing to the venipuncture site.

Care After Test
➤ Assess for the psychosocial needs of the client and family including values, beliefs, resources, and coping ability.
➤ Refer client and family to a cancer support group if results are positive.
➤ Assess for the client's ability to cope with changes in body image such as weight loss or gain, loss of hair, changes in body functions, decreased sexual function, and role changes.
➤ Refer to social services to assist with the financial and economic impact of cancer.
➤ Consult with a registered dietician

for a client with anorexia, weight loss, or special dietary needs.
➤ Provide the client opportunities to have control over care issues such as times for treatment, settings for care, and presence of significant others.
➤ Assess carefully for chronic and acute pain. Obtain pain management consultation if indicated.
➤ Assess for signs and symptoms of infection such as chills, fever, and drop in the absolute neutrophil count. Institute precautions to protect the client, such as no fresh fruits or vegetables. Remove fresh flowers and plants, and enforce good handwashing.
➤ Assess oral mucous membranes for signs and symptoms of stomatitis. Routinely give oral hygiene care.
➤ Develop and constantly update a teaching plan for the learning needs of the client and family related to diagnosis, testing, therapy, and home care.
➤ Assess the client for signs and symptoms such as bleeding from injection sites, petechia, or ecchymosis, occult blood, and decreasing platelet count related to increased risk for bleeding.
➤ Clients with impaired bone marrow function may have prolonged bleeding times. Institute safety measures such as electric razors, nonskid shoes, no intramuscular injections, no rectal temperatures, and soft toothbrushes.
➤ Encourage verbalization of fears related to cancer, prognosis, treatment, and death.
➤ Assess for occult gastrointestinal bleeding with routine stool guaiac testing. Coagulopathies may be a complication of leukemia.
➤ Review related tests such as white blood cell count with differential,

platelet count, hemoglobin, and bone marrow biopsy.

Educate Your Client and the Family

➤ Answer questions and provide emotional support until result of test is known.

➤ Inform client and family that the test result will help to support a diagnosis rather than being a diagnostic test.

➤ When white blood cells are low, teach client how to avoid infections and to prevent injury.

Lipase, Serum

lie pase • see rum

Normal Findings

ADULT AND ADOLESCENT
Values vary with methodology used.
Shihalsi/Bishop assay: 4–24 U/L
<200 U/L with triolein
<160 U/L with olive oil
20–180 IU/L
NEWBORN
9–105 IU/L
CHILD
20–136 IU/L
ELDERLY
Values are in the lower range of the adult values due to the decreased production of lipase from the pancreas.

What This Test Will Tell You

This blood test aids in the diagnosis of acute pancreatitis and differentiates acute pancreatitis from an acute abdominal disorder that may require surgery. Lipase is a pancreatic enzyme that changes fats and triglycerides into fatty acids and glycerol. The destruction of pancreatic cells, as with acute pancreatitis, releases large amounts of lipase into the blood. In acute pancreatitis the serum lipase level begins to rise within 2–6 hours, peaks in 12–30 hours, and will remain elevated up to 14 days. Lipase levels remain elevated

longer than serum amylase levels in acute pancreatitis.

Abnormal Findings

▲INCREASED LEVELS may indicate acute, recurrent, or chronic pancreatitis; pancreatic malignancy; pancreatic trauma; pancreatic pseudocyst; biliary disease such as cholelithiasis or cholecystitis; hepatic disease such as cirrhosis; diabetes mellitus; peritonitis; strangulated or infarcted bowel; gastric malignancy or perforation; or renal failure.

▼DECREASED LEVELS may indicate late pancreatic cancer or hepatitis.

ACTION ALERT!

High lipase levels are indicative of acute pancreatitis or pancreatic duct obstruction, which can lead to life-threatening complications such as adult respiratory distress syndrome.

Interfering Factors

➤ Food eaten within 8 hours of the test may interfere with the test results.

➤ The presence of calcium ions and hemoglobin may cause a decrease in the serum lipase level.

➤ Endoscopic retrograde cholangiopancreatography (ERCP) may increase lipase activity.

➤ Traumatic venipuncture can decrease lipase activity.

➤ Hemolysis of the specimen may alter test results.

➤ Drugs that may increase levels include codeine, morphine, meperidine, cholinergics, bethanechol, secretin, heparin, indomethacin, and methacholine.

➤ Protamine and calcium may decrease levels.

➤ Heavy metals, quinine, diisopropylphosphorofluoridate or ethylene diaminotetracetate (EDTA) may alter the test results.

NURSING CONSIDERATIONS

Prepare Your Client

➤ Explain that this test is important to see if there is a problem in a major gland of the body called the pancreas.

➤ Restrict food and fluids for 8–12 hours prior to the test.

➤ Consult with the primary health care provider about restricting the use of narcotics for 24 hours prior to sampling, due to their effects on smooth muscle and therefore gastrointestinal function. Explore alternative analgesics.

Perform Procedure

➤ Collect a 7-mL venous specimen in a red-top tube.

Care After Test

➤ Determine the client's level of pain, the specific location, and the duration of pain.

➤ Evaluate the effectiveness of pain relief methods, including response to pharmacologic agents. Collaborate with the primary health care provider to assure the client is receiving adequate pain control.

➤ If pancreatitis is present, restrict the client to bed rest and promote quiet and rest to decrease the client's metabolic rate and gastrointestinal stimulation, which will reduce abdominal pain.

➤ Evaluate the client's history for indications of alcohol abuse, which is often associated with pancreatitis. Refer to alcohol rehabilitation programs as indicated.

➤ Consult with a registered dietician for dietary planning as indicated.

➤ Evaluate other diagnostic tests such as serum amylase, computed tomography of the abdomen, ultrasound of the abdomen, serum calcium, serum magnesium, urine amylase, blood indices, serum carotene, chemistry profile, CBC, gamma-glutamyl transpeptidase, fasting glucose, lipid profile, serum triglycerides, serum trypsin, and stool for trypsin.

Educate Your Client and the Family

➤ If lipase levels are elevated and the client is found to have pancreatitis, instruct the client to avoid alcohol as it may lead to recurrent episodes of pancreatitis.

➤ Instruct the client to notify the primary health care provider of episodes of acute pain, jaundice, clay-colored stools, or darkened urine.

➤ Instruct the client to avoid caffeine, alcohol, and gas-forming foods (cabbage, broccoli, beans, etc.), which can exacerbate symptoms of abdominal pain, bloating, and cramping.

Lipids, Fecal

lip ids • fee kuhl

(Fecal Fat Test, Quantitative Fecal Fat, Fat Absorption, Quantitative Stool Fat Determination, Fat in Stool)

Normal Findings

RETENTION COEFFICIENT

All ages: ≥ 95%

QUANTITATIVE TEST

Adult, 60 g fat/day diet: 2–7 g/24 hours (SI units: <24 mmol/24 hours)

Adult, fat-free diet: <4 g/24 hours (SI units: <14 mmol/24 hours)

Newborn, breastfed: <1 g/24 hours (SI units: <4 mmol/24 hours)

Child, up to 6 years old: <2 g/24 hours (SI units: <7 mmol/24 hours)

RANDOM TEST

Adult: <60 droplets of fat/microscopic field

What This Test Will Tell You

This stool test aids in the diagnosis of conditions causing steatorrhea, usually resulting from malabsorption or digestive disorders. Fat content is determined by measuring the amount of fat excreted in the feces. In the healthy person most of the dietary fat is absorbed in the small intestines; however, all clients will excrete some fat in the stool from the desquamation of the mucosal cells in the small intestines. Deficiencies of bile acids or pancreatic enzymes, as well as abnormalities of the intestinal lining, will result in the increased excretion of fat in the feces.

There are two methods for collection. The random method is inexpensive, quick, simple, and less unpleasant than the 72-hour collection of stool, but it also detects triglycerides and lipolytic by-products. The 72-hour collection technique has been found to be more accurate in the measurement of fatty acids. Also, with the 72-hour collection of stool, the fat malabsorption can be assessed and the stool volume recorded.

Abnormal Findings

Any value >7 g/24 hours may indicate malabsorption or digestive problems and will result in steatorrhea (fat in the stool). Most clients with nutritionally important fat malabsorption exhibit values of at least 12 g/24 hours. Massive fat wasting occurs if the values are >60 g/day.

▲INCREASED LEVELS may indicate cystic fibrosis, pancreatic disease (cancer, chronic pancreatitis, enzyme deficiency), celiac disease, ingestion of mineral oil or castor oil, diarrhea, enteritis, hepatobiliary disease, postoperative bowel resection, bile salt deficiency, sprue, Whipple's disease, beta-lipoprotein deficiency, hypogammaglobulinemia, lymphoma, Zollinger-Ellison syndrome, regional ileitis, scleroderma, or gastrointestinal disease from radiation injury.

▼DECREASED LEVELS may indicate inadequate dietary intake of fat or be clinically insignificant.

Interfering Factors

➤ Cathartics may interfere with accurate measurement of fecal fat content because they decrease the time required for fat absorption in the small intestines.

➤ Use of glycerin suppositories, castor oil, or other laxatives will produce a false positive result.

➤ Barium, bismuth, and enemas interfere with accuracy of results.

➤ Medications including colchicine, antibiotics, calcium carbonate, alcohol, aluminum hydroxide, bisacodyl, and azathioprine may interfere with digestion of fats and therefore affect test results.

➤ If the stool specimen for the random test is obtained by digital examination, a glove lubricant may produce a false positive test result.

➤ Dietetic, low-calorie mayonnaise interferes with accuracy of results.

➤ When collecting the 72-hour stool specimen, use of coffee cans, plastic bags, or wax-coated paper containers will interfere with test results.

➤ Accidental disposal of stool or contamination with urine, menses, or other material may interfere with the results.

NURSING CONSIDERATIONS

Prepare Your Client

➤ Explain that this test is to measure the amount of fat in the stool to see if problems exist in how the body uses or eliminates fat.

➤ Instruct the client to consume at least 50–150 grams per day of dietary fat for 2–6 days before the stool collection and throughout the test. The diet should also include 100 grams of protein and 180 grams of carbohydrate. If needed, consult with a registered dietician to assist the client in achieving this level of dietary fat intake.

➤ Avoid the use of suppositories, lubricants, or mineral oil in the perianal or genital area for 3 days prior to the test and during the test.

➤ If the client is collecting stool for quantitative analysis (72-hour collection), prepare a large ($1/2$–1 gallon)

plastic or metal container with a tight-fitting lid and a method of refrigeration for the specimen during the test.

➤ Instruct your client in the appropriate procedure for stool collection.

➤ Instruct the client to record date and time each specimen is collected during the 72-hour collection.

Perform Procedure

RANDOM TEST

➤ Have the client defecate into a dry, clean bedpan or toilet seat container and transfer the stool to a clean stool specimen container.

➤ Obtain the stool specimen from the diaper of the infant or incontinent client. Be sure the stool does not contain urine.

➤ The random method is performed by obtaining a small amount of stool from a single specimen, staining the specimen with Sudan III stain, and observing the specimen microscopically before and after its treatment with acetic acid and heating.

QUANTITATIVE TEST (72–HOUR COLLECTION)

➤ Collect all stool in a dry, clean bedpan or toilet seat container. Using a wooden tongue blade, place the specimen into the large metal or plastic container supplied for stool collection.

➤ Maintain refrigeration of the stool specimen during the test.

➤ Send the specimen to the lab at the completion of the 72-hour collection time.

➤ If the lab analysis is not to be performed within 24 hours of the test completion, freeze the specimen or store it on dry ice.

Care After Test

➤ With elevated results, monitor the client's fluid and electrolyte balance to assess for depletion secondary to diarrhea.

➤ Monitor the client's skin for breakdown in the perianal area if the client has steatorrhea (fatty stools).

➤ Monitor color, consistency, and amount of stool. Fatty stools appear foamy, greasy, soft, and are very foul-smelling.

➤ With gallbladder disease, severe steatorrhea, or cystic fibrosis, instruct the client and family on a low-fat diet.

➤ After a total gastrectomy, instruct the client on a high-protein, high-calorie diet with small, frequent meals.

➤ Lactose-free or restricted diets may be indicated for the client with a lactase deficiency.

➤ Gluten-free diets may be indicated as well for the client with celiac sprue.

➤ Consult with a registered dietician to assist family and client in meeting special dietary needs.

➤ Review related tests such as triolein breath test, serum carotene, stool nitrogen levels, and stool determination of meat fibers.

Educate Your Client and the Family

➤ If the client is experiencing steatorrhea (fatty stool), instruct them to cleanse the perianal area thoroughly after each stool as the stool can irritate the skin.

➤ Encourage the use of a soothing emollient or protectant cream for the perianal area if skin irritation exists.

➤ If the test results are elevated, instruct the client in the prescribed diet and/or medications.

Lipoproteins

lie poe proe teens

(High-Density Lipoproteins, HDL, Low-Density Lipoproteins, LDL, Very Low Density Lipoproteins, VLDL)

Normal Findings

Reference values vary greatly with geographic location, age, gender, diet, method of testing, and other variables. The following are only guidelines. Check with your own laboratory for normal values.

HIGH-DENSITY LIPOPROTEINS (HDL)

Males: Average of 45 mg/dL or 24%–40% mass fraction of total lipoprotein

Females: Average of 55 mg/dL or 24%–40% mass fraction of total lipoprotein

At least 20% of the total cholesterol

level should be comprised of HDL. Ideally, HDL comprises 30% of the total cholesterol level.

LOW-DENSITY LIPOPROTEINS (LDL)

60–185 mg/dL or 28%–53% mass fraction of total lipoprotein

VERY LOW DENSITY LIPOPROTEINS (VLDL)

Up to 50% mass fraction of total lipoproteins

PREGNANT

Levels may be increased.

ELDERLY

Levels may be higher.

What This Test Will Tell You

This blood test evaluates the risk for coronary artery and peripheral vascular disease more specifically than the total cholesterol test by measuring specific lipoproteins in the blood. The test measures the blood levels of high-density lipoproteins (HDL), low-density lipoproteins (LDL), and very low density lipoproteins (VLDL). These specific lipoproteins along with total cholesterol and triglycerides often compose a lipid profile study.

High-density lipoproteins are often referred to as the "good cholesterol." Elevated HDL values are associated with a *lower* risk of coronary artery and peripheral vascular disease. HDL may protect vessels by removing excess cholesterol and preventing it from being deposited on vessel walls. HDL levels can be enhanced by exercise and moderate alcohol consumption.

Low-density lipoproteins are often referred to as the "bad cholesterol." Elevated LDL values are associated with a *higher* risk of coronary artery and peripheral vascular disease. LDL may be responsible for the deposition of cholesterol in vessel walls. LDL levels can be reduced by decreasing fat intake, especially from animal sources. The body manufactures cholesterol, however, independent of dietary intake.

Very low density lipoproteins are the main carrier for triglycerides. Elevated VLDL levels are associated with a *higher* risk of coronary artery and peripheral vascular disease.

Abnormal Findings

▲ INCREASED LEVELS *of LDL and VLDL* may indicate coronary artery disease, peripheral vascular disease, or hyperlipidemia.

▲ INCREASED LEVELS *of HDL* may indicate low risk for vessel disease, hepatitis, biliary disease, or vigorous exercise.

▼ DECREASED LEVELS *of LDL and VLDL* may indicate malnutrition, malabsorption syndromes, or effectiveness of antilipemic medications.

▼ DECREASED LEVELS *of HDL* may indicate risk for atherosclerotic vessel disease or inadequate exercise.

██████ ACTION ALERT!

HDL levels less than 35 mg/dL and/or LDL levels greater than 160 mg/dL may indicate relatively high risk for development of coronary artery and peripheral vascular disease.

Interfering Factors

➤ Medications such as oral contraceptives, phenothiazines, antilipemics, steroids, aspirin, and some antibiotics can cause increased levels.

➤ Antilipemics can cause lower levels.

➤ Recent exercise that is not routine.

➤ Recent increase or decrease in dietary fat/caloric intake.

➤ Alcohol consumption within 24 hours of the test decreases HDL levels.

➤ Smoking can cause decreased HDL levels.

➤ Using a collection tube with an anticoagulant (purple, green, or blue top) can alter results.

➤ Contrast material.

NURSING CONSIDERATIONS

Prepare Your Client

➤ Explain that this test will help determine the risk for heart disease or a heart attack, or blockage of blood vessels.

> Explain that you will need to draw blood from the vein for the test. Explain the venipuncture process clearly.

> Tell the client that foods and medications cannot be taken for 12–14 hours before the test is done. Water is permitted.

> Advise the client not to make any drastic changes in normal diet for 2 weeks preceding the blood sampling.

Perform Procedure

> Collect 5–10 mL of venous blood in a 10–15 mL red-top tube.

Care After Test

> Evaluate the client's diet for amount and sources of dietary fat.

> Evaluate the client's history for coronary and vascular disease. Especially note pain in the legs with walking, chest pain, and family deaths from heart attacks.

> Evaluate regular activity patterns for high-risk sedentary patterns.

> Evaluate other tests such as cholesterol and triglycerides.

Educate Your Client and the Family

> Explain that this test is important in determining the risk of heart disease and heart attacks.

> Teach the client with elevated cholesterol the need to reduce fat intake from animal and vegetable sources. Total fat intake should not be more than 30% of the required daily calories. Refer to a registered dietician as indicated.

> Emphasize foods that are part of a heart-healthy diet, rather than dwelling on foods that are not.

> Stress the importance of regularly scheduled exercise.

> Assist the client who weighs more than the ideal body weight to choose a reduced fat and calorie diet that incorporates personal food preferences. Be particularly attuned to including ethnic foods that the client may value.

> Emphasize to the client that there are risk factors they can control such as diet, exercise, weight, and smoking. Risk factors such as gender, family history, and diabetes cannot be eliminated, but can be minimized by addressing controllable risk factors.

Liver Biopsy, Percutaneous

lihv ur • **bie** op see • pur kyu **tay** nee us
(Needle Liver Biopsy)

Normal Findings

Normal liver pathology report: normal hepatocytes supported by a reticulin framework. Absence of cirrhosis, inflammation, infection, cysts, tumors, and abnormal vascularity.

What This Test Will Tell You

This microscopic tissue analysis diagnoses primary hepatic disease, infectious diseases of the liver, and malignancies, or monitors for rejection following transplantation. This test is indicated when less invasive means of diagnosis have failed to identify the reasons for hepatomegaly, elevated hepatic enzymes, or jaundice. Liver biopsies may also be indicated to evaluate systemic disease such as metastatic cancer and autoimmune diseases.

Abnormal Findings

Abnormalities may indicate hepatitis, biliary atresia, cholestatic liver disease, cirrhosis, malignancy, abscess, cyst, rejection (after transplantation), or systemic autoimmune disease.

ACTION ALERT!

Hemorrhage is a potential complication of percutaneous liver biopsy. Coagulation testing must precede liver biopsy. Monitor for and report any signs or symptoms of tachycardia, orthostatic hypotension, vertigo, weakness, or a drop in hematocrit or hemoglobin following this test.

Interfering Factors

➤ Failure to obtain an adequate amount of tissue, failure to obtain tissue from the affected area, or failure to place the tissue in the proper preservative may result in inadequate results.

Contraindications

➤ Infection in right upper quadrant of abdomen or right lower lobe of lungs, due to risk of infection spread.
➤ This procedure should be performed cautiously in a postoperative liver transplant client. The exact position of the liver and its blood supply should be ascertained by ultrasound prior to biopsy.
➤ This procedure is contraindicated in a client with a platelet count below 100,000; a prothrombin time greater than 15 seconds and/or a bleeding time longer than 8 minutes; a vascular tumor; or hepatic angiomas. In any of these situations an open liver biopsy should be performed under general anesthesia in the operating room.
➤ Obstructive jaundice, because leakage through biopsy site may occur due to pressure.

Potential Complications

➤ Hemorrhage
➤ Bile peritonitis
➤ Pneumothorax
➤ Infection
➤ Bowel perforation

NURSING CONSIDERATIONS

Prepare Your Client

➤ Explain that a small needle will be used to obtain a sample of liver tissue to help diagnose problems with the liver, or how well treatments are working.
➤ Explain that the test will be performed under intravenous and/or local sedation. Instruct the client there may be a brief burning sensation when the local anesthetic is administered.
➤ Restrict food and fluids for 4–8 hours before the test.
➤ Make sure baseline hematology studies have been performed, and are within acceptable limits. Record these results in the chart.
➤ Ensure that an informed consent is obtained, because of the possible complications associated with this procedure.
➤ Confirm that adults and older children have voided prior to the procedure.
➤ Record baseline vital signs, including assessment of capillary refill.
➤ Start peripheral intravenous (IV) line to be utilized for procedure.

Perform Procedure

Nurses do not perform this procedure, but should understand the process to better support and monitor the client after the procedure.

The client is placed in a supine position or left lateral position with the right hand under or above the head. Intravenous sedation is given as appropriate. Monitor vital signs according to your institution's guidelines.

The liver is percussed for point of maximum dullness and the biopsy site is marked. Note: for post-liver-transplant client or person with questionable vasculature of the area, ultrasound or other imaging may be used to determine the best site for the biopsy. A local anesthetic is injected into the biopsy area.

The biopsy is performed using a special biopsy needle attached to a syringe containing a small amount of sterile normal saline. The biopsy needle is inserted into the tissue through the intercostal space at the pre-determined site. A cooperative client is asked to take a deep breath, exhale, and hold their breath at the end of expiration. At this point, the needle is quickly inserted into the liver while negative pressure is applied with the syringe, and tissue is obtained. The needle is quickly removed and pressure applied to the site.

Care After Test

➤ The client is to remain on their right side for 4 hours following the biopsy. This applies pressure to the site. Bed rest is recommended for 24 hours following the biopsy.

➤ Monitor vital signs closely, every 15 minutes for 2 hours, every 30 minutes for 2 hours, every hour for 4 hours and every 4 hours thereafter for 24 hours.

➤ In infants and children check hematocrit before biopsy and 4 hours, 8 hours, and 24 hours post-biopsy.

➤ Regular diet may be resumed following the procedure. If client was sedated, assure they are fully awake prior to resuming diet.

➤ Client may experience mild discomfort at the biopsy site. Medicate with analgesics as necessary.

➤ Observe client closely for signs of hypovolemic shock. Assess with vital signs, capillary refill (should be 3 seconds or less), drainage on dressing, and abdominal tenderness or discomfort.

➤ Monitor for signs and symptoms of a pneumothorax, which may include tachycardia, tachypnea, decreased breath sounds, dyspnea, chest pain, and shoulder pain.

➤ Consult with a registered dietician to design a high-calorie, well-balanced diet for a client with liver disease. As appropriate, reduce sodium or protein in the diet if edema or increased ammonia levels are present.

➤ For pediatric client, supply quiet activities to maintain bed rest.

➤ Review related tests such as alanine aminotransferase (ALT), aspartate aminotransferase (AST), coagulation studies, and serum bilirubin levels.

Educate Your Client and the Family

➤ Liver biopsies are usually performed early in the workup of a specific disease. Provide support to the client and family awaiting diagnosis, and educate as needed following diagnosis.

➤ For client with severely impaired liver function, instruct family to report unusual or increased bruising and tarry stools. Instruct them to use electric razors and non-skid shoes to avoid falls and injuries.

➤ As appropriate, instruct client and family on a high-calorie, well-balanced diet. If sodium restrictions or protein restrictions are indicated, assist client and family to choose dietary selections with these limitations.

Liver-Spleen Scan

liv ur • spleen • skan
(Radioisotope Liver Scanning, Dynamic Scintigraphy)

Normal Findings

Equal distribution of the radionuclide in both the liver and the spleen, indicating that the position, shape, and size of both organs is within normal limits

What This Test Will Tell You

This nuclear scanning test detects structural abnormalities of the liver or spleen but can also detect hepatocellular disease. A radionuclide, usually technetium (Tc) sulfide, and a gamma ray camera are used to detect focal diseases such as tumors, cysts, and abscesses as well as to screen for hepatic metastasis and demonstrate hepatomegaly, splenomegaly, and infarcts of the organs. Flow studies (dynamic scintigraphy) demonstrate the vascularity and perfusion of the liver and spleen or specific focal lesion. This type of scan is also useful after a liver transplant to evaluate for infarcts in organ vessels.

Abnormal Findings

Abnormalities may reveal a primary tumor, metastasis to the liver or spleen, cysts, abscesses, cirrhosis, chronic hepatitis, or infiltrative diseases of the organs (sarcoidosis, tuberculosis, amyloidosis).

Interfering Factors

➤ Barium present in the gastrointestinal tract near the upper quadrant of the abdomen will produce defects on the scan and can be mistaken for masses.

➤ Failure of the client to lie still during the scan may interfere with adequacy of recorded images.

Contraindications

➤ Pregnancy, due to radiation exposure of the fetus.

➤ This scan may fail to detect lesions smaller than 2 cm.

➤ Cirrhosis may result in a false positive result.

Potential Complications

➤ Rare allergic reaction to the radionuclide

NURSING CONSIDERATIONS

Prepare Your Client

➤ Explain that this test is to look at two important organs called the liver and spleen to make sure there are no structural defects or masses.

➤ Restrict food and fluids for 4–6 hours prior to the test only if sedation is to be used.

➤ Explain that an intravenous (IV)

infusion is used to administer the radionuclide. Explain the venipuncture process clearly.

➤ Tell your client the scan will take approximately 1 hour to perform and that they will be asked to lie in different positions so that all surfaces of the liver can be seen.

➤ Assure the client and family there is no need to take precautions against radiation exposure because only trace doses of the radioisotope are used.

Perform Procedure

Nurses do not perform this procedure but should understand the process to prepare the client and assist the physician. The client is taken to the nuclear medicine department and radionuclide is administered intravenously. After 15–30 minutes the abdomen is scanned with the client in the various positions. The client is asked to breathe deeply to evaluate the mobility and pliability of the liver; non-movement would suggest pathology. The client is observed closely for rare allergic reactions.

Care After Test

➤ Assess client for unusual bruising or prolonged bleeding from venipuncture site. Delayed clotting is a complication of severely impaired liver function.

➤ Encourage drinking fluids unless contraindicated.

➤ Institute safety precautions for client with confusion or altered level of consciousness.

➤ Assess skin, sclera of eyes for jaundice and note findings.

➤ Consult with a registered dietician to design a high-calorie, well-balanced diet. Clients with advanced liver disease have poor absorption of nutrients due to decreased bile flow into the intestines. As appropriate, reduce sodium or protein in the diet if edema and ascites, or increased ammonia levels are present.

➤ Evaluate other liver function tests such as aspartate aminotransferase (AST), direct and indirect bilirubin levels, alkaline phosphatase, serum ammonia, and prothrombin time.

Educate Your Client and the Family

➤ Instruct the client and family to report any jaundice, the yellow discoloration of skin or whites of eyes.

➤ As appropriate, instruct client and family on a high-calorie, well-balanced diet. If sodium or protein restrictions are indicated, teach client and family to make dietary selections with these limitations.

➤ Clients with impaired liver function have prolonged bleeding times. Instruct the client and family on safety measures such as electric razors, non-skid shoes, and soft toothbrushes.

➤ Instruct the client and family to report prolonged or unusual bleeding or bruising, which can be a complication of liver disease. Also tell them to report very dark colored or tarry stools, as esophageal varices are a complication of liver disease. Nosebleeds or blood in emesis should be reported.

➤ Explain to client and family that further testing may be needed to confirm or rule out a diagnosis. This scan cannot detect lesions smaller than 2 cm.

➤ Instruct client diagnosed with liver disease, if appropriate, to avoid over-the-counter medications not approved by their physician.

Liver Ultrasonography

liv ur • ul trah soe nah grah fee

(Liver Sonogram, Liver Echogram)

Normal Findings

Homogeneous, low-level echo pattern throughout the liver, interrupted only by different echo patterns for the vascular channels. No filling defects or dilation noted.

What This Test Will Tell You

This ultrasound test investigates jaundice of unknown etiology, unexplained hepatomegaly, or suspected metastatic tumors, or further evaluates results of other hepatobiliary scans such as liver-spleen scan and liver computed tomography. Ultrasonography can demonstrate abnormalities of the liver including size, shape, locations, cysts, tumors, abscesses, and filling or dilation defects.

Abnormal Findings

Abnormalities may reveal cirrhosis, hepatic cysts, abscesses, hematomas (intrahepatic or subcapsular), biliary atresia, metastatic tumors, hepatomas (adult), or hepatoblastomas (children).

Interfering Factors

➤ Obesity may interfere with transmission of ultrasound and image.

➤ Residual barium flatus in the gastrointestinal tract may interfere with visualization of structures.

➤ Inability to follow directions and hold breath may interfere with quality of imaging.

NURSING CONSIDERATIONS

Prepare Your Client

➤ Explain to your client or family that this test is a painless examination of an important organ in the body called the liver.

➤ Explain that this test is performed in the radiology department in a darkened room so the ultrasound pictures can be seen best. This test takes approximately 15–30 minutes to perform.

➤ Instruct your client to lie still during the exam. For small children, sedation may be necessary.

Perform Procedure

Nurses do not perform this procedure but should understand the process to prepare the client and assist the physician or ultrasonography technician. The client is placed in a supine position on the exam table. A water-soluble lubricant is applied either to the right side of the abdomen or to the surface of the transducer. Scans are taken at 1-cm intervals between the costal margins and longitudinally from the right border of the liver to the left. The client is asked to take in and hold a breath periodically as pictures are taken.

Care After Test

➤ Assess client for delayed clotting, which is a complication of severely impaired liver function.

➤ Remove transducer gel from the abdomen.

➤ Assess skin, sclera of eyes for jaundice and note findings.

➤ Consult with a registered dietician to design a high-calorie, well-balanced diet. Clients with advanced liver disease have poor absorption of nutrients due to decreased bile flow into the intestines. As appropriate, reduce sodium or protein in the diet if edema and ascites, or increased ammonia levels are present.

➤ Institute safety precautions for client with confusion or altered level of consciousness.

➤ Evaluate other liver function tests such as aspartate aminotransferase (AST), direct and indirect bilirubin levels, alkaline phosphatase, serum ammonia, and prothrombin time.

Educate Your Client and the Family

➤ Instruct the client and family to report any jaundice, the yellow discoloration of skin or whites of eyes, and any prolonged or unusual bleeding or bruising, increase in abdominal size, excessive weight gain, and dark or tarry stools.

➤ As appropriate, instruct client and family on a high-calorie, well-balanced diet. If sodium restrictions or protein restrictions are indicated, teach client and family to make dietary selections with these limitations.

➤ Clients with impaired liver function have prolonged bleeding times. Instruct the client and family on safety measures such as electric razors, non-skid shoes, and soft toothbrushes.

Long Bone X-Rays
lahng • bone • eks raze
(Bone X-Ray, Skeletal X-Ray)

Normal Findings
ADULT, PREGNANT, AND ELDERLY
No evidence of fracture, tumor, infection, or congenital abnormalities.

NEWBORN AND CHILD
A thin plate of cartilage occupies the area between the shaft and the ends to allow for growth (growth plate, epiphyseal plate).

ADOLESCENT
The plate of cartilage is usually calcified by age 17 and replaced by bone tissue.

What This Test Will Tell You
Radiographic examination of the long bones of the extremities evaluates the client's pain or discomfort as well as confirms suspected injury or disease. This test also provides a mechanism for studying growth patterns through serial (repeated at timed intervals) x-ray studies, usually of the wrist; to monitor the healing of fractures; and to identify fluid in the joints. This examination can accurately identify fractures, tumors, bone infection, and bone destruction. Abnormalities identified on x-ray frequently require more extensive diagnostic evaluations through radioisotope scans or biopsy.

Abnormal Findings
Abnormalities may indicate fractures, bone spurring from persistent arthritis, osteomyelitis, growth plate abnormalities, injury, cancer, vascular insufficiency, hormonal disturbance, infection, nutritional alter-

ations, genetic abnormalities, congenital abnormalities, or metabolic disturbances.

Interfering Factors

➤ Movement during the x-ray.
➤ Incorrect positioning of the client may lead to inaccurate findings.

Contraindications

➤ This test is contraindicated during the first trimester of pregnancy due to radiation exposure of the fetus, unless the value of the test outweighs the risks of exposure.

Potential Complications

➤ Further injury to bone during positioning.
➤ Birth defects, if done during the first trimester of pregnancy. The only time that it is considered safe for women of childbearing years to have x-rays is during the menses or 10–14 days following menses. A lead shield should be used.

NURSING CONSIDERATIONS

Prepare Your Client

➤ Explain that this procedure takes a picture that can be used to identify the cause of pain, to show broken bones, or to provide information about healing or growth patterns.
➤ Explain that it is important to remain still in the position arranged by the technician in order to obtain a clear and accurate film.
➤ Immobilize and support suspected fracture.

➤ Inform client that some pain or discomfort may be felt due to the positioning.
➤ Administer pain medication prior to the procedure if indicated by suspected fracture or other injury.

Perform Procedure

➤ The radiologic technician will take x-rays.
➤ Position client using supports.
➤ Continue to talk to children when they cannot see anyone. A parent, wearing a lead shield, may in some institutions be permitted to remain with small children.

Care After Test

➤ Evaluate physical assessments such as pain sensation, strength, and movement in injured extremity.
➤ Administer analgesics as indicated.
➤ Refer child with abnormal growth problems and their family for counseling as necessary.
➤ Evaluate the client's ability to perform activities of daily living. Refer to community health services as indicated for support in the home.
➤ Evaluate related tests, such as alkaline phosphatase, bone scans, serum calcium and phosphorus, and previous x-rays of same bone.

Educate Your Client and the Family

➤ Teach client and family methods of supporting injured extremity.
➤ Teach client necessary skills for maintaining appropriate activity restrictions. This may include use of crutches, overbed trapeze, transfer techniques, sling application.
➤ Refer for genetic information if a congenital abnormality is diagnosed.

Lumbar Puncture

lum bar • punk chur

(LP, Spinal Tap, Spinal Puncture)

Normal Findings

SPINAL FLUID PRESSURE

Adult: 70–180 cm H_2O

Child, infant: 50–100 cm H_2O

What This Test Will Tell You

This fluid aspiration and pressure monitoring test measures cerebrospinal fluid pressure and is used to obtain cerebrospinal fluid (CSF) for analysis in the laboratory and microbiology. The lumbar puncture (LP) may also be performed to inject dye into the spinal column for myelograms and to instill medications such as antibiotics and anesthetics. See *Cerebrospinal Fluid Analysis* for further information.

Cerebrospinal fluid (CSF) is produced in the ventricles of the brain and circulates throughout the brain and spinal cord. It is continually being produced and reabsorbed into the bloodstream. The spinal fluid helps to protect the brain and spinal cord and to supply oxygen and nutrients and remove waste products.

Abnormal Findings

▲INCREASED *spinal fluid pressure* may indicate meningitis, subarachnoid hemorrhage, mass lesions, cerebral edema, brain abscess, encephalitis, viral infections, or impaired CSF resorption.

▼DECREASED *spinal fluid pressure* may indicate leakage of CSF, dehydration, hypovolemia, or complete spinal subarachnoid block.

ACTION ALERT!

This test should not be performed in the presence of elevated intracranial pressure due to the potential for herniation of the brain and death.

Interfering Factors

➤ The client may be in a sitting position for the lumbar puncture; however, a spinal fluid pressure can only be obtained with the client in a recumbent position.

➤ Elevations can occur if the client tenses muscles, holds breath, or performs the Valsalva maneuver.

Contraindications

➤ Do not perform this when increased intracranial pressure is suspected. A rapid decrease in intracranial pressure secondary to the lumbar puncture and removal of cerebrospinal fluid may cause the brain to shift downward (herniate) into the spinal column. The herniation could cause serious damage to the vital centers in the medulla and result in neurological damage or death.

➤ Do not perform this test on a client with primary clotting defects such as thrombocytopenia because of the risk of extradural or subdural hematoma formation.

Potential Complications

➤ Infection
➤ Headache
➤ Nausea
➤ Dizziness
➤ Bleeding into the spinal column
➤ Neurologic injury or death from herniation

NURSING CONSIDERATIONS

Prepare Your Client

➤ Explain that this procedure is to measure the cerebrospinal fluid pressure and to obtain samples of fluid for analysis. If the lumbar puncture is necessary for the injection of dye or medications, explain the purpose.

➤ Explain that the physician will place a needle into the lower back and withdraw spinal fluid.

➤ Review the potential complications of the procedure and be sure the client has signed an informed consent.

➤ Assure the client that the needle is placed far below any spinal nerves into an empty space filled with fluid, not nerves.

➤ Explain the rationale for positioning as you place the client in the side-lying position with knees curled to the chest and arms wrapped around legs. The chin should be resting on the chest. Assist the client to maintain this position throughout the procedure.

➤ Explain that the physician will numb the lumbar region of the back before placing the lumbar puncture needle.

➤ Tell your client there is no need to restrict fluids or foods before the procedure.

Perform Procedure

Nurses do not usually perform the procedure but should understand the process to prepare the client and assist the physician. Sterile technique must be maintained throughout the procedure.

Place the client in the fetal position, and reassure the client throughout the procedure. Encourage the client to breathe slowly and deeply.

After the lumbar puncture needle is in the subarachnoid space, the client will need to straighten both legs for the initial pressure reading. The reading is taken with a manometer provided in the lumbar puncture tray. The manometer is attached to the LP needle via a three-way stopcock.

Approximately 3–5 mL of fluid will be collected in a series of tubes which must be numbered sequentially. Tube 1 may be contaminated with blood and may need to be discarded. Tube 2 is usually sent to the lab for analysis of glucose, protein, and cell count. Tube 3 is used for microbiology tests such as culture and smears. Send tubes to the lab immediately.

Care After Test

➤ Place a sterile dressing over the puncture site.

➤ Have client maintain a flat position for several hours after the LP.

➤ Assess vital signs for elevated systolic pressure, widened pulse pressure, and respiratory depression, which can signal increased intracranial pressure. Decreased blood pressure may indicate shock.

➤ Report a persistent severe headache to the primary health care provider because this may require a blood patch, or injection of the client's blood into the epidural space to act as a fibrin patch for CSF leakage.

➤ Assess for pain and medicate as ordered.

➤ In head-injured clients, assure any nasal drainage is evaluated for cerebrospinal fluid content. Do not suction nasally.

➤ Encourage fluids to assist the body in replacing CSF loss.

➤ Assess for signs and symptoms of complications including changes in mental status, changes in sensory perception of lower extremities, and neck rigidity.

➤ Evaluate related tests such as cerebrospinal fluid analysis.

Educate Your Client and the Family

➤ Instruct your client to remain flat for several hours after the lumbar puncture. Loss of spinal fluid from the LP and potential leakage of CSF from the puncture site may cause headaches. Risk of CSF leakage is minimized when the client remains in a recumbent position.

➤ If increased intracranial pressure is present, instruct client on importance of avoiding the Valsalva maneuver by not coughing, sneezing, straining with bowel movements, or bending. Instruct the client to use stool softeners, sneeze with mouth open, and avoid lifting.

L

Lung Biopsy
lung • bie op see

Normal Findings
No abnormal cells or tissue

What This Test Will Tell You

This microscopic examination uses a specimen of lung tissue analyzed by culture or cytologic examination to identify pulmonary lesions, granulomas, parenchymal changes, and the etiology of pleural effusions. The sample may be obtained through the chest wall (percutaneous lung biopsy), through fiber-optic bronchoscopy, or by open lung biopsy in the operating room, which entails a thoracotomy and general anesthesia. Lung biopsies are indicated when there is diffuse pulmonary disease of unknown etiology; when malignancy, infection, or parasitic infestation is suspected; and when other, less invasive tests such as chest x-ray, computed tomography scans, and sputum analyses are inconclusive.

Abnormal Findings

Abnormalities may indicate cancer; infection with bacteria, virus, fungus, or parasites; inflammatory disorders; granulomas; tuberculosis; sarcoidosis; or fibrosis.

ACTION ALERT!

Lung biopsies may result in bleeding into lung tissue, hemothorax, pneumothorax, and infection. Carefully assess respiratory function and report problems to the primary health care provider immediately. Have suction equipment immediately available.

Interfering Factors

➤ Improper specimen collection or contamination of specimen

➤ Refrigeration of specimen

➤ Excess time elapsed between specimen collection and inoculation of culture medium (maximum is 3 hours)

Contraindications

➤ Bleeding disorders.

➤ Lung hyperinflation, especially when bullae or cysts are suspected.

➤ Inability of the client to cooperate with the procedure because of respiratory insufficiency, confusion, agitation, or other reasons, may contraindicate percutaneous or bronchoscopic biopsies. The open biopsy procedure with general anesthesia may be used instead.

Potential Complications
➤ Pneumothorax
➤ Hemothorax
➤ Hemorrhage
➤ Intercostal nerve injury
➤ Infection
➤ Cardiopulmonary arrest

NURSING CONSIDERATIONS

Prepare Your Client
➤ Explain that the test is to obtain a sample of tissue from the lung to be examined for the presence of disease.
➤ Describe the procedure used to obtain the specimen (needle biopsy, bronchoscopy, or thoracotomy).
➤ Assess complete blood count and blood clotting studies prior to the procedure to determine if client is at high risk for developing complications such as hemorrhage and infection.
➤ Confirm that a signed informed consent has been obtained from the client.
➤ Tell the client that the procedure will be performed by a physician or advanced practice nurse and that results may not be available for 2 days.
➤ Instruct the client not to eat or drink for 6–8 hours prior to the procedure.
➤ Advise the client that a sedative may be administered prior to the procedure.
➤ If a percutaneous needle biopsy is planned, explain that the client must hold as still as possible and refrain from coughing to prevent perfora-

tion of the lung by the biopsy needle.
➤ Administer premedications if ordered, such as atropine to decrease secretions and sedatives.
➤ Provide a hospital gown or assist the client to disrobe above the waist (for percutaneous lung biopsy).

Perform Procedure
Nurses do not perform this procedure but should understand the process to prepare the client and assist the primary health care provider.

PERCUTANEOUS NEEDLE BIOPSY
Assist the client to a sitting position with the arms supported on a pillow on an overbed table. The procedure may be performed at the client's bedside or in the radiology department under fluoroscopy. Cleanse the needle insertion site with an antiseptic solution. The insertion site is infiltrated with local anesthesia. Remind the client to remain as still as possible and avoid coughing.

The biopsy needle is inserted through the chest wall into the selected intercostal space. The needle is then rotated to obtain the sample and the needle is withdrawn.

Apply pressure to the biopsy site. Place the sample in the appropriate container using aseptic technique. Dress the puncture site with a pressure bandage after bleeding ceases.

BRONCHOSCOPIC BIOPSY
Remove the client's dentures. Assist the client to a supine or semi-Fowler's position as indicated. Spray local anesthetic into the nose and throat.

A tube is passed through the mouth or nose or through an endotracheal tube if indicated. Spray more local anesthetic in the trachea to inhibit the cough reflex. The specimen is obtained from the appropriate lung area using a cutting forceps, needle, or bronchial brush. The tube is withdrawn slowly.

Observe the client during the procedure for signs of respiratory insufficiency or laryngospasm. Place the sample in the appropriate container using aseptic technique.

OPEN LUNG BIOPSY

Transport the client to the operating room, where general anesthesia is administered and the client is prepped and draped. With the client in a supine position, a small incision is made into the chest wall. A piece of lung tissue is obtained and the chest is then surgically closed. Chest tubes are inserted and used for about 24 hours to re-expand and drain the pleura. Place the sample obtained in the appropriate container using aseptic technique.

Care After Test

➤ Label specimen containers, indicating the site and method used to obtain the specimen, and transport to the laboratory or pathology department immediately.

➤ Closely monitor following the procedure for signs and symptoms of hemothorax, pneumothorax, infection, and hemorrhage.

➤ Maintain patency of any chest tubes.

➤ Observe for blood-tinged sputum and/or frank hemorrhage. Report immediately.

➤ Following a percutaneous needle biopsy or bronchoscopic biopsy, the client is placed in a semi-Fowler's position to assist in maximum lung ventilation.

➤ Following an open biopsy, the client is transported to the recovery room. Care and observation are the same as for anyone who has had a thoracotomy under general anesthesia.

➤ Monitor respiratory status closely for signs of hemo- or pneumothorax, such as dyspnea, tachypnea, cyanosis, and decreased breath sounds on the biopsy side.

➤ Obtain a chest x-ray if ordered to check for complications.

➤ Observe for signs of bleeding at the biopsy site and check vital signs every 15–30 minutes for 1–2 hours until stable. Note tachycardia, thready pulse, hypotension, etc.

➤ Assess the client's comfort level and administer analgesics if indicated.

➤ Resume fluids and food after the gag reflex has returned and been verified.

➤ Evaluate related tests such as chest x-ray, computed tomography scans, sputum cultures, and complete blood counts.

Educate Your Client and the Family

➤ Describe the nursing routine of closely monitoring vital signs and respiratory status.

➤ Instruct the client to report immediately any difficulty breathing, bleeding from the puncture site, or other discomforts.

➤ Describe any activity restrictions.

➤ Teach client and family about the diagnosed condition. Refer to support groups as indicated.

Lung Scan

lung • skan

(Ventilation Scan, Ventilation/Perfusion Scan, VPS, V/Q Scan, Pulmonary Scintiphotography)

Normal Findings

All ages:

Normally functioning lung tissue

Ventilation scan: Equal gas distribution, normal gas exchange

Perfusion scan: Normal pulmonary vasculature with uniform uptake pattern

What This Test Will Tell You

This nuclear scanning test is used to detect the percentage of normal lung function, to diagnose and locate pulmonary emboli, and to assess the pulmonary vascular supply by estimating regional pulmonary blood flow. In the perfusion portion of the scan, radioactive dye is injected intravenously and carried into the pulmonary vasculature. Decreased blood flow to any part of the lung is revealed by decreased radioactivity in that area. This may indicate pulmonary embolism. However, other lung diseases such as pneumonia, tuberculosis, and emphysema also cause a defect in pulmonary blood perfusion. Therefore, although the perfusion scan accurately identifies pathological areas, it is not specific for the cause.

In the ventilation portion of the scan, radioactive gas is inhaled to produce an image of the areas where ventilation is occurring. Ventilation images are compared with the perfusion images. If there are areas in which there is ventilation but little or no perfusion, a pulmonary embolus is suspected. If ventilation is diminished in the same area as the perfusion abnormality, pulmonary parenchymal disorders are suspected, such as pneumonia, atelectasis, emphysema, and effusion.

Because this test is limited in its diagnostic specificity, it should be correlated with other pulmonary tests, such as chest x-ray, computed tomography scan, pulmonary function tests, and blood gas studies. If pulmonary embolus is strongly suspected, pulmonary angiography should be performed.

Abnormal Findings

Abnormalities may indicate pulmonary embolism or infarction, pneumonia, atelectasis, emphysema, tumors, asthma, tuberculosis, pulmonary fibrosis, or bronchiectasis.

ACTION ALERT!

Assess clients carefully for allergic reaction to contrast material, including dyspnea, itching, urticaria, flushing, hypotension, and shock. Life-threatening anaphylactic reactions can occur and need to be recognized and treated immediately.

Interfering Factors

➤ Metal objects such as jewelry or cardiac electrodes in the x-ray field distort images.

➤ Client movement causes difficulty interpreting the image.

➤ Recent examinations with radionuclides may interfere with interpretation.

Contraindications

➤ Pregnancy or potential pregnancy, due to radiation exposure of the fetus.

➤ Nursing mothers. If the V/Q scan is deemed necessary, the mother is advised to stop nursing for 3–4 days postscan.

➤ History of allergy to radioisotopes.

Potential Complications

➤ Allergic reaction to the radioisotope.

➤ Potential damage to a fetus exists with any radionuclide exposure. However, the risk from a single scan is considered to be negligible.

NURSING CONSIDERATIONS

Prepare Your Client

➤ Explain that the test is to obtain a more detailed picture of the lungs and surrounding tissue, particularly the blood supply to the lungs, than is possible with a chest x-ray. The test usually takes about 1 hour, and is performed in the nuclear medicine department.

➤ Allay any fears the client may have about radioisotope procedures. Assure the client that only small doses of isotopes are used.

➤ Ensure that an informed consent has been signed.

➤ Obtain a history of allergies from the client. Notify the radiologist if the client reports previous allergic reaction to radioisotope substances.

➤ Advise the client that it is not necessary to fast prior to the test.

➤ Check to see if a recent chest x-ray is available for comparison with the scan.

➤ Instruct the client to remove clothing and jewelry above the waist and put on a hospital gown.

➤ Administer sedation, if ordered, for client who is unable to cooperate and lie still during the procedure.

Perform Procedure

Nurses do not perform this procedure but should understand the process to prepare the client and assist the physician. Assist the client onto the x-ray table. Establish intravenous access.

Observe for signs and symptoms of allergic reaction to the radioisotope. Report these to the primary health care provider immediately and prepare for a cardiopulmonary emergency.

PERFUSION SCAN

The radionuclide is injected slowly intravenously over several respiratory cycles; half with the client sitting up, the other half with the client supine. The client is positioned under the camera and scanning with the gamma ray detector is immediately begun. Views are obtained in the supine, prone, various lateral, and oblique positions.

VENTILATION SCAN

Instruct the client to inhale the mixture of air and radioactive gas through a face mask for several minutes. The scans are performed during and after breathing the gas. Observe for signs and symptoms of allergic reaction to the radioisotope. Report these to the primary health care provider immediately and prepare for a cardiopulmonary emergency.

CARE AFTER TEST

➤ Encourage increased fluid intake to expedite excretion of the radionuclide in the urine.

➤ No special radiation precautions are required.

➤ If pulmonary embolus is strongly suspected, assess the client closely for dyspnea, cyanosis, tachypnea, tachycardia, and hypotension. Intervene with oxygen administration and other treatments as indicated.

➤ Watch for delayed allergic response to the radionuclide.

➤ Evaluate related tests such as chest x-ray, computed tomography scan, pulmonary function tests, and arterial blood gases.

Educate Your Client and the Family

➤ Advise the client that they may resume their previous diet and activity level unless otherwise indicated.

➤ Inform the client that the test will be interpreted by the radiologist and results given to their primary health care provider.

➤ Refer client who smokes to smoking cessation programs.

➤ Teach client to pace activities.

Lupus Erythematosus Test

loo pus • ehr eh thee mah toe sus • test
(Lupus Erythematosus Cell Prep, LE Prep, LE Preparation, Lupus Erythematosus Cell Test, LE Cell Test, LE Slide Cell Test)

Normal Findings

Negative

What This Test Will Tell You

This blood test screens for systemic lupus erythematosus (SLE). The test is frequently repeated over 3 days because the result may be negative one day and show many lupus erythematosus (LE) cells on a successive day. SLE is an autoimmune disease characterized by the formation of antinuclear antibodies, which react with components of the cell nuclei. The blood test traumatizes the white blood cells to expose the nuclear material, which is then incubated with the client's serum. If the client's neutrophils phagocytize the nuclear material, the LE test is considered positive. Approximately 50%–80% of clients with active LE will have a positive test.

Abnormal Findings

Positive results may indicate systemic lupus erythematosus, rheumatoid arthritis, scleroderma, drug-induced lupus, Raynaud's syndrome, chronic active hepatitis, or other rheumatic diseases.

Interfering Factors

➤ Several medications may cause false positive results: acetazolamide, aminosalicylic acid, chlorprothixene, chlorothiazide, clofibrate, griseofulvin, hydralazine, isoniazid, mephenytoin (mesantoin), methysergide, methyldopa, oral contraceptives, penicillin, phenylbutazone, phenytoin sodium, procainamide, quinidine, reserpine, streptomycin, sulfonamides, tetracyclines.

➤ Steroids may cause false negative results.

➤ Hemolysis of the blood may adversely affect test results.

NURSING CONSIDERATIONS

Prepare Your Client

➤ Explain that this test screens for diseases of the immune system, specifically a disease called lupus erythematosus.

Perform Procedure

➤ Collect 5–10 mL of venous blood in a red-top or green-top tube.

➤ Cover the puncture site with a dressing to decrease the risk of infection. Many clients having this test have a depressed immune system and are at increased risk for infection.

➤ Handle the specimen carefully to avoid hemolysis. Send the specimen to the lab immediately.

Care After Test

➤ Observe for general signs and symptoms of SLE such as oral ulcers; fever; weight loss; excessive fatigue; and erythematous rash on face (butterfly rash), neck, or extremities.

➤ During acute exacerbations of the disease, monitor your client closely for abrupt changes in condition. Monitor temperature for fever. Assess joint pain, inflammation, and limited range of motion. Record intake and output accurately. Monitor fluid retention secondary to steroid therapy. Assess for renal failure. Central nervous system involvement may indicate the need for seizure precautions.

➤ Offer emotional support to client and family members. Refer your client and family to community agencies and support groups.

➤ Evaluate other tests such as antinuclear antibodies (ANA) and antideoxyribonucleic acid (anti-DNA).

Educate Your Client and the Family

➤ Teach your client and family about the prescribed medication's actions, side effects, dose, and administration.

➤ Teach energy conservation activities and pacing techniques.

➤ Explain the importance of avoiding physical and emotional stress as well as exposure to infectious diseases.

Luteinizing Hormone Assay

loo tee ih nize ing • hor mone • a say
(LH Assay, Interstitial-Cell-Stimulating Hormone Assay)

Normal Findings

ADULT
Male: 6–30 mIU/mL (6–30 U/L)
Female:
Follicular phase: 2–15 mIU/mL (2–15 U/L)
Ovulatory phase: 30–60 mIU/mL (30–60 U/L) *This is also called midcycle. Normal may also be measured as three times the client's known baseline.*
Luteal phase: 0–15 mIU/mL (0–15 U/L)
Postmenopausal: 35–100 mIU/mL (35–100 U/L)

PREGNANT
Normally, all steroid hormone levels increase as pregnancy progresses.
CHILD
Values are dependent on development.
0–12 mIU/mL (0–12 U/L)
ADOLESCENT
Values are dependent on development.
Male: 7–19 mIU/mL (7–10 U/L)
Female: 3–29 mIU/mL (3–29 U/L)

What This Test Will Tell You

This blood test evaluates infertility, alterations in normal menstrual patterns, and endocrine function, and monitors fertility therapy. Luteinizing hormone (LH) is secreted by the anterior pituitary and together with follicle-stimulating hormone (FSH) is important for ovulation in women. In the female, LH stimulates the ovaries and maintains the corpus luteum. A dramatic rise in LH indicates ovulation has occurred and can assist in identifying when fertility is maximal. In the male, LH stimulates the testosterone secretion that is responsible for spermatogenesis. Serum LH levels are also important to diagnose endocrine abnormalities in pediatric clients exhibiting such clinical problems as precocious or delayed puberty.

Abnormal Findings

▲INCREASED LEVELS may indicate hypogonadism, precocious puberty, anorchia, menopause, complete testicular feminization syndrome, Stein-Leventhal syndrome, acromegaly, Klinefelter's syndrome (primary testicular failure), or Turner's syndrome (primary ovarian failure).

▼DECREASED LEVELS may indicate hypothalamic insufficiency, secondary gonadal dysfunction, anovulation, hypogonadotropism, pituitary insufficiency, or ovarian tumors.

Interfering Factors

➤ Medications that can decrease LH levels include steroids, oral contraceptives, progesterone, estrogen, and testosterone.
➤ Testing with radioisotopes within 1 week invalidates test results.
➤ Hemolysis of sample invalidates test results.

NURSING CONSIDERATIONS

Prepare Your Client

➤ Explain that this test is done to evaluate how well sex hormones in the body are working.

Perform Procedure

➤ Collect 7 mL of venous blood in a red-top tube.

Care After Test

➤ Evaluate reproductive history for infertile couples. Assess if either partner has previously had children as well as any history of miscarriages.
➤ Provide referrals to support groups as appropriate for couples with infertility problems.
➤ Review related tests such as serum levels of estrogen, testosterone, progesterone, and follicle-stimulating hormone.

Educate Your Client and the Family

➤ Explain to the client and family that further testing is often required.
➤ For a couple with fertility problems, explain the role of serial LH levels in determining if ovulation has occurred and indicating maximal fertility time.

Lyme Disease Test

lime • di zeez • test

(Lyme Disease Antibody Test, *Borrelia burgdorferi* Antibody Test, Lyme's Disease Test)

Normal Findings

Negative: <1:256 titer

Borderline: 1:128 titer, calls for retesting

What This Test Will Tell You

This blood test diagnoses Lyme disease by detecting antibodies to the spirochete *Borrelia burgdorferi* bacteria. This disease was first recognized in Lyme, Connecticut in 1975. It is a multisystem disease transmitted to humans through the bite of an *Ixodid dammini* tick. Approximately 4–20 days after a tick bite, an erythematic skin rash, erythema chronicum migrans (ECM), appears at the site of the tick bite, accompanied by flu-like symptoms. Weeks to months after the initial symptoms, the client may develop central nervous system (CNS), cardiovascular, and musculoskeletal abnormalities.

Abnormal Findings

Positive results may reveal Lyme disease.

Interfering Factors

➤ A high rheumatoid factor may cause a false positive result.

NURSING CONSIDERATIONS

Prepare Your Client

➤ Explain that this test is used to help diagnose Lyme disease, a sickness that results from the bite of certain ticks.

Perform Procedure

➤ Collect 5–10 mL of blood into a red-top tube.

Care After Test

➤ Early in the disease process assess your client for ECM at the site of the tick bite. Weeks to months after the tick bite, assess for neurologic and cardiac changes and symptoms of arthritis.

➤ Evaluate other test results such as rheumatoid factor, electrocardiogram, Western blot assay, and enzyme-linked immunosorbent assay (ELISA).

Educate Your Client and the Family

➤ If your client is in the early stages of the disease, explain that there may be additional symptoms weeks to months after the rash disappears. Stress the importance of taking antibiotics as ordered and keeping follow-up appointments.

➤ Prevention of the disease is important. Instruct your client and family members to wear clothing that covers all extremities and the head when in wooded areas likely to be infested with ticks, and to check themselves for ticks afterward.

Lymph Node Biopsy

limf • node • bie op see

Normal Findings

Negative

What This Test Will Tell You

This microscopic analysis determines involvement of lymph nodes in disease processes. Lymph tissue is obtained for analysis during either an open or closed (needle) biopsy. The open lymph node biopsy involves making an incision in the lymph node and surrounding tissue to dissect lymph tissue.

Abnormal Findings

Positive results may indicate carcinoma, Hodgkin's disease, sarcoidosis, fungal disease, or tuberculosis.

Interfering Factors

➤ A negative needle biopsy may indicate that the cells obtained were negative, but not prove the absence of disease because positive cells may not be present in a single sample. A positive cell biopsy is sufficient to confirm a diagnosis.

Potential Complications

➤ Bleeding may occur.
➤ Disease may be spread if the biopsy knife passes through neoplastic cells and releases cells into the lymph system.

NURSING CONSIDERATIONS

Prepare Your Client

➤ Explain that this test is to look at a part of the body involved in fighting infections called the lymph nodes.
➤ Ensure that an informed consent is obtained, because of the possible complications associated with this procedure.

Perform Procedure

Nurses do not usually perform this procedure, but should understand the process to prepare the client. The client may receive either local or general anesthesia for this procedure. A closed biopsy may be performed in the physician's office or at the bedside. The procedure involves aspirating lymph tissue through a needle inserted into lymph nodes. An open biopsy is performed in the operating room and involves making an incision to reach the designated lymph nodes.

Care After Test

➤ Apply a sterile dressing to the biopsy site.
➤ Observe for bleeding. Apply pressure to the site as needed to control bleeding.
➤ Change the biopsy site dressing as ordered.
➤ Evaluate the wound for healing and for indications of infection.
➤ Offer emotional support to your client and family members if a positive biopsy indicating cancer or other diseases is obtained.

Educate Your Client and the Family

➤ Explain to your client that the lymph node biopsy is important to help in the diagnosis of disease. Lymph nodes are the filtering system of the body, so disease can often be detected and diagnosed by examining lymph nodes.
➤ Inform your client that the dressing should be changed as ordered by

the primary health care provider to decrease the risk of infection. Stress the importance of washing hands before changing dressings and keeping the site clean.

> If a positive biopsy report is obtained, explain the disease process diagnosed. Answer client and family questions about the disease treatment.

Lymphocyte Transformation Tests
lim foe site • trans for may shun • tests
(LTTs, Immunoblast Transformation Tests)

Normal Findings
> Nonimmune tests/mitogen assay: Stimulation index >10 indicates immunocompetence.
> Antigen-specific tests: Stimulation index >3 indicates prior exposure to antigen.
> Mixed lymphocyte culture: Nonresponsiveness indicates good histocompatibility.

What This Test Will Tell You
This blood test determines immunocompetence, prior exposure to specific antigens, and organ donor–recipient antigen match. These tests introduce antigens into a blood specimen to see whether the immune system mounts a response.

Nonimmune tests are accomplished by introducing agents called mitogens that cause normally responsive lymphocytes to become immunoblasts. The lymphocytes incubate in the mitogen for approximately 72 hours. Radioactive thymidine is added to the cells. The amount of thymidine uptake indicates the extent of lymphocyte proliferation.

Antigen-specific tests are accomplished by introducing specific antigens. Observation of T-cell responses indicates whether the client has been introduced to the antigens previously.

Mixed lymphocyte culture (MLC) is used to determine histocompatibility at the D locus. Lymphocytes from the recipient are incubated for 5–7 days with lymphocytes from the living donor. The degree of lymphocyte proliferation is an indication of the body's recognition of the antigens as foreign.

Abnormal Findings
▼LOW INDEX *for mitogen assay* may reveal depressed immune system, abnormal T-cell maturation, congenital thymus defects, T-cell depleting diseases such as acquired immune deficiency syndrome (AIDS), Hodgkin's disease, immunosuppressive chemotherapy, or total lymphoid irradiation.

▲HIGH INDEX *for antigen-specific tests* may reveal exposure to specific disease antigens such as malaria, hepatitis, mycoplasmal pneumonia, periodontal disease, or viral infections.

▼LOW INDEX *for antigen-specific tests* may reveal depressed immune system, abnormal T-cell maturation, or unusual susceptibility to certain infectious diseases such as herpes simplex and *Mycobacterium avium*.

▲ HIGH INDEX *for MLC* may reveal poor tissue compatibility for transplantation.

▼ LOW INDEX *for MLC* may reveal good tissue compatibility for transplantation.

Interfering Factors

➤ Use of oral contraceptives may cause decreased response to phytohemagglutinin tests.

➤ Pregnancy may cause decreased response to phytohemagglutinin tests.

➤ Radioisotope studies within prior week may alter results.

➤ Chemotherapy may cause inaccurate test results. Obtaining baseline results before chemotherapy is started provides a method of comparing test results before and after chemotherapy.

➤ Radioisotope scan within prior week can interfere with results.

NURSING CONSIDERATIONS

Prepare Your Client

➤ Explain that this test determines the body's ability to fight infection or reject foreign materials. If this test is to monitor the client's response to therapy, explain this to your client. If this test is to determine histocompatibility for a transplant, explain that the test will help determine the best organ match to decrease the risk of organ rejection.

➤ If your client is taking birth control pills, she should consult her primary health care provider about the possible effects this medication may have on test results.

Perform Procedure

➤ Collect 5–7 mL of venous blood in a heparinized green-top tube.

Care After Test

➤ If your client is immunosuppressed, observe the puncture site for signs of infection.

➤ Offer emotional support to your client and family members. If this test is being done as part of screening for an organ transplant workup, all parties involved need the opportunity to express concerns and ask questions.

➤ Review related tests such as lymphocyte marker assay, HLA-B27 antigen, and delayed hypersensitivity skin tests.

Educate Your Client and the Family

➤ Teach an immunocompromised client to avoid young children with respiratory symptoms and large crowds.

➤ Teach your client and family members the importance of washing hands to decrease the risk of infection.

➤ Discuss with organ transplant donors and recipients the importance of keeping all appointments for screening and testing.

Magnesium, Urine and Serum

mag **nee** see um • **yur** in • and • see rum
(Serum Magnesium, Urine Magnesium, Mg^{++})

Normal Findings

URINE

Adult, pregnant, child, infant, and adolescent: 6.0–10.0 mEq/24 hours (SI units: 3.0–5.0 mmol/24 hours)

Elderly: May be normally decreased from adult values.

SERUM

Adult: 1.3–2.5 mEq/L (SI units: 0.65–1.30 mmol/L)

Pregnant: Gradual fall of about 10%–20% percent during pregnancy.

Infant: 1.2–1.8 mEq/L (SI units: 0.6–0.9 mmol/L)

Child:

5 months 6 years: 1.4–1.9 mEq/L (SI units: 0.7–0.95 mmol/L)

6–12 years: 1.4–1.7 mEq/L (SI units: 0.7–0.85 mmol/L)

Adolescent:

12–20 years: 1.4–1.8 mEq/L (SI units: 0.7–0.8 mmol/L)

Elderly: 1.2–1.9 mEq/L (SI units: 0.50–0.78 mmol/L)

What This Test Will Tell You

These blood and 24-hour urine tests determine electrolyte status and evaluate neuromuscular and renal function. Magnesium is important in the transmission of nerve impulses and in the contraction of skeletal, smooth, and cardiac muscles. Additionally, the magnesium ion Mg^{++} is essential for the use of adenosine triphosphate (ADP) as an energy source, the function of enzyme systems, and normal clotting mechanisms. Magnesium balance is interdependent with many other electrolytes, but imbalances may also reflect renal tubular dysfunction. Magnesium is the second most abundant intracellular body cation, and is essential to the absorption and metabolism of calcium. This electrolyte competes with absorption sites for calcium and phosphorus in the small intestine, resulting in an inverse relationship between the amount of dietary calcium and phosphorus and the amount of magnesium absorbed.

Abnormal Findings: Serum

▲INCREASED LEVELS may indicate renal disorders, Addison's disease, leukemia, adrenalectomy, excessive administration of magnesium, dehydration, or diabetic ketoacidosis.

▼DECREASED LEVELS may indicate malabsorption syndromes, chronic diarrhea, chronic renal failure, chronic alcoholism, acute and chronic pancreatitis, aldosteronism, hyperaldosteronism, malnutrition, colon resection, severe burns, ulcerative colitis, toxemia of pregnancy, hypercalcemia, hyperthyroidism, hypoparathyroidism, or prolonged gastric drainage.

Abnormal Findings: Urine

▲INCREASED LEVELS may indicate Bartter's syndrome, early renal disease, adrenocortical insufficiency, or alcoholism.

▼DECREASED LEVELS may indicate malabsorption syndromes, cirrhosis, pancreatitis, diarrhea, diabetic acidosis, chronic renal disease, alcoholism, diuretic therapy, or hyperaldosteronism.

ACTION ALERT!

➤ **If levels fall below 1 mEq/L, convulsions and dysrhythmias may occur.**

➤ If levels exceed 3 mEq/L, respiratory failure, cardiac arrest, coma, and/or death may occur.

➤ Carefully assess neonates of mothers receiving magnesium sulfate for treatment of toxemia of pregnancy. Assessment of the neonate includes reflexes, respiratory status, and muscle strength.

➤ If the urine magnesium levels are abnormal, check the serum level and monitor the client for signs and symptoms such as weakness, tremors, dysrhythmias, hypoventilation, convulsions, and confusion. In magnesium imbalances, the urine magnesium levels change before the serum levels do. Serum levels may remain normal even when body stores of magnesium have been depleted by as much as 20%.

Interfering Factors

SERUM

➤ Levels may be decreased with hyperbilirubinemia, prolonged nasogastric suctioning, prolonged hyperalimentation or IV therapy, exchange blood transfusions, diuretic therapy, calcium gluconate, cisplatin, corticosteroids, and insulin.

➤ Levels may be increased with the use of magnesium-containing antacids, cathartics, thiazide diuretics, ethacrynic acid, salicylates, and lithium.

➤ Hemolysis of the specimen falsely increases results.

URINE

➤ Collection of urine in a metal container will affect results.

➤ An increased blood alcohol increases the excretion of urinary magnesium.

➤ Levels are increased by thiazide diuretic therapy, aldosterone, alcohol, corticosteroids, platinum therapy, magnesium-containing antacids, and ethacrynic acid.

➤ Levels may be decreased by aminoglycosides and amphotericin B.

NURSING CONSIDERATIONS

Prepare Your Client

➤ Explain that either of these tests helps to evaluate the chemical balance of the body, especially one chemical called magnesium.

➤ If urine test is used, instruct the client on method of 24-hour urine collection.

Perform Procedure

SERUM

➤ Collect 7 mL of venous blood in a red-top tube.

URINE

➤ Use a 3-L, acid-washed, metal-free container with no preservative.

➤ Carefully follow technique for 24-hour urine collection.

Care After Test

➤ Monitor for signs and symptoms of hypomagnesemia including tremors, convulsions, hyperactive reflexes, leg and foot cramps, cardiac dysrhythmias, muscle weakness, and tetany.

➤ Monitor for signs and symptoms of hypermagnesemia including lethargy, hypotension, flushing, diaphoresis, nausea, vomiting, diminished reflexes, drowsiness, muscle weakness, and hypoventilation.

➤ Institute continuous cardiac monitoring for client with known or suspected magnesium imbalances.

➤ Institute safety precautions if neuromuscular deficits are known or suspected.

➤ Consult with the primary health care provider regarding the administration of calcium gluconate or calcium chloride for hypermagnesemia.

➤ If levels are low, maintain an environment with decreased stimuli due to neurological irritability.

> Review related tests such as serum calcium and phosphorus.

Educate Your Client and the Family
> Magnesium is found in all natural foods, so encourage a well-balanced diet with adequate servings of fresh fruits and vegetables.
> Teach client and family that high intake of phosphate-containing medications and/or foods can decrease both magnesium and calcium absorption and should be avoided. These include milk, carbonated beverages, and laxatives or enemas.
> Teach client with hypermagnesemia to eat foods containing fiber and to drink plenty of fluids to promote elimination through the bowel.

M

Magnetic Resonance Imaging

mag **net** ik • **rez** oh nans • **im** aj ing
(MRI, MR Imaging, MR Blood Flow Scanning, MRF, Nuclear Magnetic Resonance, NMR, Magnetic Resonance Angiography, MRA, MR Angiography, Magnetic Resonance Spectroscopy, MRS)

Normal Findings
Normal tissue structure
Normal tissue blood flow

What This Test Will Tell You
This magnetic radiographic test detects structural, circulatory, and metabolic abnormalities in the body. Utilizing magnetic fields, MRI (magnetic resonance imaging) is a noninvasive method that provides valuable information about soft and/or fluid-filled tissues without the use of ionizing radiation. There are no known risks associated with magnetic resonance imaging. By causing hydrogen ions in soft tissue molecules to arrange themselves in relation to the magnetic field the MR imager creates, sharp images of internal tissues and organs are produced. MRI can also differentiate normal from abnormal tissues, reveal ischemia, infarctions, and thrombi, and provide critical information about metabolism.

MRI presently has limited usefulness in evaluating bones because bones have little water, and therefore hydrogen, making visualization by magnetic imaging relatively poor. Although the test is more expensive, MRI is preferred to CT scans in some neurologic pathology such as tumors, infarcts, and demyelinating diseases because of its greater sensitivity and ability to differentiate gray from white matter in the brain. MRI is not as effective as CT scans in detecting lower spinal cord abnormalities. Magnetic resonance (MR) angiography does not show ulceration or plaque formation as well as cerebral angiography in clients with atherosclerotic cerebrovascular disease.

Abnormal Findings
Abnormalities may indicate tumors; blood clots; cysts; edema; hemorrhage; abscesses; infarctions; aneurysms; acute tubular necrosis;

acute rejection of transplanted organs; blood velocity in vessels; vascular occlusive disease; focal artery narrowing associated with migraine, arteritis, and drug abuse; multiple sclerosis; dementia; muscular disease; skeletal abnormalities; congenital heart disease; intervertebral disc abnormalities; spinal cord compression; aortic dissection; or arteriovenous malformations.

Interfering Factors

➤ Movement can diminish the quality of the image. The client must be able to lie still for the 45–90 minutes required for completing the imaging.
➤ Obesity interferes with imaging of underlying tissues and organs due to the high water (hydrogen) content of adipose tissue.

Contraindications

➤ Severe claustrophobia.
➤ Ferrous metal in the body such as aneurysm clips, heart valves, and surgical clips. The MRI magnet may cause movement of ferrous metal objects within the body. Implanted metal intravenous ports usually do not provide a safety hazard, but check with the manufacturer for specific information and guidance.
➤ This test is contraindicated in clients who have had injuries that left ferrous metal within the body, such as metal shavings in the eye. Movement of the metal could cause severe eye damage.
➤ The magnetic field may deactivate some cardiac pacemakers. Check with the manufacturer for specific information and guidance.
➤ Critical or unstable condition of the client. The client must remain unattended in the MRI unit throughout the test, which prohibits close monitoring of client's condition.

Some intravenous drip regulators are disrupted by the magnetic field. Current emergency equipment has a high risk of malfunctioning or becoming projectile in the magnetic field, so the client must be removed from the chamber in the event of a cardiac/respiratory arrest.

Potential Complications

➤ Injury resulting from internal movement of ferrous metal within the body

NURSING CONSIDERATIONS

Prepare Your Client

➤ Explain that this test does not involve any radiation and is used to help find problems in the part of the body for which the test was ordered.
➤ Caution client that they will hear noises of various rhythms and volume as the radio waves are turned on and off. Earplugs are available if desired.
➤ Assess client for a history of claustrophobia. If present, a sedative may be needed.
➤ Teach client relaxation and visualization techniques to decrease anxiety, because some people feel claustrophobic in the chamber.
➤ Assure your client there is no pain with this test.
➤ Ensure that all metal jewelry, hairpins, glasses, dental bridges, and watches have been removed. Credit cards should not be carried in a wallet, pocket, or left in the MRI unit, because their magnetic strips will be erased.
➤ Check with the policy of your imaging laboratory about parents staying with young children during imaging. Some children may lie still and cooperate with the test better if a

parent is allowed in the MRI unit during the procedure. Since there is no radiation, this does not pose a risk for the parent. Be sure the parent is stripped of all metal objects and does not have any internal ferrous metal objects that may move within the body.

➤ Alert client that tooth fillings and caps may cause a strange feeling during the test.

➤ Tell client the test takes approximately 45–90 minutes for imaging a body part or organ. Blood flow imaging of the extremities takes about 15 minutes for each arm or leg.

➤ Verify that client has voided before the test.

Perform Procedure

Nurses do not perform this test. They need to understand the test to explain it to the client and family members. The client is placed on a table and moved through a cylinder which contains a very large magnet. The magnet causes the atoms in the cells of the body to line up in parallel fashion. Radiowaves are sent through the magnetic field, causing the cellu-

lar atoms to move. This movement is sensed by the computer, which produces cross-sectional images of the body. A microphone and earphones are used to communicate with the client during the imaging. An injectable contrast medium may be used to enhance central nervous system imaging. This can be injected intravenously immediately before the test begins.

Care After Test

➤ Assess the client for signs and symptoms of the disorder for which the test was ordered.

➤ Carefully inspect the skin for signs of pressure from prolonged immobility on the hard platform the client lies on during imaging.

➤ Evaluate other related tests such as CT scan, cerebral angiography, and cardiac angiography.

Educate Your Client and the Family

➤ Your client may require treatment for a condition diagnosed with the MRI. Give specific education about the treatment or procedure prescribed.

Mammography

ma mah grah fee

(Mammogram, Xeromammograms)

Normal Findings

Negative, no tumor

What This Test Will Tell You

This x-ray test detects breast cancer. Breast cancer can often be detected by mammogram long before a nodule or lump can be palpated. Signs of breast cancer on x-ray are white

specks, asymmetric density, skin thickening, and a poorly defined mass. The American Cancer Society recommends a baseline mammogram at ages 35 and 45, and for women over 50 years of age or at risk for breast cancer, yearly mammograms. Mammograms are used when signs and symptoms of breast cancer are present including nipple or skin retraction, breast pain, nipple discharge, or skin changes of the breast. Mammograms are also particularly useful with large breasts that are difficult to examine, with a family history of breast cancer, to screen for breast cancer, and in detection of other breast diseases such as fibrocystic changes or cysts.

Abnormal Findings

The x-ray may reveal benign tumors, cancerous mass, fibrocystic changes, breast cysts, breast abscesses, or suppurative mastitis.

Interfering Factors

➤ Medullary and colloid carcinomas are difficult to diagnose with mammography.
➤ Jewelry around the neck can prevent clear visualization.
➤ Deodorant, perfume, and ointments can leave residue on the skin that interferes with the x-ray. Aluminum chlorhydrate in some of these mimics calcium clusters.
➤ Breast implants prevent total visualization.

Contraindications

➤ Pregnant clients risk fetal damage.

NURSING CONSIDERATIONS

Prepare Your Client

➤ Explain that this test is used to detect abnormalities and disease of the breast, and that mammography is the easiest method of detecting early breast cancer.
➤ Explain that this test is done by an x-ray technician, and a radiologist may ask to examine the breast.
➤ Explain to the client that this procedure uses a minimal amount of radiation.

➤ Instruct the client to undress above the waist and put on the gown provided.
➤ Explain that the procedure takes about 30 minutes and may be uncomfortable when the breast is compressed for visualization.

Perform Procedure

Nurses do not usually perform this procedure but should understand it to prepare the client and assist with the mammography. The client may be asked to identify any problem area on the breast for special visualization. One breast at a time is placed on an x-ray plate. An x-ray cone goes on top of the breast to compress it. Views from several angles are taken.

Care After Test

➤ Assess breasts for redness or bruising and document.
➤ Assess client for breast pain. Provide cool compresses or ice, or consult with primary health care provider as necessary for mild analgesics.
➤ If cancer is diagnosed, assess for signs and symptoms of metastatic cancer including bone pain, fatigue, and recurring symptoms of the tumor.
➤ Refer client and family to a cancer support group.
➤ Review related tests such as thermomammography, complete blood count, and erythrocyte sedimentation rate.

Educate Your Client and the Family

➤ Instruct your client in breast self-examination.
➤ Teach client to decrease caffeine intake.

Manganese, Serum
man gah neez • see rum

Normal Findings
All ages: 0.4–0.85 ng/mL

What This Test Will Tell You
This blood test screens for or diagnoses manganese toxicity. Manganese is a trace mineral that is essential to many metabolic functions of the body that depend upon important enzymes. Normally, only very low levels are present in the blood from dietary intake of nuts, green leafy vegetables, and cereals. However, industrial settings often present workers with exposure, which can result in toxic levels.

Abnormal Findings
▲INCREASED LEVELS indicate manganese toxicity.

▼DECREASED LEVELS are associated with prolonged parenteral nutritional therapy, dietary deficiency, altered bone formation, glucose intolerance, or high calcium and phosphorus diet.

ACTION ALERT!

Elevated levels of manganese (>1.5 ng/mL) require prompt medical intervention. Be prepared to administer calcium if ordered by primary health care provider. Manganese toxicity can lead to central nervous system failure and death.

Interfering Factors
➤ High dietary intake of calcium and phosphorus found in antacids, milk, cheese, dried fruits and vegetables, and fish can interfere with the intestinal absorption of manganese.
➤ Estrogen can increase levels.
➤ Glucocorticoids can alter distribution of manganese in the body.

➤ Hemolysis can alter test results.
➤ Use of a metal collection tube can alter results.

NURSING CONSIDERATIONS
Prepare Your Client
➤ Explain that this test is used to determine the level of an important mineral in the body called manganese.

Perform Procedure
➤ Collect 7 mL of venous blood in a 10–15 mL red-top, metal-free tube.
➤ Avoid handling that could result in hemolysis.

Care After Test
➤ Assess the client's history for magnesium exposure through work in the steel and dry-battery industries; welding; and the manufacture of pottery, glass, food additives, and varnish.
➤ Monitor client for signs and symptoms of manganese toxicity including Parkinsonian symptoms such as tremors, rigidity of large joints, muscle weakness, difficulty chewing or swallowing, depression, and mask-like facial expression.
➤ Institute safety precautions for client with muscle weakness or movement disorders.
➤ Consult with a registered dietician to assist the family and client in selecting and preparing foods if dysphagia is noted.
➤ Review related tests such as computed axial tomography, magnetic resonance imaging, serum electrolytes, and electroencephalogram.

**Educate Your Client
and the Family**

➤ Instruct client to avoid industrial exposure to manganese.

➤ Explain that manganese is an essential trace element found in green leafy vegetables, nuts, and unrefined grains.

Mediastinoscopy
mee dee as ti nah skoe pee

Normal Findings
Normal mediastinal structure and lymph nodes; no evidence of disease.

What This Test Will Tell You
In this endoscopic procedure, a lighted scope is inserted through an incision at the base of the neck (suprasternal notch) to visualize mediastinal structures and lymph nodes and to biopsy lymph nodes. The mediastinal nodes receive lymphatic drainage from the lungs, so biopsies may reveal diseases such as cancer, granulomatous infections, and sarcoidosis. Lymphomas such as Hodgkin's disease and metastatic lung cancer may also be identified. Mediastinoscopy is routinely performed to stage lung cancer prior to thoracotomy, and when x-rays, sputum cytology, bronchoscopy, computed tomography scans and lung scans have not confirmed a diagnosis.

Abnormal Findings
Abnormalities may indicate lung cancer, metastasis, Hodgkin's disease, lymphoma, granulomatous infection, sarcoidosis, mediastinal tuberculosis, or histoplasmosis.

ACTION ALERT!

Injury to blood vessels, major airways, or other mediastinal structures can result in a medical emergency requiring immediate intervention and cardiopulmonary resuscitation.

Contraindications
➤ Previous mediastinoscopy contraindicates another examination because adhesions make an adequate dissection of nodes extremely difficult.

Potential Complications
➤ Puncture of esophagus, trachea, lungs, or blood vessels

NURSING CONSIDERATIONS
Prepare Your Client
➤ Explain that this procedure is performed to look at and take samples of lymph nodes that drain the lung for study in the laboratory.
➤ Explain that this is a surgical procedure performed in the operating room and requires general anesthesia.
➤ Ensure that informed consent has been obtained and that the signed consent form is on the chart.
➤ Restrict food and fluids for 8–12 hours prior to the procedure.

Perform Procedure
This procedure is performed by a surgeon in the operating room and takes about 1 hour. The nurse should understand the process to prepare the client, assist the physician if nec-

essary, and provide postoperative care.

The client is placed under general anesthesia. A small incision is made in the suprasternal notch and the lighted scope is passed through the incision and along the course of the anterior trachea. The area, structures, and tissues are visualized. Photographs of specific areas and structures may be taken, and biopsies are performed.

The scope is withdrawn and the incision is surgically closed. Place biopsy specimens in appropriate containers. Dress the incision using aseptic technique. Label specimen containers, indicating the site and method utilized in obtaining the specimen, and transport to the laboratory immediately.

Care After Test

➤ Transport the client to the post-anesthesia recovery room according to hospital policy.

➤ Assess vital signs every 15 minutes for 1 hour, then every 30 minutes for 1 hour, then hourly for 4 hours or until stable.

➤ Monitor airway and respiratory status.

➤ Elevate head of bed to enhance gas exchange.

➤ Check especially for postoperative swelling, which can result in airway obstruction. Ensure a tracheostomy tray is readily available, as well as oxygen therapy.

➤ Observe wound for signs of bleeding or infection. If bleeding is present, apply pressure to wound, being careful not to obstruct the airway. Notify the primary health care provider and obtain assistance immediately.

➤ Report if crepitus is noted on neck or chest area. This could be due to air leaking into the subcutaneous tissue as a result of lung puncture.

➤ Evaluate related tests such as x-rays, computed tomography scans, bronchoscopy, or sputum cytology.

Educate Your Client and the Family

➤ Describe the nursing routine of closely monitoring vital signs, respiratory status, and wound status.

➤ Instruct the client to report immediately any difficulty breathing, speaking, or swallowing; hoarseness; bleeding from the incision; or other discomforts.

➤ Describe any activity restrictions.

➤ Tell the client that the pathologist will examine biopsied tissue and convey results to their primary health care provider, and that this may take at least 2 days.

M

Metyrapone

meh **teer** ah pone
(Metopirone)

Normal Findings

ALL AGES
Urinary: Urinary excretion of 17-hydroxycorticosteroids is stimulated to twice the basal level (or a rise of 8–10 mg/24 hours) with administration of metyrapone.

Blood:
11-deoxycortisol levels > 7 µg/dL
Cortisol levels < 10 µg/dL

What This Test Will Tell You

These blood and urine tests evaluate adrenal cortical function and diagnose hyperplasia or tumors of the adrenals. Metyrapone is an enzyme that can block the production of cortisol. When it is administered, cortisol levels decline, which stimulates the pituitary to secrete more adrenocorticotropic hormone (ACTH) in an attempt to increase cortisol production. In normal persons, urinary 17-hydroxycorticosteroid levels rise sharply in response to the body's attempt to increase cortisol levels that are being blocked. Because metyrapone also inhibits cortisol synthesis, levels of the cortisol precursor (11-deoxycortisol) rise in the blood.

Abnormal Findings

Abnormal results may indicate adrenal hyperplasia, Cushing's syndrome, tumor of the adrenal glands, tumor of the pituitary gland, or an ectopic ACTH-producing tumor.

ACTION ALERT!

This test may induce adrenal crisis in clients with insufficient adrenal or pituitary reserve. Observe closely for hypotension, tachycardia, emotional changes, weak or thready pulse, cold or clammy skin, increase in body temperature, nausea, or vomiting. Be prepared to administer intravenous fluids and hydrocortisone as well as to pharmacologically support circulatory function.

Interfering Factors

➤ Medications that may interfere with accuracy of test results include chlorpromazine, phenobarbital, and estrogens.

➤ Testing with radioisotopes within one week invalidates test results.

Contraindications

➤ Known or suspected adrenal insufficiency (Addison's disease), because an adrenal crisis may be precipitated

Potential Complications

➤ Adrenal insufficiency crisis

NURSING CONSIDERATIONS

Prepare Your Client

➤ Explain that these tests are performed to see how well a special gland in the body (adrenal gland) is working by measuring hormones in the blood and urine.

URINARY
➤ Explain the process for 24-hour urine collection.
➤ Explain that urine will be collected for three 24-hour periods.

BLOOD
➤ No additional preparation is required.

Perform Procedure

URINARY AND BLOOD
➤ Collect a 24-hour urine specimen to establish a baseline excretion rate of 17-hydroxycorticosteroids.
➤ Collect 7–10 mL of venous blood at 8 A.M. in a red- or green-top tube for baseline cortisol level.
➤ Administer metyrapone as ordered. Methods of testing and dosing vary widely. Dose may be repeated during test, e.g., every 4 hours for 24 hours.
➤ Continue 24-hour urine collection for 2 more days (during metyrapone administration and for 1 day following drug administration).
➤ For a blood test, give metyrapone at 11 P.M. the night before the sample is taken.

Care After Test

➤ Assess for signs and symptoms of adrenal insufficiency including weakness, nausea, vomiting, cyanosis, hypotension, hyperthermia, electrolyte imbalances, and hypoglycemia.

➤ Assess for signs and symptoms of increased adrenal function including hirsutism, atrophy of breasts, and masculinization in females.

➤ Assess adult client for thin skin, round face, mood changes, history of infections, hypertension, and edema.

➤ Observe closely for changes in mental status including depression. Protect client from self-injury.

➤ Protect client with manifestations of weakness by surveying and making changes in the client's environment.

➤ Review related tests including urine 17-ketogenic steroids, 17-ketosteroids, serum cortisol, serum electrolytes, blood glucose, adrenocorticotropic hormone (ACTH), dexamethasone suppression test, and complete blood count with differential.

Educate Your Client and the Family

➤ Inform client that they may be more susceptible to infections. Emphasize the importance of handwashing and avoiding exposure to people with known infections.

➤ Teach client with adrenal hyperplasia the importance of a low-sodium, high-potassium diet.

➤ Encourage client and family to report depression or other mental status changes promptly to the primary health care provider.

Mononucleosis Spot Test

mon oe noo klee oe sis • spot • test

(Mono-Spot Test, Monospot Test, Monotest, Mononuclear Heterophile Test, Heterophile Antibody, Heterophile Antibody Titer, HAT)

Normal Findings

HETEROPHILE ANTIBODY TITER
Negative: <1:28
MONONUCLEOSIS SPOT TEST
Negative: <1:28

What This Test Will Tell You

This blood test diagnoses infectious mononucleosis. Epstein-Barr virus (EBV) is generally accepted as the causative organism.

Heterophiles are antibodies that react to antigens other than the antigen causing the antibody formation. In humans, EBV causes heterophile antibodies to agglutinate erythrocytes of sheep and horses. When EBV heterophile antibodies react with the red blood cells of sheep at a serum dilution of 1:225 or greater, the antibody titer is considered positive for mononucleosis. The antibody titer usually increases by the third day of the illness, continues to increase for 2–3 weeks, and remains elevated for up to 6 weeks.

The spot test screens for mononucleosis. This commercially available test uses antigens derived from horse serum. The client's serum is mixed with the horse serum. If agglutination occurs, the test is considered positive. The heterophile antibody test is then performed to confirm the diagnosis of infectious mononucleosis.

Abnormal Findings

Abnormal results may reveal infectious mononucleosis, chronic Epstein-Barr virus, chronic fatigue syndrome, serum sickness, viral infections, or Burkitt's lymphoma.

HETEROPHILE ANTIBODY TITER
Elevated level: >1:56–1:224
Positive: ≥1:225
MONONUCLEOSIS SPOT TEST
Positive: ≥1:28

Interfering Factors

➤ Serum sickness and Forssman antibodies may cause false positive titers.
➤ Upper respiratory tract infections may cause false positive titers.
➤ False positive titers may result from blood transfusions if blood-group-specific substances have been added to neutralize isoagglutinins.

NURSING CONSIDERATIONS

Prepare Your Client

➤ Explain that this test is important in diagnosing mono (infectious mononucleosis).

Perform Procedure

➤ Collect 5–10 mL of venous blood in a red-top tube for the heterophile antibody test. Collect 2 mL of blood in a red-top tube for the monospot test.

Care After Test

➤ Explain to your client that a repeat blood test may be required to monitor the titer results.

➤ Assess for general signs and symptoms of infectious mononucleosis including fever, malaise, anorexia, pharyngitis, lymphadenopathy, and splenomegaly.
➤ Assess for dermatologic manifestations of mononucleosis including a macular, maculopapular, or petechial skin rash and for periorbital edema.
➤ Assess for system-specific symptoms resulting from involvement of the heart (arrhythmias, congestive heart failure), liver (hepatitis, jaundice, hepatomegaly), central nervous system (headache, photophobia, stiff neck), and respiratory system (cough, dyspnea).
➤ Encourage your client to rest and drink plenty of fluids.
➤ Encourage your client to take medications as prescribed.
➤ Evaluate any related diagnostic tests such as nasopharyngeal culture and white blood cell count.

Educate Your Client and the Family

➤ If your client has splenomegaly, discourage activities such as lifting heavy objects or contact sports that could potentially cause injury to or rupture of the spleen. Discourage using pressure with held breath (Valsalva maneuver) during bowel movements until the splenomegaly has resolved.
➤ Stress the importance of rest, plenty of fluids, and good nutrition. Unless your client has a bacterial infection, antibiotics usually are not useful.
➤ Saline gargles may be helpful in easing throat discomforts. Analgesics may be helpful in relieving generalized discomforts.

Multiple Sclerosis Screening Panel

mul ti pul · skleh roe sis · skreen ing · pan el

(MS Screening Panel, Multiple Sclerosis Panel, MS Panel, Multiple Sclerosis Expanded Evaluation)

Normal Findings

➤ Cerebrospinal fluid (CSF) IgG synthesis rate: < 8.0 mg/24 hours
➤ Albumin index: < 9.0
➤ Oligoclonal immunoglobulins: < 2 abnormal bands detected (only bands present in CSF and not in serum reported)
➤ Myelin basic protein: < 1.0 ng/mL
➤ IgG index: < 0.7
➤ IgG: < 0.1 mg/dL
➤ IgA: < 0.01 mg/dL
➤ IgM: < 0.01 mg/dL

What This Test Will Tell You

This blood and cerebrospinal fluid test aids in the detection and diagnosis of multiple sclerosis. Multiple sclerosis (MS) is a progressive neurologic disorder characterized by exacerbations and remissions. Inflammation and myelin damage occurs throughout the central nervous system.

This screening panel consists of two tests. The first test is the IgG index test, which detects IgG synthesis in the central nervous system. The second test uses electrophoresis to determine the presence of oligoclonal bands in blood and CSF samples.

Abnormal Findings

▲INCREASED LEVELS *of IgG or IgG-albumin index* may indicate multiple sclerosis, infectious disease, subacute sclerosing leukoencephalitis, neurosyphilis, or chronic central nervous system infection.

▲INCREASED LEVELS *of CSF albumin* may indicate lesions of choroid plexus, blockage of CSF flow, or damage to central nervous system.

▲INCREASED LEVELS *of IgG and normal levels of albumin* may indicate multiple sclerosis, neurosyphilis, subacute sclerosing panencephalitis, or chronic central nervous system infections.

Presence of oligoclonal bands in CSF without corresponding bands in blood may indicate multiple sclerosis, cryptococcal meningitis, idiopathic polyneuritis, neurosyphilis, chronic rubella panencephalitis, or subacute sclerosing panencephalitis.

Interfering Factors

➤ Delay in getting the specimen to the lab may yield false negative results.

Potential Complications

For lumbar puncture to obtain CSF:
➤ Bleeding into the spinal canal
➤ Neurologic injury
➤ Infection
➤ Headache, nausea, dizziness, neck pain

NURSING CONSIDERATIONS

Prepare Your Client

➤ Explain that this test is used to diagnose multiple sclerosis and other nervous system diseases.

➤ Tell your client that this test requires samples of both blood and cerebrospinal fluid. Explain the venipuncture process clearly. Explain that the primary health care provider will place a needle into the lower back and withdraw spinal fluid.

➤ Explain that the test will measure specific substances in the cerebrospinal fluid to assist the primary health care provider in making a diagnosis. The cerebrospinal fluid results will be compared with the blood results.

➤ Ensure that an informed consent is obtained, because of the possible complications associated with this procedure.

Perform Procedure

➤ Collect 7 mL of venous blood in a red-top tube.

➤ Label the sample and send immediately to the lab.

➤ Within 2 hours of the blood sample collection the lumbar puncture should be performed. Position your client in a side-lying position with knees drawn to chest and chin tucked down.

➤ Assist the primary health care provider during collection of the CSF. Approximately 3–5 mL of fluid will be collected in a tube. (See *Lumbar Puncture*.)

➤ Label the CSF tube and send it to the lab immediately.

Care After Test

➤ Evaluate the client for clinical signs and symptoms including weakness, paralysis, fatigue, sensory disturbances, gait problems, tremors, bowel and bladder difficulties, pain, and dementia.

➤ Position your client flat in bed for several hours after the lumbar puncture to decrease the risk of a headache. Assess for pain. Administer analgesics for headache and discomforts as ordered.

➤ Observe your client for complications of lumbar puncture including changes in vital signs, numbness and tingling of the lower extremities, neck rigidity, and changes in level of consciousness.

➤ Evaluate related tests such as myelin basic protein, electronystagmography, cerebrospinal fluid immunofixation, and evoked potential studies.

Educate Your Client and the Family

➤ Instruct your client to relax during the lumbar puncture by taking slow, deep breaths. Stress the importance of remaining as still as possible during the procedure.

➤ If the client has MS, inform the client and family to expect periods of exacerbations and remission. Explain that viral infections and stress may cause worsening of symptoms.

➤ Provide the client and family with information about support groups and agencies in their area.

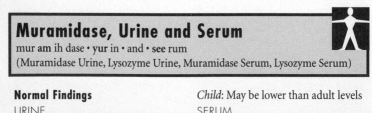

Muramidase, Urine and Serum

mur **am** ih dase • yur in • and • see rum
(Muramidase Urine, Lysozyme Urine, Muramidase Serum, Lysozyme Serum)

Normal Findings

URINE
Adult, pregnant, infant, adolescent, and elderly: <3.6 mg/24 hours

Child: May be lower than adult levels
SERUM
Adult, pregnant, infant, adolescent, and elderly:

Gel diffusion assay 0.4–1.3 mg/dL
Nephelom 0.36–0.78 mg/dL
Radioimmunoassay 0.46 ± 0.08 mg/dL
Turbidim 0.27–0.93 mg/dL
Child and infant: Levels may be somewhat lower than adult norms.

What This Test Will Tell You

These serum and 24-hour urine tests determine whether there is evidence of granulocyte and monocyte breakdown, which may indicate acute leukemia, inflammatory disease, or renal graft rejection. Muramidase is an enzyme present in saliva, sweat, tears, mucus, phagocytic cells, and the kidneys that is released into the bloodstream when monocytes and granulocytes break down. Elevated levels of muramidase are usually seen with Gram-positive bacterial destruction. In renal disease, serum levels may be normal despite elevated urine levels.

Abnormal Findings

URINE AND SERUM

▲INCREASED LEVELS may indicate acute myelomonocytic leukemia, chronic granulocytic leukemia, regional enteritis (Crohn's disease), renal homograft rejection, renal tubular disease, Hodgkin's disease, human immunodeficiency virus, otitis media, polycythemia vera, sarcoidosis, or tuberculosis.

■■■■ ACTION ALERT!

Elevated levels may indicate acute leukemia or renal graft rejection. Notify the primary health care provider immediately of increased levels so that appropriate therapy can be instituted immediately.

Interfering Factors

URINE

➤ Urine not kept on ice during and after collection will cause erroneous results.

➤ Failure to collect all urine during the test period.

➤ Urinary tract infections.

➤ Blood from menses or saliva from coughing will result in a false elevation of results.

SERUM

➤ Bacterial contamination will cause elevated results.

M

NURSING CONSIDERATIONS

Prepare Your Client

➤ Explain as appropriate that this test is helpful in the evaluation of certain leukemias, inflammatory diseases, and kidney transplant rejection.

➤ For the urine test, instruct the client in the proper technique for collection of a 24-hour urine specimen.

Perform Procedure

URINE

➤ Use a 3-L container and no preservative.

➤ Closely follow the procedure for collecting a 24-hour urine sample.

➤ Keep the collection container on ice during the collection period.

SERUM

➤ Collect 10 cc of venous blood to fill two purple-top tubes.

Care After Test

➤ When leukemia is suspected, institute safety precautions related to bleeding such as use of soft toothbrushes and electric razors, additional pressure over venipuncture sites, and avoiding intramuscular injections whenever possible.

➤ Monitor urinary output for client with suspected renal disease or transplant rejection.

➤ Verify that a serum muramidase determination was made during the urine testing period so as to confirm urine results.

➤ Observe for signs of renal graft rejection when appropriate, including fever, anemia, malaise, and graft site tenderness.

➤ Administer immunosuppressive medications as ordered by the primary health care provider.

➤ Review related tests such as blood urea nitrogen levels, serum creatinine, creatinine clearance, and white blood cell count with differential.

Educate Your Client and the Family

➤ For client with renal graft rejection, review immunosuppressive therapy with them to assure compliance. Teach family and client about any changes in therapy.

➤ Instruct client and family on how to prevent infections due to high susceptibility from disease process or from medications to suppress the immune or inflammatory responses. This includes meticulous oral hygiene and handwashing, avoiding persons with upper respiratory infections, and avoiding large crowds.

Myasthenia Gravis Test Panel

mie as thee nee ah • gra vis • test • pan el
(Acetylcholine Receptor Antibodies, Acetylcholine Receptor Modulating Antibodies, Acetylcholine Receptor [AChR] Binding Antibodies, Acetylcholine Receptor Blocking Antibodies)

Normal Findings

➤ Acetylcholine receptor (AChR) binding antibodies: ≤ 0.03 nmol/L
➤ AChR modulating antibodies: 0%–20% loss of AChR
➤ AChR blocking antibodies: 0%–20% blockade of AChR
➤ Striational antibodies: < 1:60, negative. May be positive in 55% of clients over 60 years of age. Note: Not all labs include striational antibodies testing.

What This Test Will Tell You

This blood test diagnoses myasthenia gravis and thymoma. Myasthenia gravis is an autoimmune disease in which antibodies are formed to acetylcholine receptors (AChRs) and contractile elements of striated muscles. As the number of AChRs

decreases, neuromuscular conduction is impaired, resulting in fatigue, weakness, and prolonged recovery time of skeletal muscles.

Thymomas are epithelial tumors of the thymus that contain acetylcholine receptor–like material. After removal of a thymoma, a serially rising striational antibody titer may indicate recurrence of the tumor.

Abnormal Findings

▲INCREASED LEVELS may indicate myasthenia gravis or thymomas.

ACTION ALERT!

Myasthenia gravis may leave a client's swallowing and respiratory effort severely compromised. Observe the client carefully for any evidence of difficulty with maintaining a patent airway or ventilation.

Interfering Factors

➤ Immunosuppressant therapy may suppress AChR antibody levels and cause false negative results.

➤ Amyotrophic lateral sclerosis may cause false positive results for AChR antibody tests, especially if the client has been treated with snake venom.

➤ Muscle relaxants used during surgery may elevate AChR modulating and AChR blocking antibodies, resulting in false positive findings after surgery.

NURSING CONSIDERATIONS

Prepare Your Client

➤ Explain that this test is important to help diagnose a condition called myasthenia gravis, which can cause muscle weakness and vision symptoms.

Perform Procedure

➤ Collect 10 mL of venous blood in a red-top tube.

Care After Test

➤ Assess for clinical symptoms including ptosis, diplopia, swallowing difficulties, abnormal speech, and respiratory difficulties.

➤ Ensure that the client is referred to speech therapy if speaking or swallowing difficulties are noted.

➤ Ensure your client's safety. Muscle weakness may contribute to aspiration, falls, and respiratory difficulties.

➤ Evaluate other tests such as the edrophonium (Tensilon) test and electromyography.

Educate Your Client and the Family

➤ Explain that hormonal changes during pregnancy, the menstrual cycle, and disturbances in thyroid function may make symptoms worse. Emotional stress may also cause increased muscle weakness.

➤ Explain the names, dosages, side effects, and potential risks of medications to your client and family members.

Myelin Basic Protein

mie e lin • bay sik • proe teen
(MBP)

Normal Findings

<4 ng/mL indicates absence of demyelination or remission of disease (SI units: <4 µg/L)

What This Test Will Tell You

This cerebrospinal fluid test helps diagnose neurologic disease by detecting active demyelination of nerve cells. Myelin is a lipid-protein that covers some nerve fibers along the nerve pathway in the central and peripheral nervous systems. Myelinated nerve pathways have faster nerve transmission than nonmyelinated nerve pathways because nerve impulses jump from one nonmyelinated node (node of Ranvier) to another along the myelinated pathway. Breakdown of myelin results in slower nerve impulses and destruction of nerve axons.

Abnormal Findings

Weakly positive: 4–8 ng/mL indicates chronic disease with slow demyelination, or recovery phase from acute exacerbation.

Positive: >8 ng/mL indicates active demyelination.

Elevated levels may indicate multiple sclerosis, encephalitis, leukodystrophies, metabolic encephalopathies, central nervous system lupus, cranial irradiation, intrathecal chemotherapy, or recent stroke.

ACTION ALERT!

This test should not be performed in the presence of elevated intracranial pressure due to the potential for herniation and death.

Contraindications

➤ Do not perform a lumbar puncture for CSF when increased intracranial pressure is suspected. A rapid decrease in intracranial pressure secondary to the lumbar puncture and removal of cerebrospinal fluid may cause the brain to shift downward (herniate) into the spinal column. The herniation could cause serious damage to the vital centers in the medulla and result in neurological damage or death.

➤ Do not perform lumbar puncture for CSF in clients with primary clotting defects such as thrombocytopenia because of the risk of extradural or subdural hematoma formation.

Potential Complications

➤ Infection
➤ Headache
➤ Nausea
➤ Dizziness
➤ Bleeding into the spinal column
➤ Neurologic injury or death from herniation

NURSING CONSIDERATIONS

Prepare Your Client

➤ Explain that this procedure is to measure the cerebrospinal fluid pressure and to obtain samples of fluid for analysis.

➤ Explain that the physician will place a needle into the lower back and withdraw spinal fluid.

➤ Review the potential complications of the procedure and be sure the client has signed an informed consent.

➤ Assure the client that the needle is placed far below any spinal nerves into an empty space filled with fluid, not nerves.

➤ Explain the rationale for positioning as you place the client in the side-lying position with knees curled to the chest and arms wrapped around them. The chin should be resting on the chest. Assist the client to maintain this position throughout the procedure.

➤ Explain that the physician will numb the lumbar region of the back before placing the lumbar puncture needle.

➤ Tell your client there is no need to restrict fluids or foods before the procedure.

Perform Procedure

Nurses do not perform this procedure but should understand the process to prepare the client. Sterile technique must be maintained throughout the procedure. Place the client in the fetal position. Reassure the client throughout the procedure. Encourage the client to breathe slowly and deeply.

After the lumbar puncture needle is in the subarachnoid space, the client will need to straighten their legs for the initial pressure reading. The reading is taken with a manometer, provided in the lumbar puncture tray, that is attached to the needle via a three-way stopcock. At least 3 mL of cerebrospinal fluid is collected into a sterile, additive-free tube.

Label the tube and take to the laboratory immediately. The specimen may be stored in the refrigerator or freezer if necessary.

Care After Test
➤ Place a sterile dressing over the puncture site. Maintain client in a flat position for several hours after the procedure.
➤ Assess vital signs for elevated systolic pressure, widened pulse pressure, and respiratory depression, which can signal increased intracranial pressure. Decreased blood pressure may indicate shock.
➤ Assess for pain and medicate as ordered.
➤ Encourage drinking fluids to assist the body in replacing CSF loss.
➤ Assess for signs and symptoms of complications: changes in mental status, changes in sensory perception of lower extremities, and neck rigidity.

➤ Obtain occupation and physical therapy referrals if ability to perform activities of daily living (ADLs) are compromised in the client.
➤ Evaluate the need for community health services if ADLs are affected and the family's ability to support the client in these functions is limited.
➤ Evaluate related tests such as cerebrospinal fluid analysis, cerebrospinal fluid immunofixation, evoked potential studies, and magnetic resonance imaging (MRI).

Educate Your Client and the Family
➤ Instruct your client to remain flat for several hours after the lumbar puncture. Loss of spinal fluid during the lumbar puncture and potential leakage of CSF from the puncture site may cause headaches. Risk of CSF leakage is minimized when the client remains in a recumbent position.
➤ Assist your client in learning methods of compensating for changes in abilities to carry out necessary tasks.

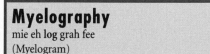

Myelography
mie eh log grah fee
(Myelogram)

Normal Findings
Normal spinal arachnoid space, no lesions or obstructions

What This Test Will Tell You
This radiologic test diagnoses abnormalities in the vertebrae and spinal cord. Injection and movement of a contrast medium (or air) within the spinal column during the radiologic procedure allows localization of tumors, herniations, and bone deformities. By visualizing abnormal flow of contrast medium or air injected into the subarachnoid space of the spinal canal, obstructions or

anatomical abnormalities can be discerned. This test may be done in conjunction with a CT (computed tomography) scan or MRI (magnetic resonance imaging) when more detailed visualization is required.

Abnormal Findings

Abnormalities may indicate herniated intervertebral disc, spinal tumor, spinal cyst, spinal adhesion, syringomyelia, bony deformity, astrocytoma, ependymoma, neurofibroma, meningioma, spinal injury, or arachnoiditis.

ACTION ALERT!

➤ If contrast material is used for this test, allergic reaction could occur, resulting in mild to life-threatening reactions. Emergency medications such as diphenhydramine, steroids, and epinephrine as well as emergency equipment should be immediately available for cardiopulmonary resuscitation.

➤ Oil-based material may cause meningeal irritation and water-soluble contrast material may cause seizure activity. Maintain appropriate positionings to avoid these complications. If they occur, maintain client's safety and comfort by keeping them in a low position. Keep oral airway at bedside, pad side rails up. Keep room dark and noise minimal.

Interfering Factors

➤ Feces and gas may decrease visualization.

➤ Oil-based contrast material may not visualize small anatomical areas or flow through severely stenotic, yet not fully obstructed, areas.

➤ Medications such as phenothiazines, amphetamines, tricyclic as well as other antidepressants, and central nervous system stimulants may lower the seizure threshold and result in seizures following the procedure in clients who receive metrizamide as a contrast material.

Contraindications

➤ Increased intracranial pressure may result in herniation during the lumbar puncture.

➤ Air, rather than iodine contrast medium, should be used in clients with allergy to iodine and/or shellfish, as well as those in traction with unstable fractures of the spine.

➤ Infection near the injection site contraindicates a myelogram because bacteria could be introduced and result in a bacterial meningitis.

➤ Multiple sclerosis is a contraindication because the procedure may cause acute exacerbation of the disease.

➤ Pregnancy is a contraindication due to radiation exposure of the unborn fetus.

➤ Renal failure or impairment would require special consideration and selection of contrast material to prevent further renal injury. The benefits should clearly outweigh the risks.

Potential Complications

➤ Allergic reaction to iodine medium (flushing, itching, urticaria, and anaphylaxis)
➤ Seizures
➤ Infection
➤ Headache
➤ Nausea
➤ Dizziness
➤ Meningitis
➤ Bleeding into the spinal column
➤ Neurologic injury or death from brain stem herniation

NURSING CONSIDERATIONS

Prepare Your Client

➤ Explain that this is an x-ray test (radiographic exam) in which air or dye is put inside the backbone (spinal column) using a needle and takes about 1 hour.

➤ Assure the client that the needle is inserted well below any nerves in the backbone.

➤ Ensure that an informed consent is obtained, because of the possible complications associated with this procedure.

➤ Ask about and inform the primary health care provider of allergies to iodine, radiopaque dyes, or shellfish.

➤ Review medications for phenothiazines, amphetamines, tricyclic as well as other antidepressants, and central nervous system stimulants, which could lower the seizure threshold. Inform the primary health care provider.

➤ Restrict food and fluids for 4–8 hours before the test. Consult with the radiology department for specific information related to the contrast material the client will be receiving. Some contrast materials specifically require adequate hydration, so prolonged periods of being without oral fluids would be contraindicated.

➤ Administer a cleansing enema as ordered the night before the test.

➤ Obtain baseline vital signs.

➤ Make sure the client has emptied both bowel and bladder before the test.

➤ Administer sedatives, narcotics, and atropine as ordered by the primary health care provider.

Perform Procedure

Nurses do not perform this procedure, but might assist in the lumbar puncture. Nurses should be familiar with the process to educate the client.

A lumbar puncture is performed (see *Lumbar Puncture*) and approximately 15 cc of cerebrospinal fluid

(CSF) is removed. An equivalent amount of contrast medium or air is injected (see *Lumbar Puncture*). Warn the client that a warm, flushed feeling may be experienced after the contrast medium is injected.

After the dye is injected, client lies on their abdomen and is strapped to a table. The table is tilted during the exam to allow the contrast medium to move within the spinal column. Radiographic (x-ray) films are taken as indicated.

If an oil-based contrast medium is used, it is withdrawn from the lumbar region after the test. Keep the head elevated to prevent migration of the oil-based contrast medium to the head, where it can cause irritation of the meninges. If a water-based contrast medium is used, it does not need to be aspirated at the end of the test.

Care After Test

➤ Monitor neurological and vital signs. Indications of impending cerebral herniation include decreased mentation, changes in pupil size and equality, increased blood pressure, decreased pulse, and irregular respirations. Irritability, neck rigidity, and fever are signs of meningitis.

➤ Assess for signs and symptoms of lumbar puncture complications: changes in mental status, changes in sensory perception of lower extremities, and neck rigidity.

➤ Assess for pain and medicate as ordered. Headaches, nausea, and vomiting may occur after this procedure.

➤ Encourage fluids to assist the body in replacing CSF loss and to maintain hydration. Contrast material has a diuretic effect. The client should void within 8 hours of the test. Evaluate intake and output for at least 8–12 hours following the test.

➤ If a water-based contrast medium was used, keep the client in a high Fowler's position for 6-8 hours after the test.

➤ If an oil-based contrast medium was used, the client will need to remain flat in bed for 6–12 hours.

➤ If air was used as the contrast material, the head is usually kept lower than the trunk for up to 48 hours.

➤ Observe for delayed signs of allergic reaction including urticaria, wheezing, tachycardia, hypotension, dyspnea, anxiety, rash, and hives.

➤ Evaluate related tests such as computed tomography, magnetic resonance imaging, and electromyography.

Educate Your Client and the Family

➤ Instruct your client in proper body mechanics to decrease the risk of further back injury.

➤ Teach client the importance of drinking more liquids to help excrete any contrast material that was used.

Myoglobin, Serum
mie oe gloe bin • see rum

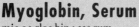

Normal Findings
All ages: 0–90 ng/mL (μ/L)

What This Test Will Tell You
This blood test helps diagnose myocardial infarction, myocardial trauma, musculoskeletal trauma, and muscular degenerative diseases. The test measures the blood levels of myoglobin, an oxygen-carrying protein found in both skeletal and cardiac muscle. Myoglobin carries oxygen within muscle cells to the energy-producing mitochondria.

Abnormal Findings
▲ INCREASED LEVELS may indicate acute myocardial infarction, myocardial ischemia, cardiac contusion, trauma, polymyositis, muscular dystrophy, skeletal muscle ischemia, cardioversion or electrical shock, skeletal muscle trauma and inflammation, lupus erythematosus, shock, acute renal failure, rhabdomyolysis, malignant hyperthermia, severe burns, or delirium tremens.

Interfering Factors
➤ Refrigeration of blood sample.

➤ Timing of sampling may miss increase in serum levels.

➤ Radioactive scans within 1 week may elevate levels.

The following will elevate levels:

➤ Vigorous exercise

➤ Intramuscular injections

➤ Hypothermia accompanied by prolonged shivering

➤ Convulsions

➤ Recent surgery, cardioversion, or anginal attack

➤ Hemolysis of sample

NURSING CONSIDERATIONS
Prepare Your Client
➤ Explain as appropriate that this test is to help diagnose muscle disease or heart damage.

➤ Determine as exactly as possible the onset of chest pain in client being evaluated for myocardial infarction. Serum myoglobin levels peak at 4–8 hours.

➤ Inform the client there is no need to restrict fluid or food before the test, but there should be no strenuous exercise for 24 hours preceding the test.

➤ Explain that multiple blood samples for the rise and fall of other enzyme levels over time will be necessary if this test is being done to evaluate for myocardial infarction.

Perform Procedure

➤ Perform a venipuncture to collect 5–7 mL of venous blood in a red-top tube.

➤ Send the sample to the laboratory immediately. Do not refrigerate.

Care After Test

➤ Evaluate the client's history for coronary and vascular disease if the test is being done to help diagnose a myocardial infarction.

➤ Assess the client for continued chest pain and response to treatment.

➤ If serum levels are greatly elevated, closely monitor renal function by assessing urinary output, and checking for fluid and electrolyte imbalances.

➤ Evaluate other tests such as lactic dehydrogenase (LDH), creatinine phosphokinase (CPK), aspartate aminotransferase (SGOT or AST), and urinary myoglobin.

Educate Your Client and the Family

➤ Instruct client with suspected heart disease to notify the nurse or physician immediately if chest pain should occur or worsen.

➤ Encourage significant others to learn cardiopulmonary resuscitation (CPR).

➤ Teach client and family how to have a heart-healthy diet, with no added salt.

➤ Instruct client on activity program appropriate to diagnosis.

Myoglobin, Urine

mie oe gloe bin • yur in

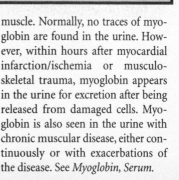

Normal Findings

All ages: No traces

What This Test Will Tell You

This urine test helps diagnose myocardial infarction, myocardial trauma, musculoskeletal trauma, and muscular degenerative diseases. The test measures the presence of myoglobin, an oxygen-carrying protein found in both skeletal and cardiac muscle. Normally, no traces of myoglobin are found in the urine. However, within hours after myocardial infarction/ischemia or musculoskeletal trauma, myoglobin appears in the urine for excretion after being released from damaged cells. Myoglobin is also seen in the urine with chronic muscular disease, either continuously or with exacerbations of the disease. See *Myoglobin, Serum*.

Abnormal Findings

▲INCREASED LEVELS may indicate acute myocardial infarction, myocardial ischemia, cardiac contusion, skeletal muscle trauma or ischemia or inflammation, trauma, polymyositis, muscular dystrophy, cardioversion or electrical shock, lupus erythematosus, shock, acute renal failure, rhabdomyolysis, diabetes mellitus, barbiturate toxicity, sepsis, or delirium tremens.

Interfering Factors

➤ Vigorous exercise may elevate levels.

➤ Large intake of ascorbic acid may cause the reagent test method to fail to detect myoglobin.

➤ Recent surgery, cardioversion, or anginal attack may affect levels.

➤ Timing of sampling may miss increase in urinary levels.

NURSING CONSIDERATIONS

Prepare Your Client

➤ Explain that this test is used to help diagnose muscle disease or heart damage or to evaluate trauma. Tailor this explanation to the specific reason the test was ordered for the client.

➤ Determine as exactly as possible the onset of chest pain in client being evaluated for myocardial infarction.

Urinary myoglobin levels generally appear 3–24 hours following myocardial infarction.

➤ Inform the client there is no need to restrict fluid or food before the test, but there should be no strenuous exercise for 24–48 hours preceding the test.

Perform Procedure

➤ Collect a clean urine sample.

➤ Label the sample and note any interfering factors or medications.

➤ Send the sample to the laboratory immediately. Do not refrigerate.

Care After Test

➤ Evaluate the client's history for coronary and vascular disease if the test is being done to help diagnose a myocardial infarction.

➤ Evaluate other tests such as lactic dehydrogenase (LDH), creatine phosphokinase (CPK), aspartate aminotransferase (SGOT or AST), and serum myoglobin.

Educate Your Client and the Family

➤ Instruct client with suspected heart disease to notify the nurse or physician immediately if chest pain should occur or worsen.

➤ Teach client and family a heart-healthy diet, with no added salt.

➤ Instruct the client on activity program appropriate to diagnosis.

Nasopharyngeal Culture

nay zoe fah rin jel • kul chur

(NP Culture, Nasopharynx Culture, NPH Culture)

Normal Findings
Negative

What This Test Will Tell You

This microbiological test diagnoses nasopharyngeal infections and screens for upper respiratory and systemic bacterial infections. Potentially pathogenic organisms cultured from nasopharyngeal specimens may not necessarily be the cause of respiratory or systemic infection. Clinical signs and symptoms of disease must also be considered when evaluating the results of the culture.

Cultures may also be performed to identify carrier states, as in the case of health care workers during outbreaks of nosocomial infections.

Abnormal Findings

➤ Always abnormal bacteria in nasopharyngeal culture may include *Mycobacterium tuberculosis*, *Corynebacterium diphtheriae*, and *Bordetella pertussis*.

➤ Frequently significant bacterial findings in nasopharyngeal culture of children include *Hemophilus influenzae* type B and *Neisseria meningitidis*.

➤ Significant nasopharyngeal culture in children with otitis media include *Streptococcus pneumoniae*, *Staphylococcus aureus*, *Hemophilus influenzae*, *Branhamella catarrhalis*, and beta-hemolytic streptococci.

➤ Frequently significant culture in presence of clinical findings include *Candida albicans*, *Neisseria meningitidis*, *Hemophilus influenzae*, *Streptococci*, coronaviruses, and rhinovirus.

Interfering Factors

➤ Use of antibiotics before the specimen is collected for culture.

➤ Transport of specimen in sodium chloride may significantly lower the yields of *Branhamella catarrhalis* and *Hemophilus influenzae*.

➤ *Bordetella pertussis* does not survive well in transport media.

Potential Complications

➤ Injury to the nasopharyngeal membranes may occur while collecting a specimen from a child or uncooperative adult. Ask for assistance of parents or other health care workers if difficulty collecting the specimen is anticipated.

NURSING CONSIDERATIONS

Prepare Your Client

➤ Explain that this test is to identify bacteria or germs that may be causing their illness. If this procedure is to determine the client's carrier status, explain that the client may have organisms that make other people ill without making the client sick.

➤ Explain that the procedure is very quick and should not be painful.

Perform Procedure

➤ Insert a flexible culture swab into the nose. Rotate the swab against the posterior pharynx.

➤ Place the swab in the culture medium. Label the container and transport to the lab immediately.

Care After Test

➤ Collaborate with the primary health care provider to treat symptoms such as fever, aches, and pains.

➤ Begin antibiotic therapy as ordered after the culture has been obtained.

➤ Evaluate other diagnostic and lab tests such as blood and sputum culture, pneumococcal antigen detection, enzyme immunoassay, chest x-rays, and bronchoscopy.

Educate Your Client and the Family

➤ Teach your client about decreasing the spread of infection by washing hands, covering mouth when coughing or sneezing, and cleaning a sick child's toys before sharing them with other children.

➤ Emphasize the importance of taking antibiotics as prescribed. Explain that antibiotics must be taken until the prescription is gone, even if there are no longer any symptoms, to be sure the infection has been fully treated and to prevent superinfections.

Nipple Stimulation Test

nip pul • stim yu lay shun • test
(NST, Breast Stimulation, BST)

Normal Findings

Negative test: No late decelerations during 3 contractions in 10 minutes, suggests fetal well-being for last 7 days.

What This Test Will Tell You

This manometric test determines how the fetus will respond to labor contractions. It is used for high-risk pregnancies and is performed after 34 weeks' gestation. This test will display on a fetal monitor how the fetus will tolerate the stress of labor by producing contractions in response to nipple stimulation. During a contraction, placental blood flow is decreased temporarily. If the fetus is healthy, it tolerates the decreased blood flow during a contraction and the fetal heart rate remains within normal limits. If the results are abnormal, other tests may be ordered, such as amniocentesis or biophysical profile, before the fetus is delivered.

Abnormal Findings

Fetoplacental insufficiency

ACTION ALERT!

This test should be performed near a childbirth unit where resuscitation equipment and cesarean section are available. Any positive test (late decelerations) should be reported to the primary health care provider immediately. Immediate evaluation of fetal well-being is indicated.

Interfering Factors

➤ Hypotension may give a false positive reading.

Contraindications

➤ Threatened preterm labor
➤ Ruptured membranes
➤ Hydramnios
➤ Previous preterm labor
➤ Previous classical cesarean delivery
➤ Placenta previa
➤ Multiple fetuses
➤ Abruptio placentae
➤ Previous hysterotomy

➤ Pregnancy of less than 32 weeks' gestation

Potential Complications
➤ Premature labor.
➤ Hyperstimulation or overstimulation of the uterus resulting in too many or too hard contractions of the uterus could result in uterine rupture.

NURSING CONSIDERATIONS
Prepare Your Client
➤ Explain that this test is to see how the baby will tolerate being born (labor contractions).
➤ Explain that this test measures the baby's heart rate (FHR) to check for any abnormal decrease during the contractions.
➤ Explain that the contractions will be similar to mild labor. Teach the client breathing exercises to control the discomfort.
➤ Instruct the client to void before the procedure.

Perform Procedure
➤ Assist the client to lie on her left side with the head of bed elevated to avoid compression of the large blood vessels by the uterus.
➤ Assess the client's vital signs and monitor the fetal heart rate and uterine activity for 10–20 minutes before beginning the test.
➤ Connect the client to the external fetal monitor to record the fetal heart rate, and apply the external uterine monitor to the fundus to record uterine contractions.
➤ Do not have the client start nipple stimulation if uterine contractions are noted during the 10–20-minute initial monitoring period. Observe for three spontaneous 40–60-second palpable contractions in 10 minutes.

➤ Monitor the fetal heart rate for any late decelerations during contractions, which may indicate an inadequate oxygen supply to the fetus.
➤ Assess the contractions. Three contractions without decelerations are needed for a valid or complete test.
➤ Instruct the client, if needed, to apply a warm washcloth to one breast for several minutes. Then she will be told to gently roll or twist the nipple of one breast for 2 minutes and stop for 5 minutes. Both breasts should be stimulated if contractions do not occur.
➤ Instruct the client to stop stimulation during contractions.
➤ If decelerations occur, stop nipple stimulation and place in left lateral position, notify the primary health care provider, and apply oxygen at 6–8 liters per mask.

Care After Test
➤ Monitor the client's blood pressure, fetal heart rate, and uterine activity until they return to the pre-stimulation state.
➤ Monitor the client for any additional contractions or any increase in frequency or intensity of contractions, which could indicate preterm labor.
➤ Instruct the client who does not have contractions produced by nipple stimulation that intravenous oxytocin may be administered in a contraction stress test. A biophysical profile may also be ordered.
➤ Ask the client if she is taking her prenatal vitamins as ordered by her primary health care provider. Stress the importance of supplemental vitamins in providing good nutrition and normal growth and development of her baby.

N

➤ Assess the client's knowledge of prenatal care including diet, activity, rest, signs and symptoms of labor, and danger signs in pregnancy. Provide instruction as indicated.

➤ Assess mother's readiness to meet parental role functions by reviewing infant care knowledge, methods of infant feeding, and ability to obtain needed supplies. Provide instruction and/or community health service referrals as indicated.

➤ Assess the client's ability to provide adequate nutrition for the fetus. Refer to social services and Women, Infants, and Children program (WIC) for assistance.

➤ Refer to a registered dietician if dietary deficiencies are suspected.

➤ Assess the client for use of cigarettes, tobacco products, alcohol, over-the-counter medications, and street drugs. Instruct the client as necessary to avoid these substances as they may cause intrauterine growth retardation.

➤ If the client reports decreased fetal movements, assess recent maternal history for maternal activity and relationship to fetal movement. Assess also her recent consumption of food or fluids and its relationship to fetal movement. Consult with the primary health care provider about instructing the client to eat, drink, and then rest. During rest, tell her to concentrate on fetal movements for 1 hour. Three fetal movements in 1 hour are reassuring.

➤ Review related tests such as nonstress test, acoustic stimulation, biophysical profile, amniocentesis, and daily fetal movement count.

Educate Your Client and the Family

➤ Teach your client the signs of preterm labor such as abdominal cramping with or without diarrhea, uterine contractions every 10 minutes or more frequently, menstrual-like cramps in the lower abdomen, low backache, increase or change in vaginal discharge, or pelvic pressure.

➤ Advise the client to lie down on her left side and notify the primary health care provider if preterm labor occurs.

➤ Instruct the client in assessing daily fetal movement. (See *Daily Fetal Movement Count*.)

➤ Advise the client to notify the primary health care provider if fetal movement decreases or stops.

➤ Educate the client about any other needs related to her care or the baby.

➤ Instruct the client about any additional tests that will be performed.

Nonstress Test

nahn stres • test
(NST, Fetal Activity Determination, Fetal Activity Acceleration Determination, FAD)

Normal Findings

Reactive: Fetal heart rate accelerations are present. Two or more accelerations of 15 beats per minute that last for 15 seconds within 10 minutes.

What This Test Will Tell You

This noninvasive monitoring test is used between 32 and 34 weeks' gestation to evaluate fetal well-being, especially in high-risk pregnancies, to determine the need for a contraction stress test. Increases (accelerations) of the fetal heart rate in response to fetal movement are measured to provide information on general well-being and the balance between the central nervous system and the autonomic nervous system of the fetus. Fetal activity may be induced by uterine contractions, external manipulation, acoustic stimulation, or be spontaneous, but is not induced by oxytocin in this test. Nonstress testing is 99% reliable in determining fetal viability and has allowed many high-risk pregnancies to continue so that the fetus is more mature at birth.

Abnormal Findings

Nonreactive: Normal accelerations are not present with fetal movement within a 40-minute period or there is a lack of fetal movement. These findings may indicate fetal hypoxia, fetal sleep cycle, or effects of drugs.

ACTION ALERT!

Any nonreactive nonstress test needs to be reported to the primary health care provider immediately and further evaluated.

Interfering Factors

➤ Fetal sleep (fetal sleep cycle averages 40 minutes)
➤ Maternal alcohol or narcotic use

NURSING CONSIDERATIONS

Prepare Your Client

➤ Explain that this test measures how the baby's heart rate changes when it moves and is one test to help ensure the baby is doing well.

➤ Explain to the mother that she will be connected to a fetal monitor and be given a button to press to record when the baby moves.

➤ Instruct the client (usually outpatient) to eat before the test because fetal activity is assisted with high maternal serum glucose.

➤ Assure the client that the test will not be uncomfortable.

Perform Procedure

➤ Have the client void and then lie in a sidelying position. Many primary health care providers prefer the left side for better uteroplacental circulation.

➤ Locate the fetal heart tones.

➤ Apply a conductive gel to the external fetal monitor and place on the client's abdomen where the fetal heart tones are heard.

➤ Give the client a button to press when she feels fetal movement. Explain the equipment to the client.

➤ Watch the fetal monitor for fetal heart rate accelerations with fetal movement.

➤ Observe for two or more accelerations of 15 beats per minute that last for 15 seconds within a 10-minute period.

➤ Stimulate fetal activity if the fetus is quiet for 20 minutes. This can be done by rubbing the mother's abdomen, making noise in the room, or by using an acoustic stimulator.

Care After Test

➤ If the test is nonreactive, report to the primary health care provider immediately.

➤ Remove the monitor and the conductive gel from the abdomen.

➤ Assess the client's knowledge of prenatal care including diet, activity,

rest, signs and symptoms of labor, and danger signs in pregnancy. Provide instruction as indicated.

➤ Assess mother's readiness to meet parental role functions by reviewing infant care knowledge, methods of infant feeding, and ability to obtain needed supplies. Provide instruction and/or community health service referrals as indicated.

➤ If the client reports decreased fetal movements, assess recent maternal history for maternal activity and relationship to fetal movement. Assess also her recent consumption of food or fluids and its relationship to fetal movement. Consult with the primary health care provider about instructing the client to eat, drink, and then rest. During rest, tell her to concentrate on fetal movements for 1 hour. Three fetal movements in 1 hour are reassuring.

➤ Review related tests including contraction stress test, pregnanediol level, obstetrical ultrasonography, serum estrogen level, daily fetal movement count, and amniocentesis.

Educate Your Client and the Family

➤ If the client has a high-risk pregnancy, reinforce the importance of keeping the appointments for regular nonstress testing.

➤ Instruct the client how to check for daily fetal movement count (DFMC).

➤ Teach the client about danger signs in pregnancy such as a gush of fluid, vaginal bleeding, abdominal pain, temperature elevation, dizziness, blurred vision, persistent vomiting, severe headache, edema, muscular irritability, difficult urination, or decreased/absent fetal movements.

➤ Instruct client to notify her primary health care provider if she has less than three movements in 1 hour. A nonstress test or biophysical profile may be ordered.

➤ Advise the client to lie down on her side and notify the primary health care provider if preterm labor is suspected.

5-Nucleotidase

5 • noo clee oe tie dase
(5-NT, 5'NT)

Normal Findings

ADULT AND ELDERLY
2–17.5 U/L
PREGNANT
Values may be slightly higher in the third trimester.
NEWBORN
Values may be slightly lower than adult.
CHILD
Values may be slightly lower than adult.

What This Test Will Tell You

This blood test helps determine the presence of hepatobiliary disease and evaluates the source of elevated alkaline phosphatase levels. 5-nucleotidase is an enzyme found in liver tissue, and to a small degree in red blood cells. Elevated alkaline phosphatase (ALP) with normal 5-nucleotidase levels indicates skeletal disease. Elevated 5-nucleotidase levels along with elevations in alkaline phosphatase (ALP), gamma-glutamyl transferase (GGT), leucine amino-peptidase (LAP), alanine amino-transferase (ALT), and aspartate aminotransferase (AST) levels are indicative of hepatobiliary disease.

Abnormal Findings

▲INCREASED LEVELS may indicate hepatitis, biliary obstruction from calculi or tumor, hepatic carcinoma or tumor, cirrhosis, necrosis of liver, hepatotoxic agents, or ischemia of liver.

Interfering Factors

➤ Hemolysis of the sample may falsely increase the level.
➤ Use of cholestatic drugs, such as phenothiazine, oral contraceptives, chlorpromazine, erythromycin estolate, estrogens, acetaminophen, aspirin, and any potentially hepatotoxic agents may elevate 5-NT levels.

NURSING CONSIDERATIONS

Prepare Your Client

➤ Explain that this test is used to diagnose liver disease.
➤ Consult with the primary health care provider about the need to withhold medications known to alter the results.

Perform Procedure

➤ Collect 7–10 cc of venous blood in a red-top tube.
➤ Handle sample gently—hemolysis may alter results.

Care After Test

➤ Assess your client for signs of liver function impairment such as ascites, unusual bruising or prolonged bleeding, tarry stools, and tremors.
➤ Assess for occult gastrointestinal bleeding with routine stool guaiac testing. Esophageal varices and mucosal bleeding are complications of liver disease.
➤ Consult with a registered dietician to design a high-calorie, well-balanced diet. People with advanced liver disease have poor absorption of nutrients due to decreased bile flow into the intestines. As appropriate, reduce sodium or protein in the diet if edema and ascites, or increased ammonia levels are present.
➤ Evaluate other liver function tests such as alkaline phosphatase, bilirubin, alanine aminotransferase (ALT), aspartate aminotransferase (AST), gamma-glutamyl transferase (GGT), prothrombin time, ammonia, and aminopeptidase.

Educate Your Client and the Family

➤ In the presence of liver disease, instruct client and family to notify staff of tarry stools, easy bruising, tremors, or the development of jaundice.
➤ Instruct client and family on high-calorie, well-balanced diet as appropriate. If sodium or protein restrictions are indicated, help client and family make dietary selections with these limitations.
➤ Clients with impaired liver function have prolonged bleeding times. Instruct client and family on safety measures such as electric razors, non-skid shoes, and soft toothbrushes.

Obstetric Ultrasonography

ob steh trik • ul trah sah nah grah fee

(Obstetric Sonogram, Obstetric Echography, Pelvic Ultrasonography in Pregnancy, Pregnant Uterus Ultrasonography, Ultrasound)

Normal Findings

Normal fetal position and size

Evidence of fetal movement and cardiac activity

Normal amniotic fluid volume

Normal size, structure, and location of the placenta

What This Test Will Tell You

This ultrasound test evaluates the female pelvis; the size, status, and location of the fetus; and the placenta. High-frequency sound waves are directed from the transducer to the uterus, placenta, and fetus. These sound waves (echoes) are returned and electronically converted to a picture of the pattern. Obstetric ultrasonography is used for diagnosing pregnancy; diagnosing an abnormal pregnancy (ectopic pregnancy); evaluating fetal age by the diameter of the head; determining fetal position; measuring fetal growth; identifying multiple pregnancies; locating the position of the placenta; identifying an abnormal placenta; diagnosing uterine and ovarian enlargements; and assisting with various diagnostic procedures such as amniocentesis, fetoscopy, and intrauterine procedures.

Abnormal Findings

Abnormalities may indicate tubal pregnancy, placenta previa, abruptio placentae, multiple fetuses, abnormal fetal position (breech, transverse), fetal anomalies, fetal death, intrauterine growth retardation, polyhydramnios, neoplasms, cysts, endometriosis, pelvic inflammatory disease, hydatidiform mole, or abscesses.

Interfering Factors

➤ Failure to fill the bladder may impair imaging.

➤ Air-filled bowel, because gas does not transmit sound waves.

➤ Recent gastrointestinal studies with barium, because it distorts sound waves.

➤ Obesity may interfere with interpretation.

➤ Dehydration prevents proper contrast between organs and body fluids.

➤ A posterior placental site may be difficult to identify.

NURSING CONSIDERATIONS

Prepare Your Client

➤ Explain that the procedure is done to obtain information about the size and position of the baby, the placenta, and the womb.

➤ Explain that the test is performed by a physician, ultrasound technician, or nurse and takes about 20 minutes.

➤ Explain that the test is noninvasive and will not be uncomfortable except for a full bladder.

➤ Assure the client that the test will not harm the fetus.

➤ Have the client drink 800–1000 mL of water or another liquid 1 hour prior to the exam to fill the bladder.

➤ Instruct the client not to void until the test is completed so that visualization is optimal.

➤ If a vaginal probe is used, do not increase the client's oral fluid intake and ensure the client has emptied her bladder.

Perform Procedure

Nurses, unless specially trained, do not usually perform this procedure but should understand the process to prepare the client and assist the physician or ultrasonographer. The client is assisted to a supine position on the examining table. A water-soluble conductive gel is applied to the abdomen to enhance ultrasound transmission and reception. The transducer is moved on the skin vertically and horizontally over the abdomen and pelvis. If a transvaginal approach is used, the transducer is covered with a clear, plastic sleeve and inserted into the vagina for imaging. Pictures are recorded with either approach. Fetal structures may be pointed out to the mother during the exam.

Care After Test

➤ Wipe off the conductive gel from the abdomen.

➤ Allow the client to void.

➤ Assess the client's knowledge of prenatal care including diet, activity, rest, signs and symptoms of labor, and danger signs in pregnancy. Provide instruction as indicated.

➤ Assess mother's readiness to meet parental role functions by reviewing infant care knowledge, methods of infant feeding, and ability to obtain needed supplies. Provide instruction and/or community health service referrals as indicated.

➤ If the client reports decreased fetal movements, assess recent maternal

history for maternal activity and relationship to fetal movement. Assess also her recent consumption of food or fluids and its relationship to fetal movement. Consult with the primary health care provider about instructing the client to eat, drink, and then rest. During rest, tell her to concentrate on fetal movements for 1 hour. Three fetal movements in 1 hour are reassuring.

➤ Review related tests including contraction stress test, pregnanediol level, nonstress test, serum estrogen level, daily fetal movement count, and amniocentesis.

Educate Your Client and the Family

➤ Teach the client about danger signs in pregnancy such as a gush of fluid, vaginal bleeding, abdominal pain, temperature elevation, dizziness, blurred vision, persistent vomiting, severe headache, edema, muscular irritability, difficult urination, or decreased/absent fetal movements.

➤ Instruct client to notify their primary health care provider if they have less than three movements in 1 hour. A nonstress test or biophysical profile may be ordered.

➤ Teach the client the signs of preterm labor such as abdominal cramping with or without diarrhea, uterine contractions every 10 minutes or more frequently, menstrual-like cramps in the lower abdomen, low backache, increase or change in vaginal discharge, or pelvic pressure.

➤ Advise the client to lie down on her side and notify the primary health care provider if preterm labor is suspected.

Obstruction Series
ob **struck** shun • **seer** ees
(Flat Plate of the Abdomen, Abdominal Plain Film, Abdominal Film, Scout Films)

Normal Findings
All ages: No evidence of bowel obstruction, abnormal calcifications, abscesses, foreign bodies, or free air

What This Test Will Tell You
This x-ray test is used as a diagnostic tool for clients suspected of having a bowel obstruction, paralytic ileus, perforation of the intestines or stomach, abdominal abscess, kidney stones, appendicitis, or foreign body ingestion. X-ray films in the standing position are examined for free air under the diaphragm, which would indicate a perforated bowel or stomach. The left lateral decubitus position is used for clients unable to stand for the x-ray. An examination of the air/fluid level in the stomach and intestines may determine a bowel obstruction or paralytic ileus.

Utilizing supine x-rays, a localized cluster of tiny bubbles is diagnostic of an abdominal abscess. Calcifications within a ureter are found in the client experiencing a kidney stone. A calcification within the right lower quadrant in the client complaining of abdominal pain may indicate appendicitis. A gas-filled, distended abdomen may signal an obstruction or an ileus.

Abnormal Findings
Abnormalities may indicate bowel obstruction, kidney stone, hepatomegaly, splenomegaly, presence of foreign bodies, paralytic ileus, abdominal abscess, perforation of the small or large intestines, appendi-colithiasis, calcification of structures, calcium deposits, abdominal aortic aneurysm, peritoneal effusion, or abnormal position of the kidneys.

Interfering Factors
➤ Retained barium from previous gastrointestinal x-rays may obscure details on the x-ray films.
➤ Failure to remove radiopaque objects such as jewelry or clothing in the x-ray field can obscure details on the x-ray films.

Contraindications
➤ Pregnancy, because x-rays may harm the fetus

NURSING CONSIDERATIONS
Prepare Your Client
➤ Explain that this test is used to find problems in the abdomen or stomach area. Assure the client that the test is not painful.
➤ Administer the bowel preparation to clear the intestinal tract if ordered by the primary health care provider.
➤ Ensure this test is performed before any studies involving barium.
➤ Remove all underclothing, dentures, jewelry, and hairpins or other objects that might obscure the anatomic details on the x-ray film.

Perform Procedure
Nurses do not usually perform this procedure, but should understand the process to prepare the client. A series of one to three x-ray images are taken of the abdomen. A supine, left lateral, and standing x-ray may be

done. If the client is unable to lie flat, assist them to a left lateral position with the right arm over head. Provide shielding for male client over the penis and testicles to prevent radiation exposure. Female ovaries cannot be protected because of their proximity to the kidneys. Tell the client to breathe out and hold their breath as the x-ray is taken. A single x-ray is taken. The x-ray is repeated in a standing or sitting position if required. The supine film will be done on an x-ray table or in bed, if portable. It requires the client to position their arms over their head. A cross table lateral view may be indicated for older persons since clarification of the abdominal aorta may hide an aortic aneurysm.

Care After Test

➤ Assess the client's patterns of bowel and bladder elimination.

➤ Consult with a registered dietician to assist the family and client in meeting special dietary needs related to alterations in bowel elimination.

➤ If foreign body ingestion is confirmed or suspected, carefully assess all stools for the object, and assess for abdominal pain or cramping, which may signal obstruction.

➤ Evaluate related tests such as barium enemas, air contrast barium enema, small bowel follow-through, liver biopsy, liver scans, intravenous pyelogram, abdominal computed tomography scan, and/or abdominal magnetic resonance imaging.

Educate Your Client and the Family

➤ If the presence of a foreign body is noted and it is determined that the client should pass the object naturally, instruct the client or family to increase roughage in the diet and to monitor all stool specimens until the object is excreted to ensure its passage from the gastrointestinal tract.

➤ Educate client about treatment plans for specific abnormal findings.

Oculoplethysmography

ok yu loe pleth iz mog rah fee
(OPG)

Normal Findings

Ear and eye pulsations occur simultaneously, or within less than 10 milliseconds.

What This Test Will Tell You

This noninvasive blood flow test determines carotid artery blood flow and diagnoses occlusive disease. Carotid artery blood flow is measured indirectly by measuring the flow in the ophthalmic artery, which is the first internal branch of the internal carotid.

Abnormal Findings

Delayed pulsations may indicate carotid occlusive disease.

ACTION ALERT!

If corneal abrasions result from the test, apply a lubricant or topical antibiotic therapy as ordered and patch the affected eye.

Interfering Factors
➤ Constant blinking will cause artifacts on the tracings.
➤ Lack of client cooperation will cause artifacts on the tracings.

Contraindications
➤ Eye surgery within 6 months of the procedure
➤ Enucleation
➤ Lens implantation
➤ Cataracts
➤ History of retinal detachment
➤ Hypersensitivity to anesthetic used in eye during procedure

Potential Complications
Scleral hematoma
Conjunctival hemorrhage
Photophobia
Scleral erythema
Corneal abrasions

NURSING CONSIDERATIONS

Prepare Your Client
➤ Tell the client that this test is used to find blockages in blood flow through the blood vessels in the neck that go to the brain.
➤ Instruct a client who wears contact lenses to remove them before the test.
➤ Tell the client the test usually takes 30 minutes.
➤ Assure the client that there is no pain with this procedure.
➤ Inform the client that the local anesthetic drops used on the eyes usually burn slightly.
➤ Assure client that any visual loss that occurs when suction is applied is temporary.

Perform Procedure
Nurses do not usually perform this procedure but should understand the process to explain it to the client. Place the client on continuous electrocardiogram monitoring. Place anesthetic drops in the client's eyes. Photoelectric probes will be placed on each ear. Eyecups that look much like contact lenses are positioned on the eyes and held in place with light suction. Tracings of blood flow in the ears and eyes are recorded on graph paper as suction is applied and released to measure blood flow. Pulsation tracings are recorded. The differences in pulse rates between the eyes, between the ears, and between the eyes and ears are measured. Delay is measured when a stenosis of the internal carotid is present.

Care After Test
➤ Assess the client for signs of corneal abrasion such as eye pain and photophobia.
➤ Evaluate related test procedures such as cerebral angiography, computed tomography (CT) scan, and magnetic resonance imaging (MRI).

Educate Your Client and the Family
➤ Instruct your client not to wear contact lenses for approximately 2 hours after the procedure.
➤ Instruct your client to refrain from rubbing eyes for approximately 2 hours after the procedure. Rubbing may cause corneal abrasion.
➤ Tell your client that mild burning of the eyes is normal as the anesthetic wears off. Severe burning is not to be expected and should be reported to the primary care provider. The anesthetic usually wears off in less than 1 hour.
➤ Encourage the client to use prescribed eye drops for irritation or sunglasses for sensitivity to the light.

Osmolality, Serum

oz moe lal ih tee • see rum

Normal Findings

ADULT, PREGNANT,
ADOLESCENT, ELDERLY
275–295 mOsm/kg H_2O
NEWBORN
266–295 mOsm/kg H_2O
CHILD
275–295 mOsm/kg H_2O

What This Test Will Tell You

This blood test helps evaluate the concentration of a client's serum as well as the client's kidneys' concentrating and diluting abilities. The number of dissolved particles (urea, glucose, electrolytes, medications, organic acids, and ethanol) compared to the volume of water is reflected in serum osmolality. An elevated level indicates more concentrated blood, while a decreased level indicates relatively more dilute blood. The level of serum osmolality is closely regulated by antidiuretic hormone. When the blood becomes more concentrated (increase in level) from a relative deficit of fluid, antidiuretic hormone levels increase, causing the body to retain fluid. Conversely, when the blood becomes less concentrated (decreased level) from a relative excess of fluid, antidiuretic hormone levels decrease, causing the body to eliminate water.

Abnormal Findings

▲INCREASED LEVELS may indicate hypernatremia, dehydration, intracellular dehydration, hypovolemia, hyperglycemia, brain trauma, hypercalcemia, diabetes mellitus, diabetes insipidus, hyperosmolar hyperglycemic non-ketotic acidosis, or renal failure.

▼DECREASED LEVELS may indicate water intoxication, syndrome of inappropriate antidiuretic hormone, Addison's disease, adrenogenital syndrome, lung cancer, adrenocortical insufficiency, hyponatremia, or acute renal disease.

ACTION ALERT!

Levels of 400–425 mOsm/kg H_2O are often accompanied by seizures and/or cardiopulmonary arrest. Carefully decrease all stimuli to the client, provide a safe environment, and institute continuous cardiac monitoring while a definitive diagnosis is made and therapy is initiated. Intravenous fluid therapy needs to be initiated and/or solutions selected need to provide more free water.

Interfering Factors

➤ Corticosteroids, insulin, mannitol, and diuretics will result in increased values by affecting fluid balance.

NURSING CONSIDERATIONS

Prepare Your Client

➤ Explain that this test helps evaluate how well the kidneys are working to keep a good water balance in the body.

Perform Procedure

➤ Collect 5–10 mL of venous blood in a red-top tube.

Care After Test

➤ Assess for signs of dehydration by noting poor skin turgor, dry and cracked tongue, dry mucous membranes, dark urine, tachycardia, slow venous filling, orthostatic hypotension, and thirst. In infants and children, crying without tears and sunken fontanel may be noted.

➤ Assess for signs of overhydration by noting edema, light to clear urine, weight gain, tachycardia, distended neck veins, distended hand veins, labored respirations, adventitious breath sounds in the lungs, and hypertension.

➤ Monitor and record all fluid intake and output.

➤ If serum osmolality is elevated, consult with the primary health care provider regarding a need for intravenous fluid therapy that provides more free water.

➤ Institute seizure precautions and monitor for increase or decrease in level of consciousness.

➤ Evaluate related tests including urine osmolality, serum electrolytes, blood urea nitrogen level, serum glucose, water load (dilution) test, and urinalysis.

Educate Your Client and the Family

➤ Instruct the client in the importance of limiting or increasing oral intake based on laboratory results and disorder.

➤ Instruct client with adrenocortical insufficiency to take steroid replacements as prescribed and wear medical alert identification. Increased dosages of steroids are needed during times of excessive physiologic or psychologic stress.

Osmolality, Urine

oz moe lal ih tee • yur in

Normal Findings

ADULT, PREGNANT, ADOLESCENT, ELDERLY

50–1400 mOsm/kg H_2O (dependent on fluid intake) (SI units: 50–1400 mmol/kg H_2O)

After 12–hour fluid restriction: At least 3 times serum level, or >850 mOsm/kg H_2O (SI units: >850 mmol/kg H_2O)

NEWBORN

100–600 mOsm/kg H_2O (dependent on fluid intake) (SI units: 100–600 mmol/kg H_2O)

After 12-hour fluid restriction: >850 mOsm/kg H_2O (SI units: >850 mmol/kg H_2O)

CHILD

50–850 mOsm/kg H_2O (dependent on fluid intake) (SI units: 50–850 mmol/kg H_2O)

After 12-hour fluid restriction: >850 mOsm/kg H_2O (SI units: >850 mmol/kg H_2O)

What This Test Will Tell You

This urine test is an indicator of a client's serum concentration as well as the kidneys' concentrating and diluting abilities. Osmolality refers to the balance between water and solutes. An elevated level indicates dehydration and hemoconcentration, whereas a decreased level indicates overhydration and hemodilution. Urine osmolality provides more specific information than a specific gravity about a client's level of hydration. Values vary based on the volume of water excreted with solutes.

Abnormal Findings

▲ INCREASED LEVELS (concentrat-

ed urine) may indicate syndrome of inappropriate antidiuretic hormone secretion, acidosis, shock, intracellular dehydration, hypovolemia, hypernatremia, liver disease, hyperglycemia, congestive heart failure, high-protein diet, or Addison's disease.

▼DECREASED LEVELS *(dilute urine)* may indicate diabetes insipidus, hyponatremia, hypokalemia, hypercalcemia, early chronic renal failure, inhibition of antidiuretic hormone release, acute tubular necrosis, excessive intravenous fluid therapy with 5% dextrose in water solution, pyelonephritis, aldosteronism, or psychogenic polydipsia.

ACTION ALERT!
➤ Levels <100 mOsm/kg H_2O may indicate severe hypervolemia and electrolyte disturbances. Monitor for respiratory distress, severe hypertension, dysrhythmias, and seizures.
➤ Levels >800 mOsm/kg H_2O may indicate severe hypovolemia and electrolyte imbalances. Monitor for signs of shock including tachycardia, hypotension, poor peripheral perfusion, cold clammy skin, dysrhythmias, and seizures.

Interfering Factors
➤ Anesthetic agents, carbamazepine, vincristine, and chlorpropamide increase values.

NURSING CONSIDERATIONS

Prepare Your Client
➤ Explain that this test is to help evaluate the water balance in the body, and the kidneys' ability to eliminate or keep the amount of water the body needs.
➤ Instruct the client not to drink fluids or eat for 8–12 hours prior to urine collection, unless only a random sample is ordered.

Perform Procedure
➤ Collect a freshly voided morning urine specimen.
➤ Collect 5–10 mL of venous blood in a red-top tube if a serum osmolality level is ordered to accompany the urine level.

Care After Test
➤ Assess for signs of dehydration by noting poor skin turgor, dry and cracked tongue, dry mucous membranes, dark urine, tachycardia, slow venous filling, orthostatic hypotension, and thirst. In infants and children, crying without tears and sunken fontanel may be noted.
➤ Assess for signs of overhydration by noting edema, light to clear urine, weight gain, tachycardia, distended neck veins, distended hand veins, labored respirations, adventitious breath sounds in the lungs, and hypertension.
➤ Monitoring and record all fluid intake and output.
➤ If serum osmolality is elevated, consult with the primary health care provider regarding a need for intravenous fluid therapy that provides more free water.
➤ Institute seizure precautions and monitor for changes in level of consciousness for increased or decreased levels.
➤ Evaluate related tests including serum osmolality, serum electrolytes, blood urea nitrogen level, serum glucose, water load (dilution) test, and urinalysis.

Educate Your Client and the Family
➤ Instruct the client on the importance of limiting or increasing oral intake based on laboratory results and disorder.

➤ Instruct client with adrenocortical insufficiency to take steroid replacements as prescribed and wear medical alert identification. Increased dosages of steroids are needed during times of excessive physiologic or psychologic stress.

Osmotic Fragility
oz **mot** ik • frah jil ih tee
(OF, RBC Fragility, Erythrocyte Fragility, Autohemolysis)

Normal Findings
All ages: Normally, hemolysis occurs in solutions of 0.30%–0.45% saline. Osmotic fragility values, the percentage of hemolyzed red blood cells, are calculated and plotted against decreasing saline tonicities (from hypertonic to hypotonic) to produce an S-shaped curve. Results are compared with the normal curve.

What This Test Will Tell You
This blood test determines how resistant red blood cells are to hemolysis, and is used most commonly in diagnosing various anemias or liver diseases. Osmotic fragility measures the susceptibility of the erythrocytes to break down when exposed to increasingly hypotonic saline solutions. When red blood cells are added to a hypotonic (less concentrated) saline solution, they take up water until they burst. If red blood cells are placed in a hypertonic (more concentrated) solution, the cells shrink. The degree of hypotonicity needed to produce hemolysis varies inversely with the red blood cells' osmotic fragility. The closer the saline tonicity is to normal (0.9%) when hemolysis occurs, the more fragile are the cells. The main factor affecting osmotic fragility is the shape of the red blood cell, which depends on the volume, surface area, and functional status of the red blood cell membrane.

Abnormal Findings
▲INCREASED LEVELS *(increased tendency to hemolysis; solutions > .50% saline)* may indicate hereditary spherocytosis; acquired immune hemolytic anemia; hereditary stomatocytosis; chemical poisoning; severe burns; spider, bee or snake venom injury; severe hypophosphatemia; or erythroblastosis fetalis.
▼DECREASED LEVELS *(increased resistance to hemolysis; solutions < .30% saline)* may indicate iron deficiency anemia, thalassemias, asplenia, liver disease, sickle-cell anemia, obstructive jaundice, or polycythemia vera.

Interfering Factors
➤ Hemolytic organisms, such as beta-hemolytic streptococcus, in the blood may cause hemolysis of the cells, regardless of the tonicity of the saline.
➤ Severe anemia will affect the test results, as there are insufficient cells available for testing.
➤ Hemolysis of the sample before testing occurs.

NURSING CONSIDERATIONS

Prepare Your Client

➤ Explain that this test is to see how strong the red blood cells are in order to help find the cause of the client's anemia.

Perform Procedure

➤ Collect 7 mL of venous blood in a green-top (heparinized) tube or secure a special heparinized tube for collecting defibrinated blood.

➤ Completely fill the tube with the correct amount and invert it gently several times to adequately mix the sample and the anticoagulant.

Care After Test

➤ Observe the client for signs and symptoms of anemia: pallor, tachycardia, dyspnea, activity intolerance, and fatigue.

➤ Encourage rest for fatigue that occurs with anemia. Plan for consistent periods of light exercise but instruct the client in seeking assistance as fatigue occurs.

➤ Consult with a registered dietician to assist the family and client in meeting special dietary needs, especially with iron deficiency anemias.

➤ Review related tests such as the erythrocyte indices, hematocrit, hemoglobin, and complete blood cell count.

Educate Your Client and the Family

➤ Instruct the client in the signs and symptoms of anemia including palpitations, rapid heart rate, difficulty breathing, pallor, fatigue, and chest or leg pain.

➤ Instruct client and family on the importance of a well-balanced diet and adequate sleep.

Educate client and family on pacing activities with frequent rest periods to conserve energy.

Ova and Parasites, Sputum
oe vah • and • pair ah sites • spyoo tum

Normal Findings

Negative for ova and parasites

What This Test Will Tell You

This sputum microbiologic test diagnoses parasitic infections. Most ova and parasitic infections are diagnosed from blood and feces. However, other tissue and body fluids are occasionally submitted to the laboratory to confirm a diagnosis. Sputum is usually examined microscopically as a wet saline or iodine mount.

Abnormal Findings

Positive results may reveal *Paragonimus westermani*, *Echinococcus*, *Pneumocystis carinii*, hookworm larvae, *Ascaris lumbricoides* larvae, *Strongyloides* or *Schistosoma* species, or *Cryptosporidium parvum*.

Interfering Factors

➤ Dilution of sputum specimen with saliva may cause false negative results.

➤ An induced sputum is recommended for *Pneumocystis carinii.* More invasive procedures such as open lung biopsy, lung needle aspiration, or bronchial brushing for collection may be recommended.

➤ Recent medication therapy for ova and parasites may cause false negative results.

NURSING CONSIDERATIONS

Prepare Your Client

➤ Explain that this test is to diagnose an infection in the lungs.

EXPECTORATION SAMPLE

➤ Explain the sputum collection process. An early morning culture is best. Instruct your client to breathe deeply and give several deep coughs to raise sputum from the lungs.

➤ Give your client a sterile container to collect the sputum. Explain that spitting saliva into the container will dilute the sputum specimen and may give false negative results.

TRACHEAL SUCTIONING SAMPLE

➤ Explain the tracheal suctioning process.

➤ Attach a sputum trap to the suction catheter to collect the specimen.

Perform Procedure

➤ Collect 5–10 mL of sputum from the client. Place the lid on the sterile collection container.

➤ Label the container and transport to the lab immediately.

Care After Test

➤ Serologic testing may be necessary to determine the effectiveness of treatment.

➤ Assess client for signs and symptoms of respiratory compromise including increased respiratory rate, nasal flaring, use of accessory muscles, and inability to maintain patent airway related to increased secretions.

➤ Administer oxygen and humidification as ordered.

➤ Suction client as indicated to maintain patent airway.

➤ Review related tests such as serologic tests for the specific organisms and stool for ova and parasites.

Educate Your Client and the Family

➤ Stress the importance of finishing any antibiotic therapy ordered.

➤ Explain the routes of acquiring infection to your client and family members. Explain the importance of hand washing, cooking food thoroughly, and wearing foot covering to avoid infection.

Oxalate, Urine
ok sa late • yur in

Normal Findings

All ages: 0–40 mg/24 hours (SI units: 0–456 µmol/24 hours)

What This Test Will Tell You

This urine test diagnoses kidney stones, the genetic disorder of primary hyperoxaluria, and systemic poisoning due to ethylene glycol. Oxalate is a by-product of metabolism that is eliminated by the kidneys. Frequently, oxalate combines with calcium, resulting in renal calculi. In the genetic disorder hyperoxaluria, oxalate may also precipitate and form deposits in soft tissues, causing damage in a variety of organ systems.

Abnormal Findings

▲INCREASED LEVELS may indicate ethylene glycol poisoning, primary hyperoxaluria, diabetes, pyridoxine deficiency, Crohn's disease, adverse reaction to methoxyflurane anesthesia, vitamin B_6 deficiency, sarcoidosis, pancreatic disease, biliary disease, small bowel disease or resection, celiac disease, some autoimmune diseases, or cirrhosis.

▼DECREASED LEVELS may indicate renal failure.

Interfering Factors

➤ Levels may be increased by foods such as rhubarb, strawberries, gelatin, beans, beets, tomatoes, cocoa, spinach, chocolate, and tea.

➤ Medications that may increase levels include vitamin C and calcium.

NURSING CONSIDERATIONS

Prepare Your Client

➤ Explain that this test is to help diagnose kidney stones or a problem with eliminating a special salt in the body called oxalate.

➤ Restrict foods that increase excretion of oxalate for at least 1 week before the urine collection.

➤ Explain procedure for 24-hour urine collection.

Perform Procedure

➤ Collect a 24-hour urine specimen using hydrochloric acid as a preservative.

➤ Keep the sample protected from light.

Care After Test

➤ Strain all urine for signs of renal calculi in client with suspected kidney stones.

➤ Encourage adequate fluid intake unless otherwise indicated to reduce the concentration of urinary crystals.

➤ Consult with a registered dietician to assist the family and client in meeting special dietary needs, such as moderating dietary intake of calcium.

➤ Review related tests such as abdominal x-ray, urinalysis, and renal sonogram.

Educate Your Client and the Family

➤ If medication is ordered to treat and prevent oxalate deposits, explain the purpose and instruct client not to stop medication without consulting the primary health care provider.

➤ Explain the role of calcium in the diet in facilitating the formation of kidney stones or deposits of oxalate in the body.

Oximetry

ok sim eh tree
(Pulse Oximetry, Oxygen Saturation, O$_2$ Sat)

Normal Findings

ADULT, PREGNANT, CHILD, AND
ADOLESCENT
95%–100%
NEWBORN
40%–90%. Decreased values persist
until the lungs are fully developed.
ELDERLY
Values for oxygen saturation
decrease as functional lung capacity
decreases with increasing age.

What This Test Will Tell You

Oximetry is a noninvasive spec-
trophotometric measurement of the
ratio of arterial hemoglobin saturated with oxygen to the total
amount of hemoglobin in the bloodstream. Normally, hemoglobin
should be completely (100%) saturated with oxygen. When 95% to
100% of the hemoglobin carries oxygen (O$_2$), the tissues are being adequately oxygenated. At O$_2$ saturation
levels below 75%, the tissues are
unable to extract enough oxygen to
carry out their vital functions. O$_2$
saturation is affected by the P$_{O_2}$, body
temperature, pH, and the chemical
and physical structure of the hemoglobin itself.

Abnormal Findings

▲INCREASED LEVELS may indicate oxygen toxicity.
▼DECREASED LEVELS may indicate respiratory insufficiency or
impaired cardiopulmonary function.

ACTION ALERT!

Saturations below 75% or downward trends
in oxygen saturation observed with oximetry monitoring indicate the need for thorough assessment of the client's oxygenation status. Vital signs and cardiovascular
and respiratory status must be assessed
and appropriate intervention instituted
immediately to prevent cardiopulmonary
arrest and death.

Interfering Factors

➤ Hypotension, hypothermia, and
vasoconstriction reduce arterial
blood flow and interfere with the
interpretation of oxygen saturation.
➤ Movement of the finger or other
area where the probe is placed may
interfere with oxygen saturation
readings.
➤ Failure to place probe properly
may result in no reading or a falsely
low reading.
➤ Very bright light surrounding the
probe may make obtaining a reading
difficult.
➤ Elevated carboxyhemoglobin,
methemoglobin, or sulfhemoglobin
may cause falsely elevated results.
➤ Hyperbilirubinemia may cause
falsely decreased results.
➤ Use of ear oximetry is considered
less reliable than finger or toe oximetry because it is impossible to keep the
earlobe capillary blood arterialized
without continuous intervention.
➤ Oximetry may be somewhat less
accurate when used on dark-skinned

or jaundiced clients because it measures oxygen saturation on the basis of light absorption through the skin.

NURSING CONSIDERATIONS

Prepare Your Client

➤ Explain that the test is to monitor how well the blood is getting oxygen.

➤ Describe to the client that the clip or probe must be kept attached to the fingertip, earlobe, etc., if continuous monitoring is being performed.

➤ Reassure the client that no discomfort is associated with the procedure.

➤ Advise the client that alarms may sound if the machine is not picking up normal readings. Reassure the client the nurse will check the equipment periodically and any time an alarm sounds.

➤ Cleanse and dry area to be utilized for monitoring.

Perform Procedure

➤ Attach probe to toe, hand, or foot for infant; finger, toe, bridge of nose, or earlobe for adult. If using the bridge of the nose (e.g., for obese persons), place probe over cartilage for best results.

➤ Turn on the pulse oximeter and allow time (at least 30 seconds) for the sensor to pick up pulsations and display results on the monitor.

➤ Set low and high alarm limits according to manufacturer's directions.

➤ Observe oxygen saturation values continuously for critically ill client or have alarms set so they can be readily heard by the nurse.

➤ If low readings or downward trends are observed, encourage the client to breathe deeply or to comply with oxygen therapy if indicated.

➤ Document results of oximetry readings hourly or more often if indicated.

➤ Observe for downward trends or improvement in oxygen saturation in response to oxygen therapy, medication administration, positioning, nursing interventions, and other therapies.

➤ Perform a thorough cardiovascular and pulmonary assessment for readings below 92% and intervene appropriately.

Care After Test

➤ Remove probe. Observe the area for signs of impaired skin integrity if the probe was in place for a prolonged period.

➤ Advise client that repeated oximetry readings or continuous monitoring may be necessary.

➤ Reassure client and family when alarms sound.

➤ Evaluate related tests such as arterial blood gases, complete blood count, (especially hemoglobin levels) chest x-ray, and cardiovascular and pulmonary assessments.

Educate Your Client and the Family

➤ Remind the client to hold the area still where the probe is attached to assure accurate readings.

➤ If lung disease is present and the client is a smoker, refer to smoking cessation programs.

Papanicolaou Smear

pah pa nee ko low • smeer

(Pap Smear, Pap Test, Cytologic Test for Cancer)

Normal Findings

Class 1: Absence of atypical or abnormal cells (normal)

What This Test Will Tell You

This microscopic analysis is used primarily for early detection of cervical, vaginal, and endometrial carcinoma. A Pap smear allows examination of cells shed into the cervical and vaginal secretions to detect early cellular changes that may occur with premalignant and malignant conditions.

Pap smears are recommended as part of a routine pelvic exam of women over age 18 once a year (earlier if client is sexually active). The American Cancer Society recommends that a Pap smear be taken annually for two negative exams and then every 3 years until age 65 in asymptomatic women. Women with a family history of cervical cancer, with venereal infections, and those whose mothers took DES (diethylstilbestrol) need more frequent testing. Gonorrhea cervical cultures are usually done with a Pap smear.

A Pap smear is used also to detect cancers of the breast (aspiration of mammary gland tissue), lung (sputum or bronchoscopy), stomach (aspirated secretions), renal system (urine sediment), prostatic secretions, and solid tumor cells from needle aspiration. Cells can also be evaluated for hormonal effect and organisms.

Abnormal Findings

Abnormal results may indicate cancer, infertility, venereal disease, inflammatory processes, parasitic conditions, or fungal conditions.

Class 2: Atypical cells, no evidence of malignancy, usually caused by inflammation

Class 3: Suggestive of but not conclusive concerning malignancy, needs to be further evaluated

Class 4: Strongly suggestive of malignancy, needs further evaluation

Class 5: Conclusive of malignancy, requires treatment

Reclassification in cervical intraepithelial neoplasia (CIN):

CIN 1: Mild and mild to moderate dysplasia (class 2 and 3)

CIN 2: Moderate and moderate to severe dysplasia (class 3 and 4)

CIN 3: Severe dysplasia and carcinoma in situ (class 4 and 5)

Interfering Factors

➤ Lubricating jelly on the speculum distorts the cells.

➤ Douching and tub bathing may wash away cells.

➤ A delay in fixing a specimen allows the cells to dry, destroys the stain, and is difficult to interpret.

➤ Menstrual flow can interfere with test results.

➤ Hormone cytology is affected by infections.

➤ Digitalis and tetracycline preparations can alter the results by affecting the squamous epithelium.

Contraindications

➤ Taking a Pap smear during a menstrual period can alter the interpretation of the sample.

NURSING CONSIDERATIONS

Prepare Your Client

➤ Explain that this test is done to detect cancer early.

➤ Obtain from the client the date of her last menstrual period; date of last Pap test; any prior abnormal Pap tests; use of hormones, contraceptives or intrauterine devices; complaints of vaginal discharge, pain, or itching; and history of surgery, chemotherapy, or radiation.

➤ Schedule the test midcycle of menses.

➤ Instruct the client regarding intercourse. Some primary health care providers prefer that clients abstain from intercourse for 24–48 hours before the test.

➤ Explain that the test takes 10 minutes and is not uncomfortable except for speculum insertion.

➤ Instruct the client to void before the examination.

Perform Procedure

Nurses, unless specially trained, do not usually perform this procedure but should understand the process to prepare the client and assist the primary health care provider. The client needs to remove clothing from the waist down. A drape is provided and her heels placed in stirrups. A speculum is inserted into the vagina.

The specimen is obtained by rotating a swab or spatula from the endocervical canal. The cells are wiped across a clean glass slide and fixed immediately according to the laboratory instructions. Label the slide with client's name, age, parity, and last menstrual period. Send the specimen to the laboratory immediately.

Care After Test

➤ Assist the client to a sitting and then standing position. Observe carefully for dizziness and provide further assistance or lay the client back as indicated.

➤ Review related tests including endometrial biopsy, colposcopy, and cervical punch biopsy.

Educate Your Client and the Family

➤ Instruct the client that she will be notified if the test is abnormal.

➤ Instruct the client when to return for the next Pap smear.

Parathyroid Hormone

pair a thie roid • hor mone
(Parathormone, PTH, Parathyroid Hormone Assay, Parathyrin, PTH-C Terminal)

Normal Findings

ALL AGES
N-terminal: 236–630 pg/mL
C-terminal: 410–1760 pg/mL
Parathormone: 20–70 mEq/L
Note: There are a variety of laboratory methods to determine results. Check your own institution's values.

What This Test Will Tell You

This blood test diagnoses problems of calcium balance and parathyroid gland function. Parathyroid hormone (parathormone, or PTH) regulates calcium and phosphorus balance in the body. Increased secretion and circulating levels of PTH result in higher serum concentration of calcium and lower serum concentration of phosphorus. Conversely, decreased levels of PTH are responsible for lower calcium and higher phosphorus serum levels. Parathyroid hormone increases serum levels of calcium by stimulating its release from bones, decreasing its urinary excretion, and increasing its intestinal absorption.

Abnormal Findings

▲INCREASED LEVELS may indicate hyperparathyroidism, ectopic parathyroid hormone–producing tumors (lung or renal carcinoma), hypocalcemia, malabsorption syndromes, parathyroid adenoma, parathyroid carcinoma, parathyroid hyperplasia, osteomalacia, rickets, chronic renal failure, or vitamin D deficiency.

▼DECREASED LEVELS may indicate hypoparathyroidism, parathyroidectomy, some autoimmune diseases, metastatic cancer, sarcoidosis, some leukemias, hypercalcemia, Graves' disease, hypomagnesemia, or vitamin D toxicity.

Interfering Factors

➤ Decreased levels may be caused by excessive intake of vitamin D or milk prior to sampling.
➤ Hyperlipidemia may result in inaccurate findings.
➤ Hemolysis may interfere with results.
➤ Testing with radioisotopes within prior week may result in inaccurate findings.
➤ Alterations in normal sleep-wake patterns of night sleeping and awakening in the early morning may alter levels.
➤ Failure to follow dietary restrictions may affect results.

NURSING CONSIDERATIONS

Prepare Your Client

➤ Explain that this test measures how well a gland in the body called the parathyroid can balance calcium and other minerals in the body.
➤ Restrict food and fluids (except water) for at least 8 hours prior to blood sampling.
➤ Ensure the client does not work a night shift, which could affect the timing of normal levels.
➤ Confer with primary health care provider if client works a night shift regularly, as this may alter the normal diurnal rhythm.

Perform Procedure

➤ Collect 5–10 mL of venous blood in a red-top tube in the morning.
➤ If your laboratory requires, collect 15 mL of venous blood in a plastic tube, pack the specimen on ice, and send to the laboratory immediately.
➤ A serum calcium level is often drawn simultaneously.

Care After Test

➤ Observe the client for signs of hypercalcemia including lethargy, bone pain, decreased muscle tone, nausea, vomiting, anorexia, constipation, flank pain, headache, thirst, and increased urinary output.
➤ Monitor intake and output carefully.
➤ Observe the client for signs of hypocalcemia including bone pain, lethargy, constipation, nausea, vomiting, cramps, shallow breathing, bronchospasm, dysrhythmias, decreased urinary output, increased abdominal girth, tetany, Chvostek's sign, and Trousseau's sign.
➤ Prepare to administer 10% calcium gluconate or calcium chloride by slow intravenous infusion in

severe cases, or oral calcium supplements for less severe cases of hypocalcemia.

➤ Evaluate vitamin D and phosphorus balance as possible causes of calcium imbalance.

➤ Consult with a registered dietician to assist the family and client in meeting special dietary needs.

➤ Monitor electrocardiogram continuously, especially with hypocalcemia.

➤ Review related tests including serum phosphorus, serum albumin, urinalysis for calculi, clotting studies, parathyroid hormone levels, electrocardiogram, and serum digoxin level.

Educate Your Client and the Family

➤ Explain that the purpose of calcium in the body is to aid muscle contraction including the heart's beating, to strengthen bones and teeth, and to help the blood to clot.

➤ If calcium is low, discuss increasing calcium-rich foods in diet. Provide a list of foods high in calcium content.

➤ If calcium is high, encourage fluids and consult with primary health care provider about an anti-ash diet to prevent kidney stones.

Partial Thromboplastin Time, Activated

par shal • throm boe plas tin • time • ak tih vay ted
(APTT, Activated Partial Thromboplastin Substitution Test, Partial Thromboplastin Time, PTT, Activated Partial Thromboplastin Time)

Normal Findings

ALL AGES
APTT: 30–40 seconds
PTT: 60–70 seconds
With heparin therapy, the APTT is usually maintained at 1.5–2.5 times the control value.

What This Test Will Tell You

This blood test assesses bleeding disorders or the effectiveness of heparin therapy by evaluating intrinsic coagulation factors necessary for blood clotting. The basis of the test is fibrin clot formation and it evaluates all the clotting factors of the intrinsic pathway except Factors VII and VIII. The time that is required to form a fibrin clot after the addition of calcium and phospholipid emulsion to a plasma sample is measured. The activated partial thromboplastin time (APTT) is a modified version of the partial thromboplastin time (PTT) that is frequently used to monitor the efficacy of heparin therapy because it is more sensitive than a PTT.

Abnormal Findings

▲ INCREASED LEVELS (prolonged time) may indicate hemophilia, vitamin K deficiency, liver disease, presence of circulating anticoagulants, disseminated intravascular coagulation (acute or chronic), or von Willebrand's disease.

▼ DECREASED LEVELS (shortened time; <50 seconds for APTT) may indicate extensive cancer (except when the liver is involved), or very early stages of disseminated intravascular coagulation.

An APTT > 70 seconds or a PTT >100 seconds indicates a high risk for spontaneous bleeding. Avoid injections, protect the client's safety, assess for indications of bleeding, and notify the primary health care provider immediately. Administer protamine sulfate as ordered to reverse heparin therapy if indicated (1 gram of protamine sulfate for every 100 units of heparin).

Interfering Factors

➤ Failure to discard the first 2–3 mL of blood drawn may contaminate the specimen with tissue thromboplastin.

➤ Failure to completely fill the collection tube with blood may cause prolonged results.

➤ Hematocrits over 50% may cause falsely prolonged results and hematocrits below 20% may falsely decrease results.

➤ Drawing the sample from an intravenous line being kept open with a heparin flush will cause falsely prolonged results.

➤ Anticoagulant therapy within 2 weeks prior to the test will invalidate the results unless the test is being used to evaluate heparin therapy.

➤ Aspirin, phenothiazines, codeine, non-steroidal anti-inflammatory drugs, antihistamines, chlorpromazine, and alcohol can prolong the results.

Potential Complications

➤ Prolonged bleeding or hematoma formation at the venipuncture site in clients with coagulopathies.

NURSING CONSIDERATIONS

Prepare Your Client

➤ Explain that this test is used to look for clotting problems or monitor how well heparin therapy is working.

➤ Inform the client who is on heparin therapy that this test may be repeated at regular intervals to assess response to treatment.

➤ If the test is to assess heparin therapy, obtain sample 30–60 minutes before the next heparin dose is due.

Perform Procedure

➤ Collect 7 mL of venous blood into a blue-top tube containing sodium citrate. Fill the tube with the correct amount and invert it several times to mix the sample and anticoagulant adequately. Do not shake the tube vigorously as this can result in hemolysis.

➤ Do not draw from a heparin block or heparinized catheter. The blood must be drawn from a peripheral vein.

Care After Test

➤ If the client is on heparin therapy, venipuncture site should be held for 5 minutes.

➤ Observe the client for signs and symptoms of bleeding. Protect client from injury.

➤ Avoid intramuscular injections or unnecessary venipunctures.

➤ Review related tests such bleeding time, prothrombin time, tissue plasminogen, hematocrit, hemoglobin, and complete blood cell count.

Educate Your Client and the Family

➤ If preoperative test results are prolonged, surgery may need to be postponed unless it is an emergency.

➤ Teach the client and family members about bleeding precautions: using a soft-bristled toothbrush, using only electric razors, avoiding constipation, avoiding aspirin and aspirin products, and avoiding constricting clothing.

➤ Teach the client and family members the signs and symptoms of bleeding: petechiae, bruising, blood in the urine or stool, vaginal bleeding, and bleeding from invasive lines.

Pelvic Floor Sphincter Electromyography

pel vik • flor • sfink tur • ee lek troe mie og rah fee
(Pelvic Floor Sphincter EMG, Voiding Electromyography)

Normal Findings

ALL AGES

The EMG signal is increased during bladder filling.

The EMG signal is silent on voluntary micturition and the signal is increased at the end of voiding.

The rectal EMG signal is normal during bowel movements.

What This Test Will Tell You

This electrodiagnostic test evaluates the neuromuscular function of the urinary, and less commonly anal, sphincters in clients with altered patterns of urinary elimination. The electromyogram (EMG) measures the electrical activity of skeletal muscles during voluntary contraction and at rest. It is useful in differentiating disturbances in neurological function (neuropathies) from muscular function (myopathies). The EMG of the urinary sphincter is frequently done in conjunction with cystometrography in order to compare perineal muscle activity with detrusor (bladder) muscle contractions. The electrical activity is transmitted to sounds and visual patterns on an oscilloscope and graph paper.

Abnormal Findings

Abnormal signal patterns may indicate neuromuscular dysfunction of the urinary tract and the lower urinary sphincter.

Interfering Factors

➤ Urinary tract infections.

➤ Muscle relaxants, anticholinergic drugs, and cholinergic agents invalidate results.

➤ Caffeine and nicotine, because they are bladder and skeletal muscle stimulants.

➤ Pain can cause false results.

Contraindications

➤ Clients who are unable to follow instructions or cooperate during such a procedure

➤ Coagulopathies, if needle electrodes are used

Potential Complications

➤ If needle electrodes are used, hematoma, infection, or inflammation can occur at needle insertion sites.

➤ This test may elevate serum enzyme levels for up to 5 days.

NURSING CONSIDERATIONS

Prepare Your Client

➤ Explain that this test is to help find out why they are having trouble with going to the bathroom.

➤ Restrict coffee, tea, colas, and other caffeinated drinks as well as smoking for 3 hours prior to the test.

➤ Assure client that the test will not shock them, and that they will not feel electricity in their bodies. Electrodes are not taking electricity to their body, but rather measuring signals from the body.

➤ Explain to the client that cooperation is essential for a period of about 30 minutes.

➤ Ensure that an informed consent, if required by your institution, is obtained, because of the possible complications associated with this procedure.

➤ Restrict sedatives, analgesics, and cholinergic or adrenergic drugs for 6–8 hours prior to testing.

➤ Explain that slight, temporary discomfort may be felt if needle electrodes are used in your institution. If it persists more than a few minutes, the client should notify the technician so that the electrode can be moved.

Perform Procedure

Nurses do not perform this procedure, but should understand the process to prepare the client and assist the physician. A urologist performs this test, which usually takes about 30 minutes.

Cleanse the perineal skin with an antimicrobial solution. Two electrodes are placed on the perineal skin at the 2 o'clock and 10 o'clock positions. Surface electrodes are usually used, but needle electrodes may be inserted. Two electrodes will monitor pelvic floor muscular activity. A third electrode is placed on the thigh as a ground. An indwelling catheter with a transducer is inserted into the bladder.

Reflexes are tested first with an empty bladder. Measurements are recorded while the client coughs and while the urethra is stimulated by gently pulling on the catheter (bulbocavernous reflex). Muscular response to voluntary contraction and relaxation of the muscle is then measured.

The bladder is filled with sterile water at room temperature at the rate of 100 mL per minute. Once the bladder is full, the catheter is removed and the client is asked to void. EMG responses are recorded.

Care After Test

➤ Observe for hematuria or signs of urinary tract infection.

➤ Monitor any needle electrode sites for evidence of inflammation, redness, infection, or bleeding.

➤ If client is experiencing incontinence, assist client in trying to establish normal patterns of elimination by setting a voiding schedule and assisting the client to the bathroom.

➤ Evaluate the integrity of the perineal skin. Provide good skin care by cleansing after each voiding or bowel movement, and using protective barriers as needed.

➤ Provide adequate oral fluids unless otherwise indicated to help establish regular filling and emptying of the bladder.

➤ Evaluate related tests such as urethral pressure measurements, urine flow studies, and cystometrography.

Educate Your Client and the Family

➤ Teach client to avoid bladder stimulants such as alcohol, coffee, tea, and chocolate.

➤ Educate client experiencing incontinence in how to establish a bladder training program, which includes taking $2-2^1/2$ quarts

(2000–2500 mL) of fluids from early morning to early evening. Fluid is needed to stimulate micturition.

➤ Teach client muscle-strengthening exercises (Kegel). These include trying to stop and start the flow of urine during micturition and alternately contracting and relaxing perineal muscles three or four times per day for 5–10-minute sessions.

➤ Refer to support groups such as Help for Incontinent Persons and the Simon Foundation for Continence.

Pelvimetry
pel **vim** eh tree
(Radiographic Pelvimetry, Pelvicephalography)

Normal Findings
Normal: Transverse diameter of mid-pelvis >10.5 cm

What This Test Will Tell You
This x-ray test is used to determine if the pelvis is adequate for a vaginal delivery. During late pregnancy and/or labor, the size of the pelvis is compared with the size and position of the fetus to identify a dangerous vaginal delivery, which would indicate a cesarean delivery. Pelvimetry may be used when a vaginal delivery is planned but the fetus is thought to be abnormally positioned, the pelvis is injured or diseased, abnormal pelvic measurements have been determined clinically, there is a prior history of a difficult delivery, or labor is dysfunctional. X-ray pelvimetry is infrequently used in modern obstetrics because of radiation risk to the fetus.

Abnormal Findings
The test may reveal cephalopelvic disproportion (CPD), breech position, transverse position, or abnormalities of the pelvic structure.

Contraindications
➤ Early pregnancy, because x-rays may injure the fetus

NURSING CONSIDERATIONS
Prepare Your Client
➤ Explain that pelvimetry will help determine if the client's pelvis is large enough for a normal (vaginal) delivery.
➤ Explain that the test is performed in the x-ray department, takes 15 minutes, and is not uncomfortable.
➤ Instruct the client to remove all clothing and wear an x-ray gown.

Perform Procedure
Nurses do not perform this procedure, but should understand the process to prepare the client and assist the physician. X-ray imaging is taken with the client in various positions—standing, supine, lateral, and semirecumbent. The client may be asked to breathe deeply and rapidly, then hold a breath while the x-ray is taken.

Care After Test
➤ Assess mother's readiness to meet parental role functions by reviewing

infant care knowledge, methods of infant feeding, and ability to obtain needed supplies. Provide instruction and/or community health service referrals as indicated.

➤ Assess the client's ability to provide adequate nutrition for the fetus. Refer to social services and Women, Infants, and Children program (WIC) for assistance.

➤ Review related tests such as the results of pelvic measurements.

➤ Provide emotional support, since this test is only performed when fetal problems exist.

Educate Your Client and the Family

➤ Explain the findings to the client and family and the test's relationship to cesarean or vaginal delivery.

Percutaneous Transhepatic Cholangiography

pur kyoo tay nee us • trans hee pat ik • koe lan jee ah grah fee (PTC, PTHC)

Normal Findings

Patent and normal biliary ducts
Normal gallbladder
Absence of tumors, obstruction, atresia, strictures, and stones

What This Test Will Tell You

This x-ray test with contrast diagnoses jaundice and detects obstructions of the biliary system caused by stones or tumors. The test allows visualization of the biliary tree (hepatic ducts within the liver, common hepatic duct, cystic duct, and common bile duct) by using contrast material injected directly into the biliary tree. Fluoroscopy and periodic x-rays are used to record images. This test is indicated when oral or intravenous administration of contrast material will not be effective due to inability of the liver cells to transport the contrast.

Abnormal Findings

The test may reveal obstruction of biliary ducts within the liver or the common bile duct due to stones, tumors, cysts, or strictures; cancer of the pancreas; congenital anomalies of the biliary tree; biliary sclerosis; or sclerosing cholangitis.

▉ ACTION ALERT!

➤ Assess clients carefully for allergic reaction to contrast material, including dyspnea, itching, urticaria, flushing, hypotension, and shock. Life-threatening anaphylactic reactions can occur and need to be recognized and treated immediately.

➤ Percutaneous access to the bile ducts may result in hemorrhage, especially in clients with liver disease and associated clotting problems. Carefully assess for hemorrhage by noting abdominal pain, increase in abdominal girth, hypotension, tachycardia, diaphoresis, and poor peripheral perfusion. Notify the primary health care provider immediately for any of these symptoms and prepare to support with intravenous fluid and/or blood products.

Interfering Factors

➤ Movement during imaging may interfere with x-rays.

> Obesity or presence of stool in the intestine may decrease the clarity of x-rays.

> Presence of barium from previous contrast studies may impair imaging.

Contraindications

> Allergy to contrast material, shellfish, or iodine, unless modifications in testing are made

> Pregnancy, due to exposure of fetus to radiation

> Inflammation or infection of the bile ducts, because infusion of the contrast material may lead to rupture of ducts and sepsis

> Coagulopathics, because of the risk of hemorrhage

Potential Complications

Allergic reaction/anaphylaxis
Infection, cholangitis
Hemorrhage

NURSING CONSIDERATIONS

Prepare Your Client

> Explain that this test is to look at the gallbladder and tiny tubes (bile ducts) in the liver to make sure there are no blockages or other problems.

> Administer antibiotics prophylactically as ordered 24–72 hours before the procedure.

> Ensure that an informed consent is signed, because of potential complications.

> Administer sedatives as ordered.

> Review coagulation studies to identify possible clotting problems. Report any abnormalities immediately to the primary health care provider.

> Check with the primary health care provider about having the client typed and cross-matched for available blood in the event of hemorrhage.

> Explain to client that a local anesthetic will be given and may cause a slight burning sensation.

> Ensure the client has no allergy to contrast material, shellfish, or iodine.

> Restrict food and fluids for 8 hours prior to the test.

> Administer bowel cleansing agents such as laxatives or enemas if ordered the night before and/or morning of the exam to prevent shadows on the x-rays.

Perform Procedure

Nurses do not perform this procedure, but should understand the process to prepare the client. An intravenous infusion is started for the procedure.

The client is placed on a tilted x-ray table. The upper right quadrant of the abdomen is cleansed and sterile drapes applied and a local anesthetic administered. Fluoroscopy is used to guide the needle as it is inserted into the liver and into the biliary tree. Bile is withdrawn through the needle to confirm placement, and contrast substance is then instilled. X-rays are taken. Observe for reaction to contrast media such as nausea, rash, dyspnea, tachycardia, and hypotension. If an obstruction is identified, a catheter is left in the biliary tract to drain bile.

Care After Test

> Monitor vital signs closely until stable; usually every 15 minutes for the first hour, every 30 minutes for the next hour, and then every 4 hours for 24 hours.

> Observe for signs of allergic reaction to the contrast material.

> Observe for signs and symptoms of hemorrhage.

> Assess for abdominal pain and referred right shoulder pain, which

P

may be related to leakage of bile or blood irritating the diaphragm. Medicate for pain in collaboration with the primary health care provider because serious complications may be masked by pain medication.

➤ Assess for tachycardia, hypotension, and elevated temperature, which may indicate infection or sepsis.

➤ Carefully assess the site of percutaneous access each time vital signs are checked, noting drainage of blood or bile fluid. Immediately report continued or more than minimal quantities.

➤ Adults and older children may be required to remain on bed rest for up to 24 hours after the test is completed.

➤ Do not restart food or fluids until ordered by the primary health care provider after danger of hemorrhage or bile leakage requiring surgery has passed.

➤ Review related tests such as endoscopic retrograde cholangiopancreatography (ERCP), serum bilirubin, urine bilirubin, aspartate aminotransferase (AST), and alanine aminotransferase (ALT).

Educate Your Client and the Family

➤ Instruct overweight client about a low-calorie, low-fat, weight reduction diet with the assistance of a registered dietician.

Percutaneous Umbilical Blood Sampling on Fetus, Serum

pur kyu tay nee us • uhm bil ih kahl • blud • sam pling • on • fee tus • see rum (PUBS, Cordocentesis)

Normal Findings

Absence of abnormal cells, isoimmunization, anemia, and infection

What This Test Will Tell You

This blood test detects a problem with a fetus during the second and third trimesters. Percutaneous umbilical blood sampling (PUBS) employs ultrasound-guided puncture of the umbilical vein to obtain fetal blood or administer fetal transfusions.

PUBS is used to exclude chromosome abnormalities before fetal surgery and to obtain blood samples for rapid chromosomal analysis. PUBS may also be used to analyze cells when a congenital anomaly is found close to term or close to the legal time limit for elective termination. It may be ordered for detection of a suspected congenital infection, isoimmunization, suspected fetal anemia, karyotyping of fetuses, and determination of acid-base balance. PUBS may be ordered when the client has a child with a chromosome problem or is a known or suspected carrier of a disease.

Abnormal Findings

Abnormalities may indicate hypoxia, lactic acidosis, hypoglycemia, TORCH infections (infections detrimental to the fetus, including toxoplasmosis, rubella, cytomegalovirus, syphilis, and herpes simplex) or isoimmunization.

This invasive procedure may result in maternal hemorrhage, fetal hemorrhage, preterm labor and delivery, or spontaneous abortion, all of which can prove to be life-threatening to the mother and/or fetus. Emergency equipment and personnel should be immediately available for cesarean section delivery as well as fetal or maternal resuscitation.

Interfering Factors
➤ The bladder may need to be full or empty to gain access to the umbilical cord. Follow directions from the primary health care provider.
➤ Fetal position may need to be manually manipulated to gain access to the umbilical cord.

Contraindications
➤ Pregnancy before 19 weeks' gestation

Potential Complications
➤ Hemorrhage
➤ Spontaneous membrane rupture
➤ Infection, chorioamnionitis
➤ Spontaneous abortion
➤ Transient fetal bradycardia
➤ Thrombosis of umbilical cord
➤ Umbilical cord hematoma
➤ Fetal death

NURSING CONSIDERATIONS
Prepare Your Client
➤ Explain that this test will provide information about the baby before birth by getting a sample of the baby's blood. Many tests can be performed on this blood sample to provide information about the baby.
➤ Explain that the test is done using ultrasound and that a needle will be

carefully guided to the cord for a blood sample.
➤ Administer any medications such as sedatives that may be ordered to decrease fetal movement.
➤ Instruct the client that a local painkiller will be given as a shot to numb her skin and abdomen. Injection of the local anesthetic is the only pain she will feel. During insertion of the needle for blood sampling, she may feel pressure.

Perform Procedure
Nurses do not perform this procedure, but should understand the process to prepare the client. Promote relaxation during the procedure by using breathing techniques if needed.

The abdomen is cleansed according to policy. Assist with the administration of a local anesthetic. A 20–22 gauge spinal needle is inserted under ultrasound into the umbilical vein. 5 mL of fetal blood is obtained in heparinized syringes.

Assist the primary health care provider by obtaining fetal hemoglobin results quickly so that an intrauterine transfusion of fresh packed Rh-negative blood compatible with the mother can be given if needed in fetuses suffering from maternal-fetal Rh incompatibility.

Care After Test
➤ Instruct the client that a complete ultrasound will be performed to check the fetus.
➤ Monitor vital signs and fetal heart rate closely until stable; usually every 15 minutes for the first hour, every 30 minutes for the next hour, and then every 4 hours for 24 hours.
➤ Monitor the mother for signs of hemorrhage (such as increased pulse, decreased blood pressure, air hunger, pale, moist skin, malaise, confusion)

and ruptured membranes (trickle or gush of fluid). Report these to the primary health care provider immediately.

➤ Administer Rh_o (D) immune globulin if indicated to the Rh-negative mother with an Rh-positive fetus.

➤ Inform the client that results of rapid chromosomal analysis may be available in 48–72 hours.

➤ Provide the client with the opportunity to meet with a genetic counselor to explain the risks of genetic defects and chromosome disorders if indicated.

➤ Instruct the client that the primary health care provider may order nonstress testing following the procedure.

➤ Ask the client if she is taking her prenatal vitamins as ordered by her primary health care provider. Stress the importance of supplemental vitamins in providing good nutrition and normal growth and development of her baby.

➤ Assess the client's knowledge of prenatal care including diet, activity, rest, signs and symptoms of labor, and danger signs in pregnancy. Provide instruction as indicated.

➤ Assess mother's readiness to meet parental role functions by reviewing infant care knowledge, methods of infant feeding, and ability to obtain needed supplies. Provide instruction and/or community health service referrals as indicated.

➤ Assess the client's ability to provide adequate nutrition for the fetus. Refer to social services and Women, Infants, and Children program (WIC) for assistance.

➤ Refer to a registered dietician if dietary deficiencies are suspected.

➤ Assess the client for use of cigarettes, tobacco products, alcohol, over-the-counter medications, and street drugs. Instruct the client as necessary to avoid these substances, as they may cause intrauterine growth retardation.

➤ If the client reports decreased fetal movements, assess recent maternal history for maternal activity and relationship to fetal movement. Assess also her recent consumption of food or fluids and its relationship to fetal movement. Consult with the primary health care provider about instructing the client to eat, drink, and then rest. During rest, tell her to concentrate on fetal movements for 1 hour. Three fetal movements in 1 hour are reassuring.

➤ Review related tests such as amniocentesis, nonstress test, biophysical profile, and nipple stimulation test.

Educate Your Client and the Family

➤ Support the client and family if test results are abnormal. Assist in obtaining genetic counseling when appropriate.

➤ Teach the client signs of complications of the test such as abdominal cramps or leaking of vaginal fluid. Instruct the client to lie on her left side and call the primary health care provider. Other signs of complications are chills, elevated temperature, and decreased fetal movement.

➤ Give instructions to the client about daily fetal movement count.

➤ Assess prenatal diet, activity and rest. Give instructions as necessary.

➤ Instruct the client about normal signs of labor such as a gush of fluid, bloody show, and contractions that increase in frequency, intensity, and duration.

➤ Instruct the client about danger

signs in pregnancy such as a gush of fluid, vaginal bleeding, abdominal pain, temperature elevation, dizziness, blurred vision, persistent vomiting, severe headache, edema, muscular irritability, difficult urination, or decreased/absent fetal movements.

➤ Tell client to notify her primary health care provider if she has less than three movements in 1 hour. A nonstress test or biophysical profile may be ordered.

➤ Teach the client the signs of preterm labor such as abdominal cramping with or without diarrhea, uterine contractions every 10 minutes or more frequently, menstrual-like cramps in the lower abdomen, low backache, increase or change in vaginal discharge, or pelvic pressure.

➤ Advise the client to lie down on her side and notify the primary health care provider if preterm labor is suspected.

P

Pericardiocentesis

pair ee kar dee oe sen tee sis
(Pericardial Fluid Tap)

Normal Findings

ALL AGES

10–50 cc clear, straw-colored fluid
Absence of red blood cells or bacteria
Less than 1,000 white blood cells/mm^3

What This Test Will Tell You

This fluid analysis test helps diagnose pericarditis, trauma, malignancies, and other systemic diseases that can result in accumulation of pericardial fluid. Normally, only a small amount of clear fluid formed from plasma is present in the pericardial sac. The pericardial fluid acts as a lubricant and reduces friction between the sac and the outside of the heart. If fluid accumulates in the sac, it compresses the heart and causes a decrease in pumping action, which decreases cardiac output. An accumulation of pericardial fluid is often referred to as a pericardial effusion.

This procedure may also be performed as an emergency measure to drain excessive pericardial fluid that

is seriously impairing cardiac function. An excessive accumulation of pericardial fluid may cause a cardiac tamponade, a critical decrease in the ability of the heart to fill or pump blood that can be life-threatening.

Abnormal Findings

Abnormalities may indicate pericardial effusion, cardiac trauma, congestive heart failure, uremia, or metastatic cancer.

ACTION ALERT!

A narrowing of the pulse pressure, as noted by decreasing systolic and diastolic pressure differences, may signify a cardiac tamponade and require an emergency pericardiocentesis.

Interfering Factors

➤ Poor aseptic technique can contaminate the specimen and result in misleading bacterial growth.

Contraindications

➤ Anticoagulation therapy or bleeding disorders pose the risk of severe bleeding, which might only worsen the amount of pericardial fluid.

➤ A client who cannot lie still during the procedure poses the risk of injuring a coronary artery or perforating the heart.

Potential Complications

➤ Infection
➤ Tearing of a coronary artery
➤ Perforation of the heart
➤ Dysrhythmias
➤ Cardiac tamponade
➤ Pneumothorax
➤ Hemothorax
➤ Hemorrhage
➤ Cardiac arrest

NURSING CONSIDERATIONS

Prepare Your Client

➤ Explain that this test is used to drain fluid around the heart either to obtain a sample of the fluid for study or to relieve the compression the fluid is causing on the heart.

➤ Ensure that an informed consent is obtained, because of the possible complications associated with this procedure.

➤ Tell the client and family the procedure usually takes only about 15–30 minutes and is most often performed in the cardiac catheterization laboratory, emergency room, or special procedure room.

➤ Check the chart to be sure the client has no history of bleeding disorders or anticoagulation therapy.

➤ Ensure a prothombin time or partial thromboplastin time has been reported.

➤ Note any current antibiotic therapy.

➤ Ask client when they last took aspirin, because it has an anticoagulation effect for up to 10 days.

➤ Explain the procedure to the client or family.

➤ Record baseline vital signs.

➤ Check with the primary health care provider about withholding food and fluids for 4–8 hours preceding the pericardial tap if possible. Ask also if medications should be administered while the client is not allowed food or fluids.

➤ Ensure the client has an intravenous access for emergency medications if required.

➤ Administer sedatives or tranquilizers as ordered before the procedure.

➤ Confirm that adults and older children have voided before the procedure.

➤ Do not remove glasses, dentures, or hearing aids unless dictated by your hospital policy. The client may need these in order to communicate and cooperate during the procedure.

Perform Procedure

Nurses do not perform this procedure, but should understand the process to prepare the client and assist the primary health care provider. The client is placed in a supine position and electrodes are attached for continuous electrocardiographic (ECG) monitoring. The skin is scrubbed surrounding the sternum and sub-xiphoid area with an appropriate antiseptic such as betadine.

The primary health care provider inserts a special pericardiocentesis needle into the sub-xiphoid area, or sometimes into the 5th–6th intercostal space at the left sternal border. Observe the ECG closely for ST segment changes or a change in QRS complexes, which indicate that the surface of the heart is being touched by the needle.

As fluid is obtained, carefully mark all appropriate containers for culture and sensitivity as well as content analysis. Samples usually go to the chemistry laboratory to evaluate protein, albumin, and lactic dehydrogenase (LDH) content; to hematology for analysis of red and white blood cells; and to bacteriology for culture and sensitivity.

Apply firm pressure to the site for 5–10 minutes if the needle is removed without leaving a catheter in place.

Care After Test

➤ Monitor vital signs closely until stable.

➤ Assess for pulsus paradoxus (a drop in systolic pressure of more than 10 mm Hg pressure during inspiration), which may signal a cardiac tamponade. Additional signs and symptoms of cardiac tamponade include dyspnea, distended neck veins, muffled heart sounds, paradoxical pulse, and shock.

➤ Inspect the puncture site for drainage of fluid, bleeding, or hematoma formation. If a catheter has been left in place, note the amount of drainage hourly.

➤ Keep a sterile dressing over the puncture site and around the catheter if present.

➤ Ensure the drainage system for a catheter is also kept sterile.

➤ Report any new or increased bloody drainage.

➤ Evaluate related tests such as blood cultures and renal profile studies.

Educate Your Client and the Family

➤ Explain to the client or family that a local anesthetic is used before a needle is inserted into the sac surrounding the heart. This may produce a brief burning sensation before the area becomes numb. Explain that a medication will be given to make the client sleepy and not well aware of the procedure, which is usually not painful. Most clients describe feelings of pressure as the needle is inserted.

➤ Explain that a catheter (long thin tubing) may be left in place if excessive amounts of fluid are found so that it can continue to drain over the next hours to days. Reassure them the catheter itself should not be painful once it is in place.

➤ Encourage significant others to take cardiopulmonary resuscitation (CPR) classes.

➤ Teach client to pace activities to conserve energy.

➤ Educate client and family on fluid, food, or activity restrictions based on diagnosis.

P

Peritoneal Fluid Analysis

pair ih toe nee al • floo id • ah nal ah sis

Normal Findings

ALL AGES

Gross appearance: Sterile, odorless, clear to pale yellow, scant (<50 mL)

RBCs: Negative or ≤100,000/mm^3
WBCs: <300/μL
Neutrophils: ≤25%
Protein: 0.3–4.1 g/dL (albumin,

50%–70%; globulin, 30%–45%; fibrinogen, 0.3%–4.5%)

Glucose: 70–100 mg/dL

Amylase: 138–404 amylase units/L

Fecal content: None

Ammonia: <50 µg/dL

Alkaline phosphatase:

Male > 18 years: 90–239 U/L

Female < 45 years: 76–196 U/L

Female > 45 years: 87–250 U/L

Elderly: May be slightly higher

Lactic dehydrogenase (LDH): 48–115 U/L or equal to serum level

Cytology: Negative for malignant cells

Bacteria: Negative

Fungi: Negative

Carcinoembryonic antigen (CEA): <2.5 mg/mL

What This Test Will Tell You

This peritoneal fluid test is often performed to determine the cause of ascites. Other purposes for this test include the detection of abdominal trauma; perforation of the bladder; bacterial peritonitis; and/or peritoneal effusion caused by pancreatitis, pancreatic trauma, or gastrointestinal perforation or necrosis.

Abnormal Findings

APPEARANCE

➤ *Milky-colored fluid* may indicate chyle caused by surgical interruption of the thoracic duct, cancer, tuberculosis, parasitic infections, cirrhosis of the liver, or adhesions of the lungs.

➤ *Bloody fluid* may indicate pancreatitis, or blood resulting from the peritoneal tap.

➤ *Bile-colored fluid* may indicate pancreatitis, ruptured gallbladder, perforated ulcer, or perforated intestine.

➤ *Cloudy or hazy fluid* may indicate peritonitis, abdominal trauma with infection, perforated intestine, infarcted intestine, strangulated intestine, appendicitis, or pancreatitis.

➤ *Increased amount of fluid* may indicate ascites, liver disease, infection, or peritonitis.

ANALYSIS

➤ *Presence of bacteria or fungus* may indicate appendicitis, pancreatitis, tuberculosis, ovarian disease, peritonitis, histoplasmosis, candidiasis, or coccidioidomycosis.

➤ *Presence of red blood cells* may indicate a tumor or tuberculosis [>100/µL (0.1 × 10^9/L)] or abdominal trauma and gross intraperitoneal bleeding [>100,000/µL (100 × 10^9/L)]. If the blood obtained clots, it is from venous blood contaminating the specimen during the peritoneal tap. If the blood does not clot, it is intraperitoneal blood.

➤ *Presence of white blood cells* may indicate peritonitis, cirrhosis, chylous ascites, or tuberculosis.

➤ *Depressed glucose levels* (<60 mg/dL) may indicate tuberculosis or cancer.

➤ *Elevated amylase levels* may indicate pancreatitis, trauma to the pancreas, cysts of the pancreas, or intestinal necrosis.

➤ *Elevated protein levels* may indicate cancer or tuberculosis.

➤ *Elevated alkaline phosphatase levels* may indicate necrosis, perforation, or strangulation of the small intestine.

➤ *Elevated LDH* may indicate cancer, tuberculosis, or pancreatic disease.

➤ *Elevated ammonia levels* may indicate necrosis, perforation, or strangulation of the small intestine, large intestine, or appendix.

➤ *Albumin content* that is elevated above serum levels may indicate liver disease. Levels lower than serum content suggest cancer.

> *Elevated CEA levels* may indicate cancer of abdominal organs.
> *Microscopic examination for cytology* may reveal cancerous cells.

> Watch the client for signs of hemorrhage, shock, increasing pain, and abdominal tenderness following the paracentesis.
> If excess fluid is aspirated (≥500 mL), watch for the signs of hypovolemic shock (color change, increased pulse rate and respiratory rate, decreased blood pressure, mental status changes, and dizziness).

Interfering Factors

> Failure to send the specimen immediately to the lab may alter the test results.
> Unsterile technique during the collection of the specimen may alter the test results.
> Injury to underlying structures (liver, pancreas, intestine, stomach, bladder) may contaminate the specimen and alter the test results.

Contraindications

> Do not perform the test if marked bowel distention is present.
> Thrombocytopenia with a platelet count < 20,000/μL, due to risk of hemorrhage.
> Prothrombin time or partial thromboplastin time > 1.5 times the control, due to risk of hemorrhage.
> This test is performed cautiously in clients who are pregnant.

Potential Complications

> Perforation of the underlying abdominal organs with the trocar needle (intestines, stomach, liver, bladder)
> Hemorrhage, especially in the client with bleeding tendencies
> Hepatic coma in the client with severe hepatic disease

> Vascular collapse if a large amount of fluid is removed or if the fluid is removed too rapidly
> Infection and peritonitis if the puncture of underlying structures occurs, if sterility of the equipment is not maintained, or if improper techniques are used

NURSING CONSIDERATIONS

Prepare Your Client

> Explain that this test is important to determine the cause of fluid buildup, pain, or other symptoms in the abdomen (stomach).
> Ensure that an informed consent is obtained, because of the possible complications associated with this procedure.
> Determine the client's baseline vital signs, weight, and abdominal girth for comparison to the post-test readings.
> Immediately prior to the test have the client void to decrease the risk of accidental bladder injury.

Perform Procedure

Nurses do not usually perform this procedure, but should understand the process to prepare the client and assist the primary health care provider. Position client in a sitting position, with the back supported and feet flat on the floor. Assist the health care provider to prepare the abdominal puncture site and administer a local anesthetic.

A scalpel is used to make a small stab wound approximately 1–2 inches below the umbilicus. A trocar and cannula are threaded through the incision and peritoneum. The trocar needle is removed, leaving the cannula in place.

Peritoneal fluid is aspirated into a 50-cc syringe or connected to plastic tubing draining to a collection receptacle. Fluid is drained slowly, and the client repositioned as necessary to facilitate drainage. No more than 1000 cc in an adult should be drained to avoid hypovolemic shock and derangements of electrolytes.

Check the vital signs every 15 minutes during the procedure and monitor for an increase in heart rate or respiration, a drop in the blood pressure, dizziness, pallor, perspiration, or increased anxiety.

Care After Test

➤ Apply a pressure dressing after the test is completed.

➤ Check the pressure dressing frequently and reinforce or reapply the dressing as needed.

➤ Monitor vital signs closely until stable; usually every 15 minutes for the first hour, every 30 minutes for the next hour, and then every 4 hours for 24 hours.

➤ Weigh the client, measure the abdominal girth, and compare the results to the pretest readings.

➤ Monitor the urine output for 24 hours following the test to assess for hematuria, which could indicate bladder trauma.

➤ Watch closely for signs of increased abdominal pain or tenderness, hemorrhage, and/or shock as they could indicate a perforation of an underlying structure.

➤ Observe the client with severe hepatic disease for signs of hepatic coma, which may result from the loss of sodium and potassium accompanying hypovolemia. Notify the primary health care provider of drowsiness, changes in behavior, slurred speech, slight tremors, or stupor, which are symptoms of hepatic coma.

➤ Administer intravenous fluids and/or albumin as ordered.

➤ Consult with a registered dietician to evaluate dietary intake and needs.

➤ Evaluate other diagnostic tests such as the complete blood cell count, electrolyte studies, serum protein levels, activated partial thromboplastin time, prothrombin time, bleeding times, and computed tomography or magnetic resonance imaging studies of the abdomen.

Educate Your Client and the Family

➤ Instruct the client to notify the nurse if there is an increase in abdominal pain, dizziness, a feeling of faintness, or an increase in anxiety.

➤ If indicated, instruct the client on the importance of fluid restriction to decrease the risk of the return of the ascites.

➤ Review with the family and client any safety needs in the home or hospital environment to assure accident-free surroundings if changes in mental status or mobility are noted.

➤ Instruct client with excessive or chronic ascites that sitting up may help make breathing easier.

Phenolsulfonphthalein Excretion Test

fee nol sul fone thal ee in • ek skree shun • test

(PSP Excretion Test)

Normal Findings

ADULT, INFANT, ADOLESCENT, AND ELDERLY

25%–35% excretion in 15 minutes

50%–60% excretion in 30 minutes

60%–70% excretion in 60 minutes

70%–80% excretion in 2 hours

CHILD

5%–10% higher than adults

What This Test Will Tell You

This urine test assesses renal tubular function and renal plasma flow. Phenolsulfonphthalein (PSP) is a dye that binds to plasma albumin and that is normally excreted quickly by the kidneys. Because albumin is a large molecule, it is excreted through the renal tubules and not through the glomerulus, giving an accurate indication of renal tubular function. The value at 15 minutes is the best indicator of renal plasma flow and proximal renal tubular function. During this test, urine specimens are analyzed for PSP content. Healthy kidneys excrete more than 85% of a measured dose of PSP (6 mg or 1 mL of PSP). Together with the creatinine clearance test, the PSP provides helpful information regarding the diagnosis of renal dysfunction.

Abnormal Findings

▲ INCREASED LEVELS may indicate multiple myeloma, hypoalbuminemia, hypoproteinemia, or hepatic disease.

▼ DECREASED LEVELS may indicate acute tubular necrosis, diffuse kidney disease, renal vascular disease, urinary tract obstruction, intravenous pyelogram radiopaque dyes, hypoalbuminemia, sulfonamides, chronic pyelonephritis, fistulas, hematuria, congestive heart failure, gout, or idiopathic hypercalcemia.

P

ACTION ALERT!

Individuals with a sensitivity to PSP, congestive heart failure, or renal insufficiency may require emergency intervention during the testing period. Keep epinephrine and emergency equipment accessible.

Interfering Factors

➤ Inability of the client to void at collection times or failure to collect urine specimens at specified intervals and to empty the bladder at each collection time.

➤ Specimens of a quantity insufficient to test (less than 40 mL).

➤ Peripheral edema or draining fistulas.

➤ Hematuria.

➤ Urinary retention.

➤ Elevated bilirubin.

➤ Ingestion of carrots, rhubarb, and beets.

➤ Inaccurate measurement of PSP dosage.

➤ Sulfobromophthalein and azo dyes.

➤ Urine levels of PSP may be lowered by intravenous pyelography, radiopaque contrast material, chlorothiazide, aspirin, phenylbutazone, penicillin, sulfonamides, and probenecid.

➤ High serum protein levels will lower urine levels of PSP.

➤ Lowered levels may be seen in hypoalbuminemia, albuminuria, and severe liver disease.

Contraindications

➤ Sensitivity to PSP
➤ Acute renal insufficiency
➤ Diminished renal function indicated by elevations of blood urea nitrogen and creatinine

Potential Complications

➤ Allergic reaction to PSP may occur; keep epinephrine available.
➤ The PSP test is used cautiously in congestive heart failure and renal insufficiency due to its requirement for increased fluids. Keep emergency equipment available.

NURSING CONSIDERATIONS

Prepare Your Client

➤ Explain that this is a test to evaluate kidney function.
➤ Explain that there is a restriction on foods and medications that may affect urine color, but to ensure adequate urine production, extra fluids must be taken before and during the test.
➤ Explain that the dye may temporarily cause the urine to turn red or pink.
➤ Withhold medications that affect urine color for the 24 hours prior to the test, such as aminosalicylic acid, amitriptyline, oral anticoagulants, cascara sagrada, chloroquine phosphate, chlorzoxazone, chlorpromazine, diuretics, ethanol, indomethacin, iron complexes, methyldopa, metronidazole, phenacetin, phenols, phenothiazines, quinine sulfate, riboflavin, rifampin, salicylates, senna, sulfasalazine, triamterene, and vitamins.
➤ Withhold foods that affect urine color for the 24 hours prior to the test, such as carrots, beets, and rhubarb.

Perform Procedure

➤ Assess and report any known drug or food allergies.
➤ Have the client void and discard urine specimen.
➤ Encourage oral intake of 600–800 mL of water.
➤ Prepare the client for intravenous injection of PSP by laboratory specimen. Note the time of injection and amount of PSP injected, usually 6 mg or 1 mL.
➤ Collect at least 40 mL of urine at 15, 30, 60, and 120 minutes. Mark each urine specimen with the time and amount of voiding. Have client empty bladder at each time of voiding. Send each specimen to the laboratory immediately or refrigerate the specimens.

Care After Test

➤ Assess for any adverse reactions to the dye.
➤ Monitor intake and output. Report urine output less than 30 mL/hour in adults or 1 mL/kg of body weight in infants and children.
➤ Monitor for signs and symptoms of kidney disease including nausea, vomiting, lassitude, fatigue, and decreased mental acuity.
➤ Review related tests including blood urea nitrogen, creatinine clearance, serum electrolytes, uric acid, urinalysis, and urine cultures as well as ultrasounds or computed tomography scans of the urinary tract.

Educate Your Client and the Family

➤ If renal disease is diagnosed, teach client and family signs of worsening kidney failure including nausea, vomiting, lassitude, fatigue, and decreased mental acuity.
➤ Explain to client and family the

importance of ongoing treatment and evaluation of renal disease and the importance of general health care.

➤ Explain the importance of not drinking too much water.
➤ Teach the client and family a low-protein, high-calorie diet.

Phenylalanine Screening

fen il al ah nine • skreen ing
(PKU Test, Guthrie Test)

Normal Findings

Newborn
BLOOD
Premature newborn: 2–7.5 mg/dL
Newborn: 1.2–3.4 mg/dL
Child: 0.8–1.8 mg/dL
URINE
No green coloration, no color change

What This Test Will Tell You

This blood and urine test detects phenylketonuria (PKU), an inherited disease that can progress to mental retardation and brain damage. In PKU, there is a deficiency of the enzyme phenylalanine hydroxylase, which is necessary to convert phenyl-alanine (an amino acid for growth) to tyrosine. Phenylalanine builds up in the body and is spilled over into urine. Without dietary restriction of phenylalanine in infants with PKU, progressive mental retardation results.

PKU testing is mandatory in most states of the United States. The Guthrie test is done 2–3 days after the newborn has ingested a sufficient amount of phenylalanine (contained in human and cow's milk).

Abnormal Findings

▲INCREASED LEVELS *in serum or positive urine testing* may indicate phenylketonuria, galactosemia, or hepatic encephalopathy.

ACTION ALERT!

A serum level ≥4 mg/dL is strongly suggestive of phenylketonuria. Ensure that exact serum phenylalanine measurements and urine testing are obtained to confirm the diagnosis.

Interfering Factors

➤ Premature infants weighing less than 5 pounds may have increased levels without having the disease due to delayed development of enzyme activity in the liver.
➤ Feeding problems (vomiting) may cause false negative results.
➤ Testing earlier than 72 hours after birth may produce false negative results.
➤ Ketonuria may produce an altered urine color reaction.
➤ Antibiotics and salicylates may influence results.

NURSING CONSIDERATIONS

Prepare Your Client

➤ Explain to the family that this is a screening test for PKU, a treatable genetic disease, and is performed on all infants. Explain the importance of detecting a disease that can result in mental retardation if left untreated.
➤ Ensure the infant has received at least 3–4 full days of milk feeding.

Perform Procedure

BLOOD

➤ Cleanse heel skin with an antiseptic.

➤ Puncture the heel with a sterile disposable lancet.

➤ Spot the blood on provided filter paper, being careful to fill the circles completely. Air dry.

➤ Mark the sample with the date and time of the infant's birth as well as date and time of collection.

➤ Note on the sample the date and time feedings were initiated.

URINE

➤ Do not perform on infants less than 6 weeks of age.

➤ Place the correct amount of 10% ferric chloride into or use a reagent strip on a diaper containing freshly voided urine. If a green color appears, PKU is strongly suspected.

Care After Test

➤ If results are positive, consult with a registered dietician to assist the family and client in meeting special dietary needs.

Educate Your Client and the Family

➤ If test results are positive for PKU, explain to the family that successful dietary treatment (restriction of phenylalanine) results in normal mental development.

➤ If test results are positive, begin diet teaching immediately to prevent brain damage to the infant. Instruct the parents to substitute Lofenalac for milk, and to feed strained foods low in protein later.

➤ Explain that the infant will be monitored with blood and urine testing.

➤ Instruct women with PKU to begin a low-phenylalanine diet before conception and maintain this diet throughout pregnancy. This decreases the risk of giving birth to a mentally retarded infant.

➤ Explain importance of repeating the test when necessary.

Phosphatidylglycerol

foss fah tie dil • gliss ur ahl

(PGL, Amniostat-FLM, Shake Test, Shake Test for Lecithin/Sphingomyelin Ratio, Phospholipid Screen, Foam Stability, Rapid Surfactant Test)

Normal Findings

➤ *Foam stability test*: Fine bubble formation or foam indicating lung maturity of fetus.

➤ *L/S ratio*: L/S > 2 indicates fetal lung maturity.

➤ *Phosphatidylglycerol* when present indicates fetal lung maturity.

What This Test Will Tell You

This amniotic fluid analysis is performed to evaluate fetal lung maturity. This is a fast way of determining the lecithin/sphingomyelin ratio (L/S ratio) in surfactant, and is usually performed around 36 weeks of gestation. This test allows for rapid decision making about fetal well-being, viability, and morbidity after birth related to lung development. The test relies on the ability of surfactant in amniotic fluid to make foam bubbles when mixed with 95% ethanol and saline.

Abnormal Findings

➤ *Positive test: formation of bubbles in 1:2 dilution* indicates fetal lung maturity.

➤ *Intermediate test: equivocal formation of bubbles* indicates questionable lung maturity.

➤ *Negative test: no formation of bubbles in a 1:1 dilution* indicates fetal lung immaturity and a high probability of respiratory distress syndrome.

➤ *L/S ratio < 2* indicates fetal lung immaturity.

➤ *Phosphatidylglycerol* when absent indicates fetal lung immaturity.

ACTION ALERT!

Absence of bubble formation, absence of phosphatidylglycerol, or L/S ratio < 2 indicate lung immaturity in the fetus. If labor progresses or delivery is imminent, ensure that resuscitation equipment and trained personnel are immediately available.

Interfering Factors

➤ Test results may be inaccurate in the event of oligohydramnios.

➤ Blood and meconium in the amniotic fluid will adversely affect the fluid analysis.

➤ Disposable plastic syringes may alter amniotic fluid cells.

Contraindications

➤ None to conduct the amniotic fluid analysis. For contraindications to obtaining the fluid, see *Amniocentesis*.

NURSING CONSIDERATIONS

Prepare Your Client

➤ Explain to the client that this test is done to help judge how well the baby's lungs have formed and if the

baby is likely to have breathing problems after birth.

➤ See *Amniocentesis* for preparation in obtaining sample.

Perform Procedure

FOAM STABILITY TEST

Nurses do not usually perform this procedure but should understand the process to prepare the client and assist the physician or advanced practice nurse. See *Amniocentesis* for how sample is obtained.

Equal amounts of 95% ethanol and saline are mixed with amniotic fluid in varying dilutions and shaken for 15 seconds. The solution is inspected after 15 minutes for the presence of bubbles, indicating a normal test and lung maturity.

L/S RATIO

Amniotic fluid is measured directly for lecithin to sphingomyelin ratio to assess fetal lung maturity.

Care After Test

➤ See *Amniocentesis*.

➤ If test is negative or intermediate, prepare for neonatal respiratory distress or cardiopulmonary arrest. Make sure trained personnel including a neonatologist, neonatal advanced practice nurse, respiratory therapist, and other personnel are present for possible intubation, ventilatory support, and resuscitation.

Educate Your Client and the Family

➤ See *Amniocentesis*.

➤ Explain that a baby's lungs are not well formed and ready to breathe until the last month of pregnancy. Some babies born early need to have a tube inserted into their lungs and a machine to help them breathe until the lungs have a chance to finish forming properly.

Phosphorus, Serum

foss for us • see rum
(Serum Inorganic Phosphorus, Phosphate, P, PO₄)

Normal Findings

ADULT, PREGNANT,
ADOLESCENT, ELDERLY
2.7–4.5 mg/dL (SI units: 0.87–1.45 mmol/L)
Levels are elevated in adolescence during periods of rapid bone growth.
INFANT
3.5–8.6 mg/dL (SI units: 1.12–2.75 mmol/L)
CHILD
4.5–5.5 mg/dL (SI units: 1.45–1.78 mmol/L)
Levels are elevated during periods of rapid bone growth.

What This Test Will Tell You

This blood test is often used in the diagnosis of renal and skeletal diseases as well as to evaluate electrolyte and acid-base imbalances. Phosphorus levels are largely determined by the metabolism of calcium and the parathyroid hormone. There is an inverse relationship between calcium and phosphorus; as one rises, the other falls. Phosphorus is important in energy production, acid-base and calcium balance, and metabolism of carbohydrates and fats. Normal phosphorus levels are dependent upon proper gastrointestinal absorption from dietary sources, appropriate renal excretion, and the regulation of calcium and parathormone.

Abnormal Findings

▲INCREASED LEVELS may indicate renal failure, renal insufficiency, acromegaly, hypoparathyroidism, hypocalcemia, bone tumors, healing fractures, skeletal disease, bone metastasis of cancer, sarcoidosis, chemotherapy, high milk intake, phosphate-containing medications, diabetic acidosis, liver disease, or high vitamin D intake.

▼DECREASED LEVELS may indicate starvation, malabsorption syndrome, respiratory alkalosis, hyperparathyroidism, hypercalcemia, chronic alcoholism, continuous dextrose intravenous fluids, acute tubular necrosis, prolonged suctioning, long-term ingestion of antacids, vomiting, extensive burns, or hyperalimentation therapy without appropriate phosphorus supplementation.

ACTION ALERT!

Serum phosphate level below 1.5 mg/dL can be associated with hypercalcemia, because phosphate levels are always closely related to calcium levels. Assess client for deep bone pain, flank pain, and muscle hypotonicity. Begin continuous cardiac monitoring for the danger of dysrhythmias and cardiopulmonary arrest while definitive therapy is initiated.

Interfering Factors

➤ Aluminum hydroxide antacids, insulin, mannitol, and epinephrine can cause low levels.
➤ Hemolysis of blood produces falsely elevated results.
➤ A high-phosphate or low-calcium diet increases level.
➤ Excessive vitamin D intake, methicillin, phenytoin, heparin, anabolic steroid therapy, and use of enemas or laxatives that contain phosphates can cause elevated levels.

➤ Hemolysis of the blood can result in elevated levels.

NURSING CONSIDERATIONS

Prepare Your Client

➤ Explain that this test helps evaluate the balance of chemicals in the body, particularly phosphorus and calcium.

➤ Restrict fluids, food, and medications for 8 hours.

Perform Procedure

➤ Collect 5 mL of venous blood in a red-top tube.

➤ Handle the specimen gently to avoid hemolysis.

Care After Test

➤ For client with decreased levels, institute precautions to protect the client from infection because hypophosphatemia interferes with normal white blood cell function.

➤ Monitor for signs of hypocalcemia as a result of high phosphorus levels. Signs include paresthesia, twitching, dysrhythmias, hypotension, and laryngospasm.

➤ For client with low levels, administer oral phosphorus supplements mixed with chilled water or juice.

Educate Your Client and the Family

➤ Instruct the client to avoid using laxatives or enemas that contain sodium phosphate because they may result in toxic levels, especially in children or people with poor intestinal function.

➤ Instruct the client to avoid excess use of antacids.

➤ Explain that foods high in phosphorus are fish, poultry, eggs, legumes, and milk products.

P

Plasma Thrombin Time

plaz mah • throm bin • time

(Thrombin Time, Thrombin Clotting Time, Serum Thrombin Time, Fibrinogen Screen)

Normal Findings

ADULT, CHILD, ADOLESCENT, ELDERLY, PREGNANT

Control values vary. Check with the laboratory where the test is being performed for their normal values.

Within 2 seconds of the 9–13-second control value and within 5 seconds of the 15–20-second control value.

For effective heparin therapy, the client's thrombin time should be approximately 1.3 times the control value.

NEWBORN

Time is prolonged in newborns, due to decreased thrombin levels at birth.

What This Test Will Tell You

This blood test screens for fibrinogen deficiency and monitors anticoagulant therapy. Plasma thrombin time measures how quickly a clot forms when a standard amount of thrombin is added to the client's blood sample compared to a normal plasma control sample. After the thrombin is added, the clotting time for each sample is compared and recorded. If fibrinogen is deficient in the client, or anticoagulant therapy is excessive, prolonged clotting times result.

Abnormal Findings

▲INCREASED LEVELS *(prolonged time)* may indicate liver disease, disseminated intravascular coagulation (DIC), anticoagulant therapy when heparin is present in the blood, multiple myeloma, acute leukemia, afibrinogenemia, amyloidosis, dysfibrinogenemia, epistaxis, factor deficiency, lymphoma, obstetric complications, polycythemia vera, shock, or stress.

▼DECREASED LEVELS *(shortened time)* may indicate thrombocytosis.

ACTION ALERT!

Prolonged thrombin time indicates a high risk for hemorrhage. Carefully assess clients with prolonged times for occult as well as overt bleeding, including testing all body fluids for blood and monitoring for hypotension, tachycardia, anxiety, dyspnea, chest pain, and changes in level of consciousness. Report abnormal findings immediately.

Interfering Factors

➤ Asparaginase; fibrin degradation products; and streptokinase, tissue plasminogen activator (TPA), urokinase, and heparin within 2 days of the test will prolong the time.

➤ Hemolyzed samples invalidate the results.

➤ Failure to discard the first 2–3 mL of blood may result in specimen contamination from tissue thromboplastin.

NURSING CONSIDERATIONS

Prepare Your Client

➤ Explain that this test helps determine how well the blood can clot.

Perform Procedure

➤ If the test is being used to monitor heparin therapy, the blood is to be drawn 1 hour before administration of the heparin.

➤ Draw 2–3 mL of blood first and discard this. Then draw 7 mL of venous blood in a blue-top tube that contains sodium citrate, an anticoagulant.

Care After Test

➤ If the client is on heparin therapy, the venipuncture site should be held for 5 minutes.

➤ Observe for signs and symptoms of bleeding.

➤ Review related tests such as the activated partial thromboplastin time, prothrombin time, platelet count, hemoglobin, hematocrit, fibrin split products, and bleeding time.

Educate Your Client and the Family

➤ If the test is prolonged preoperatively, inform client that surgery may need to be postponed unless it is an emergency.

➤ Teach the client and family members about bleeding precautions: using a soft-bristled toothbrush and electric razors, avoiding constipation, avoiding aspirin and aspirin products, and avoiding constricting clothing.

➤ Teach the client and family members the signs and symptoms of bleeding: petechiae, bruising, blood in the urine and stool, vaginal bleeding, and bleeding from invasive lines.

Plasminogen, Plasma

plaz **min** oe jen • **plaz** mah

(PMG, Profibrinolysin, Pgn, Plasminogen Assay, Blood Plasminogen Assay)

Normal Findings

ADULT, NEWBORN, CHILD,
ADOLESCENT, ELDERLY
Plasminogen ≥ 65% of normal
Quantitatively, 2.5–4.5 μU/mL
PREGNANT
The blood level in the maternal
blood at term is twice the adult level.

What This Test Will Tell You

This blood test is used most commonly in the diagnosis of disseminated intravascular coagulation (DIC) to test for the presence of a blood component that has the ability to dissolve clots. Plasminogen is an inactive precursor of the enzyme plasmin, which is responsible for dissolving clots. It is activated by plasminogen activators from plasma, endothelial cells and other tissues, urine, and bacteria. The amount of this substance is useful information when the client is on thrombolytic agents.

Abnormal Findings

▲INCREASED LEVELS may indicate metastatic prostatic cancer, intrauterine death with fetal retention, fibrinolytic treatment (streptokinase, urokinase, tissue plasminogen antigen), venous occlusion, anxiety/stress, congenital defect in release of plasminogen inhibitors, deep vein thrombosis, or infection and inflammation.

▼DECREASED LEVELS may indicate fibrinolytic therapy, disseminated intravascular coagulation, severe hepatocellular disease, treatment with aminocaproic acid, hya-line membrane disease, acquired hypofibrinogenemia, liver disease, nephrosis, postoperative coronary artery bypass grafting, thrombosis, pre-eclampsia, or eclampsia.

Interfering Factors

➤ Estrogens and oral contraceptives will elevate plasminogen levels.
➤ Aminocaproic acid inhibits fibrinolytic activity.
➤ Streptococcal antibodies, streptokinase, urokinase, and asparaginase will decrease levels of plasminogen.
➤ Prolonged tourniquet application or drawing the blood too slowly will allow stasis of the blood and alter the results.

NURSING CONSIDERATIONS

Prepare Your Client

➤ Explain that this test is to help evaluate how well the body is able to dissolve and get rid of clots after they have formed.

Perform Procedure

➤ Draw and discard a 2-mL sample and draw a 5-mL venous blood sample in a blue-top tube with sodium citrate anticoagulant. Gently invert the sample several times to mix the blood and the anticoagulant.
➤ Send to the laboratory immediately.

Care After Test

➤ Client with decreased plasminogen concentrations may be prone to develop recurrent arterial and venous thromboses. Observe closely for signs and symptoms. Arterial thrombosis is manifested by pale, cool extremities with absent or impaired pulses and sensation. Venous thrombosis is manifested by swollen, edematous extremities.

➤ Review related tests such as activated partial thromboplastin time, prothrombin time, platelet count, hemoglobin, fibrin split products, hematocrit, and bleeding time.

Educate Your Client and the Family

➤ Teach warning signs and symptoms of thrombosis including abnormal sensations (paresthesia), decreased strength and ability to move an extremity (paresis), and difficulty with language function (aphasia).

➤ Instruct the client with prolonged bleeding time to avoid taking over-the-counter medications that prolong bleeding time, such as aspirin or products containing aspirin. Client should be instructed to avoid large quantities of alcohol and its regular use. A written list of products to avoid will provide the client or family with a reference when shopping or selecting home remedies for minor ailments.

Platelet Aggregation
plate let • ag reh gay shun

Normal Findings
All ages: Normal aggregation occurs in 3–5 minutes, although findings are temperature dependent and vary with the laboratory.

What This Test Will Tell You
This blood test detects von Willebrand's disease or other clotting disorders that involve ristocetin cofactor. Platelets are nonnucleated, round or oval, flattened disk-shaped structures that are vital to the formation of a hemostatic plug in vascular injury. They gather at any site of vascular injury to form an aggregate, or plug, to stop bleeding. This test measures the rate at which platelets within a sample form an aggregate.

Abnormal Findings
▲INCREASED LEVELS may indicate hemolysis, nicotine, heparin, atheromatosis, diabetes mellitus, hyperlipemia, or polycythemia vera.

▼DECREASED LEVELS may indicate von Willebrand's disease, Bernard-Soulier syndrome, renal disease, cardiopulmonary bypass, disseminated intravascular coagulation, thrombasthenia, uremia, macroglobulinemia, liver disease, acute leukemia, pernicious anemia, myeloproliferative disorders, hypothyroidism, Swiss cheese platelets, gray platelet syndrome, multiple myeloma, sideroblastic anemia, afibrinogenemia, beta thalassemia major, Chediak-Higashi syndrome, chronic myelogenous leukemia, myeloid metaplasia, essential thrombocytopenia, homocystinuria, idiopathic thrombocytopenia purpura, plasma cell dyscrasias, scurvy, or Wiskott-Aldrich syndrome.

◾ ACTION ALERT!
Clotting abnormalities increase the risk for

bleeding and hemorrhage. Closely observe the client for signs and symptoms such as frank bleeding, hypotension, tachycardia, apprehension, dyspnea, pale and cool skin, and anxiety. Be prepared to transfuse with blood products, including appropriate clotting factors.

Interfering Factors

➤ Platelet counts less than 50,000 cells/mm^3 will result in prolonged aggregation times, as there are fewer platelets available for clumping.

➤ Aspirin within prior 7–10 days will result in prolonged aggregation times.

➤ Hemolysis caused by rough handling of the sample or by trauma at the venipuncture site will result in prolonged aggregation times because hemolyzed red blood cells contain adenosine diphosphate, which causes platelets to aggregate.

➤ Failure to use a properly anticoagulated lab tube will result in shortened aggregation times.

➤ Lipemia will affect test results.

Potential Complications

➤ Prolonged bleeding or bruising at the venipuncture site

NURSING CONSIDERATIONS

Prepare Your Client

➤ Explain that this test is used to assess the blood's ability to clot.

➤ Instruct the client to fast and/or not to eat any fats for the 8 hours before the test.

➤ Withhold aspirin and aspirin compounds for 14 days prior to the test and phenylbutazone, sulfinpyrazone, phenothiazines, antihistamines, anti-inflammatory drugs, and tricyclic depressants for 48 hours before the test, as ordered. If therapy must be continued, note this on the lab slip.

Perform Procedure

➤ Collect 7 mL of venous blood in a blue-top tube containing sodium citrate. Completely fill the tube and invert it several times to mix the sample and anticoagulant adequately. Do not shake the tube vigorously as this can result in hemolysis.

Care After Test

➤ Hold pressure at the venipuncture site for 5 minutes to prevent hematoma formation.

➤ Observe the client for signs and symptoms of bleeding.

➤ Review related tests such as prothrombin time, platelet count, hemoglobin, capillary fragility test, hematocrit, and bleeding time.

Educate Your Client and the Family

➤ Teach the client and family members about bleeding precautions: using a soft-bristled toothbrush, using electric razors rather than straight razors, avoiding constipation, avoiding aspirin and aspirin products, avoiding picking their nose, and avoiding constricting clothing. If menses is experienced, the client should maintain a pad count and note the amount of saturation of each pad.

➤ Teach the client and family members the signs and symptoms of bleeding including petechiae (small purplish spots on the skin), bruising, blood in urine or stool, vaginal bleeding, or bleeding from any other sites.

➤ Teach the client to avoid over-the-counter aspirin and aspirin-containing drugs, phenothiazines, codeine, non-steroidal anti-inflammatory drugs, and alcohol.

Platelet Count

plate let • kownt

(Phase Platelet Count, Platelets, Thrombocyte Count, Blood Platelet Count)

Normal Findings

ADULT, ADOLESCENT, ELDERLY, AND PREGNANT

$130,000-450,000/mm^3$ (SI units: $130-450 \times 10^9/L$)

NEWBORN

Cord: $100,000-290,000/mm^3$

Premature: $100,000-300,000/mm^3$

3 months: $260,000/mm^3$

Infant: $200,000-473,000/mm^3$

CHILD

1–10 years: $150,000-450,000/mm^3$

What This Test Will Tell You

This blood test evaluates platelet production and assesses the effects of cancer treatment on platelet numbers. The count may be automated but is confirmed by a visual estimate of the number of platelets from a stained blood film. The platelets' size and shape are noted. Platelets are nonnucleated, round or oval, flattened disk-shaped structures that are vital to the formation of a hemostatic plug in vascular injury. The platelet count is one of the most important screening tests of platelet function.

Abnormal Findings

▲INCREASED LEVELS (thrombocytosis) may indicate hemorrhage, infectious disorders, malignancies, iron deficiency anemia, recent surgery, recent pregnancy, recent splenectomy, inflammatory disorders, fractures, cryoglobulinemia, asplenia, asphyxiation, rheumatoid arthritis, heart disease, cirrhosis, chronic pancreatitis, tuberculosis, recovery from bone marrow depression, multiple myeloma, primary thrombocytosis, myelofibrosis with myeloid metaplasia, polycythemia vera, or chronic myelogenous leukemia.

▼DECREASED LEVELS (thrombocytopenia) may reveal bone marrow depression, hypoplastic bone marrow, pernicious anemia, infiltrative bone marrow disease such as carcinoma or leukemia, megakaryocytic thrombopoiesis secondary to folic acid or vitamin B_{12} deficiency, pooling of platelets in an enlarged spleen, increased platelet destruction due to drugs or immune disorders, recent massive blood transfusions, disseminated intravascular coagulation (DIC), Bernard-Soulier syndrome, mechanical injury to platelets, idiopathic thrombocytopenia purpura (ITP), disseminated infection, exposure to DDT and other chemicals, human immunodeficiency virus (HIV) infection, cavernous hemangioma, coronary artery bypass graft, severe burns, clostridial infections, diphtheria, Gaucher's disease, May-Hegglin anomaly, or Wiskott-Aldrich syndrome.

ACTION ALERT!

➤ With an extremely high platelet count (1 million/mm^3) from a myeloproliferative disorder, there may be bleeding because of abnormal platelet function.

➤ A decrease in platelet count to less than $50,000/mm^3$ is associated with spontaneous bleeding, prolonged bleeding time, petechiae, and ecchymosis.

➤ A platelet count less than $5,000/mm^3$ generally results in fatal bleeding from the gastrointestinal tract or central nervous system.

Interfering Factors

➤ Medications that may increase platelet count are epinephrine, oral contraceptives, and vincristine.

➤ Medications that may decrease platelet counts include antineoplastic agents, phenacetin, aspirin, phenylbutazone, quinine, quinidine, sulfonamides, penicillin, streptomycin, tetracycline, barbiturates, promethazine, thiazide diuretics, mercurial diuretics, insulin, tolbutamide, phenytoin, trimethadione, diphenhydramine, gold compounds, silver, copper, reserpine, digitoxin, vitamin K, heparin, nitroglycerin, prednisone, and novocaine.

➤ Alcohol may decrease platelet counts.

➤ Strenuous exercise and residing in elevated altitudes cause increased levels.

➤ Premenstrual women may experience decreased platelet counts.

Potential Complications

➤ Prolonged bleeding at the venipuncture site

NURSING CONSIDERATIONS

Prepare Your Client

➤ Explain that this test helps assess the blood's ability to clot.

Perform Procedure

➤ Collect 7 mL of venous blood in a lavender-top tube.

➤ Apply pressure or a pressure dressing to the venipuncture site.

Care After Test

➤ Hold pressure at the venipuncture site for 5 minutes to prevent hematoma formation.

➤ Assess client for unusual bruising or prolonged bleeding from venipuncture site. Delayed clotting is a complication of severely impaired clotting.

➤ Test all body secretions including stool, gastrointestinal aspirate, and tracheal aspirate for occult blood. Closely inspect mucous membranes for bleeding.

➤ Review related tests such as complete blood count, bone marrow biopsy, direct Coombs' (antiglobulin) test, serum protein electrophoresis, clot retraction, bleeding time, prothrombin consumption test, platelet aggregation, and platelet survival.

Educate Your Client and the Family

➤ Teach the client and family members about bleeding precautions including using a soft-bristled toothbrush, using electric razors rather than straight razors, avoiding constipation, avoiding aspirin and aspirin products, avoiding picking their nose, and avoiding constricting clothing. If menses is experienced, the client should maintain a pad count and note the amount of saturation of each pad.

➤ Teach the client and family members the signs and symptoms of bleeding including petechiae (small purplish spots on the skin), bruising, blood in the urine or stool, vaginal bleeding, and bleeding from any other sites.

➤ Teach the client to avoid over-the-counter aspirin and aspirin products, phenothiazines, codeine, non-steroidal anti-inflammatory drugs, and alcohol.

Platelet Survival

plate let • sur vie vahl

(Platelet Antibody, Blood Platelet Antibody, Platelet Antibody Detection Test)

Normal Findings

ALL AGES

Negative: Normally, half the radiolabeled platelets disappear from the circulation in 84–116 hours. The remaining radioactivity normally disappears in 8–10 days, which is believed to be the normal platelet life span. When platelets disappear within these time frames, the test results are considered to be negative. When platelets disappear in less time, the test is considered positive.

What This Test Will Tell You

This blood test diagnoses problems with platelet life span associated with drug therapy, specific disease processes, or factors associated with platelet destruction. The test measures the rate at which platelets are destroyed and produced in the peripheral circulation. Platelets are labeled with chromium-51 (^{51}Cr), a radioactive substance, and are then injected back into the bloodstream. For 8–10 days, the labeled platelets remaining in the bloodstream are counted in serial samples of peripheral blood and graphed to obtain a platelet survival curve.

Abnormal Findings

▼DECREASED LEVELS (shortened survival time) may indicate idiopathic thrombocytopenia purpura, lupus erythematosus, consumptive coagulopathy, Hodgkin's disease, lymphosarcoma, or isoimmune neonatal thrombocytopenia.

Interfering Factors

➤ The presence of antiplatelet antibodies after multiple transfusions, platelet transfusion, or repeated pregnancies may interfere with accurate determination of the test results by shortening platelet survival time.

➤ Medications that may decrease platelet survival time include aspirin, heparin, thiazide diuretics, benzenes, gold salts, quinine, quinidine, and digitoxin.

Potential Complications

➤ Prolonged bleeding at the venipuncture site

NURSING CONSIDERATIONS

Prepare Your Client

➤ Explain that this test helps determine if the blood clots normally.

➤ Check the client's history for multiple blood or blood product transfusions or multiple pregnancies and report such findings to the laboratory.

Perform Procedure

➤ A venipuncture is performed and the collected venous blood is tagged with chromium-51 and then reinjected into the client. Alternatively, a specimen from donor platelets can be obtained, tagged, and injected.

➤ A specimen is then collected in a 7-mL lavender-top tube at 30 minutes and 2 hours after the tagged platelets have been infused. The collection tube should be filled completely and inverted and gently rotated to thoroughly mix the anticoagulant. Don't shake the tube vigorously, as this can result in hemolysis.

➤ Specimens may be collected in 7-mL lavender-top tubes daily for the next 8–10 days.

➤ Apply pressure or a pressure dressing to the site after each venipuncture.

➤ Label the specimen and note a history of multiple blood or blood product transfusions or multiple pregnancies.

Care After Test

➤ Hold pressure at the venipuncture site for 5 minutes to prevent hematoma formation.

➤ Assess client for unusual bruising or prolonged bleeding from venipuncture site. Delayed clotting is a complication of severely impaired clotting.

➤ Test all body secretions including stool, gastrointestinal aspirate, and tracheal aspirate for occult blood. Closely inspect mucous membranes for bleeding.

➤ Review related tests such as prothrombin time, partial thromboplastin time, bleeding time, activated clotting time, complete blood count, bone marrow biopsy, direct Coombs' (antiglobulin) test, serum protein electrophoresis, clot retraction, prothrombin consumption test, platelet aggregation, and platelet count.

Educate Your Client and the Family

➤ Teach the client and family members about bleeding precautions including using a soft-bristled toothbrush, using electric razors rather than straight razors, avoiding constipation, avoiding aspirin and aspirin products, avoiding picking their nose, and avoiding constricting clothing. If menses is experienced, the client should maintain a pad count and note the saturation of each pad.

➤ Teach the client and family members the signs and symptoms of bleeding including petechiae (small purplish spots on the skin), bruising, blood in the urine or stool, vaginal bleeding, and bleeding from any other sites.

Plethysmography, Arterial
pleh thiz mah grah fee • ar teer ee al

Normal Findings
ALL AGES

Arterial pressure gradient less than 20 mm Hg pressure between upper and lower extremities

Normal arterial pulse waveform: steep upswing with wider downstroke containing a dicrotic notch.

What This Test Will Tell You

This noninvasive pressure monitoring test diagnoses arterial occlusive disease primarily in lower extremities, but can be used in the upper extremities as well. It may also be used to evaluate results of vascular surgical and medical therapies. The test detects a reduction in systolic arterial pressure and a change in arterial waveform. It is often performed on clients who are too high risk for angiography.

Using a variety of methods and transducers, this test is used occasionally to measure pressures in fingers, toes, and eyes.

Abnormal Findings

Abnormalities may indicate arterial thrombus or embolus, arterial vascular occlusive disease, diabetic ischemia, Reynaud's disease, or vascular trauma.

■■■■ ACTION ALERT!

Complete arterial occlusion of a limb can quickly result in loss of the affected limb. This is a medical emergency requiring antithrombolytic therapy, surgical arterial bypass grafting, or thrombectomy by catheterization.

Interfering Factors

➤ Cigarette smoking prior to testing causes arterial vasoconstriction and will affect both pressure and waveform analysis.
➤ In infants and children, crying may affect accuracy of hemodynamic pressures.
➤ Arterial occlusion above the extremity will reduce pressures along the entire limb, making it impossible to pinpoint the occlusion.
➤ Development of extensive collateral circulation may not show pressure changes that would reveal the presence of partial or complete occlusion.

NURSING CONSIDERATIONS

Prepare Your Client

➤ Explain to the client and family that this test is used to diagnose clots or other circulation problems in the arteries, the blood vessels that take blood away from the heart.
➤ Inform the client that the test can take approximately 45 minutes.
➤ Let the client know that lying still

during the procedure is very important. Muscle activity may interfere with accurate pressure readings and tracings.
➤ Assure the client that the test is not painful.
➤ Record baseline vital signs.
➤ Note any vasoactive medications the client is taking.
➤ Confirm that adults and older children have voided before the procedure.
➤ Do not remove glasses, dentures, or hearing aids unless dictated by your hospital policy. The client may need these in order to communicate and cooperate during the procedure.
➤ Remove clothing entirely from any arms and legs being tested. Pressure cuffs should not be placed over clothing, nor should clothing be rolled up because it may interfere with blood flow and pressure.

Perform Procedure

Nurses do not usually perform this procedure, but should understand the process to prepare the client and assist the diagnostician. Three blood pressure cuffs are placed on the extremities being tested. They are then inflated to lower pressures than normal blood pressure cuffs to compare the pressure throughout the arm and/or leg. The cuffs are connected to a plethysmograph, which will draw a tracing of the pressure so that the shape can also be analyzed. By analyzing the pressures and the tracings, any blockage in the arteries of the arms and legs should be detected. If a significant difference in pressure occurs between two cuffs placed on an arm or leg, the blockage is probably located closer to the body (proximal) than the cuff recording the lower pressure.

Care After Test

➤ Monitor vital signs. Compare to preprocedural findings.

➤ Check circulation in the extremities frequently for any reduction in strength of pulses, slowed capillary refill, decreased temperature, or paresthesia.

➤ Evaluate related tests such as arteriography, Doppler studies, and clotting studies.

Educate Your Client and the Family

➤ Teach client and family a heart-healthy diet, including no added salt.

➤ Instruct client taking anticoagulants to avoid taking aspirin, maintain pressure on cuts or venipuncture sites 3–5 minutes, use a soft toothbrush, and avoid activities that lead to tissue trauma such as contact sports.

➤ Teach client who is experiencing paresthesia to protect extremity from injury by testing water temperature to prevent burns, wearing properly fitting shoes, and keep walking areas free of clutter.

P

Plethysmography, Venous
pleh thiz mah grah fee • vee nus

Normal Findings

ALL AGES

No indication of venous thrombosis or occlusion

Normal venous volume changes related to respiratory pattern

Rapid return of venous volume to normal levels after deflation of proximal cuff

What This Test Will Tell You

This noninvasive pressure monitoring test diagnoses venous occlusive disease primarily in the lower extremities, but may be used for upper extremities as well. It may also be used to evaluate vascular surgical and medical therapies. The test is performed by inflating a proximal blood pressure cuff until venous blood flow is occluded. A distally placed cuff on the same extremity should detect a rapid increase in venous blood volume because venous return has been occluded by the proximal cuff. If the distal cuff fails to detect a sudden increase in venous blood volume, venous vascular occlusion is suspected. Normally, once the proximal cuff is deflated, venous vascular volume quickly returns to normal. In the presence of venous occlusion, the distal cuff shows a very slow return of normal pressures because venous blood flow cannot clear from the area.

Abnormal Findings

Abnormalities may indicate deep vein thrombosis, superficial vein thrombosis, or complete or partial occlusion of veins.

Interfering Factors

➤ Venous occlusion higher in the limb than the proximal occluding cuff will interfere with pressure interpretation.

NURSING CONSIDERATIONS

Prepare Your Client

➤ Explain to the client and family that this test will help discover clots or other problems in the veins, which return blood to the heart.

➤ Inform the client that the test can take approximately 45 minutes.

➤ Discuss with the client that lying still during the procedure is very important. Muscle activity may interfere with accurate pressure readings and tracings.

➤ Assure the client and family that the test is not painful.

➤ Record baseline vital signs.

➤ Note any vasoactive medications the client is taking.

➤ Confirm that adults and older children have voided before the procedure.

➤ Do not remove glasses, dentures, or hearing aids unless dictated by your hospital policy. The client may need these in order to communicate and cooperate during the procedure.

➤ Remove clothing entirely from any arms and legs being tested. Pressure cuffs should not be placed over clothing, nor should clothing be rolled up because it may interfere with blood flow and pressure.

Perform Procedure

Nurses do not usually perform this procedure, but should understand the process to prepare the client and assist the physician. This test can be performed at the bedside or in the noninvasive vascular lab. Two blood pressure cuffs are placed on the extremities being tested. The cuff closest to the body is inflated to a higher pressure than the lower (distal) cuff to trap venous blood in the leg. Higher pressures should be recorded in the lower cuff if no blockage is present. Once the air is let out of the cuff, the pressures should quickly return to normal if no blockage is present. The cuffs are connected to a machine (plethysmograph) that will record the pressures being measured. By analyzing the pressures, any blockage in the veins of the arms and legs should be detected.

Care After Test

➤ Monitor vital signs after the test. Compare to preprocedural findings.

➤ Continue to monitor peripheral circulation.

➤ For client with deep vein thrombosis, assess carefully for signs and symptoms of embolism such as respiratory distress and chest pain.

➤ Evaluate other related tests such as Doppler studies and venography.

Educate Your Client and the Family

➤ Teach client and family the importance of activity and of not crossing feet or ankles if vascular disease is present.

➤ Instruct client who receives anticoagulant therapy to avoid taking aspirin, maintain pressure on cuts or venipuncture sites for 3–5 minutes, use a soft toothbrush, and avoid activities that lead to tissue trauma such as contact sports.

Pleural Biopsy

plur ahl • bie op see

Normal Findings

No abnormal cells or tissues present

What This Test Will Tell You

This microscopic examination uses a specimen of pleural tissue for analysis by culture or cytologic examination to identify the etiology of pleural effusions, suspected pleural tumors, the causative organism of pleural infections, or other pleural diseases. Pleural biopsies are indicated when other, less invasive tests such as chest x-ray, computed tomography scans, and sputum analyses are inconclusive or when the pleural fluid obtained through thoracentesis is inconclusive in distinguishing between infection, malignancy, and tuberculosis.

The sample may be obtained through the chest wall during a thoracentesis (percutaneous pleural biopsy), through a fiber-optic bronchoscope inserted into the pleural space (pleuroscopy), or by open pleural biopsy in the operating room, which entails a limited thoracotomy and general anesthesia. Percutaneous or pleuroscopic needle biopsy is a relatively safe, simple diagnostic procedure useful in determining the cause of pleural effusions. The advantage of the open biopsy is that a larger specimen may be obtained.

Abnormal Findings

Abnormalities may indicate cancer; infection with bacteria, virus, fungus, or parasites; tuberculosis; inflammatory disorders; granulomas; fibrosis; or collagen vascular disease of the pleura. Report problems with respiratory function to primary health care provider immediately. Have suction equipment immediately available.

Interfering Factors

➤ Improper specimen collection or contamination of specimen
➤ Refrigeration of specimen
➤ Excess time elapsed between specimen collection and inoculation of culture medium (maximum is 3 hours)

Contraindications

➤ Bleeding disorders.
➤ Inability of the client to cooperate with the procedure because of respiratory insufficiency, confusion, agitation, etc., may contraindicate percutaneous or bronchoscopic biopsies. The open biopsy procedure with general anesthesia may be used instead.

Potential Complications

➤ Pneumothorax
➤ Hemothorax
➤ Intercostal nerve injury
➤ Infection

NURSING CONSIDERATIONS

Prepare Your Client

➤ Explain that the test is to obtain a sample of tissue from the lining of the lung to be examined for disease.
➤ Assess complete blood count and

blood clotting studies prior to the procedure to identify clients at high risk for developing complications.

➤ Describe the procedure to be utilized to obtain the specimen (needle biopsy, pleuroscopy, or thoracotomy).

➤ Confirm that a signed informed consent has been obtained from the client.

➤ Instruct the client not to eat or drink anything for 6–8 hours prior to the procedure.

➤ Explain that if a percutaneous needle biopsy is to be performed, the client must hold as still as possible and refrain from coughing to prevent perforation of the lung by the biopsy needle.

➤ Reassure the client that vital signs and respiratory status will be monitored closely during and immediately after the procedure.

➤ Administer premedications if ordered, such as atropine to decrease secretions and sedatives.

➤ Provide a hospital gown or help the client disrobe above the waist (for percutaneous pleural biopsy).

Perform Procedure

Nurses do not perform this procedure, but should understand the process to prepare the client and assist the physician.

PERCUTANEOUS NEEDLE BIOPSY

Assist the client to a sitting position with the arms supported on a pillow on an overbed table. The procedure may be performed at the client's bedside or in the radiology department under fluoroscopy. The procedural steps are similar to a thoracentesis. Pleural fluid may also be obtained during this procedure for diagnostic or therapeutic purposes. Cleanse the needle insertion site with an antiseptic solution. The insertion site is infiltrated with local anesthesia. Remind the client to remain as still as possible and avoid coughing.

The biopsy needle is inserted through the chest wall into the selected intercostal space. After some pleural fluid is removed, the needle is rotated to obtain a small piece of pleural tissue. Several specimens may be obtained from different sites. Instruct the client to expire all air and then to perform the Valsalva maneuver to prevent air from entering the pleural space while the biopsies are taken and the needle is withdrawn.

Apply pressure to the biopsy site immediately after the needle is withdrawn. Place the samples in appropriate containers using aseptic technique. Dress the puncture site with an occlusive pressure dressing after bleeding ceases.

PLEUROSCOPIC BIOPSY

Assist the client to a sitting position with the arms supported on a pillow on an overbed table. The procedure may be performed in a special endoscopy room or at the client's bedside if portable endoscopic equipment is available.

Follow procedural steps as described for percutaneous needle biopsy except that a small incision is made and the fiber-optic pleuroscope is introduced for direct visualization of the pleura and surrounding structures. The specimen is obtained through the pleuroscope using a cutting forceps or needle.

The scope is withdrawn and pressure immediately applied to the incision. The incision is closed with sutures as indicated. Place samples in the appropriate containers using aseptic technique. Dress the incision site after sutures are placed.

OPEN PLEURAL BIOPSY

Transport the client to the operating room, where general anesthesia is administered and the client is prepped and draped. With the client in a supine position, a small incision is made into the chest wall. A piece of lung tissue is obtained, chest tubes are inserted for lung re-expansion and drainage, and the chest is surgically closed. Place the samples obtained in appropriate containers using aseptic technique.

Care After Test

➤ Label specimen containers, indicating the site and method used to obtain the specimen, and transport to the laboratory immediately.

➤ Maintain patency and appropriate suction and/or water seal for any chest tubes.

➤ Following a percutaneous needle biopsy or pleuroscopic biopsy, the client is placed in a semi-Fowler's position to assist in maximum lung ventilation.

➤ Following an open biopsy, the client is transported to the recovery room.

➤ Monitor respiratory status closely for signs of hemo- or pneumothorax, such as dyspnea, tachypnea, cyanosis, decreased breath sounds on the biopsy side.

➤ Obtain a chest x-ray if ordered to check for complications.

➤ Observe for signs of bleeding at the biopsy site and check vital signs every 15–30 minutes for 1–2 hours until stable. Note tachycardia, thready pulse, hypotension, chest pain, hemoptysis, and dysrhythmias, and report to the primary health care provider immediately. Prepare for emergency interventions including cardiopulmonary resuscitation if needed.

➤ Assess the client's comfort level and administer analgesics if indicated.

➤ Resume fluids and food when the client's condition is stable.

➤ Evaluate related tests such as chest x-ray, computed tomography scans, sputum cultures, complete blood counts, and thoracentesis.

Educate Your Client and the Family

➤ Describe the nursing routine of closely monitoring vital signs and respiratory status.

➤ Instruct the client to report immediately any difficulty breathing, bleeding from the puncture site, or other discomforts.

➤ Describe any activity restrictions.

➤ Tell the client that results may not be available for 2 days.

➤ Refer client who smokes to smoking cessation classes.

Porphyrins, Urine

por fih rins • yur in

(Urine Porphyrins, Aminolevulinic Acid, ALA, Porphobilinogen, PBG, Copro-porphyrin, Uroporphyrins, Coproporphyrins)

Normal Findings

Findings apply to all age groups

UROPORPHYRINS

Male: 0–42 µg/24 hours (SI units: 0–50 nmol/24 hours)

Female: 1–22 µg/24 hours (SI units: 1–26 nmol/24 hours)

COPROPORPHYRINS

Male: 0–96 µg/24 hours (SI units: 0–146 nmol/24 hours)

Female: 1–57 µg/24 hours (SI units: 1–86 nmol/24 hours)

PORPHOBILINOGEN

1.5–2 mg/24 hours (SI units: 6.6–9 mmol/24 hours)

What This Test Will Tell You

This urine test detects the presence of porphyrins, a urinary pigment that is produced during the synthesis of heme and that may accumulate abnormally in a variety of conditions. Porphyrins are used in the synthesis of hemoglobin and of any hemoproteins that are carriers of oxygen. The porphyrins are eliminated from the body in feces and urine, mainly as coproporphyrin I and III and as uroporphyrins. In health, excretion of uroporphyrins is minimal, but the amount excreted rises during liver damage, lead poisoning, congenital porphyria (an inborn error of metabolism), and pellagra.

Porphyrins are reddish fluorescent compounds. Depending on the type of porphyrin present, therefore, the urine may be reddish or the color of port wine. This may be noted on the routine urinalysis or observation of a urine specimen. There are several porphyrins, in addition to uroporphyrins, for which the urine may be tested, including aminolevulinic acid (ALA), porphobilinogen (PBG), and coproporphyrin. The presence of these specific porphyrins may be evaluated to classify the type of porphyria the client is experiencing.

Uroporphyrinogen I synthase measures blood levels of this enzyme that converts porphobilinogen to uroporphyrinogen during heme biosynthesis. This test can detect acute intermittent porphyria (AIP) even during its latent phase and thus can identify individuals before their first acute episode.

Stool and urine tests for aminolevulinic acid (ALA) and porphobilinogen may also be ordered to support a diagnosis of porphyria, because excretion of these porphyrin precursors increases substantially during an acute episode of AIP and may increase slightly during the latent phase. Evaluation of red blood cells and hemoglobin levels may also provide information about derangements of hemoglobin synthesis.

Abnormal Findings

▲ INCREASED LEVELS may indicate porphyrias, lead poisoning, liver disease, pellagra, Hodgkin's disease, or some cancers.

ACTION ALERT!

Late signs of porphyrias may include respiratory insufficiency, sensory neuropathy, and seizures. Monitor the client carefully if urine levels of porphyrins are elevated and institute continuous cardiac monitoring if any symptoms are present.

Interfering Factors

➤ Exposure of the urine to light may invalidate results. 24-hour urine specimens must be collected in a dark container or covered with aluminum foil during the collection period for accurate result. Random samples must be sent to the laboratory within 1 hour of collection.

➤ Failure to refrigerate or keep a 24-hour sample on ice may cause inaccurate results, unless a preservative has been added to the container.

➤ Drugs such as griseofulvin, rifampin, barbiturates, aminosalicylic acid (PAS), chlorpropamide, ethyl alcohol, morphine, oral contraceptives, phenazopyridine, procaine, sulfonamides, tetracyclines, and penicillins may alter results.

➤ Menstruation and pregnancy can increase porphyrins levels.

Contraindications

➤ Clients receiving barbiturate preparations. However, if intermittent porphyria is the reason for testing, the test should be done with the client receiving these medications because these drugs may provoke an attack of porphyria.

NURSING CONSIDERATIONS

Prepare Your Client

➤ Explain that this test is to measure the amount of a pigment excreted in the urine that is necessary for normal formation of red blood cell components.

➤ Describe the collection procedure to be utilized, random urine sample or 24-hour collection of urine.

➤ Instruct the client to avoid alcohol ingestion during the collection.

Perform Procedure

➤ Collect a random sample, if indicated, and send promptly to the laboratory in a container protected from light (cover with aluminum foil or a dark plastic bag).

➤ Obtain a 24-hour urine collection the same as for any test requiring a 24-hour or timed urine collection.

➤ Keep the sample refrigerated or on ice throughout the collection period.

➤ Cover a Foley catheter bag, if the specimen is being collected from a client with an indwelling catheter, with a dark plastic bag and place in a basin of ice.

➤ Encourage the client to drink fluids during the 24 hours, unless contraindicated.

➤ Label the urine collection starting and stopping times on the urine containers and the laboratory slip.

➤ Transport the urine specimens promptly to the laboratory.

Care After Test

➤ Assess the client for symptoms of porphyria, such as neurological abnormalities, acute abdominal pain, photosensitivity, or psychiatric disturbances.

➤ Assess client for nausea, vomiting, abdominal pain, diarrhea, constipation, ileus, dysuria, muscle hypotonia, respiratory insufficiency, sensory neuropathies, seizures, skin lesions, and photosensitivity.

➤ Review related tests such as complete blood count, fecal and serum porphyrins, urinalysis for color, tests for other urinary porphyrins, urine and stool tests for uroporphybilinogen, serum uroporphyrinogen I synthase, red blood cell counts, and hemoglobin levels.

Educate Your Client and the Family

➤ Teach client with porphyria and skin manifestations to avoid sun exposure.

➤ Explain to client with porphyria they must avoid medications such as barbiturates, chlordiazepoxide, chloroquine, chlorpropamide, estrogens, ethanol, glutethimide, griseofulvin, hydantoin, imipramine, meprobamate, methyldopa, and sulfonamides.

➤ Explain to client the importance of telling all health care providers they consult that they suffer from a porphyria disorder.

➤ Explain to female client that menstruation or pregnancy can induce an acute attack.

➤ Explain to the client and family the importance of eliminating any known precipitants of an attack. These may include avoidance of alcohol and prompt treatment of infections.

Positron-Emission Tomography

poz ih tron • ee mish un • toe mog rah fee
(PET, Emission-Computed Tomography, ECT, Emission CT Scan)

Normal Findings

Normal brain metabolism and blood flow
Normal cardiac metabolism and blood flow

What This Test Will Tell You

This noninvasive nuclear scanning test assesses organ metabolism as well as blood flow. Positron-emission tomograpy (PET) is most frequently associated with studying and diagnosing cerebral function. Some work has also been done studying cardiac blood flow within the first 72 hours after myocardial infarction.

The client either inhales or is injected with a radioactively tagged substance such as glucose, oxygen, nitrogen, or carbon. These tagged substances are selected based upon the type of blood flow or metabolism that needs to be evaluated. The radionuclide of the inhaled or injected substance emits positrons, which are detected on a scanning device and translated into a color-coded computer transverse image. The image indicates levels of cellular metabolism and/or blood flow. This biochemical and physiologic data distinguishes PET testing from computed tomography and magnetic resonance imaging tests.

Metabolism in the heart and brain as well as other tissues is one very important focus of PET testing, especially to identify areas of ischemia, infarct, staging of disease, or other pathology. The effectiveness of pharmacologic agents, and chemotherapeutic agents in particular, can also be measured with PET tests by observing functional changes in targeted tissues and organs.

Abnormal Findings

➤ *Brain findings* may indicate epilepsy, cerebrovascular accident, migraine, Parkinson's disease, dementia, Alzheimer's disease, Huntington's disease, schizophrenia, or neoplasms.

> *Cardiac findings* may indicate acute myocardial infarction, size of infarct, or viability of myocardium.

> *Pulmonary findings* may indicate chronic pulmonary edema or pneumonia.

> *Breast tissue findings* may indicate tumors.

Interfering Factors

> Client anxiety may result in inaccurate results when studying the brain. The client needs to cooperate with the personnel completing the procedure.

> Sedatives may prevent the client from cooperating with instructions from the personnel completing the procedure. During cerebral evaluation the client is typically asked to perform intellectual and mental tasks to see how cerebral cellular metabolism changes.

> Caffeine, tobacco, and alcohol consumption prior to the test may interfere with the results.

> Tranquilizers interfere with glucose metabolism.

NURSING CONSIDERATIONS

Prepare Your Client

> Explain to client that this test is used to look specifically at blood flow as well as how tissues and organs within the body are functioning.

> Ensure that an informed consent is obtained if required by your institution.

> Assure your client that the level of radiation exposure is very low—about one-fourth the amount received during a computed tomography (CT) scan.

> Restrict alcohol, tobacco, sedatives, tranquilizers, and caffeine for 24 hours before a cerebral PET.

> Medications altering glucose metabolism should not be given for 3–4 hours before the test. Diabetics should have long-acting insulin, with the test scheduled during the midpoint to later stage of insulin action.

> Instruct your client to urinate before going to the scan.

Perform Procedure

Nurses do not perform this procedure, but should understand the process to prepare the client and assist in the procedure. The procedure is performed in the radiology department by three to five specially trained personnel.

Instruct client to lie still during the 45–90 minutes of scanning. Provide earplugs and blindfolds to decrease external environmental stimuli during the brain PET. Instruct them not to count or sleep during the examination, but rather to recite well-known sayings or perform thinking tasks as part of the diagnostic test, to demonstrate how brain activity changes during specific mental activities. Either the client will breathe a radioactive agent into the lungs, or it will be injected through a needle into a vein. When the medication combines with particles (electrons) in the heart or brain, rays are emitted. A (positron) scanner takes cross-sectional measurements of the rays and translates the concentration of rays into colored images.

Depending upon institutional procedures, establish one or two intravenous access sites: one for injection of the radionuclide medication, and one for taking blood samples. This test takes from 1–2 hours to complete.

Care After Test

> Instruct your client to drink fluids to flush the radioactive substance out of the body.

> Instruct client to change positions slowly and ask for assistance for the first few hours after the test due to potential for postural hypotension.

> Refer the client and family to community resources and agencies for rehabilitation support following stroke or myocardial infarction.

> Evaluate related tests such as SPECT (single-photon emission computed tomography) and brain scan.

Educate Your Client and the Family

> Instruct family and client on safety precautions for people with epilepsy, if applicable.

> Emphasize the need to wear medical alert identification.

> Instruct family on methods to communicate with aphasic or disoriented client. Talking louder does not correct the problem and may increase anxiety in client.

Postcoital Test

poest koy tahl • test

(Sims-Huhner Test, Postcoital Cervical Mucus Test, Cervical Mucus Sperm Penetration Test)

Normal Findings

6–20 active sperm per high-power field

Cervical mucus adequate for sperm transmission, survival, and penetration

What This Test Will Tell You

This fertility test measures the ability of sperm to penetrate cervical mucus and maintain motility. It evaluates the quality of the cervical mucus and the effect of vaginal and cervical secretions on sperm activity. This test is usually ordered after normal results from a semen analysis. It is performed during the middle of the ovulatory cycle, when cervical mucus is maximal and the viscosity is thin, which should be optimal for sperm penetration and survival. This test may also be used to document rape by testing the vaginal and cervical secretions for sperm.

Abnormal Findings

The test may reveal pH imbalances in the cervical mucus, absent sperm, or poorly mobile sperm, all of which may contribute to infertility.

Interfering Factors

> Specimens obtained more than 6 hours after intercourse are unreliable.

NURSING CONSIDERATIONS

Prepare Your Client

> Explain that this test is to see if the sperm can make it through the birth canal and into the womb and tubes where conception normally takes place.

> Inform the client that the test is performed by a primary health care provider in about 5 minutes.

> Explain that a vaginal speculum will be inserted and it will be the only discomfort.

> Schedule the test for mid-ovulation and instruct the client in determining ovulation.

> Instruct the client that no douching, vaginal lubrication, or bathing is permitted until after the test because these will alter the cervical mucus.

> Instruct the client to remain recumbent for 15–30 minutes after intercourse to ensure cervical exposure to semen. The client should then see her primary health care provider within 2 hours.

Perform Procedure

Nurses do not usually perform this procedure, but should understand the process to prepare the client and assist the primary health care provider. The client is placed in a lithotomy position. An unlubricated speculum is used. The specimen is aspirated by the primary health care provider and sent to the laboratory immediately. A fresh specimen is placed on a glass slide and examined.

Care After Test

> Ensure client receives referrals for fertility evaluation and counseling as indicated.

> Review related tests including semen analysis and sperm antibody assay.

Educate Your Client and the Family

> Teach client that normally the sperm has to pass through a body fluid (mucus) between the birth canal (vagina) and the womb (uterus). If sperm are not strong and active or if the woman's secretions are too acid, sperm may never reach the egg for conception (fertilization).

> Assess client's knowledge of the reproductive cycle and optimal times for fertilization.

Potassium, Serum and Urine

poe tass ee um • see rum • and • yur in
(Serum K+, Urine K+)

Normal Findings

ADULT, ADOLESCENT, AND ELDERLY
Serum: 3.5–5.1 mEq/L (SI units: 3.5–5.1 mmol/L)
Urine: 25–125 mEq/24 hours (SI units: 25–125 mmol/L) Level varies with diet.

PREGNANT
Serum: During pregnancy a fall of 0.2–0.3 mEq may occur due to increased blood volume.
Urine: 25–125 mEq/24 hours (SI units: 25–125 mmol/24 hours) Level varies with diet.

NEWBORN
Serum: 3.7–5.9 mEq/L (SI units: 3.7–5.9 mmol/L)
Urine: 17–55 mEq/24 hours (SI units: 17–55 mmol/24 hours)

CHILD
Serum: 3.4–4.7 mEq/L (SI units: 3.4–4.7 mmol/L)
Urine:
6–10-year-old male: 17–54 mEq/24 hours (SI units: 17–54 mmol/24 hours)
6–10-year-old female: 8–37 mEq/24 hours (SI units: 8–37 mmol/24 hours)
Level varies with diet.

Critical values for infants are serum levels < 2.5 or > 6.0 mEq/L, and for adults < 2.5 or > 6.5 mEq/L. Monitor carefully for dysrhythmias, rapid and irregular pulse, mental confusion, hypotension, and anorexia. Severe or rapid increases or decreases in serum potassium can result in ventricular fibrillation and respiratory paralysis. Rapid infusion of intravenous potassium can result in cardiac dysrhythmias and death.

What This Test Will Tell You

These serum and urine tests evaluate fluid and electrolyte balances and identify renal dysfunction. Approximately 98% of the body's potassium is inside the cells and 2% is in the extracellular fluid. Potassium is critical to neuromuscular function, specifically skeletal and cardiac muscle activity. Potassium, along with sodium and chloride, also regulates osmotic pressure and acid-base balance. Potassium is continuously moving in and out of the cells via the sodium-potassium pump.

Potassium is absorbed into the bloodstream from the small intestine. The kidneys play a critical role in potassium balance, and about 80% of the potassium leaving the body is excreted in urine, whereas 20% is excreted through the bowel and skin. The kidneys do not conserve potassium, so there must be an adequate potassium intake each day. Potassium levels are influenced by aldosterone, serum sodium levels, serum glucose levels, and serum pH. The average daily requirements for potassium are about 40–60 mEq per day, and the average daily intake is between 80 and 200 mEq/day.

The normal level of potassium has tight parameters that are essential to maintain normal osmotic pressure and cardiac and neuromuscular electrical conduction. A potassium deficiency can also lead to a reduction in protein synthesis.

Abnormal Findings

▲ INCREASED SERUM LEVELS may indicate acute and chronic renal failure, spironolactone or triamterene therapy, diabetic ketoacidosis, infection, severe burns, crush injury, Addison's disease, hypoaldosteronism, increased potassium intake, or transfusion of hemolyzed blood.

▼ DECREASED SERUM LEVELS may indicate diarrhea, vomiting, potassium-wasting diuretic therapy, steroids, Cushing's syndrome, renal tubular acidosis, decreased potassium intake, alkalosis, hyperaldosteronism, insulin and glucose administration, calcium administration, or ingestion of licorice.

▲ INCREASED URINE LEVELS may indicate primary renal disease, metabolic acidosis, alkalosis, dehydration, starvation, excessive potassium intake, loop or thiazide diuretic therapy, Cushing's syndrome, salicylate toxicity, primary and secondary aldosteronism, or treatment with adrenocorticotropic hormone (ACTH) or hydrocortisone.

▼ DECREASED URINE LEVELS may indicate Addison's disease, acute renal failure, severe glomerulonephritis, pyelonephritis, nephrosclerosis, dehydration, starvation, diarrhea, malabsorption disorders, or syndrome of inappropriate antidiuretic hormone secretion (SIADH).

Interfering Factors

SERUM
➤ Hemolysis will elevate levels.
➤ Exercise of forearm with tourniquet in place will elevate levels.
➤ Aminocaproic acid, mannitol, potassium supplements, isoniazid,

heparin, antineoplastic drugs, lithium, captopril, succinylcholine, epinephrine, antibiotics, potassium-wasting diuretics, and histamine will elevate serum potassium levels.

➤ Medications that decrease serum potassium levels include acetazolamide, aminosalicylic acid, amphotericin B, carbenicillin, cisplatin, potassium-sparing diuretics, glucose infusions, insulin, laxatives, lithium carbonate, high doses of penicillin G, phenothiazines, salicylates, and ion-exchange resins.

➤ White blood count over 70,000 per cubic millimeter.

➤ Platelet count over 1 million per cubic millimeter.

URINE

➤ Incomplete collection of urine specimen affects results.

➤ Medications that can increase urine potassium levels include amphotericin, corticosteroids, corticotropin, desoxycorticosterone, calcitonin, carbenicillin, carbenoxolone, glycyrrhiza, mafenide, penicillin, streptozocin, sulfates, ticarcillin, and potassium-wasting diuretics such as ethacrynic acid, furosemide, and thiazides.

➤ Medications that can decrease urine potassium levels include amiloride, general anesthetic agents, diazoxide, epinephrine, growth hormone, and norepinephrine.

➤ Diet affects potassium level.

➤ Ingestion of licorice may increase urine levels of potassium.

➤ Excessive vomiting or diarrhea affects results.

NURSING CONSIDERATIONS

Prepare Your Client

➤ Explain that the test is helpful in identifying chemical imbalances, specifically potassium.

Perform Procedure

SERUM

➤ Collect 5–10 mL of venous blood in a red-top or green-top tube.

➤ Collect blood from the arm opposite an intravenous infusion of electrolyte solution.

➤ Do not allow the client to pump the arm with a tourniquet in place.

URINE

➤ Use a clean 3-L container and no preservative.

➤ Carefully collect a 24-hour urine sample.

➤ Keep the collection container on ice or refrigerated during the collection period.

Care After Test

➤ Monitor for signs and symptoms of hypokalemia including weakness, paralysis, hyporeflexia, ileus, dizziness, thirst, increased sensitivity to digoxin, and cardiac dysrhythmias.

➤ Monitor for signs and symptoms of hyperkalemia including weakness, paralysis, irritability, nausea and vomiting, intestinal colic, and diarrhea.

➤ Monitor intake and output. Report urine output less than 30 mL/hour for adults or 1 mL/kg of body weight per hour in infants and children.

➤ Assess mental status and neurological status and provide safety and seizure precautions as indicated.

➤ Initiate continuous electrocardiogram monitoring for suspected or confirmed potassium imbalances. Monitor for dysrhythmias and check client's pulse for irregularities.

➤ Assess latest serum potassium prior to administering potassium supplements.

➤ Monitor vital signs every 4 hours and note changes in blood pressure and pulse.

➤ Review related tests including urine sodium, serum and urine osmolality, serum sodium, arterial blood gases, blood urea nitrogen, creatinine, and electrocardiogram.

Educate Your Client and the Family

➤ Teach client and family that potassium is found in most foods. Cereals, dried peas and beans, fresh vegetables, fresh or dried fruits, bananas, orange or prune juice, nuts, molasses, fresh fish, and poultry are excellent sources. Clients with hypokalemia should include these foods in their diets, and clients with hyperkalemia should limit their intake.

➤ Teach client to avoid laxative or diuretic abuse.

➤ Teach client and family the importance of taking medications as ordered and avoiding the use of salt substitutes unless approved by their health care provider.

➤ Explain to a client with renal insufficiency the importance of avoiding potassium-sparing diuretics, potassium supplements, or salt substitutes.

➤ Explain to a client taking digoxin the importance of maintaining daily potassium intake (dietary or supplement).

Pregnanediol, Urine
preg nane die ol • yur in

Normal Findings
MALE
0–1 mg/24 hours
FEMALE
Premenopausal, nonpregnant:
Proliferative phase: 0.5–1.5 mg/24 hours
Luteal phase: 2–7 mg/24 hours
Pregnant: 6–100 mg/24 hours (values vary according to weeks of pregnancy). Peak levels occur at 36th week of gestation. Normal levels return 1–2 weeks postpartum.
Postmenopausal: 0.2–1.0 mg/24 hours

What This Test Will Tell You
This 24-hour urine test evaluates ovarian function, infertility, and placental function. Pregnanediol, a metabolite of progesterone, is present in the urine in varying quantities throughout the menstrual cycle and pregnancy. Because progesterone prepares the endometrium for implantation, the levels increase rapidly after ovulation, making it useful to determine when and if ovulation occurs. Pregnanediol increases during pregnancy because the placenta produces large amounts of progesterone to preserve the pregnancy. Repeated tests can be done to monitor placental function.

Abnormal Findings
▲ INCREASED LEVELS may indicate ovulation, pregnancy, luteal cysts of ovary, metastatic cancer of the ovaries, luteinized granulosa, theca cell tumors, arrhenoblastoma of ovary, hyperadrenocorticism,

choriocarcinoma of ovary, or adrenocortical hyperplasia.

▼DECREASED LEVELS may indicate amenorrhea, threatened abortion, fetal death, pregnancy-induced hypertension (PIH), ovarian hypofunction, placental failure, breast neoplasms, or ovarian neoplasms.

Interfering Factors

➤ Oral contraceptives and progesterones decrease pregnanediol levels.

➤ Adrenocorticotropic hormones (ACTH) may increase levels.

➤ Failure to collect or refrigerate all urine during the collection period interferes with accurate results.

➤ Biliary tract obstruction and adrenal hyperplasia may increase levels.

➤ Some liver diseases may decrease levels.

➤ Contamination with stool or toilet paper may interfere with results.

NURSING CONSIDERATIONS

Prepare Your Client

➤ Explain as appropriate that the test will tell when and if she ovulates (releases an egg to prepare for pregnancy), or will give information about the placenta (the part of the womb that provides oxygen and nutrition to the baby).

➤ Explain that this is a 24-hour urine collection test.

Perform Procedure

➤ Carefully follow procedure for 24-hour urine collection. Determine if your laboratory requires the use of a preservative in the urine collection container.

➤ Record on the laboratory slip the date of the last menstrual period or the number of weeks of gestation if pregnant.

Care After Test

➤ Assess the client's knowledge of prenatal care including diet, activity, rest, signs and symptoms of labor, and danger signs in pregnancy. Provide instruction as indicated.

➤ Assess mother's readiness to meet parental role functions by reviewing infant care knowledge, methods of infant feeding, and ability to obtain needed supplies. Provide instruction and/or community health service referrals as indicated.

➤ Assess the client's ability to provide adequate nutrition for the fetus. Refer to social services and Women, Infants, and Children program (WIC) for assistance.

➤ If the test is performed to evaluate infertility, provide emotional support and information regarding need to plan coitus/insemination after ovulation.

➤ Review related tests such as contraction stress test, nonstress test, progesterone assay, and obstetrical ultrasound.

Educate Your Client and the Family

➤ Instruct the client about danger signs in pregnancy such as a gush of fluid, vaginal bleeding, abdominal pain, temperature elevation, dizziness, blurred vision, persistent vomiting, severe headache, edema, muscular irritability, difficult urination, or decreased/absent fetal movements.

➤ Tell client to notify their primary health care provider if they have less than three movements in 1 hour. A nonstress test or biophysical profile may be ordered.

➤ Teach the client the signs of preterm labor such as abdominal cramping with or without diarrhea, uterine contractions every 10 minutes or more frequently, menstrual-like cramps in the lower abdomen, low backache, increase or change in vaginal discharge, or pelvic pressure.

Progesterone Assay

proe jes teh rone • a say

(Progesterone Receptor Assay, Progesterone)

Normal Findings

PREOVULATION

<150 ng/dL

MIDCYCLE

300–2400 ng/dL—values rise 16–24 hours before ovulation.

PREGNANCY

>2400 ng/dL

What This Test Will Tell You

This blood test confirms ovulation, evaluates functioning of the placenta during pregnancy, and may be part of an infertility assessment. Progesterone, a hormone secreted by the corpus luteum, prepares the endometrium for implantation of a fertilized ovum. Progesterone production is low during the first phase (follicular) of the menstrual cycle. Progesterone levels rise during the middle of the menstrual cycle in response to luteinizing hormone (LH) and continue to rise for 6–10 days. Blood samples obtained between days 8 and 21 of the menstrual cycle should show an increase in progesterone. This test may also be used to evaluate placental function during pregnancy.

Abnormal Findings

▲ INCREASED LEVELS may indicate pregnancy, ovulation, ovarian cysts, adrenal neoplasms, ovarian neoplasms, hydratidiform mole, or congenital adrenal hyperplasia.

▼ DECREASED LEVELS may indicate amenorrhea, threatened abortion, fetal death, or pregnancy-induced hypertension (PIH).

Interfering Factors

➤ Estrogen, progesterone, and adrenocorticoids may interfere with results.

➤ Hemolysis from rough handling of sample can affect results.

➤ Recent use of radioisotopes may affect results.

NURSING CONSIDERATIONS

Prepare Your Client

➤ Explain that this test measures a hormone level and may be done at specific times of her menstrual cycle.

Perform Procedure

➤ Collect 5–7 mL of venous blood in a red-top tube.

➤ Write the date of the last menstrual period, or month of gestation if pregnant, on the laboratory slip.

Care After Test

➤ Recognize that the client may have considerable anxiety about the outcome and implications of this test. Concerns will vary and include those of the pregnant client who is anxious about her baby and the client unsure of her ability to conceive.

➤ In client with high-risk pregnancy, assess fetal well-being by evaluating heart tones and daily fetal movement counts as well as diagnostic or laboratory tests.

➤ In client with suspected PIH, evaluate vital signs carefully. Assess for systemic hypertension, headache, proteinuria, and other signs and symptoms.

➤ Collaborate with primary health care provider and refer client with confirmed infertility to community support groups, adoption agencies, foster care, and fertility specialists as indicated.

➤ Review related tests such as urine estrogen, follicle-stimulating hormone, serum luteinizing hormone, serum estrogen, serum testosterone, and serum estriol.

Educate Your Client and the Family

➤ Instruct the client about normal signs of labor such as a gush of fluid, bloody show, and contractions that increase in frequency, intensity, and duration.

➤ Instruct the client about danger signs in pregnancy such as a gush of fluid, vaginal bleeding, abdominal pain, temperature elevation, dizziness, blurred vision, persistent vomiting, severe headache, edema, muscular irritability, difficult urination, or decreased/absent fetal movements.

➤ Tell client to notify their primary health care provider if they have less than 3 movements in 1 hour. A nonstress test or biophysical profile may be ordered.

➤ Teach the client the signs of preterm labor such as abdominal cramping with or without diarrhea, uterine contractions every 10 minutes or more frequently, menstrual-like cramps in the lower abdomen, low backache, increase or change in vaginal discharge, or pelvic pressure.

➤ Advise the client to lie down on her side and notify the primary health care provider if preterm labor is suspected.

Prolactin, Serum
proe lak tin • see rum
(Lactogenic Hormone, Lactogen, HPRL, Human Prolactin, Luteotropic Hormone, LTH, Mammotropin)

Normal Findings
PREGNANT
<400 ng/mL by third trimester (SI units: <400 µg/L)
NONPREGNANT ADULT AND ADOLESCENT FEMALE
5–40 ng/mL (SI units: 5–40 µg/L)
ADULT MALE AND CHILD
<20 ng/mL (SI units: <20 µg/L)
NEWBORN
>10 times adult levels

What This Test Will Tell You
This blood test assists in the diagnosis of pituitary or hypothalamic dysfunction and the evaluation of secondary amenorrhea and galactorrhea and of their treatment. Prolactin, a hormone produced by the anterior pituitary gland, promotes breast tissue growth and is necessary for the initiation and maintenance of milk production. Prolactin levels increase in pregnancy

and in lactating women. Pituitary tumors can secrete excessive amounts of prolactin. Prolactin levels are used to monitor hypothalamic disease and to monitor treatment regimes of prolactin-secreting tumors.

Abnormal Findings

▲ INCREASED LEVELS may indicate galactorrhea, amenorrhea, hypothalamus disease, prolactin-secreting pituitary tumors, acromegaly, hypothyroidism, renal failure, anorexia nervosa, bronchogenic carcinoma, Chiari-Frommel syndrome, Forbes-Albright syndrome, or Addison's disease.

▼ DECREASED LEVELS may indicate pituitary necrosis or infarction, osteoporosis, hirsutism, or gynecomastia.

Interfering Factors

➤ Radioactive scan performed within 1 week before the test may interfere with test results.
➤ Recent surgery may affect test results.
➤ Pregnancy, postpartum, lactation, nipple stimulation, exercise, sleep, stress, and exercise may increase values.
➤ Medications that can increase levels include estrogens, methyldopa, tricyclic antidepressants, phenothiazines, antihypertensives, amphetamines, morphine, haloperidol, reserpine, procainamide, metaclopramide, and ethanol.
➤ Medications that can decrease levels include apomorphine, ergot alkaloids, and levodopa.

NURSING CONSIDERATIONS

Prepare Your Client

➤ Explain that the test measures the levels of a hormone called prolactin. It is used to diagnose problems with certain glands in the body (the pituitary and hypothalamus), especially when menstrual periods stop.
➤ Restrict food and fluids for 12 hours prior to the test.
➤ Withhold drugs that may influence levels. If they must be taken, note them on the laboratory slip.

Perform Procedure

➤ Collect 5–7 mL venous blood in a red-top tube.
➤ Collect the sample at least 2 hours after the client wakes to avoid a sleep-induced increase.

Care After Test

➤ Assess for signs and symptoms of pituitary tumors including changes in neurological function, galactorrhea, and amenorrhea.
➤ Review related tests including thyroid hormone tests, estrogen and progesterone levels, and sella turcica x-rays.

Educate Your Client and the Family

➤ Teach client and family that this hormone usually rises during pregnancy and is important in preparing the body to breast-feed.
➤ If appropriate, inform client and family that this hormone can be produced in some diseases and from certain tumors. Blood levels may be followed frequently to assess how well treatment is working.

Prostate Gland Biopsy
pross tate · gland · bie op see

Normal Findings
Absence of abnormal prostate gland cells

What This Test Will Tell You
This microscopic examination of prostate tissue excised with a needle is performed when a client has prostate nodules or possible malignant prostatic hypertrophy. The procedure can confirm prostate cancer, prostatitis, benign prostatic hypertrophy, lymphomas, and rectal or bladder carcinoma.

Prostate gland biopsy may be performed transrectally (for high prostatic lesions), transurethrally, or by a perineal approach.

Abnormal Findings
Abnormal cells may indicate benign prostatic hypertrophy, prostatic cancer, prostatic nodules, prostatitis, bladder cancer, rectal cancer, or lymphoma.

 ACTION ALERT!

Report gross amounts of blood and clots in the urine to the primary health care provider. Monitor the blood pressure and pulse for signs of hemorrhage.

Interfering Factors
➤ Inadequate tissue specimen collection
➤ Failure to place the specimen in formaldehyde

Contraindications
➤ Client with coagulation defects

Potential Complications
➤ Hematuria
➤ Bleeding into the urethra and bladder

➤ Infection

NURSING CONSIDERATIONS P

Prepare Your Client
➤ Explain that this test is to study a tiny sample of tissue from a gland called the prostate to look for any possible problems.
➤ For the transrectal approach, explain that a local anesthetic is given and a needle is used to obtain the specimen. For the transurethral approach, an endoscope is used to obtain a specimen.
➤ Assess the client for any allergies to sedatives, anesthetics, and betadine or iodine.
➤ Ensure that an informed consent is obtained, because of the possible complications associated with this procedure.
➤ Obtain any blood work ordered such as partial thromboplastin and prothrombin time for blood clotting and type, and crossmatch if ordered.
➤ Restrict food and fluids for 8 hours prior to the procedure.
➤ Administer enema until clear for client having a transrectal biopsy. Instruct the client on how to do this if biopsy is performed as an outpatient procedure.
➤ Administer antibiotics and sedatives if ordered. Antibiotics are commonly ordered for a transrectal biopsy approach to minimize the complication of infection.
➤ Record baseline vital signs before the procedure begins.

Perform Procedure
Nurses do not perform this proce-

dure, but should understand the process to prepare the client and assist the physician.

PERINEAL APPROACH

Place the client in left lateral, lithotomy, or knee-chest position. Cleanse the perineum with the ordered solution such as betadine. A local anesthetic is administered. A 2-mm incision is made into the perineum and a finger inserted into the rectum to immobilize the prostate. The biopsy needle is inserted into the prostate and rotated, pulled back 5 mm, and reinserted at another angle several times to collect tissue samples. Place specimens in a labeled specimen bottle containing a 10% formaldehyde solution. Apply pressure to the biopsy site and then apply a dressing.

TRANSRECTAL APPROACH

Place the client in left lateral position. This test may be performed without an anesthetic. A needle guide is attached to the finger that will palpate the rectum. The biopsy needle is pushed next to the guide and into the prostate. The needle is rotated to excise the tissue and withdraw the specimen. The specimen is placed in 10% formaldehyde solution in a labeled specimen container.

TRANSURETHRAL APPROACH

An endoscope is inserted through the urethra to view the prostate. A cutting loop is inserted to obtain a specimen. The specimen is placed in 10% formaldehyde solution in a labeled specimen container.

Care After Test

➤ Assess vital signs and check for bleeding every 15 minutes for 1 hour, then every 30 minutes for 1 hour, then every 4 hours.

➤ Assess the biopsy site or route for hematoma and signs of infection such as edema, redness, pain, and warmth.

➤ Check voiding, assess for hematuria, frequency, and for urine retention related to difficulty voiding or clots obstructing urine flow.

➤ Review related tests such as the prostate-specific antigen level, bone scans, cystoscopy, and serum acid phosphatase level.

Educate Your Client and the Family

➤ Instruct the outpatient client to report any elevated temperature, chills, weakness, dizziness, or bleeding to the primary health care provider.

➤ Instruct the outpatient client to apply pressure to the site for 10 minutes. Notify the physician if bleeding occurs.

➤ Instruct the client to report any problems with urinating such as frequency, having an urge to urinate but not being able to (retention), or blood in the urine.

➤ Tell the client that it may take 5 days to obtain biopsy results.

➤ Teach the client how to perform a self-examination of the testicles.

Prostate-Specific Antigen

pross tate • speh sih fik • an ti jen
(PSA)

Normal Findings

ADULT AND ELDERLY
Males < 40 years: 0–2.7 ng/mL
Males > 40 years: 0–4.0 ng/mL
ADOLESCENT
Adult levels are reached at approximately 15 years old.

What This Test Will Tell You

This blood test helps diagnose prostate cancer and monitors the progression and response to surgical, radiation, and/or hormonal therapy. It is used as an early indicator of recurrence of prostate cancer. This test measures the glycoprotein prostate-specific antigen (PSA), normally found in the cytoplasm of prostatic epithelial cells. The level is greatly increased in men who have prostatic cancer. PSA test is often used in conjunction with alkaline phosphates and prostatic acid phosphate. However, the PSA is superior in predicting disease recurrence.

Abnormal Findings

▲ INCREASED LEVELS may indicate prostate carcinoma, benign prostatic hypertrophy, or prostatitis.
▼ DECREASED LEVELS are normal, or may indicate positive response to therapy.

Interfering Factors

➤ Increases occur in men with no prostatic malignancies and benign disease.
➤ Transient increase occurs following prostate palpation/massage, cystoscopy, needle biopsy, or transurethral resection (TUR) of the prostate.

NURSING CONSIDERATIONS

Prepare Your Client

➤ Explain that this test is widely used to diagnose cancer of the prostate gland as well as to see how well treatment is working.
➤ Ask client if they have had recent digital rectal examination with palpation or massage of prostate, cystoscopy, needle biopsy, or transurethral resection. If so, test needs to be delayed 2 weeks.

Perform Procedure

➤ Collect 5 mL of venous blood in a red-top tube.
➤ Label the laboratory slip with the age of client.

Care After Test

➤ Assess for signs and symptoms of metastatic cancer including bone pain, fatigue, and recurring symptoms of the tumor.
➤ Refer client and family to a cancer support group.
➤ Refer to social services to assist with the financial and economic impact of cancer.
➤ Consult with a registered dietician for client with anorexia, weight loss, or special dietary needs.
➤ Assess carefully for chronic and acute pain. Obtain pain management consultation if indicated.
➤ Assess for signs and symptoms of infection such as chills, fever, and drop in the absolute neutrophil count. Institute precautions to protect the client, such as no fresh fruits or vegetables. Remove fresh flowers and plants, and enforce good handwashing.

➤ Assess oral mucous membranes for signs and symptoms of stomatitis. Routinely give oral hygiene care.

➤ Assess the client for signs and symptoms such as bleeding from injection sites, petechia, or ecchymosis, occult blood, and decreasing platelet count related to increased risk for bleeding.

➤ Clients with impaired bone marrow function may have prolonged bleeding times. Institute safety measures such as electric razors, nonskid shoes, no intramuscular injections, no rectal temperatures, and soft toothbrushes.

➤ Encourage verbalization of fears related to cancer, prognosis, treatment, and death.

➤ Review results of other test such as alkaline phosphatase, prostatic acid phosphatase, needle biopsy, computed tomography, radionuclide imaging, and transrectal ultrasound, which when done in parallel with PSA greatly increase the sensitivity of detection of early stages of prostatic cancer.

Educate Your Client and the Family

➤ Tell the client and family that PSA testing is not used as a mass unselected screening test due to the high rate of false negative and false positive results.

➤ Explain that if the level is elevated, further workup such as digital rectal exam and transrectal ultrasound may be done.

➤ Tell a client being tested for follow-up and/or response to therapy that a low level of PSA (less than 10 ng/mL) 6 months after treatment is a sign of a positive response to treatment.

➤ Inform the client that PSA testing has not proven to be useful for staging of prostate cancer.

➤ Tell the client that PSA values drawn 3–6 months after a radical prostatectomy are a sensitive indicator of persistent disease. The antigen will not be detected if the tumor is completely removed, so serum levels of PSA should be negative.

➤ Teach the client that PSA testing may detect evidence of recurrence before other tests such as alkaline phosphatase, prostatic acid phosphatase, and digital rectal examination are positive.

➤ Reinforce with the client that PSA test may be repeated because trends are more useful than one reading.

Protein, Blood

proe teen • blud

(Albumin, Blood; Serum Albumin; Serum Protein; Total Protein; Globulins; Alpha$_1$ Globulins; Alpha$_2$ Globulins; Beta Globulins; Gamma Globulins; Serum Protein Electrophoresis)

Normal Findings

ADULT, ADOLESCENT, AND ELDERLY
Total protein

Ambulatory: 6.0–8.0 g/dL
Recumbent: 6.0–7.8 g/dL
Albumin
3.2–5.0 g/dL

Globulins
2.3–3.4 g/dL
  alpha$_1$: 0.1–0.4 g/dL
  alpha$_2$: 0.5–1.0 g/dL
  beta: 0.7–1.2 g/dL
  gamma: 0.5–1.6 g/dL
PREGNANT
Values are the same as adult values but will decrease slightly during the third trimester.
NEWBORN
Total protein
Premature infant: 4.2–7.6 g/dL
Newborn: 4.6–7.4 g/dL
1 week: 4.4–7.6 g/dL
7 months to 1 year: 5.1–7.3 g/dL
Albumin
Premature infant: 3.0–4.2 g/dL
Newborn: 3.5–5.4 g/dL
Infant: 4.4–5.4 g/dL
Globulins
  alpha$_1$: 0.1–0.3 g/dL
  alpha$_2$: 0.3–0.5 g/dL
  beta: 0.2–0.6 g/dL
  gamma: 0.2–1.2 g/dL
CHILD
Total protein
1–2 years old: 5.6–7.5 g/dL
>3 years old: 6.0–8.0 g/dL
Albumin
4.0–5.9 g/dL
Globulins
  alpha$_1$: 0.1–0.4 g/dL
  alpha$_2$: 0.4–1.0 g/dL
  beta: 0.5–1.0 g/dL
  gamma: 0.3–1.0 g/dL
Albumin/globulin ratio: ≥1.0

What This Test Will Tell You

This blood test helps diagnose hepatic, gastrointestinal, and renal disease; protein abnormalities; cancer; and blood dyscrasias. This test measures serum albumin and globulins, which are the body's major blood proteins. Albumin is formed in the liver and comprises 50%–60% of the total serum protein. Its primary function is to maintain serum colloid osmotic pressure. The globulin molecules are much larger than the albumin molecules. Both albumin and globulin are used as measures of nutrition because malnourished clients have severely decreased serum protein levels. The alpha$_1$, alpha$_2$ and beta globulins produce antibodies, are preservers of chromosomes, and along with globulins, transport blood components such as bilirubin, calcium, lipids, metals, oxygen, steroids, thyroid hormones, and vitamins. The gamma globulins are an important part of the body's immune system.

The albumin to globulin ratio is useful when the total protein remains within normal limits but albumin has leaked out of vessels into tissues. Globulins have a weaker osmotic pull.

Abnormal Findings

▲ INCREASED LEVELS *of protein* may indicate dehydration, diabetic acidosis, chronic infections, chronic inflammatory diseases, wound drainage, multiple myeloma, renal disease, or sarcoidosis.

▲ INCREASED LEVELS *of albumin* may indicate dehydration.

▲ INCREASED LEVELS *of alpha$_1$ globulins* may indicate acute infections, malignancies, pregnancy, or tissue necrosis.

▲ INCREASED LEVELS *of alpha$_2$ globulins* may indicate acute infections, acute myocardial infarction, nephrotic syndrome, chronic inflammatory disease, malignancy, trauma, or burns.

▲ INCREASED LEVELS *of beta globulins* may indicate biliary cirrhosis, nephrotic syndrome, hypothyroidism, diabetes mellitus, or malignant hypertension.

▲ INCREASED LEVELS of gamma globulins may indicate chronic liver disease, chronic infections, autoimmune diseases, rheumatoid arthritis, or systemic lupus erythematosus.

▼ DECREASED LEVELS of protein may indicate malabsorption syndromes, Crohn's disease, sprue, Whipple's disease, nephrotic syndrome, glomerulonephritis, ascites, malnutrition, hypervolemia, capillary membrane leak, malnutrition, hyperthyroidism, uncontrolled diabetes mellitus, hepatic dysfunction, surgical or traumatic shock, or toxemia during pregnancy.

▼ DECREASED LEVELS of albumin may indicate protein malnutrition, severe malabsorption, intestinal obstruction, diffuse liver disease, rheumatic fever, third space loss, advanced malignancies, congestive heart failure, chronic renal failure, severe burns, systemic lupus erythematosus, or inflammatory bowel disease.

▼ DECREASED LEVELS of alpha$_1$ globulins may indicate alpha$_1$ antitrypsin deficiency.

▼ DECREASED LEVELS of alpha$_2$ globulins may indicate hemolytic anemia or pancreatitis.

▼ DECREASED LEVELS of beta globulins may indicate hypocholesterolemia.

▼ DECREASED LEVELS of gamma globulins may indicate congenital hypogammaglobulinemia, agammaglobulinemia, nephrotic syndrome, or lymphocytic leukemia.

Interfering Factors

➤ Drugs that may increase protein levels include anabolic steroids, androgens, clofibrate, corticosteroids, dextran, epinephrine, growth hormone, heparin sodium, heparin calcium, insulin, phenazopyridine, progesterone, and thyroid hormones.

➤ Drugs that can decrease protein levels include ammonium ions, estrogens, cytotoxic agents, hepatotoxic drugs, oral contraceptives, and allopurinol.

➤ A high-fat diet before the test may alter the test results.

➤ Hemolyzed specimens may alter the test results.

➤ Falsely elevated total protein levels will be present for up to 48 hours after the use of sulfobromophthalein contrast material.

➤ Dialysis will alter the protein values.

➤ Prolonged application of a tourniquet above the venipuncture site will increase the protein in the blood sample.

➤ A specimen obtained above an intravenous (IV) infusion site may show a low value as the result of local hemodilution.

➤ Upright posture for several hours after rising increases protein concentration significantly over levels found early in the day.

➤ Bed rest for prolonged periods causes a decreased serum total protein.

➤ IV infusion rates sufficient to cause hemodilution will lower the serum total protein level.

➤ Venous stasis due to occlusion caused by disease or peripheral vascular collapse can cause elevated levels.

➤ Hyperglycemia may cause falsely elevated levels.

NURSING CONSIDERATIONS

Prepare Your Client

➤ Explain that the test is important to help check nutritional status, liver and kidney function, water balance, and to diagnose some diseases.

➤ Instruct the client that foods high in fat content should be avoided for 24 hours before the test.

Perform Procedure

➤ Collect 5–7 mL of venous blood in a red-top tube.

➤ Note client's activity level before the sampling on the laboratory slip.

Care After Test

➤ Observe for signs and symptoms of abnormalities in blood protein such as recurring infections, peripheral edema, hepatomegaly, brittle hair, decreased body weight, and dehydration.

➤ Consult with a registered dietician to assist the family and client in meeting special dietary needs.

➤ Evaluate other diagnostic tests such as the serum protein electrophoresis, urine protein, hematocrit, hemoglobin, red blood cell count, calcium, bilirubin, antibodies, plasma protein S, plasma protein C, and/or immunoelectrophoresis.

Educate Your Client and the Family

➤ If the test results indicate a protein deficiency, encourage the increased consumption of protein-rich foods such as meat products, eggs, cheese, and beans.

➤ If the test results are increased and indicate dehydration, encourage the client to increase fluid consumption unless contraindicated by the medical diagnosis.

➤ Teach client and family to notify staff of edema, weight gain, and shortness of breath, all signs of fluid retention into tissue spaces.

Protein C, Plasma

proc teen · see · plaz mah

Normal Findings

Normal range is 50%–150% of the general population mean. Test is standardized by individual laboratories.

What This Test Will Tell You

This blood test evaluates and diagnoses specific clotting disorders, including venous thrombosis and purpura fulminans. Protein C, a vitamin-K–dependent protein produced in the liver, circulates in the plasma. This protein acts as an anticoagulant by suppressing the coagulation activity of activated Factor V and Factor VIII.

Abnormal Findings

▼ DECREASED LEVELS may indicate protein C deficiency, leading to thromboembolism or purpura fulminans.

Interfering Factors

➤ Anticoagulant therapy interferes with accurate results.

➤ Hemolysis of the sample affects results.

NURSING CONSIDERATIONS

Prepare Your Client

➤ Explain that this test is important to help understand why the blood may not be clotting normally in the body.

➤ Check current and recent medications, including aspirin use, that might affect clotting.

Perform Procedure

➤ Collect 3 mL of venous blood in a blue-top tube. Be careful to process specimen according to the laboratory's specifications. Specimen may require gentle mixing of the tube after sample is collected, or may need to be transported on ice.

➤ Label the sample and note any interfering factors, especially medications that can alter clotting activity.

Care After Test

➤ Observe the client closely for signs and symptoms of abnormal clotting including swelling, pain, and discoloration of extremities. Assess for a positive Homan's sign.

➤ Administer anticoagulants as ordered.

➤ Perform range-of-motion exercises and activity as ordered to prevent venostasis.

Educate Your Client and the Family

➤ Educate parents of neonates with a rare homozygous deficiency of protein C known as purpura fulminans. This condition results in death in the perinatal period from thrombosis. Support family as necessary, making them aware of grief counseling as well as genetic counseling as appropriate.

➤ Teach client diagnosed with the more commonly found heterozygous deficiency of protein C about susceptibility to venous thromboembolism continuing throughout life. This condition may require long-term anticoagulant therapy or protein C supplement from plasma fractions.

Protein Electrophoresis, Serum

proe teen • ee lek troe for ee sis • see rum
(Protein, Blood; Total Protein; Albumin, Blood; Serum Albumin; Globulins; Alpha$_1$ Globulin; Alpha$_2$ Globulin; Beta Globulins; Gamma Globulin)

Normal Findings

See data at top of next page.

PREGNANT

Alpha-1 globulin level may be slightly increased. Serum albumin falls rapidly during the first months of pregnancy. The level decreases more slowly in the last two trimesters. Normal levels return approximately 8 weeks following delivery. Alpha and beta globulins may be slightly increased while gamma globulins may be slightly decreased.

ELDERLY

Gamma globulins and albumin levels decrease with increasing age.

What This Test Will Tell You

This blood test helps diagnose hepatic disease, protein deficiency,

Normal Findings for Protein Electrophoresis

	Adult/Adolescent	Newborn	Child
Total protein	6–8.4 g/dL	4.6–7.4 g/dL	6.6–8.4 g/dL
Albumin	3.5–5.0 g/dL	3.5–5.4 g/dL	4.0–5.9 g/dL
52%–68%, all ages			
Globulin	1.5–3.5 g/dL		
alpha-1	0.1–0.4 g/dL	0.1–0.3 g/dL	0.1–0.4 g/dL
alpha-2	0.5–1.0 g/dL	0.3–0.5 g/dL	0.4–1.0 g/dL
beta	0.7–1.1 g/dL	0.2–0.6 g/dL	0.5–1.0 g/dL
gamma	0.5–1.6 g/dL	0.2–1.2 g/dL	0.3–1.0 g/dL

hematologic disorders, renal impairment, and gastrointestinal diseases. It measures serum albumin and globulins, which are the body's major blood proteins. These proteins are separated according to their size, shape, electric charge, and rate of movement.

Albumin comprises more than 50% of the total serum protein. It helps maintain serum colloid osmotic pressure and functions as a carrier protein for a variety of hormones and drugs. Insufficient albumin levels indicate altered colloid osmotic pressure, resulting in fluid seeping out of blood vessels into tissue spaces (edema).

The alpha-1, alpha-2, and beta globulins are necessary for transportation of lipids, hormones, and metals through the blood. The gamma globulins, known as antibodies, are an important part of the body's immune system.

Abnormal Findings

▲ INCREASED LEVELS of:

➤ *Total serum protein* may indicate dehydration, infection, diabetes mellitus, diabetic acidosis, chronic inflammatory diseases, multiple myeloma, or monocytic leukemia.

➤ *Albumin* may indicate multiple myeloma or dehydration.

➤ *Globulins* may indicate autoimmune disorders, diabetes mellitus, bacterial endocarditis, chronic syphilis, tuberculosis, multiple melanoma, Hodgkin's disease, chronic inflammatory disease, malignancy, acute inflammation, nephrotic syndrome, or lipoprotein disorders.

▼ DECREASED LEVELS of:

➤ *Total serum protein* may indicate malnutrition, malabsorption syndrome, Crohn's disease, nephrosis, glomerulonephritis, hypertension, diabetes mellitus, hyperthyroidism, toxemia, ascites, burns, increased capillary membrane leak, severe shock, or congestive heart failure.

➤ *Albumin* may indicate malnutrition, renal disease, collagen vascular diseases, autoimmune disorders, metastatic cancer, hyperthyroidism, hypertension, liver disease, acquired immune deficiency syndrome (AIDS), cholecystitis, or diarrhea.

➤ *Globulins* may indicate infection, chronic inflammatory disease, malnutrition, renal disease, liver disease, cancer, blood dyscrasias, or coagulopathies.

Interfering Factors

➤ Tests must be performed on serum samples. The use of plasma alters results.

➤ Acetylsalicylic acid, bicarbonate, corticosteroids, isoniazid, neomycin, phenucemude, sulfonamides, tolbutamide, chlorpromazine, and contrast material may alter results.

➤ Oral contraceptives increase alpha-1 levels and decrease albumin results.

➤ Hemolysis of the sample may alter results.

➤ Recent dialysis may alter protein values.

NURSING CONSIDERATIONS

Prepare Your Client

➤ Explain that this test is performed to check protein levels in the blood.

➤ Check with your laboratory to determine if a fasting blood sample is required.

Perform Procedure

➤ Collect 7–10 ml of venous blood in a red-top tube.

➤ Observe the venipuncture site closely for hematoma formation or bleeding. Coagulopathies are common in many conditions for which this test is performed. Apply a pressure dressing to the venipuncture site.

Care After Test

➤ Assess your client for ascites or peripheral edema, especially if albumin level is decreased. Position to facilitate venous return and to maximize diaphragmatic expansion.

➤ Assess urinary output. Altered protein levels are associated with renal disease and systemic diseases that can affect renal function.

➤ Consult with a registered dietician to design a high-calorie, well-balanced diet with particular attention to protein intake. As appropriate, reduce sodium in the diet if edema and ascites are present.

➤ Institute special skin care and breakdown precautions if indicated. Many of the conditions diagnosed by this test can result in impaired skin integrity.

➤ Assess the client's ability to perform activities of daily living. Refer to social services for home care support as indicated.

➤ Evaluate other related tests such as aspartate aminotransferase (AST), direct and indirect bilirubin levels, alkaline phosphatase, serum ammonia, serum albumin, serum aldosterone, electrolytes, blood urea nitrogen, serum creatinine, transferrin levels, and prothrombin time.

Educate Your Client and the Family

➤ Explain the importance of a well-balanced diet, including protein intake.

➤ Teach client and family to notify staff or primary care provider of edema, weight gain, and shortness of breath, which are signs of fluid retention into tissue spaces.

➤ Teach client and family dietary restrictions or recommendations as indicated.

➤ Teach family skin care for edematous tissues to prevent breakdown.

Prothrombin Consumption Time

proe **throm** bin • kun **sum** shun • **time**
(PCT)

Normal Findings

All ages: More than 80% consumed after 1 hour

What This Test Will Tell You

This blood test identifies clotting disorders related to deficiencies of platelets or clotting factors needed to form thromboplastin. When normal blood coagulates, prothrombin is changed quickly to thrombin by the interaction of plasma thromboplastin, which originates from platelets and Factors VIII, IX, XI, and XII. Only minuscule amounts of prothrombin remain in the serum after activation of the intrinsic coagulation pathway.

The prothrombin consumption time (PCT) measures the residual prothrombin in the serum of the sample. When there is a deficiency of any of the factors required to make thromboplastin, prothrombin is incompletely consumed and therefore present in the sample 1 hour after clotting.

Abnormal Findings

▼DECREASED TIMES (shortened PCT) may indicate thrombocytopenia, uremia, anticoagulant therapy, platelet disorders such as idiopathic thrombocytopenia purpura, disseminated intravascular coagulation (DIC), or hemophilia.

 ACTION ALERT!

Deficiencies in clotting factors indicate an increased risk for bleeding and hemorrhage. Closely observe the client for signs and symptoms such as frank bleeding, hypotension, tachycardia, apprehension, dyspnea, pale and cool skin, and anxiety. Be prepared to transfuse with blood products, including appropriate clotting factors.

Interfering Factors

➤ Traumatic venipuncture, hemolysis, not placing the sample on ice, and not sending the specimen to the laboratory immediately can result in false elevations.

➤ Anticoagulants including warfarin and aspirin can result in decreased levels.

Potential Complications

➤ Prolonged bleeding at the venipuncture site.

NURSING CONSIDERATIONS

Prepare Your Client

➤ Explain that this test helps determine if the blood clots normally.

Perform Procedure

➤ Collect 7 mL of venous blood in a red-top tube.

➤ Do not draw from a heparin lock or heparinized catheter. The blood must be drawn from a peripheral vein.

➤ Label the sample and note heparin or any other anticoagulants (warfarin, aspirin, etc.). Send it to the laboratory immediately.

Care After Test

➤ Hold pressure at the venipuncture site for 5 minutes to prevent hematoma formation.

➤ Assess client for unusual bruising or prolonged bleeding from venipuncture site. Delayed clotting is a complication of severely impaired clotting.

➤ Test all body secretions including stool, gastrointestinal aspirate, and tracheal aspirate for occult blood. Closely inspect mucous membranes for bleeding.

➤ Review related tests such as prothrombin time, partial thromboplastin time, bleeding time, activated clotting time, complete blood count, platelet count, platelet survival, bleeding time, factor assays, and activated partial thromboplastin time.

Educate Your Client and the Family

➤ Teach the client and family members about bleeding precautions including using a soft-bristled toothbrush, using electric razors rather than straight razors, avoiding constipation, avoiding aspirin and aspirin products, avoiding picking their nose, and avoiding constricting clothing. If menses is experienced, the client should maintain a pad count and note the amount of saturation of each pad.

➤ Teach the client and family members the signs and symptoms of bleeding including petechiae (small purplish spots on the skin), bruising, blood in the urine or stool, vaginal bleeding, and bleeding from invasive lines.

➤ Teach client to avoid over-the-counter aspirin/salicylate drugs, phenothiazines, codeine, nonsteroidal anti-inflammatory drugs, and alcohol.

Prothrombin Time
proe throm bin • time
(PT, ProTime, Factor II)

Normal Findings

Each laboratory establishes a normal value or control based on the method and reagents used to perform the test. A value within ±2 seconds of the control set by each laboratory is considered within the normal range.

ADULT, PREGNANT, ADOLESCENT, ELDERLY

9.6–15 seconds or 85%–100%
Anticoagulated condition = 1¹/₂ to 2¹/₂ times the control

NEWBORN
<17 seconds

CHILD
11–14 seconds

What This Test Will Tell You

This blood test screens for lack of coagulation factors necessary for blood clotting. Prothrombin time measures the time required for a fibrin clot to form in a citrated plasma sample after addition of calcium ions and tissue thromboplastin (Factor III) and compares this with the fibrin clotting time in a control sample of plasma. The test indirectly measures prothrombin and is an excellent screening test for overall assessment of the extrinsic coagulation pathway. It is the test of choice for monitoring anticoagulant therapy.

Abnormal Findings

▲INCREASED LEVELS (prolonged times) may indicate afibrinogenemia, hypofibrinogenemia (<100 mg/dL), idiopathic familial hypoprothrombinemia, factor deficiency (I, II, V, VII, X), idiopathic myelofibrosis, alcoholism, biliary obstruction, disseminated intravascular coagulation (DIC), dysfibrinogenemia, celiac disease, circulating anticoagulants, snakebite, cirrhosis, colitis, congestive heart failure, chronic diarrhea, pancreatic carcinoma, fistula, hemorrhagic disease of the newborn, hepatic abscess or biopsy, hypernephroma of the kidney, hypervitaminosis A, acute leukemia, malabsorption, obstetric complication, chronic pancreatitis, polycythemia vera, Reye's syndrome, salicylate poisoning, sprue, toxic shock syndrome, vitamin K deficiency, or vomiting.

▼DECREASED LEVELS (shortened time) may indicate pulmonary embolus, arterial occlusion, myocardial infarction, deep vein thrombosis, multiple myeloma, peripheral vascular disease, spinal cord injury, or transplant rejection.

ACTION ALERT!

For prolonged prothrombin times (>20 seconds if not receiving anticoagulation therapy; >30–40 seconds with anticoagulation therapy), prepare to administer vitamin K intramuscularly immediately. Assess for bleeding by checking all body fluids for occult blood, monitoring for neurological status changes, and evaluating for hypotension or tachycardia.

Interfering Factors

➤ Hemolyzed or lipemic specimens or specimens received in the laboratory 3 or more hours after collection may cause prolonged results.

➤ Failure to properly fill the collection tube with blood may cause prolonged or decreased times.

➤ Drawing the sample from an intravenous line being kept open with a heparin flush will cause falsely prolonged results. Heparin can lengthen prothrombin time for up to 5 hours.

➤ Diets excessively high in green leafy vegetables can increase the absorption of vitamin K, which shortens the prothrombin time.

➤ A minimum of 100 g/dL of fibrinogen must be present for the prothrombin time to be accurate.

➤ Failure to discard the first 2–3 mL of blood drawn may contaminate the specimen with tissue thromboplastin, which will alter the results.

➤ Drugs that increase the prothrombin time include acetaminophen, allopurinol, aspirin, anabolic steroids, bishydroxycoumarin (Dicumarol), cathartics, chloral hydrate, chloramphenicol, chlorthalidone, cimetidine, corticotropin, diazoxide, disulfiram, diuretics, ethacrynate sodium, ethacrynic acid, glucagon, guanethidine sulfate, heparin, indomethacin, kanamycin, levothyroxine, mefenamic acid, methyldopa hydrochloride, methylphenidate hydrochloride, mithramycin, monoamine oxidase inhibitors, nalidixic acid, neomycin sulfate, nortriptyline hydrochloride, oxyphenbutazone, phenprocoumon, phenylbutazone, phenyramidol, phenytoin sodium, quinidine, quinine, reserpine, streptomycin sulfate, long-acting sulfonamides, tetracyclines, thyrotropin, tolbutamide, vitamin A, and warfarin sodium.

➤ Drugs that decrease the prothrombin time include antacids, antihistamines, ascorbic acid, barbiturates, caffeine, cholestyramine, colchicine, digitalis, diphenhydramine, estrogens, ethchlorvynol, glutethimide, griseofulvin, heptabarbital, menadiol sodium diphosphate, menadione, meprobamate, oral contraceptives, estrogens, phenobarbital, phytonadione, pyrazinamide, rifampin, sodium benzoate, tetracycline, theophylline, vitamin K, and xanthines.

Potential Complications
➤ Prolonged bleeding at the venipuncture site

NURSING CONSIDERATIONS
Prepare Your Client
➤ Explain that this test helps determine if the blood clots normally. If appropriate, explain that this test helps monitor how well medication is keeping blood from clotting too much.
➤ A baseline prothrombin time should be drawn before starting anticoagulant therapy.
➤ Inform the client on oral anticoagulant therapy that this test may be repeated at regular intervals to assess response to treatment.

Perform Procedure
➤ Draw a venous blood sample. (If the laboratory requires it, first draw 2 mL of venous blood into a syringe and discard, leaving the needle in place.) Collect 7 mL of venous blood into a blue-top tube containing sodium citrate and citric acid. Completely fill the tube and invert it several times to mix the sample and anticoagulant adequately. Do not shake the tube vigorously as this can result in hemolysis.
➤ Apply pressure or pressure dressing to the venipuncture site.
➤ Label the sample and note any anticoagulants. Send it to the laboratory immediately.

Care After Test
➤ If a coagulation defect is suspected, hold the venipuncture site for 3–5 minutes after the needle is removed. Observe the site for excessive bleeding or ecchymosis.
➤ Evaluate obtained results. Oral anticoagulant therapy usually maintains the prothrombin time at $1^1/_2$ to 2 times the lab control value. Persons with cardiac disease may be maintained at 2 to $2^1/_2$ times the control.
➤ Assess client for unusual bruising or prolonged bleeding from venipuncture site. Delayed clotting is a complication of severely impaired clotting.
➤ Test all body secretions including stool, gastrointestinal aspirate, and tracheal aspirate for occult blood. Closely inspect mucous membranes for bleeding.
➤ Review related tests such as platelet count, complete blood count, bleeding time, prothrombin consumption time, peripheral blood smear examination, and activated partial thromboplastin time.

Educate Your Client and the Family
➤ Teach the client and family members about bleeding precautions including using a soft-bristled toothbrush; using electric razors rather than straight razors; avoiding constipation; avoiding enemas, rectal thermometers, and suppositories; avoiding picking their nose; and avoiding constricting clothing.
➤ Teach the client and family members the signs and symptoms of bleeding including petechiae (small purplish spots on the skin), bruising, blood in the urine or stool, vaginal

bleeding, and bleeding from invasive lines. If menses is experienced, the client should maintain a pad count and note the amount of saturation of each pad.

➤ Teach the client to avoid over-the-counter aspirin and aspirin products, phenothiazines, codeine, non-steroidal anti-inflammatory drugs, and alcohol.

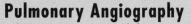

Pulmonary Angiography
pul mo **nair** ee • **an** jee **og** rah fee
(Pulmonary Arteriography, Arteriogram, Angiogram)

Normal Findings
Normal pulmonary circulation: contrast medium should circulate evenly throughout the pulmonary vasculature.

What This Test Will Tell You
This x-ray test with contrast diagnoses pulmonary embolism and visualizes the pulmonary vessels for defects. The invasive radiologic procedure involves insertion of a catheter into the vascular system followed by injection of iodine radiopaque contrast dye to allow visualization of pulmonary blood vessels. This test may be indicated when chest x-rays, computed tomography scans, or lung scans suggest pulmonary embolism or other pulmonary vascular abnormality, especially to verify and locate an embolism prior to surgical embolectomy.

Abnormal Finding
Abnormalities may indicate pulmonary embolism, pulmonary stenosis, pulmonary infarction, congenital lesions of the pulmonary vasculature, aneurysms, tumors, or emphysema.

ACTION ALERT!
Life-threatening complications such as cardiac arrhythmias, anaphylactic reactions, myocardial rupture, or arterial occlusion may occur during pulmonary angiography. Have emergency resuscitation equipment readily available.

Interfering Factors
➤ Movement by client who is unable to cooperate or hold still during the examination makes it difficult to obtain satisfactory films.
➤ Small peripheral emboli or abnormalities may not be visible with angiography.

Contraindications
➤ Pregnancy or potential pregnancy, due to radiation exposure of fetus, unless benefit outweighs risk.
➤ History of allergy to iodine or shellfish contraindicates use of iodine contrast media.
➤ Bleeding disorders.

Potential Complications
➤ Allergic/anaphylactic reaction to iodine dye
➤ Congenital defects in offspring due to exposure of the reproductive organs to x-rays
➤ Cardiac dysrhythmias
➤ Arterial occlusion

➤ Pulmonary artery or myocardial perforation

➤ Acute renal failure due to contrast media

➤ Infection

NURSING CONSIDERATIONS

Prepare Your Client

➤ Explain that this test is to look at the blood vessels in the lungs in order to find blood clots or other problems.

➤ Routinely ask any woman of childbearing years if there is any possibility she could be pregnant before performing x-ray studies. X-ray studies on pregnant women are performed only if it is deemed the benefits outweigh the risks.

➤ Obtain a history of allergies to seafood, iodine, and contrast dye. Notify the radiologist if the client reports allergies to any of these substances.

➤ Inform the client that the test will be performed in the x-ray department by a radiologist and takes about 1 hour.

➤ Check that the primary health care provider has obtained informed consent. Verify that a signed consent form is on the chart.

➤ Note recent coagulation studies, prothrombin time (PT), partial thromboplastin time (PTT), and platelet count. Report abnormal findings to the radiologist.

➤ If the client is on intravenous anticoagulant therapy, consult with the primary health care provider about how long the medication should be discontinued prior to the procedure.

➤ Tell the client that a local anesthetic will be used to numb the area where the catheter will be inserted. This may produce a brief burning sensation before the area becomes numb.

➤ Explain that the catheter is inserted into a vein in the groin or arm and is passed through the veins to the heart and vessels of the lungs.

➤ Explain that when the dye is injected, they may experience a warm flush, nausea, or salty taste, which may last 2–5 minutes.

➤ Inform the client that coughing is not abnormal after the procedure.

➤ Withhold food and fluids for 8–12 hours prior to the procedure.

➤ Explain to the client the importance of lying motionless during the procedure so the pictures will be clear.

➤ Administer sedatives as ordered prior to the procedure.

➤ Record baseline vital signs.

➤ Transport the client to the radiology department.

Perform Procedure

Nurses do not perform this procedure, but should understand the process to prepare the client. The client is assisted onto the x-ray table in the supine position. Electrocardiographic monitoring electrodes are attached away from the chest wall for continuous monitoring. Intravenous access is established for administration of emergency drugs if necessary. The femoral or antecubital vein site is cleansed with antiseptic solution and draped with sterile towels. Local anesthetic is injected over the site, and the long catheter is introduced into the vein and threaded into the pulmonary vasculature. The contrast material is injected and rapid serial x-ray films are taken while the contrast material is circulating through the pulmonary blood vessels. Monitor the client for cardiac arrhythmias and hypersensitivity throughout the procedure. The catheter is removed, pressure applied for at least 10 minutes to stop bleeding, and a pressure dressing is applied over the insertion site after bleeding has stopped.

Care After Test

➤ Assess vital signs, color, motion, sensation, and pulses in affected extremity and insertion site every 15 minutes for 1 hour, every 30 minutes for the next hour, and then every hour until stable.

➤ Observe the insertion site for signs of bleeding or hematoma. If bleeding or hematoma formation occurs, reapply pressure to the area and notify the vascular laboratory or primary health care provider.

➤ Observe site for signs of infection including inflammation, exudate, and tenderness. Report to the primary health care provider immediately and prepare to institute antibiotic therapy.

➤ Discontinue cardiac monitoring and intravenous fluids if ordered.

➤ Observe for a delayed allergic reaction to the contrast dye including tachycardia, hypotension, dyspnea, skin rash, or urticaria.

➤ Resume previous diet beginning with clear liquids and advancing as tolerated.

➤ Enforce bed rest or activity restrictions for 6–12 hours as ordered to minimize bleeding or hematoma formation.

➤ Resume anticoagulant therapy if indicated.

➤ Evaluate related tests such as lung scans, computed tomography scans, and chest x-rays.

Educate Your Client and the Family

➤ Explain the nursing routine of monitoring vital signs and the arm or leg where the catheter was inserted.

➤ Tell the client to report immediately any bleeding, numbness of the extremity, or other discomforts.

➤ Describe the need for and effects of anticoagulant therapy if indicated.

➤ Tell the client that the test will be interpreted by the radiologist and results given to the primary health care provider.

➤ Teach client to pace activities to conserve energy if indicated.

Pulmonary Function Tests

puhl moe nair ee • funk shun • tests

Normal Findings

All ages: 75%–125% of the predicted value is considered normal. The predicted values are derived from prediction equations or nomograms based on age, height, weight, and sex, and vary greatly with these factors.

What This Test Will Tell You

These tests determine the presence, nature, and extent of pulmonary dysfunction caused by either obstructive or restrictive diseases. Lung capacities, volumes, diffusion capacity, and flow rates are clinically measured by various devices connected to a computer to measure and record values. The obtained data allow determination of the presence of pulmonary disease or abnormality of lung function, extent of abnormalities, severity of impairment, progression of the disorder, and appropriate treatment. Pulmonary function tests (PFTs) can help identify whether a client has an obstructive defect, a diffusion defect, a restrictive defect, or a combination of these. They may be used preoperatively to assess the client's ability to tolerate anesthetics. They may also be part of periodic examination of workers in industries in which a lung hazard exists or in epidemiologic study of populations to provide clues to the causes of pulmonary diseases.

Abnormal Findings

Abnormal values may indicate obstructive lung disease such as emphysema, asthma, chronic bronchitis, bronchiectasis, or allergic inflammatory response; restrictive lung disease such as kyphoscoliosis, pulmonary fibrosis, neuromuscular diseases, abdominal distention or obesity, inflammatory changes of the lung tissue or pleura, tumors or pulmonary edema; diffusion defect abnormalities such as respiratory distress syndrome, pulmonary edema, and collagen vascular disease; congenital chest wall deformities; cystic fibrosis; bronchopulmonary dysplasia; and scleroderma.

ACTION ALERT!

If bronchorestrictors are used during pulmonary function testing, carefully observe the client for respiratory distress. Assure bronchodilators and emergency medications and equipment are immediately available in the event that respiratory distress occurs.

Interfering Factors

➤ Client's inability to cooperate because of age or confusion makes testing difficult or impossible.
➤ Inadequate client effort due to fatigue, pain, etc., may produce inaccurate data.
➤ Inadequate seal around the mouthpiece yields invalid data.
➤ Sedation, gastric distention, or pregnancy may alter results by lowering PFTs even in the absence of lung disease.
➤ Bronchodilators and narcotics should not be administered immediately prior to testing as this may obscure true results.

Contraindications

➤ Inability to cooperate due to pain with deep inspirations and expirations or due to confusion.
➤ Inhalation tests using bronchoconstrictors are contraindicated in known asthmatics because they may precipitate life-threatening asthma attacks.
➤ Acute respiratory distress, because the tests are fatiguing and may further stress a compromised respiratory system.

Potential Complications

➤ Respiratory distress if bronchoconstrictors are used or if spontaneous bronchoconstriction occurs during testing.

NURSING CONSIDERATIONS

Prepare Your Client

➤ Explain to client that the test is performed to find out how their lungs are working.
➤ Advise the client to refrain from smoking or eating a heavy meal for 4–6 hours prior to testing.
➤ Withhold bronchodilators, sedatives, and narcotics for 2 hours prior to the test.
➤ Tell the client to wear nonrestric-

tive clothing and that dentures may be left in during testing.

➤ Record the client's age, height, and weight on the test requisition since they will be used to predict normal range.

➤ Assess for signs and symptoms of respiratory distress.

➤ Practice breathing patterns with the client to help them prepare for the test and to obtain the most accurate results (i.e., normal breathing, rapid breathing, and forced deep inspiration and forced deep expiration). This is especially important in children.

➤ Reassure the client that the test is painless.

Perform Procedure

➤ PFTs done in the pulmonary function laboratory cover the entire range of respiratory volumes and capacities. PFTs done at the bedside or in an ambulatory care setting are modified to the more portable and easily performed studies.

➤ Position the client sitting or standing and apply a nose clip so all air movement is through the mouth.

➤ The client is instructed to breathe in and out through a mouthpiece, according to the specific test being performed. The mouthpiece is connected to a computerized machine which calculates and records values.

➤ If indicated, the client inhales a dose of bronchodilator and specific tests are repeated to determine the client's response to bronchodilator therapy and aid in diagnosis of obstructive lung disease.

➤ If indicated, a short-acting bronchoconstrictor is inhaled and specific tests are repeated to determine any cause-and-effect relationship in the client with inhalant allergies. Observe for respiratory distress and

have medication readily available to reverse the effects if necessary.

Care After Test

➤ Resume previous diet, activity level, and bronchodilator therapy.

➤ Observe for signs and symptoms of chronic respiratory disease such as barrel chest, cyanosis, and clubbing of fingernails.

➤ Observe for signs of respiratory distress such as nasal flaring, use of accessory muscles for breathing, posturing, and tachypnea.

➤ Administer only low-flow oxygen for clients with chronic obstructive pulmonary disease to avoid respiratory arrest related to obliteration of hypoxic drive.

➤ Evaluate related tests such as arterial blood gases, chest x-rays, computed tomography (CT) scans, or lung scans.

Educate Your Client and the Family

➤ Assess for fatigue, which may occur after testing in people with lung disease. Provide rest until symptoms or complaint of fatigue passes. Teach client how to pace activities.

➤ If test results indicate restrictive or obstructive lung disease, advise the client to refrain from or to stop smoking. Refer to smoking cessation programs if indicated.

➤ Teach the client about bronchodilator therapy if indicated.

➤ If tests were performed as part of preoperative assessment, educate the client about the importance of postoperative deep breathing, coughing, and other pulmonary hygiene measures.

➤ Enhance nutritional intake by teaching oral hygiene practices and rest periods before small, frequent meals.

Pulmonary Function

Total lung capacity (TLC): The total volume of the lungs when maximally inflated. It is the sum of the tidal volume, inspiratory reserve volume, expiratory reserve volume, and residual volume.

Increased TLC	*Decreased TLC*
Overdistention of the lungs associated with chronic obstructive lung disease	Restrictive disease

Tidal volume (VT or TV): The volume of air inhaled and exhaled with a normal breath.

Increased TV	*Decreased TV*
Emphysema	Fatigue
Lung hyperinflation	Restrictive lung disease
	Atelectasis
	Tumors
	Pulmonary congestion
	Pneumothorax

Inspiratory reserve volume (IRV): The maximal volume that can be inhaled following a normal inhalation. It represents forced inspiration over and beyond the tidal volume.

Increased IRV	*Decreased IRV*
Not clinically significant	Exercise
Improvement in lung function	Asthma
	Emphysema
	Airway obstruction

Expiratory reserve volume (ERV): The maximal volume that can be exhaled after normal exhalation.

Increased ERV	*Decreased ERV*
Not clinically significant	Obesity
Improvement in lung function	Pregnancy
	Ascites
	Heart enlargement
	Pleural effusion
	Kyphoscoliosis
	Thoracoplasty

Residual volume (RV): The volume of air left in the lungs after forced exhalation. The RV is determined mathematically using data from other tests. RV normally increases with aging.

Increased RV	Decreased RV
Aging	Not clinically significant
Emphysema	Improvement in lung function
Chronic air trapping	
Bronchial obstruction	
Young asthmatics	

Forced expiratory volume (FEV): The volume expired during specified time intervals of 0.5, 1, 2, and 3 seconds and are labeled FEV_1, etc.

Increased FEV	Decreased FEV
Not clinically significant	Obstructive lung diseases
Improvement in lung function	Emphysema
	Asthma

Functional residual capacity (FRC): The air left in the lungs at the end of a normal exhalation. (FRC = ERV + RV)

Decreased FRC	Increased FRC
Restrictive diseases	Air trapping
Respiratory distress syndrome	Obstructive airway disease

Inspiratory capacity (IC): The amount of air that can be inspired after normal exhalation. It is a useful measurement for determining a client's ability to be weaned from mechanical ventilation. (IC = TV + IRV)

Increased IC	Decreased IC
Not clinically significant	Chronic air trapping
Improvement in lung function	Emphysema
	Asthma
	Bronchial obstruction

Vital capacity (VC): The maximal amount of air that can be exhaled after maximal inhalation. (VC = TV + IRV + ERV)

Increased VC	Decreased VC
Physical fitness	Restrictive disease
	Obstructive disorders
	Respiratory center depression
	Neuromuscular diseases
	Pregnancy
	Pain

Forced vital capacity (FVC): The total volume exhaled forcefully and rapidly after maximal lung inhalation.

Increased VC	Decreased FVC
Not clinically significant	Restrictive lung disease
Improvement in lung function	Obstructive lung diseases

▶

Minute volume or minute ventilation (MV): The volume of air inhaled and exhaled in 1 minute.

Increased MV	Decreased MV
Not clinically significant	Fatigue
Improvement in lung function	Restrictive lung disease

Maximal inspiratory pressure (MIP): The greatest negative or subatmospheric pressure that can be generated during inspiration against an occluded airway.

Increased MIP	Decreased MIP
Not clinically significant	Restrictive lung diseases
Improvement in lung function	Obstructive lung diseases

Maximal expiratory pressure (MEP): The highest positive pressure that can be generated during a forceful expiratory effort against an occluded airway.

Increased MEP	Decreased MEP
Not clinically significant	Obstructive lung diseases
Improvement in lung function	

Peak expiratory flow rate (PEFR) or peak flow: The maximal flow rate attained during a forced vital capacity maneuver. Home testing of peak flow with a device called a peak flow meter is commonly performed by clients with asthma or lung transplants. It may also be performed by the nurse at the bedside for clients with asthma or neuromuscular diseases.

Increased PEFR	Decreased PEFR
Not clinically significant	Air trapping
Improvement in lung function	Asthma
	Respiratory compromise related to neuromuscular disease
	Rejection of lung transplant

Diffusion capacity of the lung: Client is given controlled amounts of carbon monoxide to inhale. The amount exhaled is compared to the amount inhaled to give a D_LCO, or diffusion capacity for carbon monoxide, which detects impairment of the alveolar membrane in diffusion gases.

Increased D_L	Decreased D_L
Not clinically significant	Respiratory distress syndrome
Improvement in lung function	Congestive heart failure
	Pulmonary edema
	Collagen vascular disease

Inhalation tests: Methacholine or histamine are inhaled to help diagnose reactive airway diseases such as asthma. By measuring forced expiratory volume after the inhalation of a bronchoconstricting agent, air trapping that occurs in reactive airway disease can be measured.

Increased FEV	Decreased FEV
Not clinically significant	Obstructive lung diseases
Improvement in lung function	Emphysema
	Asthma

Pyruvate Kinase
pie roo vate • kie nase
(PK, Erythrocyte PK)

Normal Findings
ALL AGES
Ultraviolet assay: 2–8.8 U/g Hgb
Low substrate assay: 0.9–3.9 U/g Hgb
There should be strong fluorescence at time 0, followed by no fluorescence at 30 minutes. Any fluorescence present at 30 minutes indicates a decreased pyruvate kinase activity. Normally, fluorescence disappears within 10–20 minutes.

What This Test Will Tell You
This blood test diagnoses and classifies congenital or acquired hemolytic anemias. Pyruvate kinase is important to the red blood cell's formation of adenosine triphosphate (ATP), which assists in maintaining normal red blood cell (RBC) membrane function. The RBC that is deficient in pyruvate kinase is a rigid, poorly formed cell that is prematurely destroyed (hemolyzed) by the spleen and the liver.

Abnormal Findings
▼DECREASED LEVELS may indicate congenital nonspherocytic hemolytic anemia, myocardial infarction, carrier of Duchenne muscular dystrophy, metabolic liver disease, or drug toxicity.

Interfering Factors
➤ Hemolyzed specimens will alter the results.
➤ Presence of white blood cells in the specimen tested interferes with results.
➤ Failure to notify the laboratory of recent blood transfusions may interfere with accurately determining serum levels.

P

NURSING CONSIDERATIONS
Prepare Your Client
➤ Explain that this test is used to detect problems in red blood cell formation.
➤ Check the client's history for recent blood transfusions and note this on the laboratory slip.

Perform Procedure
➤ Collect 7 mL of venous blood in a lavender-top tube. The collection tube should be filled properly, inverted, and gently rotated thoroughly to mix the anticoagulant. Don't shake the tube vigorously, as this can result in hemolysis.
➤ Label the sample, noting recent blood transfusions, and send it to the laboratory immediately.

Care After Test
➤ Observe the client for signs and symptoms of anemia. Mild anemia is manifested by paleness, fatigue, slight dyspnea, palpitations, and sweating associated with exercise. Moderate anemia will increase the symptoms of mild anemia. Severe anemia signs and symptoms include headache, dizziness, irritability, dyspnea on exertion and with rest, discomfort similar to angina, tachycardia, and tachypnea.
➤ Encourage rest for fatigue that occurs with anemia. Plan for consistent periods of light exercise but instruct the client to get assistance

with the activities of daily living including self-care and home maintenance.

➤ Instruct the client to maintain the usual patterns of sleep and to maintain an optimal nutritional status.

➤ Evaluate other tests such as osmotic fragility, Coombs' antiglobulin tests, red blood cell survival test, hematocrit, reticulocyte count, Heinz bodies, platelet count, bone marrow aspiration, bilirubin, haptoglobin, and complete blood count.

Educate Your Client and the Family

➤ Instruct the client in the signs and symptoms of anemia including pallor, tachycardia, dyspnea, activity intolerance, palpitations, and fatigue.

➤ Instruct the client about slowly increasing activity after blood transfusions, as the blood does not become fully oxygenated for 12–36 hours. Vigorous activity prior to this for the anemic client can cause undue fatigue and exhaustion.

Radioactive Iodine Uptake
ray dee oe ak tiv • ie o dine • up tayk
(RAI)

Normal Findings
ADULT AND ELDERLY
Normal size and position of thyroid gland. Evenly concentrated iodine uptake.
2 hours: 1%–13% absorption
6 hours: 2%–20% absorption
24 hours: 15%–35% absorption

What This Test Will Tell You
This nuclear medicine test and thyroid scan evaluate the size, position, and function of the thyroid gland. Radioactive isotopes can be traced through the body with special scanning machines. Abnormal tissue appears different on the scan because the isotope is metabolized differently. Areas of increased uptake (hot spots) are generally associated with benign adenomas, whereas areas of decreased uptake (cold spots) more often suggest malignancy.

Abnormal Findings
▲INCREASED LEVELS may indicate hyperthyroidism, Graves' disease, benign adenomas, cirrhosis, thyroiditis, or renal failure.
▼DECREASED LEVELS may indicate hypothyroidism, myxedema, or Hashimoto's thyroiditis.

Interfering Factors
➤ Medications that can decrease iodine uptake include iodine-containing drugs, thyroid medications, antithyroid drugs, corticosteroids, antihistamines, nitrates, tolbutamide, adrenocorticotropic hormone, diuretics, phenylbutazone, thiopental sodium, and warfarin.

➤ Enriched breakfast cereals and diuresis may lower iodine uptake.
➤ Clients with overall poor iodine stores will have elevated uptake, and clients with increased stores related to taking iodine medications will have decreased uptake, making results difficult to interpret accurately.
➤ Drugs such as thyroid-stimulating hormone, estrogens, barbiturates, lithium, and phenothiazines may cause an increased iodine uptake.
➤ Diarrhea or vomiting after iodine administration, intestinal malabsorption, and contrast material can decrease absorption and interfere with test results.
➤ Renal failure may increase iodine uptake.

Contraindications
➤ This test is contraindicated during pregnancy, in lactating women, and in infants and children.
➤ Iodine allergies.

Potential Complications
➤ Radioactive exposure to thyroid gland, which is greater in ^{131}I than in ^{123}I or ^{125}I

NURSING CONSIDERATIONS
Prepare Your Client
➤ Explain that this test will help identify problems in a gland called the thyroid.
➤ Assess for allergy to iodine.
➤ Review the dietary history and instruct client not to consume iodine-containing products such as

seafood, iodized salt, enriched cereals, and cabbage for at least 1 week prior to testing.

➤ Explain that the small amount of radioactive material is not a threat to the client or family.

➤ Check with your laboratory to see if fasting for 8 hours prior to the test is necessary.

➤ Explain that several scans at varying intervals are required and that timing of these scans is critical.

Perform Procedure

➤ A dose of tasteless radioactive iodine is administered orally, or alternately iodine may be administered intravenously.

➤ After a specified time the amount of iodine absorbed by the thyroid gland is measured by use of a scanner and compared to total amount administered.

➤ Instruct the client to return to nuclear medicine at designated times to measure uptake over time. Emphasize the importance of being on time.

➤ Client may eat 1 hour after iodine administration.

Care After Test

➤ Monitor urine for radioactive iodine excretion. Use gloves when handling urine. Some policies require flushing the toilet 2 times for disposal. Check your own institution's policy for hazardous waste disposal.

➤ Encourage adequate oral intake of fluids to promote urinary excretion.

➤ Review related tests including triiodothyronine and thyroxine levels.

Educate Your Client and the Family

➤ Teach client that thyroid hormone replacements must be taken for life if hypofunction is found, or if thyroid is removed surgically.

➤ Teach client how to meet rest and nutritional needs required by a hyperfunctioning thyroid. This includes frequent rest intervals and a high-calorie, high-protein diet.

➤ If a thyroid abnormality is diagnosed, provide the client with emotional support and appropriate teaching.

Radioallergosorbent Test

ray dee oe al ur goe sor bent • test
(RAST)

Normal Findings

All ages: Negative—no detectable specific IgE antibody

What This Test Will Tell You

This blood test identifies reactions to respiratory and food allergy stimulants. Radioallergosorbent tests (RASTs) measure the quantity of allergen-specific immunoglobulin-E antibodies. This test provides an alternative to skin testing and is often used for children with extrinsic asthma, hay fever, or atopic eczema. Although more expensive than conventional skin testing, RAST tests provide precise information on many common allergies without causing hypersensitivity reactions.

Abnormal Findings
A positive RAST test may indicate an allergy to a particular allergen and immediate hypersensitivity to the allergen, such as grasses, trees, molds, weeds, house dust mites, venoms, animal danders, foods, antibiotics, and insects.

Interfering Factors
➤ Radioactive scan within 1 week of venous sampling

NURSING CONSIDERATIONS
Prepare Your Client
➤ Explain that this is a test for allergies.

Perform Procedure
➤ Collect 4–10 mL of venous blood in a red-top tube for each group of six RAST tests.

Care After Test
➤ Monitor for signs and symptoms of allergies. Collaborate with the primary health care provider to provide symptomatic relief if needed.
➤ Review related tests such as results of skin testing and eosinophil and basophil counts.

Educate Your Client and the Family
➤ Explain that a positive RAST test indicates allergy and what the client is allergic to (the allergen).
➤ Review self-care measures to decrease exposure, such as avoiding certain foods or environmental allergens, putting plastic covers over mattresses and pillows, cleaning frequently, changing furnace filters, laundering, and damp dusting.
➤ When appropriate, teach client and family correct use of inhalers.

Raji Cell Assay
rah jee • sel • a say
(Raji Cell Immune Complex Assay, RIA, Immune Complex Detection by Raji)

Normal Findings
Negative, no Raji cells present

What This Test Will Tell You
This blood test helps diagnose autoimmune diseases by detecting the presence of circulating immune complexes. In this test, the client's serum is incubated with lymphoblastoid B-cells (Raji cells) to determine the extent of immune complex binding with complement C3c and C3d receptors on the Raji cell membrane surface. A transient elevation of immune complexes reflects a normal antigen-antibody response. However, prolonged elevation of immune complexes may indicate a chronic infection or autoimmune disorder. When immune complexes remain elevated for long periods, they are deposited in organs and tissues, which activates complement and results in inflammation. The kidney is frequently affected by this immune response.

Abnormal Findings
Positive results may indicate autoimmune disorders, chronic infectious diseases, viral infections, parasitic infections, microbial infections, metastasis, drug reactions, cryoglobulinemia, celiac disease, cirrhosis,

Crohn's disease, sickle-cell anemia, dermatitis herpetiformis, or ulcerative colitis.

Interfering Factors

➤ Improper timing of blood sampling may fail to yield positive results. If clinical signs and symptoms are not severe at the time of sampling, the test may not detect disease. High levels of immune complexes are more likely to be detected.
➤ Cryoglobulins, cold agglutinins, rheumatoid factors, and monoclonal proteins may cause invalid results.
➤ Antilymphocyte antibodies and antinuclear antibodies may cause false positive results.

NURSING CONSIDERATIONS

Prepare Your Client

➤ Explain that this test helps detect diseases where the body forms compounds called antigens against some of its own tissues.

Perform Procedure

➤ Collect 5–10 mL of venous blood in a red-top tube.

Care After Test

➤ Assess the client for signs and symptoms of renal involvement including changes in renal function tests and urine output. Frequently, the kidneys are compromised in immune complex disorders.
➤ Evaluate related tests such as blood urea nitrogen level, serum creatinine, creatinine clearance, rheumatoid factor, lupus erythematosus test, viral cultures, ova and parasite tests, liver function tests, and sickle-cell test.

Educate Your Client and the Family

➤ If your client has glomerulonephritis, teach them methods to manage symptoms such as monitoring input and output, adhering to dietary and fluid intake instructions, controlling fluid weight gains, taking medications as prescribed, and resting as needed.
➤ If client has an infectious process, teach the doses, side effects, and reason for taking the prescribed medication.
➤ If client has a chronic illness, offer emotional support to your client, family, and significant others. Instruct them in management of symptoms. Give them information about support organizations in your area.

Renal Angiography

ree nal • an jee og rah fee
(Renal Arteriogram)

Normal Findings

Normal, symmetrical, and equal circulation of radiopaque contrast material without obstruction through the renal vasculature and throughout the renal tissue.

What This Test Will Tell You

This radiographic examination shows the renal vasculature and parenchyma and helps identify renal vascular disorders and the condition of renal tissue. This study helps identify renal tumors, renal artery stenosis, renal aneurysms, arteriovenous fistulas, and destruction of renal tissue from infection, and in assessing renal trauma. It is also used to assess renal transplant donors and recipients before and after transplantation. This procedure is extremely helpful in the differential diagnosis of a variety of kidney problems.

Abnormal Findings

Abnormalities may indicate renal artery stenosis from atherosclerosis or other abnormalities, aneurysms, traumatic injury, abscess, cyst, tumor, renal failure, arteriovenous fistula, renal infarction, renal vascular hypertension, anatomic vascular anomalies, or renal hematoma.

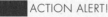 ACTION ALERT!

Assess clients carefully for allergic reaction to contrast material, including dyspnea, itching, urticaria, flushing, hypotension, and shock. Life-threatening anaphylactic reactions can occur and need to be recognized and treated immediately.

Interfering Factors

➤ Retained stool, flatus, or contrast material in the gastrointestinal tract may affect visualization.

Contraindications

➤ Allergy to contrast material or shellfish
➤ Pregnant, due to radiation exposure of the fetus
➤ Bleeding or clotting disorders
➤ End-stage renal disease

Potential Complications

➤ Embolus or clot formation
➤ Allergic reaction to contrast material
➤ Vessel damage from needle puncture

➤ Hemorrhage or hematoma formation at catheter insertion site
➤ Infection at the insertion site or sepsis

NURSING CONSIDERATIONS

Prepare Your Client

➤ Explain that this test helps identify problems in the blood vessels and tissues of the kidneys.
➤ Assess for allergies to contrast materials or shellfish and report to radiologist.
➤ Ensure that an informed consent is obtained, because of the possible complications associated with this procedure.
➤ Restrict food and fluids for 8 hours prior to the test.
➤ Explain to the client that they will have to lie still on a procedure table during the procedure.
➤ Locate the peripheral pulses and mark them with a pen to assist in postprocedure monitoring.
➤ Instruct the client that they may experience a burning or flushed feeling when the dye is injected.
➤ Have the client void just prior to the procedure or before sedation.
➤ Administer any ordered sedation.

Perform Procedure

Nurses do not perform this procedure, but should understand the process to prepare the client and assist the physician. The client is positioned supine on a special x-ray table in the catheterization laboratory. A peripheral intravenous infusion is initiated. A local anesthetic is administered near the insertion site by the radiologist. Warn the client first that this may cause a burning sensation before the area is numbed.

The radiologist inserts an intra-arterial catheter into the femoral artery and advances it with the help of fluoroscopy to the aorta, and administers test doses of contrast material. The catheter is replaced with a renal catheter, and radiopaque contrast material is injected near or directly into the renal arteries. Then a series of x-ray films are taken to evaluate the renal vessels during arterial and venous filling, and to evaluate the renal parenchyma.

When the test is completed, the catheter is removed and a pressure dressing is applied. Direct pressure or pressure with a C-clamp is applied for a period of at least 15 minutes.

Care After Test

➤ Assess vital signs every 15 minutes for the first hour, then every 30 minutes for the next hour, and then every hour for 24 hours. Assess the catheter insertion site and the integrity of the neurovascular status distal to the catheter insertion site. Note paresthesia, delayed capillary refill, cool extremities, diminished or absent pulses, and pallor in the affected extremity.

➤ If there is any evidence of bleeding or hematoma formation, or changes in the character or quality of the circulation, sensation, or motion of the extremity distal to the catheter insertion site, increase frequency of monitoring and notify the primary health care provider.

➤ Monitor the catheter insertion carefully for any evidence of bleeding or hematoma formation. Apply direct pressure, use a sandbag for pressure, or apply ice as needed to control local bleeding or hematoma formation.

➤ Maintain bed rest for 6–8 hours following the procedure to assure adequate clot formation and discourage bleeding or hematoma formation.

➤ Monitor intake and output. Encourage fluids since the contrast material has a diuretic effect.

➤ Assess for any delayed reactions to the contrast material including rashes, hives, and shortness of breath.

➤ Review related tests such as serum creatinine, creatinine clearance, blood urea nitrogen, serum electrolytes, urinalysis, renal ultrasound, and abdominal x-ray.

Educate Your Client and the Family

➤ Explain to the client the importance of drinking 2 quarts (2000 mL) of fluids a day to excrete contrast material and replace fluids lost from diuretic effect of contrast material.

➤ Instruct the client to report any changes in sensation or motion of extremity below the catheter insertion site.

Renal Biopsy

ree nal • bie op see

(Percutaneous Renal Biopsy, Kidney Biopsy)

Normal Findings

Healthy kidney tissue evidencing a Bowman's capsule, the glomerular tuft, the capillary lumen, and normal tubular sections

What This Test Will Tell You

This excision and microscopic examination of renal tissue provides kidney tissue that can be examined to assist in the differential diagnosis of kidney disease, to evaluate rejection of transplanted kidneys, or to assess the kidney's response to medical therapies. This procedure has replaced open kidney biopsies and is generally performed after renal ultrasound and computed tomography scans. The goal of the biopsy is to obtain adequate tissue from both the cortex and medulla for microscopic examination. Many times renal ultrasound or computer tomographic scans can provide a differential diagnosis without performing a biopsy.

Abnormal Findings

Abnormalities may indicate nephrosis, nephrotic syndrome, renal failure, renal malignancy, glomerulonephritis, Goodpasture's syndrome, lupus nephritis, diabetic nephropathy, Kimmelstiel-Wilson disease, or renal transplant rejection.

ACTION ALERT!

The risk of renal hemorrhage with this procedure is significant. Monitor carefully for signs of bleeding including tachycardia, diaphoresis, hypotension, thirst, hematuria, and anxiety.

Interfering Factors

➤ Inadequate tissue sample
➤ Improper handling of the tissue sample

Contraindications

➤ Coagulopathy, due to the risk of hemorrhage
➤ Operable renal tumors, because they may be seeded throughout other tissues with needle biopsy
➤ Severe hypertension
➤ Hydronephrosis, because the renal pelvis may be punctured and a persistent leak of urine may occur
➤ Urinary tract infection, because the infection may be spread
➤ Kidney abscess
➤ Advanced renal failure
➤ One functioning kidney, due to the possibility of renal injury leading to renal failure
➤ Uncooperative client, because complications such as a laceration or accidental perforation of adjacent tissues may occur

Potential Complications

➤ Hemorrhage.
➤ Hematoma formation.
➤ Infection.
➤ Accidental puncture of blood vessels or other organs. Organs include bowel, liver, lung, and spleen. Blood vessels include aorta, inferior vena cava, and renal arteries.

NURSING CONSIDERATIONS

Prepare Your Client

➤ Explain to the client and family that this is a relatively safe procedure in which kidney tissue can be obtained to look under a microscope for any problems or abnormalities.

➤ Verify that an intravenous pyelogram or renal scan has confirmed bilateral renal function.

➤ Ensure that an informed consent is obtained, because of the possible complications associated with this procedure.

➤ Assess prothrombin and partial thromboplastin time and hemoglobin and hematocrit.

➤ Restrict food and fluids for 8 hours prior to the test.

➤ Explain that clients usually experience a sense of pressure and discomfort during the procedure.

➤ Have the client void just prior to the procedure.

Perform Procedure

Nurses do not perform this procedure, but should understand the process to prepare the client and assist the physician. The client is positioned prone with a pillow or other support under the abdomen to align the spine straight. Inform the client before local anesthesia is administered that a burning sensation may be experienced before the area becomes numb. A small incision is made by the radiologist or nephrologist with sterile technique in an anesthetized area midway between the last rib and iliac crest. A biopsy needle is inserted as the client is instructed to take a deep breath. The client is then asked to hold a breath in while a specimen is collected.

When the needle is removed, direct pressure is applied to the biopsy site for 5–20 minutes and a pressure dressing is then applied. The sample is then sent to the laboratory where it is examined under light,

electron, and immunofluorescent microscopy so as to make the differential diagnosis of a renal disease or to monitor a disease's progress or responses to therapy.

Care After Test

➤ Monitor vital signs closely until stable; usually every 15 minutes for the first hour, every 30 minutes for the next hour, and then every 4 hours for 24 hours.

➤ Assess carefully for signs and symptoms of bleeding, hematoma formation or hemorrhage by assessing wound site for evidence of bleeding, decrease in blood pressure, increase in pulse rate, pallor, or back, shoulder, or flank pain. Monitor for signs of perforation of bowel or liver by assessing for abdominal rigidity, abdominal pain, and decreased bowel sounds.

➤ Instruct client to remain on bed rest in the supine (lying on back) position for 12–24 hours.

➤ Monitor the urine for presence or absence of bleeding. A very small amount of blood may be present in the urine for up to 8 hours after the procedure. Inspect the urine for obvious amounts of blood, and dipstick each sample to quantify bleeding, which may be obscure.

➤ Encourage oral fluids up to 1000 mL for 8 hours and increased fluids for at least 24 hours to prevent clot formation in the bladder of any blood that may be present.

➤ Collaborate with the primary health care provider about ordering a postprocedural hematocrit and hemoglobin to evaluate overt bleeding.

➤ Review related tests including complete blood count, blood urea nitrogen and creatinine, urinalysis, renal ultrasonography, and computed tomography (CT) scan.

Educate Your Client and the Family
➤ Explain to the client the importance of maintaining bed rest for the ordered period.
➤ Explain to the client the importance of drinking more than 2 quarts (2000 mL) of fluid each day to prevent urinary tract infections.

➤ Instruct the client to avoid for the next 2 weeks activities that could increase intra-abdominal pressure or traumatize the area (for example, contact sports, horseback riding, straining for bowel elimination, or heavy lifting).
➤ Instruct the client to report any signs of infection such as fever, chills, elevated pulse, urinary frequency, or burning on urination.

R

Renal Scan
ree nal • skan
(Renal Scanning, Kidney Scan, Renocystogram, Renogram Scan, Renogram, Nuclear Imaging of the Kidney, Triple Renal Study, Diuretic Renal Scan, Radiorenography, Renography, Radionuclide Renal Imaging, DMSA Renal Scan, DTPA Renal Scan)

Normal Findings
When radionuclide contrast material is injected, it should circulate bilaterally, symmetrically, and without delay through the kidneys, ureters, and bladder.

What This Test Will Tell You
This nuclear scanning test assesses renal tissue, plasma flow, structure, and functions. Depending on the type of radiopharmaceutical used, renal scans can evaluate acute or chronic renal diseases, renal transplant rejection, renal trauma, masses, cysts, lesions, urinary perfusion and excretion, and renovascular hypertension. These scans also evaluate renal structure, renal blood flow, nephron and collecting system function, and they may be useful in evaluating the urinary tracts of clients who are allergic to contrast materials.

Abnormal Findings
Abnormalities may indicate renovascular hypertension, tumors, urinary obstruction, pyelonephritis, impaired renal function, renal arterial atherosclerosis, traumatic injury, glomerulonephritis, abscesses, transplant rejection, congenital structural or functional defects, acute tubular necrosis, or cysts.

Interfering Factors
➤ Dehydration
➤ Radiographic contrast material within the last 24 hours

Contraindications
➤ Pregnancy, due to radiation exposure of fetus
➤ Allergy to contrast material

Potential Complications
➤ Allergic reaction including anaphylaxis

NURSING CONSIDERATIONS

Prepare Your Client

➤ Explain that this procedure is to look at the kidneys and urinary tract system.

➤ Inform client that a radioactive material is used to better study the urinary tract. Explain to the client and family that the dose is very small, so the radiation hazard is extremely low.

➤ Inform the client that the only discomfort associated with the procedure is the starting an IV (peripheral) and staying in one position for a certain period during scanning.

➤ Ensure that an informed consent is obtained, because of the possible complications associated with this procedure.

➤ Confer with the primary health care provider about administration of Lugol's solution if ^{131}I orthoiodohippurate is used to minimize thyroid uptake of the nuclear isotope.

➤ Explain that the procedure can vary in length from 1 to 4 hours.

➤ Encourage client to drink an adequate amount of fluids.

➤ Have the client void prior to the procedure.

Perform Procedure

Nurses do not perform this procedure, but should understand the process to prepare the client and assist the physician or nuclear medicine technologist. During this procedure, one or more intravenous radiopharmaceuticals are injected. Once the intravenous material has been injected, a number of x-ray films are taken at specified intervals and excretion of the radionuclide is recorded using a gamma radiographic scan. The client will be directed to assume either a prone, supine, or sitting posi-

tion while the gamma ray detector is positioned over the kidney region. A variety of agents can be used for the scanning including technetium-99m (^{99m}Tc) DTPA, technetium-99m (^{99m}Tc) DSMA, and orthoiodohippurate tagged with iodine-131 (^{131}I).

Based on that information, renogram curves are graphed for each kidney and ureter. These renograms are compared to normal reference curves to evaluate renal function.

Diuretics may be administered during this test. First, images are recorded, then a diuretic is administered and images are taken again to record the effect of diuretic therapy.

Care After Test

➤ Monitor the client carefully for signs and symptoms of allergic reactions, including anaphylaxis, to radionuclide.

➤ Handle urine with gloves for 24 hours following the procedure and wash the gloves prior to removal.

➤ Instruct the client to flush the toilet immediately after voiding and to carefully wash hands after voiding for 24 hours after the procedure.

➤ Pregnant caregivers should avoid caring for a client who has received a radionuclide material within the last 24-hour period.

➤ Encourage drinking at least 2000 mL of fluid a day unless contraindicated.

➤ Review related tests including renal computed tomography scanning, renal ultrasound, urinalysis, and blood urea nitrogen and creatinine.

Educate Your Client and the Family

➤ Instruct the client to flush the toilet immediately after use and then to carefully wash hands for 24 hours following the procedure.

➤ Instruct the client to drink at least 2 quarts (2000 mL) of fluids each day, unless contraindicated.

➤ For client with renal transplants, reinforce previous teaching concerning immunosuppressive therapy and prevention of infection.

Renin Assay

ren in • a say
(Plasma Renin Activity, PRA)

R

Normal Findings

ADULT UNDER AGE 40
Unrestricted diet: 0.3–4.3 ng/mL/hr (SI units: 0.6–4.3 µg/L/hr)
Restricted Na diet: 1.0–24.0 ng/mL/hr (SI units: 1.0–24.0 µg/L/hr)
OVER AGE 40
Unrestricted diet: 0.3–3.0 ng/mL/hr (SI units: 0.3–3.0 µg/L/hr)
Restricted Na diet: 1.0–10.8 ng/mL/hr (SI units: 1.0–10.8 µg/L/hr)
PREGNANT
Levels will normally be higher during pregnancy.
NEWBORN
<16.6 ng/mL/hr (SI units: <16.6 µg/L/hr)
CHILD, ADOLESCENT
3–6 years: <6.7 ng/mL/hr (SI units: <6.7 µg/L/hr)
6–9 years: <4.4 ng/mL/hr (SI units: <4.4 µg/L/hr)
9–12 years: <5.9 ng/mL/hr (SI units: <5.9 µg/L/hr)
12–18 years: <4.3 ng/mL/hr (SI units: <4.3 µg/L/hr)

What This Test Will Tell You

This blood test is used for differential diagnosis of essential, renal, or renovascular hypertension as well as primary hyperaldosteronism. Renin is an enzyme released by the kidneys to increase sodium and total body fluid. By activating the renin-angiotensin system, angiotensinogen is converted to angiotensin I, which is later converted to angiotensin II in the lungs. Together, angiotensin and aldosterone help increase blood pressure through sodium retention and vasoconstriction.

Abnormal Findings

▲INCREASED LEVELS may indicate hypertension of renal origin, Addison's disease, salt-losing nephropathy, hemorrhage, renin-producing renal tumors, hypokalemia, or cirrhosis.

▼DECREASED LEVELS may indicate primary aldosteronism, salt-retaining steroid therapy, antidiuretic hormone therapy, Cushing's syndrome, or essential hypertension.

ACTION ALERT!

Monitor for signs and symptoms of Addison's crisis, an emergency situation that can be fatal. These include sudden and profound weakness; severe pain in the back, abdomen, and legs; severe hyperthermia followed by hypothermia; shock; and renal failure.

Interfering Factors

➤ Hypovolemia will increase results.
➤ Levels will be higher early in the day, during pregnancy, in an upright position, and with low-salt diets.
➤ Licorice may interfere with accu-

rate results.

➤ Drugs such as diuretics, antihypertensives, estrogen, and oral contraceptives will increase levels of renin.

➤ Failure to take the specimen to the lab immediately or to keep on ice may result in inaccurate measurements.

NURSING CONSIDERATIONS

Prepare Your Client

➤ Explain that this test helps measure renin, a hormone or body chemical that helps control blood pressure.

➤ Restrict food and fluids for 8 hours prior to the test.

➤ Instruct client on a regular diet containing 180 milliequivalents (mEq) of sodium and 100 mEq of potassium, which they should consume for 3 days prior to the test.

➤ Check with your laboratory to see if client should be kept sitting upright or standing for 2 hours prior to sampling, or recumbent for 1 hour prior to sampling.

Perform Procedure

➤ Obtain 7–12 mL of venous blood in a lavender-top tube and transport immediately on ice.

➤ Note the client's position, the time, and any medications on the laboratory slip.

➤ A second, nonfasting specimen with exercise may be ordered.

Care After Test

➤ Consult with a registered dietician to assist the family and client in adapting the diet to the appropriate and recommended sodium content.

➤ Consult with the primary health care provider about obtaining ophthalmology consult for client with hypertension to screen for retinal disease.

➤ Review related tests such as plasma aldosterone levels and the renal vein renin assay.

Educate Your Client and the Family

➤ Teach appropriate self-care when a diagnosis is confirmed.

➤ Teach client the importance of taking medications that help control blood pressure even though symptoms may have disappeared.

Respiratory Syncytial Virus Antigen

ress pih rah tor ee • sin sish ahl • vie rus • an ti jen
(RSV Antigen, Enzyme Immunoassay Test for RSV)

Normal Findings

All ages: Negative for RSV antigen

What This Test Will Tell You

This analysis of respiratory tract secretions allows rapid diagnosis of respiratory syncytial virus by direct examination of nasopharyngeal secretions, tracheal aspirates, or other suitable specimens such as biopsy specimens of the lung. Respiratory syncytial virus (RSV) is the most important cause of pneumonia and bronchiolitis in infants and small children. The virus causes a wide range of respiratory illness, the most common being a cold with profuse rhinorrhea. RSV is an unusual cause of significant respiratory illness in adults, but is being seen with more frequency in immunosuppressed populations.

RSV is recovered almost exclusively from the respiratory tract. The extremely contagious virus sheds for 2–3 weeks, so rapid methods of detection are clinically important for both initiation of treatment and prevention of nosocomial spread among hospitalized children. The enzyme immunoassay test of nasopharyngeal specimens, which involves rapid detection of an antigen-antibody reaction, is the preferred diagnostic method. Additional testing may include viral culture confirmation (which may take 2–3 weeks), or serum RSV antibody titers (which may not rise in very young children).

Abnormal Findings

Positive findings indicate respiratory syncytial virus is the causative organism or one of the causative organisms of the illness.

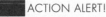ACTION ALERT!

RSV can produce life-threatening bronchiolitis and pneumonia in infants and children with congenital heart or pulmonary disease. Closely monitor for signs and symptoms of respiratory distress. Rapid deterioration resulting in cardiopulmonary arrest is possible in this population of children.

Interfering Factors

➤ Failure to place the specimen on ice for transport to the laboratory
➤ Freezing of specimens
➤ Delay in delivering specimens to the laboratory
➤ Initiation of antiviral therapy prior to obtaining specimens

Potential Complications

➤ Secretions collected by tracheal suctioning may produce transient hypoxia and require administration of supplemental oxygen.

NURSING CONSIDERATIONS R

Prepare Your Client

➤ Explain to the client or parent that this test is to detect possible infection with a severe cold virus so that medication may be given to help treat the breathing problems and cold symptoms.
➤ Describe the procedure of specimen collection and answer any questions. Explain that aspiration of secretions from the nasopharynx or trachea is necessary.
➤ Check to see if the client is receiving antiviral medication at the time of the collection, because these may cause false negative results.

Perform Procedure

➤ Obtain the specimen by aspirating the nasopharynx or throat with a suction catheter attached to an in-line suction trap or with a soft rubber bulb.
➤ Collect at least 0.5 mL of secretions.
➤ If secretions are collected with a soft rubber bulb, expel the specimen into a sterile specimen container, avoiding contamination.
➤ Place the suction trap or container in wet ice immediately.
➤ Label the container and transport to the laboratory without delay. Do not freeze.

Care After Test

➤ Observe for symptoms of hypoxia and administer oxygen after collection of specimens if indicated.

> Observe for symptoms of respiratory tract infection such as fever, rhinorrhea, malaise, or pulmonary congestion.

> Report symptoms to the primary health care provider and institute antiviral therapy, such as aerosolized ribovarin, if indicated.

> Evaluate related tests such as chest x-ray, white blood count, sputum culture and sensitivity, and RSV antibody titers.

Educate Your Client and the Family

> Instruct the client or parents to dispose of tissues in an appropriate receptacle.

> Explain that RSV is extremely contagious. Describe isolation precautions or protection of siblings if appropriate.

> Instruct client and family on the importance of compliance with antiviral therapy.

> Teach deep breathing, coughing, and other pulmonary hygiene measures if indicated.

Reticulocyte Count

reh tik yu loe site • kownt
(Retic Count)

Normal Findings

ADULT, ADOLESCENT, AND ELDERLY
Female: 0.5%–2.5%
Male: 0.5%–1.5%
PREGNANT
Reticulocyte count is elevated during pregnancy
NEWBORN
Cord blood: 3.0%–7.0%
Neonate: 0.1%–1.5%
1 day old: 3%–7%
3 days old: 1%–3%
7 days old: 0%–1%
1 month old: 0.2%–2%
1.5 months old: 0.3%–3.5%
2 months old: 0.4%–4.8%
2.5 months old: 0.3%–4.2%
3 months old: 0.3%–3.6%
4–12 months old: 0.2%–2.8%
CHILD
0.5%–3.1%

What This Test Will Tell You

This blood test evaluates anemias and assesses the effectiveness of the bone marrow in producing healthy red blood cells. In the healthy person, the red blood cell has a life span of 120 days; approximately 1% of the older red blood cells are lost daily. The bone marrow continues to produce replacement cells (reticulocytes) as needed to maintain the red blood cell count in the normal range. Reticulocytes are nonnucleated, immature red blood cells that remain in the peripheral blood for 24–48 hours while maturing.

Abnormal Findings

▲INCREASED LEVELS may indicate acquired autoimmune hemolytic anemia, Di Guglielmo disease, chronic erythemic myelosis, erythroblastosis fetalis, hemolytic anemias, chronic hemorrhage, polycythemia, hereditary herocytosis, leukemia, malaria, metastatic cancer, myxoma of left atrium of the heart, paroxysmal nocturnal hemoglobinuria, acute posthemorrhagic anemia, sickle-cell disease, thalassemia major, thrombotic thrombocytopenia purpura, or transfusion therapy.

▼DECREASED LEVELS may indicate red cell aplasia, aplastic anemia, pernicious anemia, iron deficiency anemia, folic acid deficiency, renal disease, endocrine disease, anemia of chronic disease, sideroblastic anemia, hypoplastic anemia, alcoholism, megaloblastic anemia, chronic infection, myxedema, cirrhosis of the liver, or radiation therapy.

Interfering Factors

➤ The reticulocyte count will be increased during hemolysis, pregnancy, immune reactions, the recovery phase of aplastic anemias, and in infancy.

➤ Medications that can cause a false positive result include adrenocorticotropic hormone, antimalarials, antipyretics, furazolidone, levodopa, phenacetin, and sulfonamides.

➤ Medications that can cause a false negative result include azathioprine, chloramphenicol, dactinomycin, sulfonamides, and methotrexate.

NURSING CONSIDERATIONS

Prepare Your Client

➤ Explain that this test detects anemia (too few red blood cells) or monitors the treatment for anemia.

Perform Procedure

➤ Collect 7 mL of venous blood in a lavender-top tube. The collection tube should be completely filled,

inverted, and gently rotated to thoroughly mix the anticoagulant. Don't shake the tube vigorously as this can result in hemolysis.

➤ Do not leave the tourniquet on for more than 1 minute.

➤ For young child or infant, collect blood from a finger, heel, or earlobe stick into a pipette capillary tube.

Care After Test

➤ Observe the client for signs and symptoms of anemia including pallor, dyspnea, chest pain, and fatigue.

➤ Encourage rest periods for client experiencing fatigue related to anemia.

➤ Evaluate client's ability to perform activities of daily living.

➤ Refer to community health care services as needed if client is unable to perform basic daily needs.

➤ Obtain a dietary consult to assist the client and family in choosing a well-balanced diet, including foods high in iron and vitamin B_{12}.

➤ Review related tests such as hemoglobin, hematocrit, red blood cell indices, hemoglobin electrophoresis, ferritin level, total iron-binding capacity (TIBC), bone marrow and liver biopsies, iron absorption and excretion studies, osmotic fragility, Coombs' (antiglobulin) tests, red blood cell survival test, hematocrit, platelet count, bone marrow aspiration, serum bilirubin, haptoglobin, and the complete blood count.

Educate Your Client and the Family

➤ Instruct the client in the signs and symptoms of anemia: paleness, rapid heartbeat, fainting, tiring easily, palpitations, and fatigue.

➤ Instruct the client about slowly increasing activity after blood transfusions, as the blood does not become fully oxygenated for 12–36 hours. Vigorous activity prior to this time for the anemic client can cause undue fatigue and exhaustion.

Retinol
ret in ahl
(Serum Vitamin A, Serum Carotene)

Normal Findings
VITAMIN A
All ages: 65–275 IU/dL, or 0.15–0.60 mg/mL (SI units: 0.5–2.1 mmol/L)
CAROTENE
Adult and elderly: 50–300 mg/dL (SI units: 0.9–5.6 mmol/L)
Pregnant: May be slightly elevated due to the increased intake of vitamin A during pregnancy.
Newborn: 0–40 mg/dL (SI units: 0–0.8 mmol/L)
Child: 40–130 mg/dL (SI units: 0.8–2.4 mmol/L)
Adolescent: Value range is the same as the adult range, but may be in the lower range of normal due to the decreased intake of foods rich in vitamin A (yellow or orange vegetables and fruits, green leafy vegetables).

What This Test Will Tell You
This blood test screens for fat malabsorption syndromes and biliary tract disease, helps diagnose the cause of vitamin A deficiency skin disorders, and evaluates the cause of xerophthalmia. Carotene is a fat-soluble vitamin that is absorbed from the intestines, stored in the liver, and converted to vitamin A as needed. Absorption of vitamin A requires the presence of adequate amounts of dietary fats and bile salts. Because low values may indicate poor dietary intake or malabsorption, this test is frequently used to screen for malabsorption.

Abnormal Findings
▲ INCREASED LEVELS may indicate excessive intake of vitamin A or carotene, myxedema, pancreatitis, pregnancy, oral contraceptive use, nephritis, hypercholesterolemia, or hyperlipidemia.
▼ DECREASED LEVELS may indicate low-fat diet, poor dietary intake, infectious hepatitis, hepatic disease, pancreatic insufficiency, malabsorption, celiac disease, cystic fibrosis, obstructive jaundice, steatorrhea, or kwashiorkor.

Interfering Factors
➤ A diet high in vitamin A or carotene will cause elevated test results (yellow and green vegetables and fruits, milk, milk products, egg yolks, fish oils, and liver).
➤ Ingestion of mineral oil will interfere with carotene absorption, resulting in lower serum values.
➤ Hemolysis of or shaking the specimen may interfere with the test results.
➤ Failure to protect the specimen from light after collection may result in falsely low results.
➤ A low-fat diet may cause a

decrease in the test results.

➤ Falsely elevated levels may be associated with pregnancy, the use of oral contraceptives, hyperlipidemia, hypercholesterolemia, diabetes, nephritis, and hypothyroidism.

NURSING CONSIDERATIONS

Prepare Your Client

➤ Explain that this test is important to identify how well the body is using and storing vitamin A.

➤ Restrict food and fluids (except water) for 8 hours prior to the test.

➤ Explain that all vitamin supplements containing vitamin A should be omitted for 24 hours prior to the test.

➤ Instruct the client to eliminate carotene-rich or vitamin A–rich foods for 2–3 days prior to the test. These include yellow and green vegetables and fruits, milk, milk products, egg yolks, fish oils, and liver.

➤ If the primary health care provider wishes to evaluate the client's ability to absorb carotene, instruct the client about a high-carotene diet.

Perform Procedure

➤ Collect 7 mL of venous blood in a red-top tube.

➤ Place the specimen in a bag to protect it from light.

➤ Handle the specimen gently to prevent hemolysis, which could alter the test results.

Care After Test

➤ If dietary insufficiency is discovered, consult with a registered dietician to assist the family and client to increase dietary intake of vitamin A.

➤ Evaluate the client's vision, as vitamin A is essential for normal vision and the prevention of night blindness.

➤ Evaluate other diagnostic tests such as electroretinogram, cholesterol levels, blood glucose levels, serum lipid levels, thyroxine levels, and liver enzymes.

Educate Your Client and the Family

➤ If the client's vitamin A level is low, instruct the client regarding foods rich in vitamin A and carotene (fish, eggs, meat, poultry, green leafy vegetables, and yellow fruits and vegetables).

➤ If vision is impaired, or xerophthalmia is present, emphasize the importance of follow-up with an ophthalmologist.

Retrograde Pyelography

ret roe grade • pie eh log rah fee
(Retrograde Urograms, Retrograde Ureteropyelography)

Normal Findings

Symmetrical and equal flow of contrast material through the calyxes, pelvises, and ureters.

What This Test Will Tell You

This radiographic test assesses the urinary collecting system including the calyxes, renal pelvises, and ureters in order to identify any obstructions in urine flow. The test is helpful in evaluating the collecting system when an intravenous pyelogram cannot be performed or when the intravenous pyelogram does not provide adequate diagnostic information. Indications for a retrograde pyelogram include unilateral ureteral obstruction and severely decreased renal plasma flow. This type of study will also help delineate renal calculi, tumors, ureteral strictures, or other filling defects.

Abnormal Findings

The x-ray may reveal ureteral calculi, tumors, strictures, congenital anomalies, or obstructions.

███████ ACTION ALERT!

Assess clients carefully for allergic reaction to contrast material, including dyspnea, itching, urticaria, flushing, hypotension, and shock. Life-threatening anaphylactic reactions can occur and need to be recognized and treated immediately.

Interfering Factors

➤ Retained barium for gastrointestinal x-rays

Contraindications

➤ Severe allergy to radiopaque dye, unless modifications in testing are made

Potential Complications

➤ Urinary tract infections or sepsis, due to instrumentation and possible seeding of bacteria
➤ Bladder perforation
➤ Allergic reactions to the radiopaque dye
➤ Disruption of urinary flow in the ureters, due to temporary edema

NURSING CONSIDERATIONS

Prepare Your Client

➤ Explain that this is an x-ray procedure to help evaluate the urinary collecting system from the kidneys to the bladder.

➤ Assess for allergies to contrast dye.
➤ Ensure that an informed consent is obtained, because of the possible complications associated with this procedure.
➤ Administer laxatives or enemas as ordered to cleanse the bowel and increase the quality of imaging.
➤ Restrict food and fluids for 8 hours prior to the test if general anesthesia is planned. Do not restrict food or fluids if no anesthesia is planned.
➤ Assess baseline vital signs.
➤ Explain to client that without anesthesia, the procedure may be somewhat uncomfortable and they may experience an urgency to void.
➤ Explain to the client that the procedure takes about 60–90 minutes.

Perform Procedure

Nurses do not perform this procedure, but should understand the process to prepare the client and assist the physician. The client is positioned with feet in stirrups. A urologist performs this test during a cystoscopy by catheterizing the ureters and then injecting radiopaque dye into the ureters. Once the renal pelvises have been drained, contrast material is injected into the catheter(s). A series of x-rays are taken. Then the catheters are removed, and further x-rays are taken during their removal and approximately 10 minutes after the catheter(s) are removed.

Care After Test

➤ Monitor vital signs closely until stable; usually every 15 minutes for the first hour, every 30 minutes for the next hour, and then every 4 hours for 24 hours.
➤ Assess patterns of urinary elimi-

nation for alterations, particularly urinary retention.

➤ Monitor temperature and signs of symptoms of infections including fever, chills, hypotension, and tachycardia.

➤ Encourage drinking 2–3 quarts (2000–3000 mL) of fluid per day unless contraindicated.

➤ Monitor for any signs or symptoms of a delayed allergic reaction to the contrast material including rash, hives, dyspnea, and increased heart rate.

➤ Review related test including blood urea nitrogen, creatinine, intravenous pyelogram, renal scan, renal computed tomography scan, and renal arteriogram.

Educate Your Client and the Family

➤ Teach the importance of fluid intake, if permitted, to help the body eliminate the contrast material.

➤ If renal calculi are present, teach the client dietary modifications that may help reduce stone formation including getting enough fluids, and acidification or alkalinization of urine as indicated.

Rheumatoid Factor

roo mah toid · fak tur

(RF, RA, RA Latex, RF with Titer)

Normal Findings

ADULT, INFANT, CHILD, ADOLESCENT, PREGNANT
Negative: < 60 IU/mL by nephelometric testing; < 1:20 titer
ELDERLY
May be slightly elevated

What This Test Will Tell You

This blood test helps diagnose rheumatoid arthritis by measuring the serum level of rheumatoid factor, the IgG, IgA, and IgM autoantibodies that react with the crystallizable fraction of IgG. Rheumatoid factor (RF) is not specific to rheumatoid arthritis; however, the levels are usually higher in these clients. Although this is a frequently ordered diagnostic test, recent studies have revealed limitations in the test's specificity, sensitivity, and predictive values. False positive and false negative results occur, making it important to consider clinical findings when ordering this test. Synovial fluid may also be tested for RF, and the results often correlate strongly with blood specimen results. However, RF may be positive in synovial fluid and negative in serum.

Abnormal Findings

Positive results may indicate rheumatoid arthritis, systemic lupus erythematosus, dermatomyositis, scleroderma, liver cirrhosis, early rheumatoid arthritis, bacterial endocarditis, advanced age, mononucleosis, tuberculosis, leukemia, hepatitis, syphilis, chronic infection, or juvenile rheumatoid arthritis.

Interfering Factors

➤ Gold therapy decreases the RF titer.

➤ Indicate on the lab slip if mononucleosis or Epstein-Barr virus is clinically suspected. Heterophile antibodies may lead to in vitro production of RF by human B cells.

➤ Elderly clients may have false positive results.

NURSING CONSIDERATIONS

Prepare Your Client

➤ Explain that this test is used to diagnose a form of arthritis called rheumatoid arthritis.

Perform Procedure

➤ Collect 5–10 mL of venous blood into a red-top tube.

Care After Test

➤ Evaluate your client for joint stiffness, pain, edema, warmth, and erythema resulting from rheumatoid arthritis. Morning stiffness and fatigue are two classic signs of rheumatoid arthritis.

➤ Ensure client is referred for physical therapy as indicated by their ability to perform activities of daily living or manage symptoms of pain.

➤ Refer to community agency resources if activities of daily living cannot be performed independently.

➤ Review related tests including complete blood count (CBC), erythrocyte sedimentation rate (ESR), C-reactive protein (CRP), antinuclear antibody (ANA), blood cultures, sputum cultures, lupus erythematosus test, and radiographic studies.

Educate Your Client and the Family

➤ If the client is diagnosed with rheumatoid arthritis, explain that daily range-of-motion and muscle strengthening exercises are important in maintaining flexibility of the joints.

➤ Pain control is a major goal for clients with rheumatoid arthritis. Instruct your client and family members about the use of warm or cold applications to control pain. The client will need to determine which is most effective to ease individual discomforts. Inform your client that resting the affected joint will ease pain.

➤ If anti-inflammatory medications have been prescribed, instruct your client to take the medication with food.

➤ Offer emotional support to your client and family members. Refer them to local support and educational groups.

Rh Typing

R • H • tie ping
(Blood Typing, Rh Antigen Typing, Rh Factor)

Normal Findings

Each client's blood is classified as either Rh-positive or Rh-negative.

What This Test Will Tell You

The Rh blood typing test indicates the presence or absence of the Rh antigen D, which is found on the surface of the red blood cell. Rh factor is important to determine before transfusion to prevent blood incompatibility. Hemolytic reactions may follow transfusion of mismatched blood, although Rh-incompatible blood may also start a less serious reaction within several days to 2 weeks of the transfusion when the client presents with fever, an unexplained drop in the hemoglobin level, and jaundice. Rh reactions are most likely to occur in women sensitized by red blood cell antigens via prior pregnancies or in persons who have received more than five blood or blood-product transfusions.

Abnormal Findings

Not applicable

 ACTION ALERT!

The Rh-negative (Rh−) client with evidence of fetal Rh-positive (Rh+) blood in her circulatory system will need an injection of Rh_0(D) immune globulin (RhoGAM) within 72 hours of delivery to prevent maternal isoimmunization. (See *Erythrocyte Distribution.*)

Interfering Factors

➤ Hemolyzed specimen invalidates the results.
➤ Drawing specimen from an extremity into which blood products or dextran is infusing invalidates the results.
➤ Medications that may result in a false-positive Rh test include levodopa, methyldopa, and methyldopate hydrochloride.
➤ Rh factor may be changed or suppressed by leukemia, cancer, multiple transfusions, transplantation, or septicemia.

NURSING CONSIDERATIONS

Prepare Your Client

➤ Explain that this test determines one part of blood type, which is used to match the appropriate blood donor in the event of transfusion. If appropriate, explain that blood will be drawn to determine the amount of medicine needed to protect a developing baby from blood incompatibility in future pregnancies.

Perform Procedure

➤ Collect 7–10 mL of venous blood in a red-top tube.

Care After Test

➤ If the client is receiving a blood transfusion as a result of the Rh typing, monitor closely for signs and symptoms of blood incompatibility including chills, fever, urticaria, tachycardia, dyspnea, nausea, vomiting, tightness in the chest, chest and back pain, hypotension, bronchospasm, angioedema, pulmonary edema, congestive heart failure, and shock.
➤ Evaluate other tests such as the hemoglobin, hematocrit, direct and indirect Coomb's (antiglobulin)

tests, blood typing (ABO compatibility), and serum bilirubin.

Educate Your Client and the Family
➤ Instruct the client about slowly increasing activity after blood transfusion, for the blood does not become fully oxygenated for 12–36 hours. Vigorous activity by the anemic client too soon can result in undue fatigue and exhaustion.
➤ Encourage your client to carry a blood type identification card at all times to protect them in an emergency.

Riboflavin
rie boe flay vin
(Urine Vitamin B_2)

Normal Findings
ALL AGES
Male: 0.51 mg/24 hours (SI units: 1.3 nmol/24 hours)
Female: 0.39 mg/24 hours (SI units: 1.0 nmol/24 hours)
PREGNANT
Levels may be slightly decreased due to the increased demand during pregnancy.

What This Test Will Tell You
This urine test detects vitamin B_2 deficiency by measuring the urine levels.

Abnormal Findings
▼DECREASED LEVELS may indicate periods of high metabolic demand (pregnancy, lactation, wound healing), inadequate intake of milk and protein, prolonged diarrhea, chronic alcoholism, anorexia, liver disease, stress, malabsorption, hypothyroidism, neuropathy, anemia, malignancy, pellagra, or phototherapy of infants with jaundice.

Interfering Factors
➤ Failure to collect all urine during the 24-hour testing period will alter test results.
➤ Failure to protect the urine specimen from light may alter test results.
➤ Contamination of the specimen with stool or toilet tissue may alter test results.
➤ Consumption of riboflavin-rich foods (milk products, organ meats, fish, green leafy vegetables, legumes, whole grains) may cause a falsely elevated test result.

NURSING CONSIDERATIONS
Prepare Your Client
➤ Explain that this test is important to determine if the client has enough vitamin B_2, also called riboflavin.
➤ Explain that vitamin B_2 levels can vary daily and that the test may need to be repeated.
➤ Assess the client's normal dietary intake, especially of foods rich in B_2.
➤ Explain that the test will require a 24-hour urine collection.
➤ Explain the correct method for a 24-hour urine collection, including protection of the specimen from light.
➤ Instruct the client to maintain a normal diet before the test.

> Obtain a large (approximately 1-gallon) opaque plastic container with a tight-fitting lid for the collection of the urine specimen.

Perform Procedure
> Collect all urine for 24 hours.
> Protect the specimen from light.

Care After Test
> Evaluate and assess for a sore mouth, sore throat, photophobia (sensitivity to light), seborrheic dermatitis of the face, trunk or scrotum, or excessive fatigue, and report to the primary health care provider as these symptoms may indicate a riboflavin deficiency.
> Consult with a registered dietician to assist the family and client in meeting vitamin B_2 dietary needs.

> Review related tests such as serum glutathione, complete blood count with differential, serum protein, and serum electrolytes.

Educate Your Client and the Family
> Instruct the client regarding dietary sources of vitamin B_2 (milk products, organ meats, fish, green leafy vegetables, legumes, and whole grains).
> Instruct the client that milk should be kept in opaque containers to prevent photodegradation of the riboflavin.
> Explain that an adequate ongoing intake of riboflavin-rich foods is needed to correct a vitamin B_2 deficiency.

R

Rotavirus Antigen, Fecal
roe tah vie russ • an ti jen • fee kal
(Orbivirus; Rotavirus; Reovirus-like Agent; Duovirus; Gastroenteritis Virus; Rotavirus Antigen, Feces)

Normal Findings
All Ages: No evidence of rotavirus in the specimen. The detection of rotavirus in neonates less than 2 weeks old is inconclusive.

What This Test Will Tell You
This enzyme immunoassay test of the stool helps diagnose the cause of diarrhea, most often in infants and children. Rotavirus is a member of the reovirus group and is considered the most frequent cause of infectious diarrhea in infants and young children.

Abnormal Findings
Presence of the rotavirus in stool

indicates infectious gastroenteritis.

ACTION ALERT!
Rotavirus infections are easily transmitted by the fecal-oral route and precautions, most importantly handwashing, must be taken to prevent the spread of the virus.

Interfering Factors
> Improper collection techniques such as failure to use a clean, dry collection container or failure to collect enough stool sample may alter the test results.
> Use of collection containers with metal ions, detergents, blood, or preservatives may alter results.
> The presence of urine, toilet tis-

sue, or blood may alter results.

➤ Failure to transport the warm stool specimen to the laboratory may alter results.

➤ The virus is maximally present in the specimen during the first 3 days of infection and is greatly diminished by the eighth day.

NURSING CONSIDERATIONS

Prepare Your Client

➤ Explain to the client (or parent if the client is a child or infant) that the test is important to help find the cause of diarrhea.

➤ Explain that the test will require the collection of a stool specimen.

➤ Instruct the client or family to notify the nurse as soon as the specimen is obtained so the warm specimen can be taken to the laboratory.

Perform Procedure

➤ Obtain a clean, dry, preservative-free cardboard or plastic container.

➤ If a rectal swab is to be performed, obtain a sterile, preservative-free swab container.

STOOL COLLECTION

➤ Obtain approximately 5 mL of stool and place it in the specimen collection container.

➤ Label and transport the specimen to the laboratory while the specimen is still warm. If immediate transport is not possible, place on ice and transport as soon as possible.

RECTAL SWAB

➤ Place the client in a left lateral position with the hips and knees flexed.

➤ Insert the sterile swab at least 2.5–3 cm into the rectum.

➤ Rotate the swab side to side and leave it in place for a few seconds to allow for absorption. The swab must be heavily coated with stool to provide reliable results.

➤ Place the swab into a sterile container.

Care After Test

➤ Monitor consistency and amount of stool.

➤ Monitor for the signs and symptoms of dehydration and electrolyte depletion.

➤ Provide fluids to the client to avoid dehydration from diarrhea and vomiting.

➤ Monitor the client's skin for breakdown in the perianal area and use a soothing emollient or protectant to prevent excoriation due to the diarrhea.

➤ Review related tests such as serum electrolytes, stool cultures, and stool for ova and parasites.

Educate Your Client and the Family

➤ Instruct the client or family to cleanse the area around the anus thoroughly after each stool to decrease skin irritation.

➤ For the infant, instruct the parent/caregiver to change the diaper as soon as soiled to decrease skin irritation.

➤ Teach your client and family that the virus spreads from contaminated human feces to hands to food or drink and thus to another person (the fecal-oral route). Discuss the necessity of good handwashing after handling any contaminated materials.

Rubella Antibody

roo bel ah • an ti bod ee

(Hemagglutination Inhibition Reaction, Hemagglutination Inhibition, HAI, HI, German Measles Test, 3-Day Measles Test)

Normal Findings

Susceptible to rubella: titer < 1:8
Past rubella exposure: titer of 1:10–1:32
Immunity: titer of 1:32–1:64
Definite immunity: titer > 1:64

What This Test Will Tell You

This blood test determines serum rubella antibody titer in women of childbearing age. Rubella is a viral infection that has few complications or side effects in children and adults. However, the disease causes spontaneous abortion, stillbirth, or serious deformities (congenital rubella syndrome) in the fetus if the mother contracts the virus during pregnancy, especially during the first 2 months of gestation.

The rubella titer rises rapidly after infection. The acute titer should be obtained 3 days after the rash appears. A convalescent titer should be taken 2 weeks later. A fourfold or greater rise in antibody titer in the two samples indicates a recent rubella infection. A serologic titer that remains the same or declines indicates the client was infected with rubella in the past.

Abnormal Findings

The test may reveal rubella.

Interfering Factors

➤ Recent rubella vaccination

NURSING CONSIDERATIONS

Prepare Your Client

➤ Explain that this test is important to see if they can still catch 3-day measles (rubella infection).
➤ If this is a serologic test, instruct client to return for another specimen collection in 2 weeks.

Perform Procedure

➤ Collect 3–10 mL of venous blood in a red-top tube.

Care After Test

➤ Assess your client for a rash if active disease is suspected.
➤ Evaluate other laboratory tests such as IgM and IgG ELISA (enzyme-linked immunosorbent assay).

Educate Your Client and the Family

➤ Explain the importance of rubella immunization for children 15 months of age or older and women of childbearing age who do not have rubella immunity. Immunization of this population will help prevent infection of pregnant women.
➤ Discuss with your childbearing-age client the importance of knowing her rubella immunity. If she is not immune, encourage her to get a rubella vaccine and to avoid pregnancy for 3 months after the vaccine.
➤ If your client is pregnant and does not have immunity, tell her to avoid children with respiratory infections as this may be a symptom of the initial stage of rubella.

Schilling Test

shil ing • test

(Vitamin B_{12} Absorption)

Normal Findings

ADULT, CHILD, AND
ADOLESCENT

7%–40% of the original dose of radioactive vitamin B_{12} appears in the 24-hour urine specimen in Stage I and in Stage II. Not performed during pregnancy or on infants.

ELDERLY

Values may be slightly reduced from the adult values due to the reduced rate of excretion of vitamin B_{12}.

What This Test Will Tell You

This urine test determines the vitamin B_{12} absorption in the diagnosis of pernicious anemia and malabsorption syndromes related to lack of intrinsic factor. Vitamin B_{12} taken orally in the diet cannot be absorbed from the gastrointestinal tract without the presence of intrinsic factor, which is produced by the gastric mucosa. Normally, any excess vitamin B_{12} absorbed from the gastrointestinal tract is excreted in the urine.

This test is performed by administering radioactive B_{12} orally, followed by an intramuscular injection of nonradioactive B_{12} to saturate binding sites. If the radioactive B_{12} is absorbed from the gut in the presence of normal amounts of intrinsic factor, it should be eliminated in the urine due to its excess quantity. If inadequate amounts of radioactive B_{12} are found in the urine, that demonstrates that the tagged B_{12} was never absorbed from the gut.

Abnormal Findings

▼DECREASED LEVELS may indicate pernicious anemia, intestinal malabsorption (Crohn's disease, ileal disease or resection, bacterial overgrowth after antibiotic therapy), postgastrectomy, cystic fibrosis, hypothyroidism, or liver disease.

ACTION ALERT!

Anaphylactic reaction is possible to the radionuclide used. Assess for dyspnea, hives, itching, anxiety, hypotension, and tachycardia.

Interfering Factors

➤ If the client has received radioactive nuclear material within 10 days of the testing, the test results may be altered.

➤ Clients with diabetes, kidney disease, liver disease, pancreatic insufficiency, hypothyroidism, or those who are elderly may have a reduced rate of excretion of the vitamin B_{12}.

➤ Contamination of the urine specimen by toilet tissue, stool, or blood may alter the test results.

➤ Use of laxatives may alter the test results as they decrease the rate of vitamin B_{12} absorption.

➤ Clients who have had a partial gastrectomy will have altered test results due to the lack of intrinsic factor.

➤ Repeating the Schilling test in less than 5 days may alter the test results due to the residual effects of the previous doses of radioactive medications.

➤ Incomplete collection of the urine during the specified time frame can alter the test results.

➤ Improper storage of the urine during the test may alter the test results.

➤ Failure to fast prior to the test may interfere with the test results.

Contraindications

➤ Do not perform this test if the client is pregnant as the radioactive medications may harm the fetus.
➤ Do not perform this test if the client is lactating.
➤ Do not perform this test on infants.

Potential Complications

➤ Possible anaphylactic reaction to the radionuclide

NURSING CONSIDERATIONS

Prepare Your Client

➤ Explain that this test is used to determine the body's ability to absorb vitamin B_{12}, which is needed to form red blood cells.
➤ Restrict food and fluids, except for water, for 8–12 hours prior to the test.
➤ Instruct the client to avoid the use of laxatives during the test period and for at least 24 hours prior to the test.
➤ Explain that the test is performed in 2 steps, with the client receiving an oral medication first and an injection 2 hours later. Results will come from a 24-hour urine collection.
➤ Check the client's history for exposure to radioactive materials within 10 days before the test.
➤ If bone marrow studies are ordered, be sure that they are completed prior to starting the Schilling test.
➤ Obtain a 3-L urine container without preservatives.
➤ Monitor the client's kidney function prior to the test. If the blood urea nitrogen or creatinine levels are elevated, collaborate with the pri-

mary health care provider as to whether to extend the urine collection from 24 hours to 48 hours.

Perform Procedure

➤ Resume normal diet once the injection has been given.

STAGE I

➤ Instruct the client to void and discard the urine.
➤ Administer 0.5 µg vitamin B_{12} tagged with radioactive cobalt orally.
➤ Observe the person carefully for up to 60 minutes after the oral medication for possible anaphylactic reaction to the radionuclide.
➤ Begin the 24-hour urine collection with the urine specimen kept on ice or in the refrigerator.
➤ After 2 hours give 1000 µg of non-radioactive vitamin B_{12} intramuscularly.
➤ Use rubber gloves when handling urine for 24 hours following the procedure due to the radioactive contamination of the urine. Be sure to wash the gloves with soap and water before removing them and follow by washing ungloved hands with soap and water.
➤ Instruct the client to thoroughly wash hands with soap and water after each voiding.
➤ Collect all urine for 24 hours. If the client has an elevated blood urea nitrogen or creatinine, the collection may extend to 48 hours.
➤ Label and send the entire specimen to the laboratory.

STAGE II

➤ If indicated, the second stage will be performed about 1 week after the first stage of the test.
➤ Instruct the client to void and discard the urine.
➤ Administer 0.5 µg of radioactive vitamin B_{12} orally and 60 mg of

intrinsic factor orally to the fasting client.

➤ Begin the 24-hour urine collection and store the specimen on ice or in the refrigerator.

➤ 2 hours after the test begins, administer 1000 μg of nonradioactive vitamin B_{12} intramuscularly.

➤ Collect all urine for the 24- or 48-hour period.

➤ Continue all handwashing procedures and precautions as discussed in Stage I.

Care After Test

➤ Encourage rest periods for client experiencing fatigue related to anemia.

➤ Evaluate client's ability to perform activities of daily living.

➤ Refer to community health care services as needed if client is unable to perform basic daily needs.

➤ Consult with a registered dietician to design optimal nutritional dietary plan.

➤ Review related tests such as hemoglobin, hematocrit, reticulocyte count, red blood cell indices, globin chain analysis, hemoglobin electrophoresis, peripheral blood smear for Heinz bodies, serum bilirubin, and urine bilirubin.

Educate Your Client and the Family

➤ If the test results indicate pernicious anemia, instruct the client that they will require vitamin B_{12} injections on a regular schedule (weekly at first, then monthly for maintenance). Teach client or family how to perform injections.

➤ Teach client to continue light physical activity if experiencing fatigue, but to rest when needed and not to plan too strenuous or prolonged activities.

➤ Inform client that maintaining regular patterns of sleep, rest, and activity are important to prevent fatigue.

➤ Stress the importance of a well-balanced diet to provide optimal energy stores.

Sella Turcica X-ray
sel ah • tur si kah • eks ray

Normal Findings

ADULT AND ELDERLY
Normal varies greatly. May be round or oval, deep or shallow. 58% appear oval.

CHILD AND ADOLESCENT
Normal varies greatly. May be round or oval, deep or shallow. May have a biconcave appearance. 70% appear round.

What This Test Will Tell You

This radiographic test helps diagnose tumors of the pituitary. Radiographs of the sella turcica, a bony area at the base of the skull, may be evaluated for size, shape, and depth and correlated with other clinical findings.

Interfering Factors

➤ There are great variations of normal among both children and adults, making inferences from this test difficult.

➤ Foreign objects such as hair pins, prosthetic eyes, dentures, and jewelry interfere with imaging.

Abnormal Findings

Double-contoured appearance may indicate a tumor (pituitary adenoma), unilateral enlargement may indicate intracavernous aneurysm of the internal carotid artery, general enlargement may indicate hydrocephalus, and decreased size may indicate prolonged cerebrospinal fluid shunting.

Contraindications

➤ Generally not performed during pregnancy or in newborns

NURSING CONSIDERATIONS

Prepare Your Client

➤ Explain that this test is to look for any problems in a gland, located in the brain, called the pituitary gland.

➤ Inform client they will be asked to remain very still while x-rays are taken in several positions, and that the test is painless.

➤ Remove all clothing, jewelry, glasses, hearing aids, and objects in the hair from the neck up.

Perform Procedure

➤ The radiologic technician takes several x-rays of the skull from different views, including axial, half-axial, posteroanterior, and lateral.

Care After Test

➤ Observe for signs and symptoms of pituitary dysfunction including visual disturbances, growth disorders in children, hypertension, polycythemia, osteoporosis, and amenorrhea and masculinization in females.

➤ Review related tests such as adrenocorticotropic hormone (ACTH), growth hormone, and prolactin hormone levels.

Educate Your Client and the Family

➤ Explain the importance of other endocrine tests being performed, since this test is of little value alone.

➤ If hormone replacement therapy is prescribed, instruct client or family on the importance of taking medication regularly and consulting the primary health care provider promptly when illness or stress are experienced.

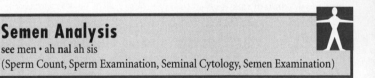

Semen Analysis
see men • ah nal ah sis
(Sperm Count, Sperm Examination, Seminal Cytology, Semen Examination)

Normal Findings

Sperm count: 20 million to 200 million/mL

Sperm motility: 60%–80%

Sperm morphology: >70% normally shaped

Liquification time: 20–30 minutes after collection

pH of fluid: 7.1–8.0

Appearance: white, gray-white, gelatinous

Odor: musty

Volume: 0.7–6.5 mL

What This Test Will Tell You

This body fluid analysis is used to evaluate male infertility, confirm success of a vasectomy, and collect evidence for rape cases. Semen contains spermatozoa in seminal fluid. For fertility testing, sperm is collected after 2–3 days of sexual abstinence and examined for volume, sperm count, motility, and morphology. Semen analysis should be done two or more times because the sperm count varies from day to day. A semen analysis is also performed to verify sterilization 6 weeks postvasectomy and in rape cases to detect semen on the body or clothing.

Abnormal Findings

▼DECREASED LEVELS may reveal infertility, vasectomy, orchitis, testicular atrophy, testicular failure, and Klinefelter's syndrome. A sperm count less than 20 million/mL is associated with infertility.

Interfering Factors

➤ Cimetidine, estrogens, methyltestosterone, and antineoplastic agents may decrease semen levels.
➤ An incomplete specimen from faulty collection diminishes the volume of the specimen.
➤ Delayed delivery of the specimen can decrease the number of sperm.
➤ Exposure of the specimen to extremes of temperature or direct sunlight may affect results.
➤ Toxic chemicals in the specimen container or condom alter results.

NURSING CONSIDERATIONS

Prepare Your Client

➤ Explain that the test measures sperm and is used to evaluate infertility or check the effectiveness of a vasectomy. For rape victims, explain that collection of fluid will help gather evidence for prosecuting the crime.
➤ Explain that the test is performed on the sperm sample in the laboratory.

FERTILITY TESTING
➤ Instruct the client to abstain from sexual activity for 2–3 days before collecting a sperm sample. Discourage prolonged abstinence because the quality and motility of sperm cells may decrease.
➤ Instruct the client not to drink alcohol for several days before the test.
➤ Explain that the best specimen requires masturbation in the health care provider's office.
➤ Instruct client who is collecting the sperm specimen at home to deliver the specimen to the laboratory within 1 hour.
➤ Instruct the client not to expose the specimen to extreme temperatures or direct sunlight.
➤ Instruct client collecting the specimen in a condom to wash the condom with soap and water, rinse, and allow it to dry before using. Powders and lubricants applied to the condom may be spermicidal. Instruct the client to tie the condom after collection, place it in a jar, and deliver it to the laboratory.

RAPE VICTIM SEMEN COLLECTION
➤ Explain how vaginal fluid or other samples will be collected, and, if appropriate, that clothing will also be sent to the laboratory.
➤ Provide emotional support.

Perform Procedure

INFERTILITY TESTING
➤ Provide a clean container for specimen collection by masturbation in a laboratory or medical office. Alternatively, collection of the specimen can occur at home through masturbation or interruption of sexual intercourse. The specimen needs to be trans-

ported to the laboratory within 1 hour.

RAPE VICTIM SEMEN COLLECTION

➤ Prepare client for insertion of an unlubricated vaginal speculum.

➤ Send clothing in a paper bag (plastic causes semen stains to mold) to the laboratory.

➤ The specimen is obtained by aspiration, saline lavage, or a vaginal smear.

➤ Label all slides and lab slips carefully. You may be questioned about the specimen's integrity.

➤ Send the specimen to the laboratory immediately.

Care After Test

➤ Explain when and how to obtain test results. Results are usually available in 24 hours.

➤ Refer a rape victim to an appropriate counselor.

➤ Review related tests for infertility including levels of thyroid-stimulating hormone, thyrotropin-releasing hormone factor, and adrenocorticotropic hormone.

Educate Your Client and the Family

➤ Teach client that infertility may be related to either the male or female partner.

➤ Provide information to client and partner on infertility support groups.

Sialography

sie ah log rah fee
(X-Ray of the Salivary Ducts)

Normal Findings

Absence of tumors, calculi, strictures, or inflammatory processes

What This Test Will Tell You

This x-ray with contrast is used to diagnose pathology in the client who has pain, tenderness, or swelling in the area associated with the salivary glands. The test examines the salivary ducts including the parotid, submaxillary, submandibular, and sublingual as well as related glandular structures.

Abnormal Findings

Abnormalities may indicate calculi, strictures, tumors, and inflammatory disease.

Interfering Factors

➤ Metal objects in the hair or on the face and head as well as dentures may interfere with imaging.

Contraindications

➤ Allergy to contrast material, unless procedure is modified.

➤ Oral infections.

➤ Hyperthyroidism, which the iodinated dye may exacerbate.

➤ Pregnancy, unless benefit outweighs risk. Shielding of the abdomen is used to prevent radiation exposure of the fetus.

Potential Complications

➤ Allergic reaction to the iodinated dye is possible but rarely occurs as the dye is not given intravenously.

NURSING CONSIDERATIONS

Prepare Your Client

➤ Explain that this test is to identify the cause of the client's symptoms of pain, tenderness, or swelling in the salivary ducts.

➤ Explain that the test requires the injection of the dye into the client's mouth.

➤ Remove jewelry, hairpins, and dentures as they may obscure the x-ray visualization.

➤ Instruct the client to rinse their mouth with an antiseptic solution to decrease the risk of bacteria entering the ductal structures.

Perform Procedure

Nurses do not perform this procedure, but should understand the process to prepare the client and assist the radiologist. X-rays are taken first to rule out calculi of the salivary glands and ductal system that would impair drainage. Inform the client that there may be a feeling of slight pressure when the contrast medium is injected into the ducts. The client is then placed in a supine position, contrast medium is injected directly into the desired duct using a special cannula, and more x-rays are taken. Next, the client is given a sour substance to stimulate salivation and another set of x-rays are taken to evaluate the ductal drainage.

Care After Test

➤ Encourage drinking fluids to help eliminate the contrast material.

➤ Consult with the primary health care provider regarding heat or cold therapy for comfort to inflamed or painful areas.

➤ Administer analgesics if ordered and evaluate effectiveness.

➤ Review related tests such as x-rays of the face or head.

Educate Your Client and the Family

➤ Instruct the client to thoroughly rinse the mouth and brush the teeth following this test to help get rid of dye.

Sigmoidoscopy

sig moy dos koe pee

(Proctoscopy, Anoscopy, Proctosigmoidoscopy)

Normal Findings

All ages: Anus, rectum and sigmoid colon of normal structure with patent lumen

What This Test Will Tell You

This endoscopic test evaluates changes in bowel habits, chronic constipation, bright red blood in the stool or mucus in the stool as a part of an annual physical examination, and can be used to biopsy gastrointestinal tissue. This test visualizes the anus, rectum, and sigmoid colon. The sigmoidoscopy may be used therapeutically for the reduction of a sigmoid volvulus (torsion of a loop of the intestine), removal of polyps, and removal of hemorrhoids. The test can be performed with a rigid or flexible sigmoidoscope.

Abnormal Findings

Abnormalities may reveal benign or

malignant tumors, polyps, bowel obstruction, ulcerative colitis, diverticulosis, diverticulitis, Crohn's disease, pseudomembranous colitis, intestinal ischemia, irritable bowel syndrome, granulomatous colitis, malabsorption syndrome, or celiac sprue.

■ ACTION ALERT!

➤ Monitor the client carefully for increasing temperature, severe abdominal pain, and/or rigidity of the abdomen following the procedure. These symptoms may indicate peritonitis from perforation of the internal organs.

➤ Do not give laxative or enema preparations to pregnant clients in preparation for this examination as they may stimulate labor.

➤ Do not give laxative or enema preparations to the client with ulcerative colitis as this could cause a worsening of the client's condition.

➤ Monitor activated partial thromboplastin time, prothrombin time, and bleeding time before performing this test. Prolonged coagulation indicates an increased risk of hemorrhage.

Interfering Factors

➤ Retained barium from previous gastrointestinal x-rays makes visualization impossible.

➤ Previous surgical intervention or radiation therapy to the bowel may inhibit the passage of the sigmoidoscope or make the tissues susceptible to damage.

➤ Incomplete evacuation of stool or improper bowel preparation may prevent visualization.

➤ Rectal bleeding can obstruct the lens system of the sigmoidoscope and prevent adequate visualization.

➤ Placement of tissue and cell specimens in the solution without a preservative can cause false results.

➤ Use of fixative sprays may distort the cells.

Contraindications

➤ Uncooperative client who does not remain still may be injured by the sigmoidoscope.

➤ Diverticulitis makes colon more readily irritated and/or perforated.

➤ Painful anorectal conditions such as fissures, fistulas, or hemorrhoids may be worsened.

➤ Severe rectal bleeding will obscure visualization through the scope, and the insertion of the scope could increase the bleeding.

➤ Suspected or actual perforated colon lesions may be worsened by the insertion of the sigmoidoscope.

Potential Complications

➤ Perforation of the intestinal wall and peritonitis is an infrequent complication.

➤ Hemorrhage from injury to the intestinal lining or at the site of a biopsy or polyp removal.

NURSING CONSIDERATIONS

Prepare Your Client

➤ Explain that this test is used to look at the lower intestines to help determine the cause of bright red blood or mucus in the stools, constipation, or changes in bowel habits.

➤ Explain the procedure, noting bowel preparation, dietary restrictions, and client positioning during the test. Preparations commonly include enemas and a light breakfast.

➤ If the client has had a barium study within 3 days prior to the test, notify the primary health care provider.

➤ Instruct the client to ingest only a light breakfast (such as juice and coffee) on the morning of the sigmoidoscopy, or restrict intake as ordered by the primary health care provider.

➤ Check the client's coagulation results prior to the test and be sure the results are posted on the client's chart. Report abnormal coagulation results to the primary health care provider.

➤ Record baseline vital signs before the test.

➤ Ensure that an informed consent is obtained, because of the possible complications associated with this procedure.

➤ Explain that during the procedure the client may feel discomfort and the urge to defecate as the sigmoidoscope is inserted, but there should be no severe pain.

Perform Procedure

Nurses do not perform this procedure, but should understand the process to prepare the client. The client is positioned in a left lateral decubitus or knee-to-chest position. The blood pressure, heart rate, and oxygen saturation are monitored prior to the administration of analgesics or sedatives and every 5 minutes during the procedure. After dilation with a well-lubricated finger of the examiner, the scope is inserted into the rectum and advanced as far as possible without excessive resistance. Air is introduced through the scope and into the rectum to expand the lower intestinal tract and increase visualization. Tissue samples are obtained as clinically indicated.

Care After Test

➤ Inform the client that they may experience flatulence or gas pains

following the procedure because the intestine was inflated with air to improve visualization.

➤ Observe the client for abdominal distention, increased abdominal tenderness, or excessive rectal bleeding.

➤ Explain that slight rectal bleeding may be experienced if biopsies were taken.

➤ If a sedative was utilized assess for side effects such as hypotension, decreased respirations, or bradycardia.

➤ Warn client they may have gas pains or be passing flatus rectally. Ambulation may help relieve pain and expel air more quickly.

➤ Monitor vital signs every 30 minutes for 2 hours following the procedure.

➤ Encourage the client to rest for several hours following the procedure. If the procedure is done on an outpatient basis the client should rest at least 1 hour before leaving.

➤ Evaluate related tests such as abdominal ultrasound, abdominal computed tomography (CT) scan, abdominal magnetic resonance imaging (MRI) scan, barium enema, colonoscopy, and kidney, ureter, and bladder (KUB) x-rays.

Educate Your Client and the Family

➤ Educate the client on the prescribed treatments such as dietary restrictions, surgery, or medicines (if applicable) for the identified disease.

➤ Instruct the client and family to notify the primary health care provider if severe rectal bleeding, severe abdominal discomfort that does not decrease after passing gas or walking, or rigidity of the abdomen should occur.

Skin Tests, Delayed Hypersensitivity

skin • tests • dee lade • hie pur sen sih tiv ih tee

(DHST, Anergic Skin Test Battery, Anergy Panel, Delayed Cutaneous Hypersensitivity, DCH, Cutaneous Delayed Type Hypersensitivity, Delayed Type Hypersensitivity, DTH, Delayed Hypersensitivity, DH, Late Cutaneous Response, LCR, Cutaneous Late-Phase Reaction, LPR, Multitest)

Normal Findings

ADULT, CHILD, ADOLESCENT, AND PREGNANT

Multitest: positive; induration, swelling, or redness at test site

Test for disease exposure: induration < 5mm

NEWBORN

Infants during the first year of life lack sufficient contact with antigens for sensitization to occur.

ELDERLY

Results may vary widely.

What This Test Will Tell You

This skin test determines cutaneous sensitivity to a single antigen or group of antigens. A small amount of antigen, to which the client has previously been sensitized, is injected intradermally. Mononuclear cells infiltrate the site, causing edema, redness, and induration. The diameter of the induration is an index of the hypersensitivity.

The Multitest, a combination of 7 antigens (tetanus toxoid, diphtheria, streptococcus, old tuberculin, candida, trichophytin, *Proteus mirabilis*) and a glycerol control is used to measure cell-mediated immunity in clients. Cell-mediated response, as scored by the Multitest, has been shown to decrease with malnutrition and advancing cancer. Thus significant changes in Multitest scores indicate changes in the client's risk for serious infection. Multitest scores are being explored as a prognostic marker and method of evaluating T-cell response in acquired immune deficiency syndrome (AIDS) clients.

Skin testing is also commonly used to determine exposure to infectious organisms such as tuberculosis, blastomycosis, coccidioidomycosis, histoplasmosis, trichinosis, and toxoplasmosis.

Abnormal Findings

▲ INCREASED LEVELS may indicate previous sensitization to antigen being tested.

▼ DECREASED LEVELS (anergy) may indicate congenital immunologic deficiency, ataxia-telangiectasia, Nezelof's syndrome, severe combined immunodeficiency, Wiskott-Aldrich syndrome, AIDS, sarcoidosis, chronic lymphocytic leukemia, carcinoma, immunosuppressive medication, rheumatoid diseases, uremia, alcoholic cirrhosis, biliary cirrhosis, lymphomas, infections, influenza, mumps, measles, viral vaccines, typhus, active tuberculosis, disseminated mycotic infection, leprosy, or scarlet fever.

ACTION ALERT!

Assess clients carefully for allergic reactions following injection, including dyspnea, itching, urticaria, flushing, hypotension, and shock. Life-threatening anaphylactic reactions can occur and need to be recognized and treated immediately.

Interfering Factors

➤ Steroid and immunosuppressants

used in prior 4–6 weeks may cause false negative results.

➤ If the test is being performed to determine infection, testing before antibodies are formed will yield a false negative result.

➤ Improper dilutions will yield errors in the results.

➤ Bacterial contamination may cause cross-reactivity with antigens, yielding inaccurate results.

➤ If the antigen is injected too deeply, a false negative reading will result.

➤ If the antigen is not injected deep enough it will leak out, causing false negative results.

➤ Results may be read improperly.

➤ Improper storage of the testing compound, such as exposure to light and heat, will decrease reactivity.

➤ Test solutions should not be stored in the syringes for long periods before injection. The antigen may be adsorbed on the container wall, leading to false negative results.

Contraindications

➤ Known active disease, such as tuberculosis, or previous positive skin tests

Potential Complications

Some clients may have a severe reaction to the antigen. This usually occurs with a second or more concentrated dose. Reactions may include erythema, large induration, blisters, and necrosis. Fever and anaphylaxis are uncommon systemic side effects.

NURSING CONSIDERATIONS
Prepare Your Client

➤ Explain that this test is used to check for different types of allergies, illnesses, or the ability to fight infection.

➤ Explain the procedure to your client. Tell your client that a small amount of antigen will be injected under the skin using a small needle.

➤ Assess the client for active infection with the disease being tested.

Perform Procedure

➤ Cleanse the inner aspect of the forearm with alcohol and let it dry.

➤ Inject the prescribed amount and dilution of antigen solution intradermally into the inner aspect of the forearm.

➤ Record the client's name, date, name of test, site of injection, and date to read results. Clearly mark the location of injection(s) by circling site on arm with indelible ink.

➤ Inform your client when erythema and induration will be measured. Purified protein derivative (PPD) is read in 48–72 hours. Multitest should be read at 24 hours and 48 hours.

➤ Report medications your client is taking that may interfere with results, such as steroid and immunosuppressant drugs.

Care After Test

➤ Assess client carefully for allergic reactions. Be prepared to administer diphenhydramine or epinephrine as ordered.

➤ Assess your client for malnutrition, which will decrease the immune response. Discuss nutritional needs with your client and family. Assist your client and family in contacting support groups available in the area.

➤ Encourage immunosuppressed client to avoid people with known infection, young children with respiratory symptoms, and large crowds.

➤ Evaluate other diagnostic tests such as lymphocyte count, complete blood counts, radiographic studies, and cultures.

Educate Your Client and the Family

➤ Inform your client that a positive skin test result does not always indicate active disease. It does indicate exposure to the infectious agent and that the body has formed antibodies against the disease.

➤ Stress the importance of the client's returning to the office or health care center for the skin test results to be read on the indicated day(s). Failure to read the results as prescribed will lead to inaccurate interpretation of results.

➤ Teach client and family ways to avoid antigens for which client tests positive, if test was to determine exposure.

➤ Instruct client who is at high risk for tuberculosis exposure to wash hands and use approved masks.

Skull X-Ray

skul • eks ray
(Skull Radiography, Skull Radiographs)

Normal Findings

All ages: Normal structure

What This Test Will Tell You

This x-ray gives diagnostic information about abnormal structure of the skull resulting from trauma, disease, birth abnormalities, or bone defects. Skull x-rays are frequently done to demonstrate the location of fractures. The actual fracture is not always readily visible on the radiographic study, however. Indications of a fracture are air, cerebrospinal fluid, or blood inside the epidural space. X-rays also show malformed bone, which may be due to birth abnormalities or facial bone destruction resulting from infection or neoplasm. Another structure shown, the calcified pineal gland, is usually midline. Deviation of this structure from midline indicates a space-occupying lesion. This test is also useful in detecting increased intracranial pressure.

Abnormal Findings

Abnormal structure may indicate skull fracture, increased intracranial pressure, chronic subdural hematoma, oligodendroglioma, meningioma, space-occupying lesions, pituitary tumor, osteomyelitis, acromegaly, Paget's disease, craniostenosis, or compression fracture from birth injury/difficult delivery.

ACTION ALERT!

➤ Any client exhibiting elevated systolic pressure and widening pulse pressure, slow bounding pulses, and decreased respiratory rate may have severely increased intracranial pressure. This is a medical emergency and needs to be reported to a primary health care provider and treated immediately.

➤ Clients who have experienced trauma may have a spinal cord injury. Maintain proper body alignment and support the neck.

Interfering Factors

➤ Movement of the client during

radiography will result in shadowed or unclear film.

➤ Improper positioning of the client will hinder radiographic interpretation.

➤ Metal hairpins, dental bridges, or glasses will obstruct visualization of skull structures.

Contraindications

➤ X-rays are discouraged during the first trimester of pregnancy. If x-rays are necessary, the woman should wear a lead apron.

Potential Complications

➤ The client may experience some pain during the radiographic procedure due to manipulation of the head into various positions.

NURSING CONSIDERATIONS

Prepare Your Client

➤ Explain that this test assists in making a diagnosis. The particular diagnostic information depends on the client history and condition.

➤ Explain that the procedure takes about 15 minutes.

➤ Inform your client that several pictures will be taken of the skull at various angles. Tell them it is very important to move into the positions the x-ray technician chooses and to remain very still during the taking of the pictures in order to get the clearest possible pictures for making a diagnosis.

➤ Inform your client that the x-rays do not cause pain. Pain may be experienced if the client's positions for the picture taking cause pressure on an injury or a painful neck or back joint.

➤ Tell your client to remove metal objects such as hairpins, jewelry, denture bridges, and glasses from the

head and neck. These objects will block the x-rays from photographing the skull structures.

Perform Procedure

Nurses do not perform this procedure. The procedure is performed by radiologic personnel. The client is positioned on a radiographic table or is seated in a chair. Sandbags or foam pads may be used to stabilize the client's head. Several skull, facial, and sinus pictures will be taken with the client in various positions. The films will be developed and checked for quality before the client leaves the radiology department. If one or more films are not of adequate quality for diagnostic purposes, the pictures will be taken again.

Care After Test

➤ Assess the client for manifestations of skull fracture. The signs and symptoms are dependent on the location of the fracture.

➤ Assess the client for increased intracranial pressure. Classic signs include elevated systolic pressure and widening pulse pressure, slow bounding pulse, and decreased respiratory rate. If indicated, oxygen administration/hyperventilation, fluid restriction, and medications such as mannitol (a hyperosmotic diuretic) may be ordered to decrease intracerebral pressure.

➤ Evaluate related tests such as cerebrospinal fluid and computed tomography scan.

Educate Your Client and the Family

➤ Teach methods for preventing head injury such as the use of helmets when motorcycling or bicycling and wearing seat belts in automobiles.

> Instruct parents to use car seats appropriate for the size and age of their child.
> Instruct client to wear protective headgear in high-risk sports such as contact sports, horseback riding, and sky diving.
> Instruct client in high-risk occupation such as construction, lumbering, or mining to wear protective headgear.

Small Bowel Biopsy

smahl • bow el • bie op see
(Small Intestine Biopsy)

Normal Findings

All ages: Normal small bowel biopsy sample consisting of fingerlike villi, crypts, columnar epithelial cells, and round cells

What This Test Will Tell You

This test is used to obtain a small sample of the intestinal mucosa for further microscopic evaluation. The normal structure of the intestinal mucosa contains fingerlike villi, crypts, columnar epithelial cells, and round cells. Variations in this normal structure may cause malabsorption or diarrhea. The biopsy sample verifies the diagnosis of some diseases such as Whipple's disease, or helps to confirm other disease processes such as sprue.

Abnormal Findings

Abnormalities may indicate eosinophilic enteritis, giardiasis, coccidiosis, infectious gastroenteritis, intraluminal bacterial overgrowth, folate and vitamin B_{12} deficiency, radiation enteritis, malabsorption, celiac sprue, tropical sprue, Whipple's disease, abetalipoproteinemia, or lymphoma.

ACTION ALERT!

> Monitor the client carefully for increasing temperature, severe abdominal pain, and/or rigidity of the abdomen following the procedure. These symptoms may indicate peritonitis from perforation of the internal organs.
> Monitor client's activated partial thromboplastin time, prothrombin time, platelet count, and bleeding time before performing this test. Prolonged coagulation should be reported to the primary health care provider prior to the test.

Interfering Factors

> Previous surgical intervention or radiation therapy to the esophagus, stomach, or small intestines may inhibit the passage of the biopsy tubing or make the tissue susceptible to damage.
> Incorrect handling of the specimen may alter the tissue sample and result in incorrect test results.
> Failure to fast before the biopsy may alter the specimen.
> Placement of tissue and cell specimens in the solution without a preservative can cause false results.
> Use of fixative sprays may distort the cells.

Contraindications

> Aspirin or anticoagulant therapy, which may contribute to hemorrhage
> Coagulation abnormalities, as there is a hemorrhage risk

> Uncooperative clients, whose behavior may not allow for the proper positioning of the tube

> Perforated stomach or duodenal lesions

Potential Complications

> Aspiration

> Hemorrhage from injury to the intestinal lining or at the site of a biopsy or polyp removal

> Vomiting

> Perforation of the small intestine and peritonitis

> Bacteremia with transient fever and pain

NURSING CONSIDERATIONS

Prepare Your Client

> Explain that this procedure is performed to obtain a small specimen of the gut (small bowel) lining, which will be analyzed to help find any problems.

> Ensure that an informed consent is obtained, because of the possible complications associated with this procedure.

> Restrict food and fluids for 8 hours prior to the test.

> Record baseline vital signs before the test.

> Check the client's coagulation results prior to the test and be sure the results are posted on the client's chart. Report abnormal coagulation results to the primary health care provider.

> Withhold aspirin, aspirin-containing drugs, and anticoagulants as ordered. If there are no orders to withhold these drugs, consult the primary health care provider regarding the need to withhold them.

Perform Procedure

Nurses do not perform this procedure, but should understand the process to prepare the client. Position the client upright. The client's throat is sprayed with a local anesthetic to decrease gagging during the tube insertion. The capsule is placed in the pharynx, the client's neck is flexed, and the physician instructs the client to swallow as the tube is advanced 50 cm. The client is placed on the right side and the physician advances the tube another 50 cm. Placement of the tube in the stomach is checked via fluoroscopy. The tube is advanced another 5–10 cm to pass the tube through the pylorus. Talking to the client about food will stimulate the pylorus, which will help to pass the tube. Tube passage through the pylorus is confirmed with fluoroscopy. The client is kept on the right side and the tube allowed to pass into the second and third portions of the small intestines by peristalsis. The capsule position is verified again by fluoroscopy.

Once the capsule has passed the ligament of Treitz, the biopsy sample can be taken. The client is placed supine, and using a 100-mL glass syringe on the end of the tube, suction is applied to close the capsule and cut off the tissue sample. Suction is maintained while removing the tube. Once the tube is removed, the suction is released and the specimen is placed in a biopsy bottle with fixative, labeled, and transported to the laboratory immediately.

Care After Test

> Resume the pretest diet after confirming that the gag reflex has returned to normal and the client can swallow without difficulty.

> Observe the client for abdominal distention, increased heart rate,

decreased blood pressure, and increased abdominal tenderness or bleeding, which may indicate bowel perforation or peritonitis.

➤ Instruct the client to notify the nurse if severe abdominal pain, a feeling of faintness, or any rectal bleeding should occur.

➤ Monitor vital signs closely until stable; usually every 15 minutes for the first hour, every 30 minutes for the next hour, and then every 4 hours for 24 hours.

➤ Encourage the client to rest for several hours following the procedure. If the procedure is done on an outpatient basis, the client should rest at least 1 hour before leaving.

➤ Evaluate related tests such as abdominal ultrasounds, abdominal computed tomography scans, abdominal magnetic resonance imaging, obstruction series, small bowel follow-through, stool for guaiac, and kidney, ureter, and bladder (KUB) x-rays.

Educate Your Client and the Family

➤ Educate the client on the prescribed treatments such as dietary restrictions, surgery, intervention, or medicines (if applicable) for the identified disease.

➤ Instruct the client or family to notify the primary health care provider if dark tarry stools, severe abdominal discomfort, or rigidity of the abdomen should occur.

Small Bowel Follow-Through

smahl • bow el • fahl oe throo
(SBF, SBFT, Small Bowel Enema, Small Bowel Series, Radiography of the Small Intestine, Fluoroscopy of the Small Intestine)

Normal Findings

All ages: Normal size and contours, patency, filling, and positioning of the structures of the small intestines. No evidence of intrinsic obstruction or extrinsic compression of the small intestines. Mucosa is smooth and regular without lesions or narrowing. Barium flows smoothly without leakage into the abdominal cavity.

What This Test Will Tell You

This radiographic test with contrast material detects abnormalities of the small intestines. The small intestine is imaged through the use of contrast material and timed x-rays, allowing evaluation and diagnosis of a variety of congenital, mechanical, or acquired abnormalities of the small intestine.

Abnormal Findings

The test may reveal tumors, obstruction, adhesions, inflammatory small bowel disease (Crohn's disease), small bowel perforation, malabsorption syndromes such as Whipple's disease or sprue, neuropathy of the bowel, congenital abnormalities (malrotation, small bowel atresia, Meckel's diverticulum), tuberculosis, ileus, intussusception, parasite infestation, duodenal diverticulum, or foreign bodies.

Interfering Factors

➤ Retained barium from previous gastrointestinal x-rays may obscure the x-ray films.

➤ Failure to follow restrictions on diet, smoking, and/or medications may interfere with the test results.

➤ Failure to remove radiopaque objects in the x-ray field can impair x-ray imaging.

➤ Excessive air in the small bowel can obscure important details of the image.

➤ Poor performance of the client or severe debilitation may prevent the client from assuming the multiple positions required for the test.

➤ Chronic narcotic use and anticholinergic agents can delay peristalsis of the gastrointestinal (GI) tract.

➤ Fear, excitement, nicotine, or nausea may increase the motility of the GI tract.

➤ Severe or poorly controlled diabetes mellitus may cause decreased GI motility and alter the test results.

Contraindications

➤ Complete bowel obstruction, as the contrast material would complicate the bowel obstruction and increase the client's discomfort

➤ Unstable vital signs

➤ Perforation of the GI tract, as the leakage of contrast into the abdominal cavity would lead to peritonitis

➤ Ileus, because the ingestion of the contrast would increase the discomfort and abdominal distention associated with the ileus

Potential Complications

➤ Aspiration of the contrast material.

➤ Constipation or bowel obstruction as a result of unexpelled barium. When obstruction is already present, barium may cause a complete blockage.

NURSING CONSIDERATIONS
Prepare Your Client

➤ Explain that this test is used to look at part of the gut (the small intestines) and see if there are problems in how the gut is formed or working.

➤ Ensure that an informed consent is obtained, because of the possible complications associated with this procedure.

➤ Inform the client that the procedure requires several hours for completion and encourage the client to carry reading material or paperwork to occupy the time while waiting. If the client is hospitalized for the test, arrange for transportation back to the nursing unit between the serial films.

➤ Instruct the client to maintain a low-residue diet for 2–3 days before the test (for example, decrease vegetables, grains, nuts, and fruits).

➤ Restrict food and fluids for at least 8 hours before the test.

➤ Assure the client that the test is not painful.

➤ Instruct the client to avoid smoking for 8 hours before the test as well as during the test because smoking can increase the GI motility.

➤ Administer the bowel preparation only if ordered by the primary health care provider.

➤ If the client has a hyperactive bowel, administer atropine as ordered to decrease the peristalsis.

Perform Procedure

Nurses do not perform this procedure, but should understand the process to prepare the client. Either the client drinks the contrast substance or it is administered by a nasogastric tube. Barium sulfate, a chalky, thick substance that is radiopaque, is generally used for contrast material. However, if there is concern about a leakage into the abdominal cavity or possible perforation of the GI tract, a water-soluble contrast such as Gastrograffin is used. Following the ingestion of the contrast material, the client is assisted to the supine, erect, and lateral side positions as ordered by the radiologist. X-ray films are taken at intervals of 30–60 minutes for 6–8 hours after the ingestion of the contrast. This test is usually scheduled in conjunction with an upper GI series.

For a small bowel enema, the contrast material is injected directly through a tube placed in the small bowel. X-rays are taken as the contrast material passes through the small intestines.

Care After Test

➤ Assess for diarrhea in the client who received a water-soluble contrast material because the radiopaque material is an osmotic diuretic.

➤ Administer a cathartic such as milk of magnesia as ordered to prevent hardening of the barium, which could lead to a fecal impaction.
➤ Encourage the client to drink more fluids, unless otherwise indicated, to improve the passage of the barium through the GI tract.
➤ Encourage the client to rest for several hours following the procedure.
➤ Evaluate related tests such as abdominal ultrasounds, abdominal computed tomography (CT) scans, abdominal magnetic resonance imaging (MRI) scans, barium enema, and/or abdominal x-ray films.

Educate Your Client and the Family

➤ Educate the client on the prescribed treatments such as dietary restrictions, surgery, or medicines (if applicable) for the identified disease.
➤ Instruct the client or family to monitor the stool to ensure that it returns to normal consistency within 3 days. Explain that it is normal for the stool to be clay-colored for the first day or so after the x-ray as the barium is being expelled.

Sodium, Serum and Urine

soe dee um • see rum • and • yur in
(Serum Sodium, Urine Sodium, Na+)

Normal Findings

SERUM
Adult, pregnant, elderly, adolescent: 135–145 mEq/L (SI units: 136–145 mmol/L)
Newborn: 133–146 mEq/L (SI units: 133–146 mmol/L)
Child: 138–145 mEq/24 hours (SI units: 138–145 mmol/24 hours)

URINE
Adult, pregnant, elderly, adolescent: 40–220 mEq/24 hours (SI units: 40–220 mmol/24 hours)
Urinary values vary with dietary intake of sodium.
Newborn: Full-term, 7–14-day-old

newborns have sodium clearances of about 20% of adult levels.

Males, 6–10 years: 41–114 mEq/day (SI units: 41–115 mmol/day)
Females, 6–10 years: 20–69 mEq/day (SI units: 20–69 mmol/day)

What This Test Will Tell You

These serum and urine tests for sodium levels evaluate fluid and electrolyte balance as well as renal or adrenal disorders. Sodium is the main cation of the extracellular fluid and is a critical factor in acid-base balance and the water balance between blood and body tissues.

Approximately 95% of the body's physiologically active sodium is in the extracellular fluid. Sodium does not move easily across the cell wall membrane and therefore plays a critical role in water distribution and extracellular fluid (ECF) volume. A low sodium level (hyponatremia) is associated with a diluted ECF and water moving into the cells, whereas a high sodium level (hypernatremia) is associated with a concentrated ECF and water moving out of the cells. Low sodium levels will result in increased aldosterone secretion, whereas an elevated sodium level will result in decreased aldosterone secretion.

Sodium is absorbed into the bloodstream via the small intestine. Its excretion via the urine is controlled by the kidneys, with a small amount lost through the skin. Urine sodium levels are helpful in determining early changes in sodium levels. Both urine and serum levels are required to completely understand whole body sodium concentrations.

Abnormal Findings

▲ INCREASED SERUM LEVELS may indicate water deprivation, increased insensible water loss, watery diarrhea, corticosteroid therapy, excessive sodium intake or administration, hypernatremic dehydration, excessive diuresis or diaphoresis, severe vomiting, impaired renal function, fever, draining intestinal wounds, hyperaldosteronism, bicarbonate therapy, clonidine, estrogens, oral contraceptives, Cushing's disease, coma, head trauma, diabetes insipidus, anabolic steroids, or osmotic diuresis.

▼ DECREASED SERUM LEVELS may indicate diuretic therapy, water intoxication, salt-losing nephritis, loss of gastrointestinal fluids, adrenal insufficiency, renal insufficiency, uremia, excessive administration of 5% dextrose and water, excessive water intake, hypotonic tube feedings, hyponatremic dehydration, syndrome of inappropriate antidiuretic hormone secretion (SIADH), burns, congestive heart failure, prolonged diarrhea, nasogastric suctioning, excessive cathartics, cirrhosis with ascites, paracentesis, hypoalbuminemia, Addison's disease, sprue, starvation, polyuria, or malabsorption syndromes.

▲ INCREASED URINE LEVELS may indicate dehydration, increased salt intake, syndrome of inappropriate antidiuretic hormone, adrenocorticosteroid insufficiency, diuretic therapy, fever, diabetic ketoacidosis, head trauma, salicylate intoxication, toxemia, or starvation.

▼ DECREASED URINE LEVELS may indicate acute renal failure, diarrhea, corticosteroid therapy, fluid retention, hypernatremia dehydration, congestive heart failure, diaphoresis, diuresis, shock, severe/prolonged vomiting, Cushing's disease, or cirrhosis.

Levels of sodium must always be considered in relationship to level of hydration and serum osmolality. With severe or rapid hyponatremia (serum sodium below 120 mEq/L), hypovolemic shock, seizures, and death can occur. Severe or rapid hypernatremia (serum sodium above 155 mEq/L) can result in seizures and hypermania. Also evaluate for dyspnea and hypertension with fluid overload, which can lead to respiratory distress and cardiopulmonary arrest.

Interfering Factors
SERUM

➤ Adrenocorticotropic hormone (ACTH), steroids, carbenicillin, clonidine, corticosteroids, diazoxide, estrogens, guanethidine, lactulose, licorice, methoxyflurane, methyldopa, oral contraceptives, oxyphenbutazone, phenylbutazone, reserpine, sodium bicarbonate, calcium, and sodium-containing anticoagulants can result in elevated serum sodium levels.

➤ Amitriptyline, ammonium chloride, amphotericin B, captopril, carbamazepine, chlorpropamide, cisplatin, clofibrate, cyclophosphamide, diuretics, heparin, imipramine, indomethacin, lithium, nonsteroidal anti-inflammatory agents, tolbutamide, vasopressin, and vincristine can cause low serum sodium levels.

➤ Hemolysis of the blood specimen will invalidate serum results.

➤ Dietary intake will influence results.
URINE

➤ Caffeine, calcitonin, captopril, carbonic anhydrase inhibitors, cisplatin, diuretics, dopamine, heparin, lithium, niacin, high doses of progesterone, sulfates, tetracycline, and vincristine can result in elevated urine levels.

➤ Corticosteroids, diazoxide, epinephrine, levarterenol, and propranolol can result in decreased urine levels.

➤ Sodium values are influenced by the amount of dietary sodium intake.

➤ Failure to collect all urine voided during the 24-hour period.

➤ Failure to keep urine specimen on ice or refrigerated during collection period.

NURSING CONSIDERATIONS

Prepare Your Client

➤ Explain that this test is helpful in evaluating the balance of chemicals in the body, particularly sodium. Explain how sodium balance is regulated by the kidneys and two glands near the kidneys called the adrenals.

Perform Procedure
SERUM

➤ Collect 5–7 mL of venous blood in a red-top tube.

➤ Avoid collecting blood near a vein where saline or electrolyte solutions are infusing.
URINE

➤ Collect 24-hour urine specimen without preservatives.

➤ Keep specimen refrigerated or on ice during the collection period.

➤ Instruct the client that all urine voided in the next 24-hour period must be added to the collection container.

Care After Test

➤ Monitor intake and output. Report urine output less than 30 mL/hour in adults, less than 1 mL per kg body weight per hour in infants and children.

➤ Monitor urine specific gravity every 8 hours and as indicated. Urine specific gravity less than 1.010 indicates hypervolemia and could indicate hyponatremia; specific gravity over 1.030 indicates hypovolemia and could indicate hypernatremia.

➤ Monitor vital signs every 4 hours and note changes in blood pressure and pulse.

➤ Weigh daily; assure the clothing, time of day, and scales are consistent.

➤ Assess breathing sounds every 4 hours for presence of rales.

➤ Inspect neck veins for jugular vein distention every 4 hours.

➤ Assess for dependent edema in ankles or sacral area.

➤ Assess mental status and neurological status and provide safety and seizure precautions as indicated.

➤ Monitor for signs and symptoms of hyponatremia including fatigue, weakness, confusion, stupor, anorexia, apprehension, headache, nausea, vomiting, diarrhea, and abdominal pain.

➤ Monitor for signs and symptoms of hypernatremia including dry mucous membranes, fever, sweating, increased thirst, oliguria, flushed skin, agitation, restlessness, and decreased reflexes.

➤ Assess medication use, specifically diuretics, lithium, steroids, and sodium-containing medications.

➤ Anticipate and manage stressful situations.

➤ Monitor client receiving intravenous (IV) solutions containing sodium for fluid overload and/or hypernatremia.

➤ For client with dry sticky mucous membranes, provide mouth care every 2 hours.

➤ With hyponatremia, increase high-sodium foods including bacon, ham, cheese, celery, cold cuts, pickles, olives, catsup, and tomato juice.

➤ With hypernatremia, decrease high-sodium foods.

➤ Review related tests including serum and urine osmolality, serum potassium, hemoglobin and hematocrit, blood urea nitrogen.

Educate Your Client and the Family

➤ Teach the client to avoid or increase dietary sodium depending on diet prescription. High-sodium foods include bacon, ham, cheese, celery, cold cuts, pickles, olives, catsup, and tomato juice.

➤ Teach client on diuretics the signs and symptoms of sodium deficit (fatigue, confusion, loss of appetite, headache, nausea) and fluid deficit (dry mouth, thirst, dark urine).

➤ Instruct client and family on the importance of reading all labels on food and over-the-counter drugs for sodium content. Over-the-counter drugs that are high in sodium include laxatives, pain relievers, sedatives, and cough syrups.

Somatotropin

so **mat** oe **troe** pin

(Growth Hormone, Human Growth Hormone, hGH)

Normal Findings

ADULT, ADOLESCENT, AND ELDERLY

Male: 0–8 ng/mL (SI units: 0–8 µg/L)
Female: 0–30 ng/mL (SI units: 0–30 µg/L)

NEWBORN

10–40 ng/mL (SI units: 10–40 µg/L)
Preterm infant may be higher.

CHILD

0–6 ng/mL (SI units: 0–16 µg/L)

What This Test Will Tell You

This blood test is used to confirm hypo- or hyperpituitarism. Somatotropin (growth hormone) increases serum glucose and fatty acid levels, and promotes protein synthesis and amino acid uptake. Challenge or stimulation tests may detect growth hormone deficiency.

Abnormal Findings

▲ INCREASED LEVELS may indicate gigantism (in children), acromegaly (in adults), pituitary or hypothalamic tumor, diabetes mellitus, or anorexia nervosa.

▼ DECREASED LEVELS may indicate dwarfism (in children), pituitary insufficiency, or pituitary tumor.

Interfering Factors

➤ Oral contraceptives, estrogens, arginine, levodopa, insulin, hypoglycemia, starvation, fasting, amphetamines, and beta-adrenergic blockers will cause increased levels.

➤ Corticosteroids, phenothiazines, hyperglycemia, and obesity will cause decreased levels.

➤ Radioactive scans within 1 week and hemolysis will interfere with accurate determinations.

➤ Exercise, sleep, stress, and nutritional status interfere with accurate determinations.

NURSING CONSIDERATIONS

Prepare Your Client

➤ Explain to the client that this test helps evaluate growth patterns in children and metabolism in adults.

➤ Restrict food and fluids (except water) for 8–10 hours prior to the test.

➤ Assure the client is quiet and resting for 1 hour prior to testing.

Perform Procedure

➤ Collect 5–10 mL of venous blood in a red-top tube between 6 A.M. and 8 A.M. on 2 consecutive days.

➤ Transport immediately because hGH rapidly metabolizes.

Care After Test

➤ Evaluate growth in a child using standard pediatric growth charts.

➤ Assess the need for counseling for child with severe abnormalities of growth.

➤ Review related tests such as growth hormone stimulation test and insulin levels.

➤ Teach client to give own insulin injections if indicated.

Educate Your Client and the Family

➤ Stress the importance of additional testing to confirm a diagnosis.

➤ Explain that increased levels of growth hormone decrease the body's ability to handle glucose. Educate client regarding signs and symptoms of hyperglycemia, including increases in thirst, urination, and hunger.

➤ In children, a lack of growth hormone is treated medically by injections of growth hormone so the child develops normally. Parents will need detailed instructions about the injections and follow-up care. Refer to support groups whenever available.

Somatotropin Suppression Test
soe mat o troe pin • suh preh shun • test
(Growth Hormone Suppression Test, GHST, SST, hGH Suppression Test)

Normal Findings
All ages: 0–3 ng/mL (SI units: 0–3 µg/L) 30–120 minutes after glucose administration

What This Test Will Tell You
This blood test detects diseases of growth hormone production, including gigantism in children and acromegaly in adults. Growth hormone is needed for tissue repair and growth of cells. In its absence, repair of tissue damage is slow and bones grow slowly. Children that do not grow at sufficient rates may be suspected to have a growth hormone deficiency. With too much growth hormone, the bones may continue to grow, resulting in gigantism.

Abnormal Findings
Levels greater than or equal to 5 ng/mL (5 µg/L) may indicate acromegaly in adults or gigantism in infants and children.

Interfering Factors
➤ Eating, stress, exercise, and sleep can increase levels.
➤ A decreased growth hormone response to glucose may be seen with obese individuals, high-carbohydrate diets, and hypothyroidism.
➤ Radioactive scans up to 1 week prior to testing.

➤ Hemolysis.
➤ Medications that may decrease levels include corticosteroids, beta blockers, histamines, chlorpromazine, and phenothiazines.
➤ Medications that may increase levels include levodopa, beta blockers, amphetamines, arginine, glucagon, estrogens, histamine, oral contraceptives, and niacin.

NURSING CONSIDERATIONS
Prepare Your Client
➤ Explain that this test is to look for any problems with a hormone needed for growth and healing.
➤ Restrict food, fluids, and activities for 10–12 hours prior to the test.
➤ Keep the client relaxed and lying down for at least 30 minutes prior to testing.
➤ Inform client that testing needs to be done between 6 and 8 A.M. because the time of day may affect hormone levels.
➤ Confer with primary health care provider to determine if medications affecting results should be withheld.

Perform Procedure
➤ Collect 6–10 mL of blood into a red-top tube between 6 and 8 A.M. before giving glucose.

➤ Have client ingest slowly a prescribed amount of glucose (usually 100 grams). IV glucose may be used for a client unable to drink the glucose solution.

➤ Draw 6–10 mL of venous blood into a red-top tube at 1 hour and 2 hours after ingestion of glucose.

➤ Send each blood sample to the laboratory immediately after its collection.

Care After Test

➤ Assess for signs and symptoms of acromegaly including thickened soft tissue and bones; coarse facial features; and enlargement of lower jaw, lips, tongue, feet, and hands.

➤ Assess for signs and symptoms of growth disorders. Record and plot on standardized growth charts the height, weight, head circumference, and chest circumference of infants and toddlers.

➤ Assess for body image problems associated with a growth disorder and refer for counseling if needed.

➤ Review related tests including serum growth hormone, growth hormone stimulation test, x-rays of long bones, sella turcica x-ray, and pituitary hormone studies.

Educate Your Client and the Family

➤ Teach client and family the importance of hormonal therapy, and instruct them not to discontinue therapy without medical clearance.

➤ Assist client and family in understanding that medical management and therapy will be lifelong.

Sperm Antibody Assay

spurm • an ti bod ee • a say

(Sperm Agglutination and Inhibition, Infertility Screen, Antisperm Antibody Test, Sperm Antibodies)

Normal Findings

Negative

What This Test Will Tell You

This blood or fluid analysis determines if the male or female has antibodies against sperm cells, which can result in decreased fertility. Antisperm antibodies may be found in seminal plasma attached to sperm or in the male or female bloodstream.

Abnormal Findings

Positive results may reveal infertility or blocked efferent ducts in the testes.

Interfering Factors

➤ Heavy coffee consumption and heavy tobacco smoking may decrease sperm motility.

➤ Improper specimen collection or failure to deliver it to the lab quickly may alter results.

NURSING CONSIDERATIONS

Prepare Your Client

➤ Explain that this test is to try to diagnose problems with fertility caused by the body's making antibodies to destroy sperm.

➤ Explain to the male client that the

testing will be done on semen and he may also need to have a blood sample collected. Explain to the female that she will need to have a blood sample collected.

➤ Instruct the male to avoid ejaculation for 3 days prior to collecting a semen specimen.

➤ Inform the male that the specimen may be obtained at home via masturbation or intercourse with a condom.

➤ Instruct the client who collects the specimen at home to take it to the laboratory within 2 hours.

Perform Procedure

SERUM ANTIBODY TESTING

➤ Collect 7–10 mL of venous blood in a red-top tube.

SEMEN ANALYSIS FOR ANTIBODIES

➤ Instruct the male where and when to collect a semen specimen if he did not bring a fresh specimen with him.

➤ Write the semen collection time on the laboratory slip and send it to the laboratory immediately.

Care After Test

➤ Ensure client receives referrals for fertility evaluation and counseling as indicated.

➤ Assess the client's knowledge of the reproductive cycle and optimal times for fertilization.

➤ Review related tests including semen analysis and postcoital (Sims-Huhner) tests.

Educate Your Client and the Family

➤ Teach clients that infertility may be related to either the male or female partner.

Sputum Culture and Sensitivity

spyu tum • kuhl chur • and • sen sih tiv ih tee
(Sputum C&S, Sputum Culture)

Normal Findings

All ages

Negative for pathogenic organisms; no growth of pathogenic organisms

What This Test Will Tell You

This microscopic analysis diagnoses infectious diseases of the respiratory tract and tests for antimicrobial sensitivity to determine the effects of various antibiotics on the identified microorganism. This test involves the direct microscopic inspection of a sample of sputum for Gram stain, culture, and sensitivity studies. The sputum is initially Gram stained to identify the organism as gram-posi-

tive or gram-negative. This provides guidelines to begin appropriate antimicrobial therapy. The sputum is then incubated for 24 and 48 hours on the appropriate culture medium and studied by a microbiologist to allow further identification of the infecting organism. Once the organism is identified, its sensitivity or resistance to various antimicrobial agents is tested and appropriate antibiotic therapy may then be prescribed.

Sputum cultures for both fungus and mycobacterium tuberculosis require special laboratory methods and may take 6–8 weeks to complete.

Abnormal Findings

Positive results may indicate bacterial pneumonia, chronic bronchitis, viral pneumonia, bronchiectasis, or pulmonary tuberculosis or other mycotic infections.

ACTION ALERT!

Suctioning to obtain a sample for culture and sensitivity can produce hypoxia and bradycardia. These conditions can be serious and deteriorate to cardiopulmonary arrest quickly. Administration of oxygen therapy or resuscitation should be anticipated, with appropriate emergency equipment readily available.

Interfering Factors

➤ Contamination of the specimen causes inaccurate results.

➤ Antibiotic or sulfonamide therapy begun before samples are obtained may cause false negative results.

➤ Delay in delivering specimens to the laboratory causes inaccurate results.

➤ Specimens should not be refrigerated.

➤ Sputum from deep in the bronchial tree must be produced by cough or suction. Nasopharyngeal drainage or saliva causes inaccurate results.

Contraindications

None

Potential Complications

➤ Hypoxia with suctioning
➤ Dysrhythmias with suctioning

NURSING CONSIDERATIONS

Prepare Your Client

➤ Explain to the client that this test is to detect possible infections of the respiratory system and to find the best medicine to treat it.

➤ Describe the procedure for sputum collection and emphasize that the specimen must come from deep in the lungs; saliva and nasopharyngeal drainage are not sputum and will not provide information needed for adequate treatment.

➤ Advise the client that an early morning specimen is best, after sputum has collected in the lungs overnight.

➤ Give the client a sterile specimen container the night before sputum is to be collected so that it will be available when the client awakens.

➤ Instruct the client to rinse the mouth with water before coughing up sputum to decrease the chance of contamination with normal germs in the mouth.

➤ Teach the client to breathe deeply and cough from the diaphragm to obtain the best sample.

➤ Check to see if client is receiving antibiotics at the time of the collection, because these may cause false negative results.

➤ Inform the client that it will take 24–48 hours before results are available. Cultures for *Mycobacterium tuberculosis* may take up to 8 weeks to obtain.

➤ Increase fluid intake the night before, unless contraindicated, or have the client breathe humidified air to help liquify secretions and aid in coughing up sputum.

Perform Procedure

➤ The material from the first deep productive cough of the morning should be expelled without contaminating the inside of the sterile container or lid by touching it with the mouth or hands. A volume of 1–3 mL of sputum is satisfactory.

➤ Obtain the specimen from the

lungs: saliva and nasal drainage are not sputum. A specimen of sputum must be coughed up or suctioned from deep within the bronchi.

➤ Collect an early morning specimen, after secretions have collected overnight.

➤ Determine the procedure by which the specimen will be collected (coughing or tracheal suctioning).

➤ If the client is unable to produce sputum, contact respiratory therapy for postural drainage and chest percussion to stimulate production of acceptable sputum.

➤ Label the container and transport to the laboratory immediately. Do not refrigerate.

➤ If pulmonary infection is strongly suspected, therapy may begin after obtaining cultures but before confirmation by culture results.

Care After Test

➤ If tuberculosis is suspected, a nucleic acid probe can provide more immediate results and should be performed.

➤ Observe for symptoms of hypoxia and administer oxygen after collection of sputum specimens if indicated.

➤ Observe for symptoms of respiratory tract infection such as fever, pro-ductive cough, pulmonary congestion, or dyspnea. Report to primary health care provider immediately.

➤ Provide pulmonary toileting therapy by encouraging deep breathing and coughing, as well as performing postural drainage and cupping.

➤ Institute antibiotic therapy if ordered.

➤ Evaluate related tests such as chest x-ray, nucleic acid probe, and white blood cell count.

Educate Your Client and the Family

➤ Instruct client to cover their mouth and nose when coughing or sneezing and to dispose of tissues in an appropriate receptacle.

➤ Inform the client that results will not be available for 1–2 days (unless testing for tuberculosis) and that antibiotic therapy may be started before laboratory confirmation of infection.

➤ Instruct client on the importance of complying with antibiotic therapy, especially completing the prescribed course of treatment.

➤ Teach deep breathing, coughing, and other pulmonary hygiene measures if indicated.

➤ Refer to a smoking cessation program if appropriate.

Sputum Cytology
spyu tum • sie tahl oe jee

Normal Findings

All ages: Normal epithelial cells; no inflamed, malignant, suspiciously malignant, or atypical cells present

What This Test Will Tell You

This microscopic analysis detects pathologic cell changes within the pulmonary system due to malignancies or inflammatory conditions. It involves the microscopic study of the number and type of cells of the respiratory tract and/or sputum to detect the presence of cells abnormal for that specimen, including tumor or pretumor cells or evidence of an infective or inflammatory process. Cytologic studies will commonly be reported as inflammatory, benign, atypical, suspicious for malignancy, or positive for malignancy. Any abnormalities of cells must be correlated to clinical data for diagnosis.

Abnormal Findings

Cell abnormalities may indicate malignancy; premalignant or atypical cell changes related to chronic inflammation; infection with bacteria, viruses or parasites; or lipid or aspiration pneumonia.

ACTION ALERT!

Suctioning to obtain a sample for culture and sensitivity can produce hypoxia and bradycardia. These conditions can be serious and deteriorate to cardiopulmonary arrest quickly. Administration of oxygen therapy or resuscitation should be anticipated, with appropriate emergency equipment readily available.

Interfering Factors

➤ Nasopharyngeal drainage or saliva causes inaccurate results. Sputum from deep in the bronchial tree must be produced by coughing or suctioning.

➤ Delay in delivering specimens to the laboratory may cause a deterioration of tumor cells.

➤ Incidence of false negatives is about 15% even with careful examination of multiple deep cough specimens.

Contraindications

➤ Obtaining specimen by tracheal suctioning is contraindicated in clients with thrombocytopenia. Caution should be used when suctioning clients with bradycardia.

Potential Complications

➤ Sputum collected by tracheal suctioning may produce transient hypoxia, requiring administration of supplemental oxygen.

NURSING CONSIDERATIONS

S

Prepare Your Client

➤ Explain to the client that this test is to detect abnormal cells that may be present in the lungs.

➤ Sputum for cytologic studies may be obtained by coughing, by tracheal suctioning, or during bronchoscopy. If the specimen is obtained during bronchoscopy, follow the nursing considerations for that procedure.

➤ Describe the procedure for sputum collection and answer any questions. Emphasize that the specimen must come from deep in the lungs; saliva or nasal drainage are not sputum.

➤ Advise the client that an early morning specimen is best, after sputum has collected in the lungs overnight.

➤ Advise the client that several specimens will be obtained at different times. It is common practice to collect sputum specimens on three separate mornings.

➤ Give the client a sterile specimen container the night before sputum is to be collected so that it will be available when the client awakens.

➤ Instruct the client to rinse the mouth with water before coughing up sputum to decrease the chance of contamination with normal flora in the oral cavity.

➤ Increase fluid intake the night before or have the client breathe humidified air to help liquify secretions and aid in coughing up sputum.

Perform Procedure

➤ Collect an early morning specimen, after secretions have collected overnight. Usually three samples are obtained on three different occasions.

➤ Determine the procedure by which the specimen will be collected (coughing or tracheal suctioning).

➤ If the client is unable to produce sputum, contact respiratory therapy for postural drainage and chest percussion or aerosol therapy to stimulate production of acceptable sputum.

➤ The material from the first deep productive cough of the morning should be expelled without contaminating the inside of the sterile container or lid by touching it with the mouth or hands. A volume of 3–5 mL of sputum is satisfactory.

➤ Use a wide-mouthed sterile container or sterile container to which 50% alcohol has been added, depending on laboratory procedure.

➤ Instruct the client to alert the nurse as soon as the specimen has been obtained so it may be sent to the laboratory immediately.

➤ Label the container with the name, date, specimen source, specimen number, diagnosis, and clinical symptoms on the laboratory requisition and transport to the laboratory immediately.

Care After Test

➤ Observe for symptoms of hypoxia or dysrhythmias and administer oxygen after collection of sputum specimens if indicated.

➤ Evaluate related tests such as chest x-rays, computed tomography (CT) scans, bronchoscopy, thoracentesis, culture reports, pleural fluid analysis, and pleural or lung biopsies.

Educate Your Client and the Family

➤ Explain to the client that results will be interpreted by the pathologist, who will relay results to their primary health care provider. Cytologic studies may take 2 or more days for final interpretation.

➤ Teach deep breathing, coughing, and other pulmonary hygiene measures if indicated.

➤ Refer to smoking cessation programs if indicated.

➤ Teach client how to pace activities to reduce fatigue and how to enhance nutrition.

➤ Explain the importance of a well-balanced diet with adequate protein intake.

Stool Culture
stool • kul chur
(Stool for Culture and Sensitivity, Stool for C&S)

Normal Findings

All ages: Negative for pathogens; no growth other than normal flora

What This Test Will Tell You

This stool specimen analysis is frequently ordered for clients with persistent or bloody diarrhea accompanied by fever or for clients with known exposure to enteric pathogens. Pathogenic organisms that cause gastrointestinal disease include *Salmonella*, *Staphylococcus aureus*, *Shigella*, *Campylobacter*, *Vibrio cholerae*, *Clostridium difficile*, *Vibrio parahaemolyticus*, *Clostridium botulinum*, *Clostridium perfringens*, *Escherichia coli*, *Bacillus cereus*, *Yersinia enterocolitica*, and *Aeromonas hydrophilia*.

Abnormal Findings

Positive results may indicate gastroenteritis related to bacterial, parasitic, and/or protozoan infections.

Interfering Factors

➤ If the client has received barium, mineral oil, or laxatives, bacterial growth may be inhibited.

➤ Improper collection technique may lead to a contaminated specimen.

➤ Antibiotic therapy may decrease the bacterial growth in the specimen.

➤ Failure to transport the specimen to the laboratory promptly may decrease the bacterial growth.

➤ Urine mixed with the stool may decrease the bacterial growth.

➤ If an enema must be administered to collect the specimen, only normal saline or tap water should be used to prevent interference with the bacterial growth within the specimen.

NURSING CONSIDERATIONS

Prepare Your Client

➤ Explain that the test will help find the reason for the client's symptoms of diarrhea, gas, or stomach pain.

➤ Collect a stool specimen on 3 consecutive days.

➤ Question the client regarding dietary pattern, recent antibiotic therapy, or recent out-of-the-country travel.

➤ Instruct the client to avoid mixing urine or toilet paper with the specimen.

Perform Procedure

➤ Instruct the client to obtain the stool specimen in a clean bedpan or specimen container.

➤ If the client is nonambulatory or incontinent, collect the specimen in a clean bedpan or from the client's diaper. Be sure that the specimen has not been contaminated with urine.

➤ To collect a specimen from the rectum, insert a sterile applicator past the anal sphincter, rotate the applicator gently and allow 30 seconds for the applicator to absorb the organisms, remove the applicator, and place it in a sterile container. This method is far less effective in obtaining an adequate specimen for analysis.

➤ Place a 1-inch diameter stool specimen into a sterile container using a sterile wooden tongue blade.

➤ Label the specimen including the date and time of collection, suspected cause of enteritis, and current antibiotic therapy.

➤ Send the specimen immediately to the laboratory. If there is to be a delay of 2–3 hours, the specimen must be put into a transport medium such as buffered saline-glycol or alkaline peptone water.

Care After Test

➤ Monitor the client's temperature if a pathogenic organism is suspected.

➤ Place the client in isolation if the test is positive for *Salmonella*, *Shigella*, *Campylobacter*, *Yersinia*, *Vibrio*, or *Clostridium*.

➤ Monitor consistency and amount of stool.

➤ Monitor for signs and symptoms of dehydration and electrolyte depletion if the client is having diarrhea.

Educate Your Client and the Family

➤ If food poisoning is suspected, instruct the client on correct cooking and storage of food.

➤ If the client is experiencing diarrhea as the result of the pathogenic organism, instruct the client to consume small amounts of clear liquids with electrolytes, to increase the amount of the clear liquids as tolerated, and to progress to soft, bland foods as tolerated.

➤ Instruct the client to avoid milk and milk products for at least a week after the diarrhea stops.

➤ If the diarrhea has caused irritation of the skin in the anal area, instruct the client or family to cleanse the area thoroughly, apply a repellent cream, and use witch hazel compresses or sitz baths to relieve the irritation.

➤ Instruct the client and family about the importance of minimizing the risk of transmission of pathogenic organisms through meticulous handwashing, maintaining good personal hygiene, and restricting the use of the client's glasses, plates and utensils.

➤ Instruct the client to report any increase or changes in abdominal pain, persistent vomiting, blood in the stools, diarrhea that continues for more than 7–10 days, and fainting or extreme weakness.

Stool for Occult Blood

stool • for • ah kult • blud

(Occult Blood, Fecal or Stool for Guaiac, Blood in Stool, Fecal Blood, Hemoquant®, Hemoccult®, Hema-Chek®, ColoScreen Self Test®, EZ-Detect Test®)

Normal Findings

All ages: Negative, <2–2.5 mL/day

What This Test Will Tell You

This test diagnoses gastrointestinal bleeding or screens for the early stages of colorectal cancer by identifying red blood cells in the stool. A small amount of blood (2–2.5 mL/day) is normally present in the stool. Occult blood (not visible to the unaided eye) may be present in the stool for several weeks following a gastrointestinal (GI) bleed. Bright red blood in the stool indicates that the bleeding is occurring in the lower GI tract. Black or tarry stools indicate blood loss in excess of 50 mL in the upper GI tract.

Abnormal Findings

Positive results may indicate gastrointestinal bleeding, colonic polyps, colon carcinoma, hemorrhoids, peptic ulcer, stress ulcer, recent GI surgery, gastritis, esophagitis, diverticulosis, Crohn's disease, ulcerative colitis, variceal bleeding, necrotizing enterocolitis, or nasopharyngeal bleeding.

ACTION ALERT!

A strongly positive test is indicative of bleeding within the gastrointestinal tract. Assess the client for shock manifested by tachycardia, hypotension, chest pain, anxiety, diaphoresis, and tachypnea. Notify the primary health care provider immediately, institute continuous cardiac monitoring, and prepare to resuscitate with fluids and/or blood products.

Interfering Factors

➤ A diet high in meats, poultry, fish, and green leafy vegetables may cause a false positive test result.

➤ Consumption of fruits/vegetables high in peroxidase (such as broccoli, turnips, horseradish, cauliflower, radishes, cantaloupe) may cause a false positive test result for up to 4 days after ingestion.

➤ Medications that can lead to bleeding in the intestinal tract and result in positive findings include aspirin and other salicylates, heparin, warfarin, large doses of iron, colchicine, steroids, and non-steroidal anti-inflammatory medications.

➤ Vitamin C (ascorbic acid) greater than 500 mg/day may cause a false negative result.

➤ Colchicine, iron, rauwolfia derivatives, iodine, bromides, and boric acid may cause a false positive test result.

➤ Urine or soap solution in the fecal specimen may affect the test results.

➤ A positive result will be obtained if the specimen is contaminated with menstrual blood or povidone-iodine.

➤ Ingestion of 2–5 mL of blood such as from bleeding gums or recent dental procedures can cause abnormal results.

➤ Long-distance runners may have occult blood in the feces after a vigorous run.

➤ Liquid stool may cause a false negative result when filter paper is used.

➤ Menstrual bleeding and hemorrhoids will produce positive results in the absence of GI bleeding.

NURSING CONSIDERATIONS

Prepare Your Client

➤ Explain that the test is important to identify any bleeding problems in their stomach or the intestinal tract.

➤ Instruct the client to limit the consumption of red meat, poultry, fish, and green leafy vegetables for 3 days prior to the test.

➤ Instruct the client to avoid peroxidase-containing foods (broccoli, turnips, horseradish, cauliflower, radishes, cantaloupe) for 3 days prior to the test.

➤ Instruct the client to avoid mixing urine with the stool specimen.

➤ Advise the client to avoid salicylates and non-steroidal anti-inflammatory (NSAIDs) agents as well as alcohol for 1 week prior to the test.

➤ If the client is menstruating when the sample is to be obtained, instruct the client to be sure that the specimen is not contaminated by menstrual fluid as this would interfere with the test results.

Perform Procedure

HEMOCCULT® TEST CARDS, HEMOQUANT® AND HEMA-CHEK®

➤ Obtain a small amount of stool and open the front flap of the guaiac-impregnated slide.

➤ Using a wooden applicator, apply a small smear of stool to each box. Be sure to obtain each sample from a different part of the stool specimen. Close the slide cover.

➤ The slide must be treated within 48 hours of collection.

➤ Open the back flap of the slide and apply 2 drops of the developer to each box and to the quality monitor.

➤ Read the results after 30 seconds and within 2 minutes. The appearance of a blue color is considered a positive result.

➤ Repeat the test on consecutive stool specimens if ordered.

COLOSCREEN SELF TEST® OR EZ-DETECT TEST®

➤ Flush the toilet at least three times to remove any detergent or cleaner residue. Flush any urine that is voided.

➤ Instruct the client to defecate into the toilet.

➤ Float the test pad on the water in the toilet bowl.

➤ Observe the test pad for a positive response, a blue-green color change (2 minutes for the EZ-Detect Test and 0–30 seconds for the ColoScreen Self Test).

Care After Test

➤ Resume the client's usual diet and medications following the completion of the test.

➤ If the test result is positive, assess each stool, especially noting dark, tarry appearance.

➤ Assess for symptoms of blood loss including tachycardia, tachypnea, fatigue, chest pain, hypotension, orthostatic hypotension, pale skin and mucous membranes, anxiety, and diaphoresis.

➤ Review related tests such as hemoglobin, hematocrit, fibrinogen, partial thromboplastin time, platelets, prothrombin time, sigmoidoscopy, barium enema, and colonoscopy.

Educate Your Client and the Family

➤ Encourage the client to report any abnormal stools, especially those that are dark black or tarry. However, if the client is receiving an iron supplement, instruct them that the black or tarry appearance of the stool is normal.

➤ Teach client with significant bleeding and anemia to pace activities to decrease fatigue.

➤ Instruct client to eat foods high in iron or take iron supplements if appropriate.

Stool for Ova and Parasites

stool • for • oe vah • and • pair ah sites
(Stool for O&P; Parasite Screen, Stool)

Normal Findings

All ages: Negative—no parasite, ova, or larvae present

What This Test Will Tell You

This microscopic stool analysis is performed when the client has diarrhea of unknown origin and a parasitic infestation is suspected. The parasites are identified at various stages of development from ova (egg) through the mature stages of development. Amoeba, flagellates,

tapeworms, hookworms, and roundworms are the most common parasites found in the stool.

Abnormal Findings

Positive results may indicate tapeworms, pinworms, roundworms, amoeba, protozoa, or hookworms.

Interfering Factors

➤ The presence of urine, toilet tissue, soap, or disinfectants in the specimen may alter the test results.

➤ Collection of too few stools may fail to detect whether the organisms are parasites, larvae, or ova because they may not be continuously present in the stool specimen.

➤ Failure to transport the warm stool specimen to the laboratory quickly may alter the test results.

➤ Refrigeration or exposure to extreme cold may alter the test results.

➤ Exposure of the specimen to excessive heat may alter the test results.

➤ Collection from a toilet bowl rather than a dry container will alter the test results.

➤ Use of castor oil, mineral oil, bismuth compounds, antacids, iron, magnesium compounds, antidiarrheals, antibiotics, barium enemas, or hypertonic saline enemas may interfere with the microscopic analysis and decrease the number of parasites present.

➤ Antimicrobial or antiamebic therapy within 5–10 days prior to the specimen collection may cause a false-negative result.

NURSING CONSIDERATIONS

Prepare Your Client

➤ Explain that this test is important to identify an infection of parasites (worms) that may be causing the client's symptoms.

➤ Collect stool specimens for 3 consecutive days.

➤ Assess client's recent medication history for interfering agents and for recent diagnostic testing that included enemas or barium.

➤ Question the client about recent out-of-the-country travel or well water consumption.

➤ Instruct the client to avoid mixing urine or toilet tissue with the specimen.

➤ Clarify with the laboratory whether a preservative is needed for the specimen. If a preservative is to be used, obtain the preservative of 5% formalin or other preservative the lab may supply.

Perform Procedure

➤ Instruct the client to collect the stool specimen in a clean, dry bedpan or specimen container.

STOOL COLLECTION

➤ Obtain a clean container of plastic, waxed cardboard, or glass with a tight-fitting lid for the collection of the stool specimen.

➤ Use a sterile tongue blade to transfer at least 2 tablespoons of the stool specimen from the bedpan or collection container into the specimen container.

➤ Be careful not to contaminate the inside of the specimen container.

➤ Label the specimen including the date and time of collection, any recent antibiotic therapy, any recent out-of-the-country travel by the client, and the suspected diagnosis of the client.

COLLECTION FOR PINWORM EGGS

➤ Obtain clear cellophane tape and a tongue blade.

➤ Collect the specimen about 2 hours after client has fallen asleep or in the early morning before the bath or bowel movement.

➤ Wrap clear cellophane tape around a tongue blade with the gummed side away from the tongue blade.

➤ Press the tape to 3–4 separate places in the perianal area close to the anus.

➤ Do not insert the tongue blade into the anus.

➤ Remove the tape from the tongue blade and gently press the gummed side of the tape against a glass slide.

➤ Place the slide in a container and transport it to the lab.

COLLECTION FOR TAPEWORM

➤ Collect the entire stool specimen in a clean, dry bedpan or specimen container.

➤ Send the entire stool specimen to the lab for analysis to identify the head of the tapeworm.

➤ Use caution when handling the sample, as parasitic infections are very contagious.

Care After Test

➤ Monitor consistency and amount of stool.

➤ Monitor for the signs and symptoms of dehydration and electrolyte depletion if the client is having diarrhea.

➤ Monitor the white blood cell count for eosinophilia, which may be caused by parasitic infection.

➤ Monitor the client for pathologic changes in other parts of the body, as helminths may migrate from the intestinal tract (examples are peritonitis due to bowel perforation or pneumonitis due to migration to the lungs).

➤ Monitor the client for megaloblastic anemia, which may be caused by tapeworms.

➤ Instruct the client to resume medication discontinued before the test.

➤ Evaluate other tests such as stool for occult blood, stool for culture and sensitivity, hematocrit, hemoglobin, mean cell volume, mean cell hemoglobin, mean cell hemoglobin concentration, red blood cell counts, and white blood cell counts and differentials, especially eosinophil levels.

Educate Your Client and the Family

➤ If pathogenic infection is suspected in relation to the ingestion of contaminated food or fluids, instruct the client to cook food correctly and to the proper temperature, or to boil water before drinking if contamination of water is suspected.

➤ For clients with well water, assist them in making arrangements to have their water analyzed for contamination.

➤ If the client is experiencing diarrhea as the result of the parasitic infection, instruct the client to consume small amounts of clear liquids with electrolytes, to increase their consumption of the clear liquids as tolerated, and to progress the diet to soft, bland foods as tolerated.

➤ Instruct the client to avoid milk and milk products during diarrhea episodes.

➤ If the diarrhea has caused irritation of the skin in the anal area, instruct the client or family to cleanse the area thoroughly, to apply a repellent cream, and to use witch hazel compresses or sitz baths to relieve the irritation.

➤ Instruct the client and family about the importance of minimizing the risk of transmission of pathogenic organisms through meticulous handwashing and maintaining good personal hygiene.

➤ Instruct the client to report any increase or changes in abdominal pain, or blood in stools, diarrhea that continues for more than 7–10 days, fainting, extreme weakness, or perianal itching.

Sweat Test

swet • test

(Sweat Electrolytes, Iontophoretic Sweat Test)

Normal Findings

Sodium: <50 mEq/L
Chloride: <50 mEq/L

What This Test Will Tell You

This electrolyte evaluation test is used primarily to rule out or confirm the diagnosis of cystic fibrosis by quantitatively measuring electrolyte concentrations (sodium and chloride) in sweat. Cystic fibrosis is a hereditary disease, usually diagnosed in early childhood, involving the exocrine function of multiple glands. Characterized by chronic pulmonary disease, pancreatic insufficiency, abnormally high sweat electrolyte levels, and sometimes cirrhosis of the liver. This is a serious and fatal multisystem disease. The sweat test is very reliable for the diagnosis of cystic fibrosis after the neonatal period.

Abnormal Findings

▲ INCREASED LEVELS (sodium >90 mEq/L, chloride >60 mEq/L) indicate cystic fibrosis, and may also indicate Addison's disease, fucosidosis, glucose-6-phosphatase deficiency, congenital adrenal hyperplasia, nephrotic syndrome, familial hypoparathyroidism, or hereditary nephrogenic diabetes insipidus.

Indefinite findings (sodium 50–90 mEq/L, chloride 50–60 mEq/L) need to be repeated and followed until more conclusive results are obtained.

ACTION ALERT!

To prevent electric shock, use only battery-powered equipment.

Interfering Factors

➤ Failure to obtain an adequate sample of sweat prevents proper testing. This may occur in small infants.
➤ Failure to cleanse the test area properly may cause false elevations.
➤ Failure to seal the test area properly causes evaporation and may falsely elevate levels.
➤ Drainage from wounds affects results.

Potential Complications

➤ Do not perform iontophoresis on the chest, because the current can induce cardiac arrest, especially in small children.
➤ This procedure should always be performed on the extremities on the right side of the body because of the slight electrical current used and the potential for interference with cardiac conduction.
➤ The test should be stopped immediately if client complains of a burning sensation. This may indicate that the positive electrode is improperly positioned.

NURSING CONSIDERATIONS

Prepare Your Client

➤ Explain that this test is to measure the amount of salt in the sweat and diagnose cystic fibrosis.
➤ Assure the family and child that the test is not painful, although the child may feel a slight tingling sensation during the procedure.
➤ This test will take up to 90 minutes to perform.

S

Perform Procedure

Nurses do not usually perform this procedure, but should understand the process to prepare the client and assist the technician. The flexor surface of the right arm (right thigh in small infants) is cleansed with distilled water and dried. A gauze pad saturated with pilocarpine solution to stimulate diaphoresis is placed on the positive electrode. A gauze pad saturated with normal saline or bicarbonate solution is placed on the negative electrode. Both electrodes are secured with straps to the area to be iontophoresed. Lead wires are connected to the analyzer and are given a current of 4 milliamperes in 15 to 20 seconds. This process (iontophoresis) is continued at 15–20 second intervals for 5 minutes.

When iontophoresis is completed, the electrodes are removed, the gauze pads are discarded, and the area is cleansed with distilled water and then dried. Using forceps, a previously weighed dry gauze pad or filter paper is placed on the area where the pilocarpine was iontophoresed. This pad is covered with a piece of plastic or paraffin seal and the edges sealed with waterproof tape. This is left in place for approximately 40–60 minutes. At the end of the time, the pad is removed with forceps and placed in a specimen bottle. This is weighed and the dry weight of the pad is subtracted to determine the amount of the sweat specimen obtained.

Care After Test

➤ Wash the iontophoresed area with soap and water and dry.

➤ The area may be slightly red; reassure the family the redness should disappear within a few hours.

➤ Consult with a registered dietician to assist the family and client in meeting special dietary needs.

➤ Assess for respiratory compromise by noting cough, wheezing, tachypnea, dyspnea, vomiting related to coughing, history of recurrent pulmonary infections, and clubbing of fingers in older children.

➤ Assess for gastrointestinal manifestation of cystic fibrosis by noting frequent, bulky, foul-smelling stools; protuberant abdomen; wasted buttocks; and failure to gain weight.

➤ Review related tests such as pulmonary function studies, fecal fat, chest x-ray, and trypsin content of stools.

Educate Your Client and the Family

➤ If the diagnosis of cystic fibrosis is confirmed, there is great need for education about the disease and the treatment needed to optimize the child's health. The child should be followed by a pediatric health care team familiar with this disease.

➤ Instruct the family on the need to have siblings screened for cystic fibrosis.

➤ Teach the family the importance of genetic counseling.

➤ Teach the family to perform pulmonary care procedures, leg percussion, and postural drainage if indicated.

Syphilis Detection Test

sif ih lis • dee tek shun • test

(Fluorescent Treponemal Antibody Test, FTA, Serologic Test for Syphilis, STS, Venereal Disease Research Laboratory, VDRL, Rapid Plasma Reagin, RPR, Fluorescent Treponemal Antibody Absorption Test, FTA-ABS, Hemagglutination Treponemal Test for Syphilis, HATTS)

Normal Findings

Negative or nonreactive

What This Test Will Tell You

This blood or cerebrospinal fluid test is ordered to diagnose syphilis, a disease caused by the spirochete organism *Treponema pallidum*. Various laboratory methods detect two groups of antibodies to *T. pallidum*. One antibody, reagin, is directed against a lipoid agent from the infection. The other antibody works against *Treponema*.

The rapid plasma reagin (RPR) test is a new, more sensitive test, but it tests for a nonspecific antibody. When an RPR or Venereal Disease Research Laboratory (VDRL) test is positive, the fluorescent treponemal antibody absorption test (FTA-ABS) may be ordered to confirm the diagnosis because it is more specific.

Abnormal Findings

Positive results indicate syphilis.

Interfering Factors

➤ Alcohol ingestion within 24 hours may alter the results.

➤ Excess chyle in the blood may alter the results.

➤ Hemolysis of the sample may interfere with accurate results.

➤ Systemic lupus erythematosus may alter the results.

➤ Many conditions may cause false positive results for VDRL and RPR tests. The conditions include acute bacterial and viral infections, mycoplasma pneumonia, malaria, autoimmune diseases, pregnancy, and narcotic addiction.

NURSING CONSIDERATIONS

Prepare Your Client

➤ Explain that this is a test for syphilis, a sexually transmitted disease.

➤ Instruct the client to abstain from alcohol for 24 hours before the test.

Perform Procedure

BLOOD TEST

➤ Collect 7 mL of venous blood in a red-top tube.

CEREBROSPINAL FLUID ANALYSIS

➤ Assist the primary health care provider with a lumbar puncture for the diagnosis of late-stage syphilis in the cerebrospinal fluid.

Care After Test

➤ Assess for signs and symptoms of primary syphilis including presence of a chancre (painless, eroded papule with a raised and indurated border).

➤ Assess for signs and symptoms of secondary syphilis including alopecia, lymphadenopathy, lesions in the mucous membranes and skin, and neurological changes.

➤ Discuss with client all sexual contacts and arrange testing.

Educate Your Client and the Family

➤ Instruct the client about the importance of completing antibiotic therapy if they tested positive.

➤ Teach client that primary symptoms may go away even without treatment, but the disease will continue to be present and cause lifelong problems if left untreated.

➤ Educate client on the proper use of condoms.

Terminal Deoxynucleotidyl Transferase

tur min ahl · dee ok see noo clee o tie dil · trans fur ase

(TDT, TdT)

Normal Findings

All ages:

0%–2% in bone marrow

Negative in peripheral blood

0–10 IU/10^{13} cells in blood

What This Test Will Tell You

This test of the bone marrow and blood is used to make a differential diagnosis of leukemia. High levels of TDT are used to help differentiate acute lymphocytic leukemia (ALL) from acute nonlymphocytic leukemia (ANLL). It may be helpful in determining the prognosis, the early diagnosis of a relapse, and the response to therapy.

Abnormal Findings

▲ INCREASED LEVELS may indicate acute lymphocytic leukemia, acute lymphoblastic leukemia, lymphoblastic lymphoma, chronic myelogenous leukemia "blast crisis," or acute nonlymphocytic leukemia.

▼ DECREASED LEVELS may indicate remission or positive response to therapy.

Interfering Factors

➤ Failure to obtain a representative sample of marrow may result in inaccurate findings.

➤ Bone marrow regeneration, neuroblastoma, and thrombocytopenia purpura may give false positive results.

Potential Complications

➤ Bleeding at bone marrow puncture site

➤ Perforation of underlying tissues

➤ Hemorrhage

➤ Infection

NURSING CONSIDERATIONS

Prepare Your Client

➤ Explain that this test is performed to help diagnose problems in the bone marrow and white blood cells. If appropriate, explain also that this test is done to help determine the type of leukemia, decide how helpful therapy for the leukemia has been, or see if there has been a relapse.

➤ Warn the client that during this test, a brief sharp sensation may be felt.

Perform Procedure

BLOOD SAMPLING

➤ Collect two 7-mL samples of venous blood in 2 green-top tubes.

BONE MARROW ASPIRATION

➤ Ensure that an informed consent is obtained, because of the possible complications associated with this procedure.

➤ Collaborate with the primary health care provider to determine the need for sedation.

➤ Position client as comfortably as possible. For sternal aspiration, the client is positioned with pillow under the thoracic spine. For iliac crest aspiration, the client is in a side-lying position on abdomen. For tibial aspiration, the client is in a prone position.

➤ A local anesthetic is administered before the aspiration is undertaken. Caution the client that a brief stinging sensation may be felt when the anesthetic is administered.

➤ The physician or advanced practice nurse will insert a needle through the bone until bone marrow is reached. The plunger on the syringe is pulled back to withdraw a small amount of bone marrow into the syringe.

➤ Assist with procedure to assure collection of 2 mL of bone marrow aspirate in heparinized syringe.

➤ Keep sample at room temperature.

➤ Apply adhesive bandage or small pressure dressing.

Care After Test

FOR VENOUS SAMPLING

➤ Observe the venipuncture site closely for hematoma formation or bleeding. Coagulopathies are common in leukemias. Apply a pressure dressing to the venipuncture site.

➤ Assess for occult bleeding with routine stool guaiac testing.

FOR BONE MARROW ASPIRATION

➤ Assess vital signs and bleeding at site.

➤ Explain to client the need to rest in bed for an hour before resuming normal daily activities.

➤ Apply pressure and ice packs to site to control bleeding.

➤ Administer mild analgesic as ordered for pain.

FOR BOTH METHODS

➤ Refer client and family to a cancer support group.

➤ Assess for the client's ability to cope with changes in body image such as weight loss or gain, loss of hair, changes in body functions, decreased sexual function, and role changes.

➤ Refer to social services to assist with the financial and economic impact of cancer.

➤ Consult with a registered dietician for client with anorexia, weight loss, or special dietary needs.

➤ Provide the client opportunities to have control over care issues such as times for treatment, settings for care, and presence of significant others.

➤ Assess carefully for chronic and acute pain. Obtain pain management consultation if indicated.

➤ Assess for signs and symptoms of infection such as chills, fever, and drop in the absolute neutrophil count. Institute precautions to protect the client, such as no fresh fruits or vegetables. Remove fresh flowers and plants, and enforce good hand-washing.

➤ Assess oral mucous membranes for signs and symptoms of stomatitis. Give oral hygiene care frequently with a soft toothbrush or sponge-tip applicator.

➤ Develop and constantly update a teaching plan for the learning needs of the client and family related to diagnosis, testing, therapy, and home care.

➤ Assess the client for signs and symptoms such as bleeding from injection sites, petechia, or ecchymosis, occult blood, and decreasing platelet count related to increased risk for bleeding.

➤ Clients with impaired bone marrow function may have prolonged bleeding times. Institute safety measures such as electric razors, non-skid shoes, no intramuscular injections, no rectal temperatures, and soft toothbrushes.

➤ Encourage verbalization of fears related to cancer, prognosis, treatment, and death.

➤ Evaluate other blood tests such as platelet and complete blood count with differential.

Educate Your Client and the Family

➤ Provide answers to questions and emotional support while awaiting results of test.
➤ Teach client the need to avoid situations that put them at risk for infection.

➤ Clients with leukemia may have prolonged bleeding times. Instruct the client and family on safety measures such as electric razors, non-skid shoes, and soft toothbrushes.
➤ As appropriate, instruct client and family on a high-calorie, well-balanced diet.

T

Testosterone, Serum, Plasma

tes tos teh **rone** • see rum • **plaz** mah
(Total Testosterone)

Normal Findings

Female: 26–95 ng/dL (SI units: 1.0–3.0 nmol/L)
Male: 300–1200 ng/dL (SI units: 10.5–42 nmol/L)
Female child: 26–95 ng/dL (SI units: <1.5 nmol/L)
Male child: 300–1200 ng/dL (SI units: <3.5 nmol/L)
Prepuberty female: <40 ng/dL (SI. units: <40 nmol/L)
Prepuberty male: <100 ng/dL (SI units: <100 nmol/L)

What This Test Will Tell You

This blood test assists in the diagnosis of precocious puberty in males, hypogonadism, pituitary gonadotropin dysfunction, impotency, cryptorchidism, male infertility, and female ovarian and adrenal tumors. Testosterone is the hormone produced by the Leydig cells of the testes that induces puberty and maintains male secondary sex characteristics. Testosterone is also secreted by the adrenal glands in men and by the ovaries and the adrenal glands in women. Testosterone production increases in puberty from the stimulation of the luteinizing hormone (LH) from the anterior pituitary. Production begins to decrease at age 40. Excessive production of testosterone produces masculine characteristics in females and premature puberty in boys.

Abnormal Findings

▲ INCREASED LEVELS may indicate adrenal hyperplasia, idiopathic sexual precocity, adrenocortical hyperplasia, polycystic ovaries, adrenal tumor, adrenogenital syndrome with virilization, arrhenoblastoma, central nervous system lesions, hirsutism, ovarian tumor, Stein-Leventhal syndrome with virilization, or testicular tumors.

▼ DECREASED LEVELS may indicate primary or secondary hypogonadism, Klinefelter's syndrome, cryptorchidism, orchidectomy, male climacteric, hypopituitarism, impotence, anemia, cirrhosis, Down syndrome, testicular cancer, or prostatic cancer.

Interfering Factors

➤ Exogenous sources of estrogens and androgens can interfere with test results.

➤ Thyroid and growth hormones increase free testosterone.

➤ Pituitary hormones may alter results.

➤ Hemolysis from improper handling of the sample may affect results.

➤ Male testosterone levels peak in the early morning and after exercise, and decrease after immobilization and glucose loading.

➤ Radioactive scanning within 7 days before the test invalidates the results.

➤ Medications that may increase levels include anticonvulsants, barbiturates, estrogens and oral contraceptives, and cimetidine.

➤ Medications that may decrease levels include halothane, phenothiazines, spironolactone, tetracycline, androgens, dexamethasone, digoxin (males), digitalis, estrogens (males), and ethanol glucose.

NURSING CONSIDERATIONS

Prepare Your Client

➤ Explain that this test helps to evaluate how much of the male sex hormone, testosterone, the body is making.

➤ Explain that this test is performed by collecting a blood sample.

Perform Procedure

➤ Collect 7 mL of venous blood. Use a red-top tube if serum is to be collected or a green-top (heparinized) tube if plasma is to be collected. The sample is stable for up to 1 week without refrigeration or preservatives. Frozen samples are stable for 6 months.

➤ Write the client's age, sex, and hormone therapy history on the laboratory slip.

➤ Handle the sample gently to prevent hemolysis.

Care After Test

➤ Evaluate client for signs and symptoms of feminization of males (loss of hair, small genital size, gynecomastia) or virilization of females (facial hair, decreased breast size).

➤ Evaluate related tests including levels of thyroid-stimulating hormone, thyrotropin-releasing hormone factor, and adrenocorticotropic hormone.

➤ Provide support for client experiencing body image disturbances.

Educate Your Client and the Family

➤ Teach client the importance of hormone therapy if ordered, and of taking medications regularly.

Thiamine, Serum And Urine

thie ah min • see rum • and • yur in
(Urine Vitamin B$_1$ or Serum Vitamin B$_1$)

Normal Findings

ALL AGES
Serum: 5.3–7.9 µg/dL
Urine: 100–200 µg/24 hours (SI

units: 300–600 nmol/24 hours)
PREGNANT
Values may be slightly decreased due to the higher demand.

What This Test Will Tell You

This blood or urine test measures levels of vitamin B_1 and screens for deficiency. Vitamin B_1 is a water-soluble vitamin which, in the presence of folic acid, is absorbed in the duodenum and excreted in the urine. Vitamin B_1 helps to metabolize fats, proteins, and carbohydrates. Beriberi, a deficiency of vitamin B_1, usually results from inadequate dietary intake; impaired absorption; impaired utilization as in hepatic disease; or conditions that increase the metabolic demand such as pregnancy, fever, surgery, and high carbohydrate intake.

Abnormal Findings

▲INCREASED LEVELS may indicate leukemia, polycythemia vera, or Hodgkin's disease.

▼DECREASED LEVELS may indicate inadequate dietary intake, malabsorption syndrome, alcoholism, liver disease, beriberi, thyrotoxicosis, hyperthyroidism, hemodialysis, chronic diarrhea, diuretic therapy, depression, increased metabolic demands (fever, pregnancy), excessive consumption of raw fish and tea, congestive heart failure, pyruvate carboxylase deficiency, maple syrup urine disease, or Wernicke's encephalopathy.

Interfering Factors

➤ Use of barbiturates will cause a decreased serum thiamine level.
➤ Diet high in freshwater fish or tea made from tea leaves may decrease thiamine levels as these foods contain thiamine antagonists.
➤ Failure to collect all urine or keep it refrigerated/iced during the test period may alter the test results.
➤ Failure to protect the urine specimen from prolonged exposure to light may alter the test results.
➤ Contamination of the urine specimen with stool, blood, or toilet tissue may alter the test results.

NURSING CONSIDERATIONS

Prepare Your Client

➤ Explain that the test is important to determine if the client has too little vitamin B_1.
➤ Check the client's diet history to rule out inadequate intake of vitamin B_1.
➤ For the serum test, restrict food and fluids for 8 hours prior to the test.
➤ For the urine test, explain the correct procedure for the collection of the 24-hour specimen to the client or family.

Perform Procedure

SERUM
➤ Collect 7 mL of venous blood in a red-top tube.
➤ Place the specimen immediately into a paper bag to protect the specimen from light.
URINE
➤ Carefully follow 24-hour urine collection technique.
➤ Collect all urine in a light-protected container. Be sure the specimen remains on ice or is refrigerated.

Care After Test

➤ Assess for signs and symptoms of thiamine deficiency including congestive heart failure, tachycardia, distended neck veins, cardiomegaly, hepatomegaly, symmetrical motor and sensory dysfunction, peripheral neuritis, nystagmus, ataxia, confusion, impaired memory and cognition, abdominal pain, edema, irritability, pallor, and seizure activity.

> Institute safety precautions for client with mental status changes or risk of seizure activity.

> Evaluate the client's ability to perform activities of daily living if neuromuscular functional impairment is noted. Refer to community health services as needed.

> Consult with a registered dietician to assist the family and client in meeting special dietary needs.

> Review related tests such as electromyography, electroencephalogram, alanine aminotransferase (ALT), aspartate aminotransferase (AST), and blood chemistries.

Educate Your Client and the Family

> If the client's results indicate a deficiency in vitamin B_1, advise the client that beef, pork, organ meats, fresh vegetables, legumes, wheat, and whole grains are good dietary sources.

> Instruct the client to decrease their intake of freshwater fish and tea made from tea leaves, as they contain thiamine antagonists.

> Explain that an adequate ongoing intake of thiamine-rich foods is needed to help prevent a vitamin B_1 deficiency.

Thoracentesis and Pleural Fluid Analysis

thor a sen tee sis • and • ploo ral • floo id • ah nal ah sis
(Pleural Tap)

Normal Findings

ALL AGES

> Negative for abnormal cells
> Amount: <20 mL
> Color: Clear
> pH: 7.37–7.43
> Specific gravity: <1.016
> Protein: <3 g/dL
> Fibrinogen: None
> Red blood cells: <1000/mm^3
> White blood cells: <1000/mm^3, consisting mainly of lymphocytes
> Lactate dehydrogenase: Equal to serum level
> Glucose: Equal to serum level
> Amylase: Equal to serum level
> Gram stain and culture: No organisms present
> Cytological examination: No abnormal cells
> Triglycerides, cholesterol, immunoglobulins, carcinoembryonic antigen (CEA), complement: Equal to serum level

What This Test Will Tell You

This fluid analysis is performed whenever a pleural effusion needs to be drained due to compromise of cardiopulmonary function, or is of unknown etiology and needs to be diagnosed. Diagnostic thoracentesis involves the insertion of a needle into the pleural space in order to aspirate fluid to determine the nature and cause of a pleural effusion. Removal of pleural fluid may also be done for therapeutic purposes, such as to relieve pulmonary compression causing dyspnea or pain.

The fluid collected may include laboratory analysis for chemistry, bacteria, and cytology. Exudates have a specific gravity >1.017 with a high concentration of protein and lactate dehydrogenase (LDH). Transudates have a protein count no higher than in the serum and do not clot. Color, density, and viscosity are noted. In empyema, pleural fluid appears purulent with a foul-smelling odor. With a chylothorax, the aspirant appears milky white.

Elevations in the white blood cell (WBC) count and differential on the pleural fluid help to identify bacterial infections or tuberculosis. Gram stain and bacteriologic culture are performed to identify bacterial pneumonias or empyema. If tuberculosis is suspected, cultures for acid-fast bacilli are performed. Cytologic analysis of effusions are performed if malignant effusions are suspected. Pleural effusions may also be tested for levels of immunoglobulins, complement components, carcinoembryonic antigen (CEA), and other contents.

Abnormal Findings

Abnormalities may indicate malignancy, empyema, infection, pneumonia, congestive heart failure, lymphoma, tuberculosis, rheumatoid disease, pulmonary infarction, cirrhosis, hypoalbuminemia, nephrotic syndrome, peritoneal dialysis, myxedema, systemic lupus erythematosus, pancreatitis, ruptured esophagus, trauma, collagen vascular disease, gastrointestinal disease, chylothorax, or hypoproteinemia.

ACTION ALERT!

Thoracentesis may result in bleeding into lung tissue, hemothorax, pneumothorax, and infection. If performed as low as the 10th rib, laceration of either the spleen or the liver may occur. Emergency equipment and intravenous fluid therapy should be readily available in the event that bleeding or respiratory distress occur.

Interfering Factors

➤ Blood in the sample due to traumatic thoracentesis makes analysis for true blood content as in a hemothorax difficult.
➤ Undetected hypoglycemia or hyperglycemia.
➤ Contamination of the sample with skin cells and pathogens.
➤ Delay in sending specimen to the laboratory or refrigeration of specimen.

Contraindications

➤ Bleeding disorders
➤ Inability of the client to cooperate with the procedure because of respiratory insufficiency, confusion, or agitation

Potential Complications

➤ Pneumothorax
➤ Hemothorax
➤ Intercostal nerve injury
➤ Infection
➤ Bradycardia
➤ Hypertension
➤ Seeding the needle tract with tumor
➤ Air embolism

NURSING CONSIDERATIONS
Prepare Your Client

➤ Explain to the client that the test is to obtain a sample of fluid from the space between the lung and the chest wall. If the test is also being done therapeutically to relieve compression on the lung, explain that the test will remove a buildup of fluid that is making breathing difficult.
➤ Explain to the client that the area in which the thoracentesis needle is to be inserted will be numbed but the client will still feel some pressure.
➤ Review the complete blood count

and blood clotting studies prior to the procedure to identify clients at high risk for developing complications such as bleeding.

➤ Ensure that an informed consent is obtained, because of the possible complications of this procedure.

➤ Emphasize to the client that they must hold as still as possible and refrain from coughing to prevent perforation of the lung by the thoracentesis needle. The procedure usually takes less than 30 minutes.

➤ Administer a cough suppressant before the procedure if indicated.

➤ Assist the client to disrobe above the waist and provide a hospital gown.

➤ Obtain the most recent chest x-ray films so that the location of the fluid may be determined.

Perform Procedure

Nurses do not perform this procedure, but should understand the process to prepare the client and assist the physician. The procedure is performed at the bedside or in the radiology department under fluoroscopy and takes about 30 minutes.

Assemble needed supplies: sterile gloves, injectable lidocaine, thoracentesis tray, collection bottles with heparin, sterile 4 × 4 gauze pads, tape, and antiseptic solution. Assist the client to a sitting position with the arms supported on a pillow on an overbed table. Cleanse the needle insertion site with an antiseptic solution.

The insertion site is infiltrated with local anesthesia. Tell the client that the local anesthetic may produce a temporary burning sensation, but it should produce numbing in a few seconds. Remind the client to remain as still as possible and avoid coughing.

The needle is inserted through the chest wall into the selected intercostal space until the parietal membrane is penetrated. Explain to the client that the local anesthetic should prevent pain at the site, but pressure may still be felt as the catheter or introducer is passed.

Fluid is withdrawn with a syringe and a three-way stopcock. A short catheter may be inserted into the pleural space for fluid aspiration to decrease the risk of puncturing the visceral pleura. Approximately 50 mL of fluid are obtained for analysis. Monitor the client's pulse for reflex bradycardia. For therapeutic purposes, large volumes (no more than 1 L in adults) may be collected by connecting the catheter to a gravity-drainage or vacuum system. Instruct the client to exhale fully before the needle is withdrawn to minimize the possibility of air entering the pleural space. Apply pressure to the needle insertion site immediately after the needle is withdrawn.

Place samples in the appropriate containers using aseptic technique. Dress the puncture site with an occlusive pressure dressing. Label specimen containers indicating the site and method utilized in obtaining the specimen, and transport to the laboratory immediately.

Care After Test

➤ Position the client on the unaffected side for 1 hour to allow the pleural puncture to seal.

➤ Monitor respiratory status every 15–30 minutes for up to 2 hours until stable for signs of hemothorax, pneumothorax, or tension pneumothorax such as dyspnea, tachypnea, hemoptysis, cyanosis, decreased breath sounds on the affected side, and crepitus around the puncture site.

➤ Obtain a chest x-ray if ordered to check for complications.

➤ Observe for signs of bleeding at the needle insertion site and check vital signs every 15–30 minutes for 1–2 hours until stable. Note tachycardia, thready pulse, hypotension, diminished breath sounds, or other abnormal vital signs and report to the primary care provider immediately.

➤ Assess for ipsilateral shoulder pain, which is a sign of diaphragmatic perforation.

➤ Assess the client's comfort level and administer analgesics if indicated.

➤ Resume food and fluids and previous activity level in 1 hour or when the client's condition stabilizes.

➤ Evaluate related tests such as chest x-ray, computed tomography (CT) scans, sputum cultures and cytology, bronchoscopy, complete blood counts, or pleural and lung biopsies.

Educate Your Client and the Family

➤ Describe the routine of closely monitoring vital signs and respiratory status.

➤ Instruct the client to report immediately any difficulty breathing, bleeding from the site, or other discomforts.

➤ Explain any activity restrictions.

Thorn Test
thorn • test
(ACTH Test)

Normal Findings

ADULT
A 50% or greater decrease in the eosinophil count 4 hours after ACTH has been administered

What This Test Will Tell You

This blood test evaluates adrenal cortex function, measures the effectiveness of therapy, and evaluates adrenal cortical response to stress prior to surgery. After a baseline eosinophil count is obtained, ACTH (adrenocorticotropic hormone) is administered intramuscularly. In persons whose adrenal cortex is functioning normally, a decrease in the eosinophil count will result because cortisol decreases eosinophils.

Abnormal Findings

No change or only a slight decrease (<20%) in eosinophil count may signify adrenal insufficiency (Addison's disease).

ACTION ALERT!

Severe adrenal cortical dysfunction can be associated with life-threatening fluid and electrolyte imbalances. Immediate correction of fluid and electrolyte imbalances as well as replacement steroid therapy is indicated.

Interfering Factors

➤ Oral contraceptives, estrogen, and steroids may interfere with test results.

➤ Obesity or strenuous physical

activity can cause an elevated serum ACTH level.

NURSING CONSIDERATIONS

Prepare Your Client

➤ Explain that this test helps find any problems with a gland called the adrenal gland.

➤ Inform the client that strenuous physical activity and food should be avoided for 12 hours prior to the test.

Perform Procedure

➤ Obtain a baseline venous blood sample for serum ACTH by collecting 7–10 mL in a red-top tube, and for an eosinophil count by collecting 7 mL in a lavender-top tube.

➤ Administer ACTH (generally 25 mg intramuscularly), noting the exact time of administration on the laboratory slip.

➤ Send first two samples to lab immediately.

➤ Collect another 7-mL venous blood sample in a lavender-top tube 4 hours later for an eosinophil count, and send to lab.

Care After Test

➤ Observe for signs and symptoms of adrenal cortical insufficiency such as muscle weakness, fatigue, weight loss, anorexia, nausea, diarrhea, constipation, hypotension, hypoglycemia, hyponatremia, hyperkalemia, mental status changes, and increased pigmentation.

➤ Review related tests such as serum glucose, blood and urine cortisol levels, serum electrolyte studies, and urine studies including 17-ketosteroids, 17-hydroxycorticoids, and 17-ketogenic steroids.

Educate Your Client and the Family

➤ If adrenal cortical insufficiency is diagnosed, teach the client about cortisone therapy, which is likely to be prescribed.

➤ Teach client to inject hydrocortisone, which will be necessary during times they are unable to tolerate oral medications or during periods of acute stress such as trauma. Emphasize the importance of always seeking medical attention promptly so the primary health care provider can properly adjust dosages for stress, injury, or illness.

➤ Instruct the client and family to always have a portable emergency kit available that contains a syringe of dexamethasone; alcohol wipes for skin preparation; written information with diagnosis, medication prescription and dosage schedule; and emergency contacts including phone numbers.

➤ Instruct client to wear medical alert identification.

➤ Teach client that the cortisone replacement therapy must be maintained for life and failure to take medication will cause a crisis that may lead to death.

Throat Culture
throte • kul chur

Normal Findings
Negative

What This Test Will Tell You
This microbiological test differentiates streptococcal throat infections from viral and other throat infections. Approximately 5% of adult and 10%–15% of pediatric sore throats are caused by streptococcal infection. A positive rapid-identification strep test may be done in the lab or primary health care provider's office and justifies immediate initiation of treatment. All negative rapid tests should be confirmed by throat culture.

Abnormal Findings
Positive results may indicate beta-hemolytic streptococcus, *Hemophilus influenzae*, *Corynebacterium diphtheriae*, gonococcus, or meningococcus.

Interfering Factors
➤ Improper technique when collecting the specimen will yield false negative results.
➤ Antibiotic therapy and antiseptic mouthwash may cause false negative results.
➤ Contamination of the specimen may cause overgrowth of nonpathogenic organisms.

NURSING CONSIDERATIONS
Prepare Your Client
➤ Explain that this test is to help decide the best medicine for the sore throat.
➤ Tell your client to refrain from rinsing mouth with antiseptic mouthwash before the procedure.

Perform Procedure
➤ Depress your client's tongue with a tongue blade. A flashlight may be used to visualize the back of the throat.
➤ Rub the sterile swab for specimen collection over each tonsilar area and back of throat. If there are white patches visible, be sure to swab those areas. Do not touch the lips, tongue, or inside cheeks during the procedure.
➤ Place the swab in the transport medium. Label the specimen, indicate medications your client is taking that may interfere with results, and send specimen to lab.

Care After Test
➤ Assess for clinical signs and symptoms such as fever, abrupt onset of symptoms, patches on the throat, red rash over trunk and body creases, and elevated white blood cell count.
➤ Inform your client of results if a rapid test is used. If a culture is indicated, tell your client that results will be available in 48–72 hours.
➤ If antibiotic therapy is indicated, instruct your client to take the full prescription. Failure to take all the medication may cause superinfection or complications such as severe kidney disease (glomerulonephritis) or rheumatic fever.
➤ Evaluate other diagnostic tests such as white blood cell count, nasopharyngeal culture, and sputum culture.

Educate Your Client and the Family
➤ Inform family members they may need to be tested for strep infection.

Frequently more than one family member is infected.

➤ Tell your client and family that strep is spread through droplets from coughing or sneezing. Instruct your client to cover mouth when coughing or sneezing.

➤ Stress the importance of washing hands well to prevent spread of infection.

➤ Inform client and family members that the client is considered contagious until 36–48 hours after antibiotic therapy is completed.

➤ Teach client and family that a follow-up visit to the primary health care provider is important to determine if the antibiotic therapy was effective.

Thyroid Biopsy
thie roid • bie op see

Normal Findings
ADULT, ADOLESCENT, AND ELDERLY
Normal cytological features

What This Test Will Tell You
This microscopic examination of thyroid tissue is generally performed to differentiate between benign and malignant thyroid nodules. This test should always include additional diagnostic testing as it may result in false positive or false negative findings.

Abnormal Findings
Abnormal cells may indicate malignancy, benign tumors, subacute granulomatous thyroiditis, Hashimoto's thyroiditis, or hyperthyroidism.

█████ ACTION ALERT!
Monitor client closely for upper airway edema or tracheal puncture, which may lead to a respiratory emergency. Be prepared to establish an artificial airway emergently.

Interfering Factors
➤ The major limitation is the small amount of tissue obtained, which

may not be representative of the entire lesion.

Contraindications
➤ Coagulopathy

Potential Complications
➤ Hemorrhage
➤ Tracheal puncture
➤ Airway obstruction
➤ Laryngoparalysis
➤ Respiratory arrest

NURSING CONSIDERATIONS
Prepare Your Client
➤ Explain that this test is done to discover any problems with a gland in the neck called the thyroid gland.
➤ Ensure that an informed consent is obtained, because of the possible complications associated with this procedure.

Perform Procedure
Nurses do not perform this procedure, but should understand it to prepare the client and assist the primary health care provider.

The client is positioned supine with a pillow under the shoulders to situate the trachea and thyroid gland prominently anterior. A local anesthetic is injected, which may temporarily cause a burning sensation. Instruct the client not to swallow, which could potentially cause damage from needle movement. Once the biopsy needle has obtained a specimen, the needle is withdrawn and the sample is placed immediately in formaldehyde. Apply pressure to the site until bleeding has ceased, and apply an adhesive dressing.

Care After Test

➤ Monitor closely for upper airway obstruction, hematoma formation, and bleeding every 15 minutes for the first hour, every 30 minutes for the next hour, and then every 4 hours for at least 8 hours.
➤ Elevate the head of the bed and do not hyperflex the neck.
➤ Instruct the client to support the back of the head when lifting it off the pillow to avoid strain on the biopsy site and pain.
➤ Review related tests such as thyroid scan, radioactive iodine uptake (RAI), thyroid-stimulating hormone levels, thyroxine levels, and triiodothyronine levels.

Educate Your Client and the Family

➤ Instruct client to avoid strenuous activity for 24 hours following the test.
➤ Instruct client not to do any lifting greater than 5 pounds for 24–48 hours following the biopsy.
➤ Instruct client on spacing active periods with rest periods and eating a high-calorie, high-protein diet if findings indicate a malignancy that produces thyroid hormone.
➤ Emphasize the importance of additional testing as prescribed.

Thyroid Scan

thie roid • skan
(Thyroid Scintiscan)

Normal Findings

ADULT, ADOLESCENT, AND ELDERLY
Evenly distributed concentration of radioactive iodine. Normal size, position, and shape of the thyroid gland.

What This Test Will Tell You

This nuclear medicine test evaluates thyroid size, position, and function, diagnoses abnormalities, and is often used in the differential diagnosis of masses in the neck or mediastinum. A thyroid scan measures the uptake of radioactive iodine by the thyroid.

The scanned radioactivity of the gland is transformed onto a film or plotted on a computed tomography (CT) scan, outlining the gland and demonstrating any areas of abnormality. Benign adenomas usually appear as nodules of increased uptake (hot spots or functioning nodules), whereas malignant areas usually appear as areas of decreased uptake (cold spots or nonfunctioning nodules).

Abnormal Findings

▲INCREASED LEVELS of uptake

can indicate benign adenomas, Graves' disease, or localized toxic goiter.

▼ DECREASED LEVELS of uptake can indicate carcinoma, cysts, Hashimoto's disease, lymphoma, nonfunctioning adenoma, nonfunctioning goiter, or localized thyroiditis.

Interfering Factors
➤ Contrast material used in client during last 6 months may interfere with accurate imaging.

Contraindications
➤ Thyroid scans are contraindicated during pregnancy, and generally not performed in infancy or childhood.

Potential Complications
➤ Radiation-induced tumor formation

NURSING CONSIDERATIONS
Prepare Your Client
➤ Explain that this test is used to discover any abnormal areas of a gland in the neck called the thyroid gland.
➤ Instruct the client not to consume iodine-containing items such as seafood, iodized salt, enriched cereals, cabbage, cough medicine, and vitamins for at least a week before the test.
➤ Reassure the client and family that the small amount of radioactive material used should not offer any of them any danger.

Perform Procedure
➤ Radioactive iodine capsule or oral liquid, or intravenous radionuclide are administered in the nuclear medicine department.
➤ A thyroid scan performed with

iodine is generally done along with a radioactive iodine uptake study. Usually the neck area is scanned at 6 and 24 hours. Scan time is approximately 20–30 minutes.
➤ If radioactive technetium is used, scanning is done at 2 hours.

Care After Test
➤ Assess for signs of hypothyroidism including hypothermia, bradycardia, weight gain, thick and dry skin, thin hair, hypotension, cold extremities, mask-like expression, fatigue, slowed mental processes, myalgia, weakness, and constipation.
➤ Assess for signs of hyperthyroidism including nervousness, apprehension, tachycardia, diaphoresis, flushed skin, tremor in hands, constipation, diarrhea, weight loss, weakness, amenorrhea, and cardiac dysrhythmias.
➤ Institute safety measures if weakness is noted.
➤ Review related tests such as levels of serum thyroxine, protein-bound iodine, thyrotropin-releasing hormone, thyroid-stimulating hormone, and triiodothyronine suppression test.

Educate Your Client and the Family
➤ Teach client that thyroid hormone replacement must be taken for life if hypofunction is found or if the thyroid is removed surgically.
➤ Teach client how to meet rest and nutritional needs required by a hyperfunctioning thyroid. This includes frequent rest periods and a high-calorie, high-protein diet.
➤ Instruct client on iodized salt sources for treatment of goiter.

Thyroid-Stimulating Hormone

thie roid • stim yu lay ting • hor mone
(TSH)

Normal Findings

ADULT, CHILD, ADOLESCENT,
ELDERLY, AND PREGNANT
0.4–6.0 µU/L (SI units: 0.4–6.0
mU/L)
NEWBORN
3–18 µU/L (SI units: 3–18 mU/L)
<25 µU/L by day 3 (SI units: 25
mU/L)

What This Test Will Tell You

This blood test measures the circulatory level of thyroid-stimulating hormone (TSH) to aid in the diagnosis
of hypothyroidism and differentiate
primary from secondary hypothyroidism. The role of TSH is to stimulate the thyroid gland to release
stored hormones. TSH is produced
by the anterior pituitary gland but is
also influenced by the parathyroid
gland. If thyroxine and T_3 levels are
too high as in hyperthyroidism, the
secretion of TSH decreases. In primary hypothyroidism, TSH levels
rise in response to low levels of thyroid hormone.

Abnormal Findings

▲INCREASED LEVELS (6–10 µU/L)
may indicate hypothyroidism. Values
greater than 10 µU/L may indicate
primary hypothyroidism.
▼DECREASED LEVELS (0.1–0.4
µU/L) may indicate secondary
hypothyroidism, hyperthyroidism,
Graves' disease, or thyroiditis. Levels
<0.1 are indicative of hypothy-
roidism.

Interfering Factors

➤ Aspirin, corticosteroids, heparin,
dopamine, and triiodothyronine may

decrease values.
➤ Lithium, TSH therapy, and potassium iodide will increase values.
➤ Radioactive scans performed
within 1 week of venous sampling
may interfere with results.
➤ Pregnancy, postmenopausal state,
hydatidiform mole, and choriocarcinoma may result in elevated TSH
levels.
➤ Levels are increased in newborns
due to hypersecretion of TSH. Levels
should be in the adult range by 14
days of life.
➤ Hemolysis may yield inaccurate
results.

NURSING CONSIDERATIONS

Prepare Your Client

➤ Explain that this test is used to
find any problems in a gland in the
neck called the thyroid gland.

Perform Procedure

➤ Collect 5 mL of venous blood in a
red-top or green-top tube.
➤ Perform a heelstick on newborns.

Care After Test

➤ Assess for signs of hypothyroidism
including hypothermia, bradycardia,
weight gain, thick and dry skin, thin
hair, hypotension, cold extremities,
mask-like expression, fatigue, slowed
mental processes, myalgia, weakness,
and constipation.
➤ Institute safety measures if weakness is noted.
➤ Review related tests such as levels
of serum thyroxine, protein-bound
iodine, thyrotropin-releasing hormone, thyroid-stimulating hormone,

and triiodothyronine suppression test.

Educate Your Client and the Family

➤ Teach client that thyroid hormone replacement must be taken for life if hypofunction is found or if the thyroid is removed surgically.

➤ Explain the importance of additional endocrine testing.

Thyroid-Stimulating Immunoglobulin, Serum

thie roid • stim yu lay ting • im yoo noe glob yu lin • see rum
(Long-Acting Thyroid Stimulator, TSI, TSIg)

Normal Findings

All ages: Negative; ≤10 µU/mL (Levels >10 µU/mL present in only 5% of healthy people.)

What This Test Will Tell You

This blood test aids in diagnosing and monitoring treatment of thyroid disorders, including thyrotoxicosis and Graves' disease. This immunoglobulin is an autoantibody that acts against the thyroid cell plasma membrane and mimics thyroid-stimulating hormone (TSH). Production of TSI stimulates the thyroid gland to produce and excrete excessive amounts of thyroid hormones, resulting in a clinical picture of hyperthyroidism. TSH is suppressed through the normal feedback mechanism.

Abnormal Findings

Presence of TSI indicates Graves' disease, hyperthyroidism, or malignant exophthalmos.

Interfering Factors

➤ Administration of radioactive iodine within 48 hours will alter test results.

➤ Hemolysis of blood sample.

➤ 5% of normal persons may have positive TSI results without the clinical presence of disease.

NURSING CONSIDERATIONS

Prepare Your Client

➤ Explain that this test helps to find problems that may be present in a gland in the body called the thyroid gland, and tells whether the body is actually making antibodies to attack this gland.

Perform Procedure

➤ Collect 5–7 mL of venous blood into a red-top tube.

➤ Avoid hemolysis of sample.

Care After Test

➤ Assess for signs of hyperthyroidism including nervousness, apprehension, tachycardia, diaphoresis, flushed skin, tremor in hands, constipation, diarrhea, weight loss, weakness, amenorrhea, and cardiac dysrhythmias.

➤ Institute safety measures if weakness is noted.

➤ Review related tests such as levels of serum thyroxine, protein-bound iodine, thyrotropin-releasing hormone, thyroid-stimulating hormone,

and triiodothyronine suppression test.

Educate Your Client and the Family
➤ Educate the client regarding Graves' disease once the diagnosis is confirmed.

➤ Teach client how to meet rest and nutritional needs required by a hyperfunctioning thyroid. This includes frequent rest periods and a high-calorie, high-protein diet.

Thyroid Ultrasound
thie roid • ul tra sownd

Normal Findings
All ages: Ultrasound waves uniformly reflected throughout the gland. Normal pattern and image of thyroid for size, depth, and dimension.

What This Test Will Tell You
This ultrasound test differentiates cysts from tumors or reveals the depth of nodules. Identification of fluid-filled cysts allows for needle aspiration without surgery. Solid or mixed nodules usually require surgery for diagnosis and treatment.

Abnormal Findings
Abnormalities may include cysts, adenomas, tumors, goiters, and carcinomas.

Interfering Factors
➤ Abnormalities smaller than 1 cm may escape detection.

NURSING CONSIDERATIONS
Prepare Your Client
➤ Explain that this test is done to find any problems in a gland in the neck called the thyroid gland.
➤ Explain that this test uses harmless and painless sound waves to evaluate the thyroid gland.

Perform Procedure
Nurses do not usually perform this procedure, but should understand it to assist the ultrasound technician. Place the client supine on an examining table with the neck hyperextended. Transducer gel is applied liberally to the neck and the transducer is passed over the thyroid while images are recorded.

Care After Test
➤ Assess for signs of hypothyroidism including hypothermia, bradycardia, weight gain, thick and dry skin, thin hair, hypotension, cold extremities, mask-like expression, fatigue, slowed mental processes, myalgia, weakness, and constipation.
➤ Assess for signs of hyperthyroidism including nervousness, apprehension, tachycardia, diaphoresis, flushed skin, tremor in hands, constipation, diarrhea, weight loss, weakness, amenorrhea, and cardiac dysrhythmias.
➤ Institute safety measures if weakness is noted.
➤ Review related tests such as levels of serum thyroxine, protein-bound iodine, thyrotropin-releasing hormone, thyroid-stimulating hormone,

and triiodothyronine suppression test.

Educate Your Client and the Family

➤ Teach client that thyroid hormone replacement must be taken for life if hypofunction is found or if the thyroid is removed surgically.

➤ Teach client how to meet rest and nutritional needs required by a hyperfunctioning thyroid. This includes frequent rest periods and a high-calorie, high-protein diet.

➤ Instruct client on iodized salt sources for treatment of goiter.

Thyrotropin-Releasing Hormone

thie ro troe pin • ree lees ing • hor mone
(Thyrotropin-Releasing Hormone Stimulation, TRH, Thyrotropin-Releasing Factor, TRF)

Normal Findings

ADULT, ADOLESCENT, AND ELDERLY

TSH should promptly increase to approximately two times the baseline level, normally within 30 minutes. This response is generally greater in females.

What This Test Will Tell You

This blood test differentiates primary, secondary, and tertiary hypothyroidism by assessing the responsiveness of the anterior pituitary gland to the administration of thyrotropin-releasing hormone (TRH). Normally, thyrotropin-releasing hormone (released by the hypothalamus) stimulates the anterior pituitary gland to release thyroid-stimulating hormone (TSH). In primary hypothyroidism, where the thyroid gland itself is dysfunctional, a two- to threefold rise in TSH occurs when TRH is administered. In secondary hypothyroidism, where the anterior pituitary is dysfunctional and never properly releases TSH to stimulate the thyroid, there is no rise in TSH when TRH is administered.

Finally, in tertiary hypothyroidism, where the hypothalamus is dysfunctional and never releases TRH to stimulate the pituitary to release TSH for normal thyroid function, there is a delay in the rise of TSH when TRH is administered.

Abnormal Findings

▲ INCREASED LEVELS (exaggerated TSH response) may indicate primary hypothyroidism, or tertiary hypothyroidism if the response is slow.

▼ DECREASED LEVELS (low or no TSH response) may indicate hyperthyroidism and secondary hypothyroidism.

Interfering Factors

➤ Thyroid hormone therapy will alter results.

➤ Pregnancy increases the response to TRH.

➤ Antithyroid medications, estrogens, oral contraceptives, corticosteroids, aspirin, levodopa, and thyroxine can all interfere with accurate results.

➤ Hemolysis may interfere with results.

NURSING CONSIDERATIONS

Prepare Your Client

➤ Explain that this test is used to help discover any problems in a gland in the neck called the thyroid gland.

➤ Thyroid medications are usually discontinued for 4–6 weeks prior to sampling.

Perform Procedure

➤ Collect 5 mL of venous blood in a red-top tube to obtain a baseline TSH blood level.

➤ Generally a 500-μg bolus of TRH is given intravenously and blood samples are collected in red-top tubes at varying intervals over several hours.

➤ Multiple injections of TRH may be required to induce a response in tertiary hypothyroidism.

➤ Check for the specific procedure with the laboratory.

Care After Test

➤ Assess for signs of hypothyroidism including hypothermia, bradycardia, weight gain, thick and dry skin, thin hair, hypotension, cold extremities, mask-like expression, fatigue, slowed mental processes, myalgia, weakness, and constipation.

➤ Institute safety measures if weakness is noted.

➤ Review related tests such as levels of serum thyroxine, protein-bound iodine, thyrotropin-releasing hormone, thyroid-stimulating hormone, thyroid ultrasound, thyroid scan, and triiodothyronine suppression test.

Educate Your Client and the Family

➤ Teach client that thyroid hormone replacement must be taken for life if hypofunction is found or if the thyroid is removed surgically.

Thyroxine

thie rok sin

(Total T_4, L-Thyroxine Serum Concentration, Neonatal Thyroxine, Neonatal Screen for Hypothyroidism)

Normal Findings

ADULT, ADOLESCENT, AND ELDERLY

Total levels: 5–13.5 μg/dL (SI units: 64–174 nmol/L)

PREGNANT

Values will be increased during pregnancy.

NEWBORN

Total levels: 10.1–20 μg/dL; possible critical value: <7.0 μg/dL

Filter paper method:

1–5 days: >5μg/dL equivalent

6–8 days: >4 μg/dL equivalent

9–11 days: >3.6 μg/dL equivalent

12–120 days: >3 μg/dL equivalent

CHILD (UP TO 10 YEARS)

Total levels: 5.5–14 μg/dL

What This Test Will Tell You

These blood tests are used to help diagnose hypothyroidism, especially as a screen in neonates, and to monitor the response to therapy. Thyroid hormone is required for normal growth and development of the brain, bones, and other vital organs and tissues. The total thyroxine (T_4) test is frequently used within the first week of life to identify congenital hypothyroidism. Approximately 95% of thyroxine is bound to protein, while about 5% of the circulating thyroxine is free or unbound.

Abnormal Findings

▲ INCREASED LEVELS may indicate hyperthyroidism, acute and subacute thyroiditis, or early hepatitis.

▼ DECREASED LEVELS may indicate cretinism, hypothyroidism, myxedema, chronic or subacute thyroiditis, nephrosis, cirrhosis, hypoproteinemia, or malnutrition.

ACTION ALERT!

Thyroxine values that suggest hypothyroidism in a newborn require immediate medical intervention for more definitive testing and treatment. Left untreated, hypothyroidism in the neonate can result in permanent mental retardation.

Interfering Factors

➤ Estrogen therapy, estrogen-secreting tumors, oral contraceptives, heroin, methadone, and pregnancy can increase T_4 levels.

➤ Steroids, androgens, heparin, salicylates, phenytoin, sulfonamides, chronic liver disease, and nephrosis can decrease T_4 levels.

➤ Thyroid medications will interfere with T_4 results. If baseline results are desired, medications should be discontinued 4–6 weeks prior to testing.

NURSING CONSIDERATIONS

Prepare Your Client

➤ Explain that this test is to discover if there are any problems with a gland in the neck called the thyroid gland.

➤ Explain to the family of a newborn that this is a routine screening test.

Perform Procedure

➤ Collect 5 mL of venous blood in a red-top tube.

NEONATAL SCREENING

➤ Follow directions closely on neonatal screening kit.

➤ Cleanse the skin of heel with an antiseptic and puncture with a sterile lancet.

➤ Hold the foot below the level of the heart to facilitate bleeding.

➤ Place one side of the filter paper against heel until the blood is visible on the front side of the paper and fills the circle.

➤ Air-dry for 1 hour and send to laboratory.

Care After Test

➤ Assess for signs of hypothyroidism including hypothermia, bradycardia, weight gain, thick and dry skin, thin hair, hypotension, cold extremities, masklike expression, fatigue, slowed mental processes, myalgia, weakness, and constipation.

➤ Assess for signs of hyperthyroidism including nervousness, apprehension, tachycardia, diaphoresis, flushed skin, tremor in hands, constipation, diarrhea, weight loss, weakness, amenorrhea, and cardiac dysrhythmias.

➤ Institute safety measures if weakness is noted.

➤ Review related tests such as levels of serum thyroxine, protein-bound iodine, thyrotropin-releasing hormone, and thyroid-stimulating hormone, and triiodothyronine suppression test.

Educate Your Client and the Family

➤ Teach client and family that thyroid hormone replacement must be taken for life if hypofunction is found or if the thyroid is removed surgically.

➤ Teach client how to meet rest and nutritional needs required by a hyperfunctioning thyroid. This includes frequent rest periods and a high-calorie, high-protein diet.

Thyroxine-Binding Globulin
thie rok sin • bine ding • glob yu lin
(TBG)

Normal Findings

ADULT, ADOLESCENT, AND ELDERLY

Normal ranges vary dramatically in different laboratories. Check with your laboratory for normal ranges.
Electrophoresis: 10–25 µg/dL (SI units: 130–322 nmol/L)
Radioimmunoassay: 1.3–2 mg/dL

PREGNANT

Values will be increased.

NEWBORN

Radioimmunoassay: 2.0–7.6 mg/dL or 20–76 mg/L

CHILD

Radioimmunoassay: 2.5–5.0 mg/dL or 25–50 mg/L

What This Test Will Tell You

This blood test determines congenital abnormalities of thyroxine-binding globulin (TBG) or confirms abnormalities of thyroxine-binding proteins. TBG is important in the regulation of T_4 levels. If TBG levels are inaccurate, then determinations of total T_3 and T_4 are not accurate. Instead, levels of free T_3 and free T_4 need to be relied upon. Performing a thyroxine level on the same blood sample as the TGB will allow for a differential diagnosis between true thyroid disorders and related problems.

Abnormal Findings

▲INCREASED LEVELS may indicate hypothyroidism or genetic or idiopathic hepatic disease.

▼DECREASED LEVELS may indicate hyperthyroidism, nephrotic syndromes, or liver disease.

Interfering Factors

➤ Oral contraceptives, estrogen therapy, and phenothiazines increase TBG levels.

➤ Anabolic agents, aspirin, prednisolone, phenytoin, and androgens decrease TBG levels.

➤ Estrogen-secreting tumors elevate levels.

NURSING CONSIDERATIONS

Prepare Your Client

➤ Explain that this test will help find any problems in a gland in the neck called the thyroid gland.

Perform Procedure

➤ Collect 2–5 mL of venous blood in a red-top tube.

➤ In an infant, use a heelstick method of collecting the venous sample.

Care After Test

➤ Assess for signs of hypothyroidism including hypothermia, bradycardia, weight gain, thick and dry skin, thin hair, hypotension, cold extremities, masklike expression, fatigue, slowed mental processes, myalgia, weakness, and constipation.

➤ Assess for signs of hyperthyroidism including nervousness, apprehension, tachycardia, diaphoresis, flushed skin, tremor in hands, constipation, diarrhea, weight loss, weakness, amenorrhea, and cardiac dysrhythmias.

➤ Institute safety measures if weakness is noted.

➤ Review related tests such as levels of serum thyroxine, protein-bound iodine, thyrotropin-releasing hormone, thyroid-stimulating hormone, and triiodothyronine suppression test.

Educate Your Client and the Family

➤ Teach client and family that thyroid hormone replacement must be taken for life if hypofunction is found or if the thyroid is removed surgically.

➤ Teach client how to meet rest and nutritional needs required by a hyperfunctioning thyroid. This includes frequent rest periods and a high-calorie, high-protein diet.

Tolbutamide Tolerance

tol **byoo** tah mide • tol ur ans

Normal findings

All ages: Glucose decreases by about 50% of baseline value within 30 minutes and then gradually returns to the pretest level within 1 1/2–3 hours.

What This Test Will Tell You

This blood test diagnoses certain tumors of the pancreas and rules out functional hyperinsulinism by measuring the insulin and glucose responses to the injection of the hypoglycemic agent tolbutamide. The injection of tolbutamide stimulates the beta cells of the pancreas and certain tumors (insulinomas) to secrete insulin. Upon release of insulin, glucose levels will decrease rapidly and then return to the pretest levels in approximately 1 1/2–3 hours. Abnormal insulin secretion can be demonstrated indirectly by monitoring the glucose levels. The fall in blood glucose is more dramatic in insulinomas than in functional hypoglycemia. With the latter, the blood glucose level fails to recover within 3 hours if an insulinoma is present.

Abnormal Findings

▲ INCREASED LEVELS may indicate diabetes mellitus.

▼ DECREASED LEVELS may indicate insulinoma, severe liver disease, acute pancreatitis, malnutrition, azotemia, or idiopathic hypoglycemia in children.

ACTION ALERT!

➤ Do not perform this test if the fasting blood sugar is below 50 mg/dL because of the danger of developing severe hypoglycemia.

➤ Assess for signs and symptoms of hypoglycemia including diaphoresis, cold skin, tachycardia, hypotension, weakness, restlessness, nervousness, anxiety, and deterioration of mental status. If these should develop during the test, stop the tolbutamide infusion immediately, send a STAT blood glucose level, and prepare to administer intravenous glucose immediately.

➤ Assess clients carefully for allergic reaction to tolbutamide including dyspnea, itching, urticaria, flushing, hypotension, and shock. Life-threatening anaphylactic reactions can occur and need to be recognized and treated immediately.

Interfering Factors

➤ A diet deficient in carbohydrate in the 3 days prior to the test may alter the test results.

➤ Smoking before and during the test may alter the test results.

➤ Use of caffeine, beta-adrenergic blocking agents, oral antidiabetic agents, heroine, catecholamines, benzodiazepines, monoamine oxidase inhibitors, thyroid hormones, and sulfonamides may worsen the hypoglycemic response.

➤ Oral contraceptives, estrogen, progesterone, and corticosteroids may decrease the expected amount of drop in glucose level.

Contraindications

➤ Fasting blood sugar less than 50 mg/dL

➤ Hypersensitivity to tolbutamide or other sulfonylureas and sulfonamides

Potential Complications

➤ Hypoglycemia
➤ Anaphylaxis

NURSING CONSIDERATIONS

Prepare Your Client

➤ Explain that this test is used to see if there are any problems with a gland in the body called the pancreas that helps regulate how the body uses sugar.

➤ Instruct the client to eat a high-carbohydrate diet for 3 days before the test.

➤ Restrict food and fluids for 8–12 hours prior to the test.

➤ Encourage the client to bring reading material or other activities as the test will take approximately 3 hours.

➤ Question the client regarding a history of adverse reactions to tolbutamide, sulfonylureas, or sulfonamides.

➤ Describe the signs and symptoms of hypoglycemia (extreme hunger, restlessness, irritability, weakness, sweating, nervousness) and ask the client to report them immediately should these symptoms be experienced.

Perform Procedure

➤ Insert a heparin lock to maintain the patency of and access to a vein in order to prevent multiple venipunctures.

➤ Collect the fasting blood sample of 10 mL venous blood in a gray-top tube. If hypoglycemia is suspected, have sample tested before proceeding. (See Action Alert! for this test.)

➤ Prepare the tolbutamide with 20 mL of sterile saline and shake well to dissolve any crystals. The adult dose is 25–40 mg/kg body weight with a maximum of 1 gram to be given over 2–3 minutes. For newborns the dose is 25 mg/kg intravenously diluted in 10 mL of sterile saline and given over 2–3 minutes.

➤ Draw blood samples at 15, 30, 45, 60, 90, 120, 150, and 180 minutes after the infusion of the tolbutamide.

➤ Document the collection time on the lab slips for each sample.

➤ Monitor the client closely for any signs or symptoms of hypoglycemia (extreme hunger, restlessness, irritability, weakness, sweating, or nervousness).

➤ If the client should experience hypoglycemia, notify the primary health care provider, stop the test, draw a blood sample, and give intravenous glucose to reverse the hypoglycemic reaction.

Care After Test

➤ Discontinue the heparin lock after the last blood sample has been drawn unless otherwise indicated.

➤ Instruct the client to eat a balanced meal after the completion of the test.

➤ Continue to assess for signs or symptoms of hypoglycemia for up to 2 hours.

➤ Review related tests such as serum insulin, fasting blood sugars, 2-hour postprandial blood sugars, oral glucose tolerance test, serum adrenocor-ticotropic hormone (ACTH), serum C-peptide, serum electrolytes, plasma glucagon, insulin antibodies, insulin assay, vasoactive intestinal polypeptide, chemistry profile, creatinine clearance, quantitative glucose, and qualitative glucose.

Educate Your Client and the Family

➤ If the test results indicate diabetes, begin diabetic teaching.

➤ If the test results indicate an insulinoma, instruct the client regarding the prescribed diet. Teach them to increase the amount of starches, breads, potatoes, and rice in their diet, as these are slowly absorbed carbohydrates and help to prevent hypoglycemic episodes.

➤ Discuss the importance of regular balanced meals and snacks that are eaten at approximately the same times each day.

TORCH Test
torch test
(TORCH Screen, TORCH Titer)

Normal Findings

Maternal: IgG and IgM titer antibodies—negative

Infant under 2 months: IgG and IgM titer antibodies—negative

What This Test Will Tell You

This blood test screens for congenital infection of an infant. TORCH is an acronym for toxoplasmosis, other infectious diseases such as syphilis and listeriosis, rubella, cytomegalovirus, and herpes simplex. The IgG and IgM titers of the mother and infant are compared. If the infant's IgG titer is higher than the mother's and the infant has an IgM titer, TORCH infection of the infant is likely. Infants should be less than 2 months of age when the test is performed. The effect of these congenital infections may be severe, causing congenital abnormalities, spontaneous abortion, or fetal death.

Abnormal Findings

Positive results may reveal rubella, cytomegalovirus, toxoplasmosis, herpes simplex, syphilis, or other viruses.

Interfering Factors
➤ If antibody production does not begin early enough in the infection, a false negative is possible.
➤ Rheumatoid factors may cause false negative results.
➤ Competing levels of IgG may cause false negative IgM levels.

NURSING CONSIDERATIONS
Prepare Your Client
➤ Explain that this test screens for possible infection of the baby for a variety of diseases.

Perform Procedure
➤ Collect 10 mL of venous blood in a red-top tube from the mother.
➤ When collecting a specimen from the infant after birth, collect 3 mL of venous or cord blood in a red-top tube.

Care After Test
➤ Evaluate the infant for signs and symptoms of congenital anomalies or infection.

➤ Evaluate related tests such as hemagglutination inhibition and complete blood count with differential. Enzyme immunoassays are useful for documenting past infections or immunity. IgM enzyme-linked immunosorbent assay tests demonstrate recent infection with toxoplasmosis and rubella. Virus isolation is preferred for cytomegalovirus and herpes simplex.

Educate Your Client and the Family
➤ Instruct the mother about the importance of avoiding infection with the specific diseases during pregnancy. Infection during the first trimester results in the most severe complications. TORCH infections that cross the placenta may cause congenital deformities, spontaneous abortion, or stillbirth.
➤ Tell the client that if the TORCH screen is positive, more testing will be required to determine the specific infectious organism.

Total Erythrocyte Porphyrins
toe tahl • eh rith roe site • por fi rins
(Erythrocyte Total Porphyrins, Erythropoietic Porphyrins, Protoporphyrin, Coproporphyrin, Uroporphyrin)

Normal Findings
Total porphyrin level: <60 µg/dL (SI units: <1.08 µmol/L)
Protoporphyrin: 16–60 µg/dL (SI units: <0.30–1.08 µmol/L)

What This Test Will Tell You
This blood test identifies metabolic disorders of the red blood cells and accelerated erythropoiesis. Porphyrins are important pigments for energy storage and utilization. Disorders of porphyrins may be either genetically determined or acquired and result from metabolic defects in heme biosynthesis.

Abnormal Findings

▲ INCREASED LEVELS may indicate protoporphyria, intoxication porphyria that can be caused by heavy metals such as lead, exposure to halogenated solvents, or iron deficiency anemia.

NURSING CONSIDERATIONS

Prepare Your Client

➤ Explain that this test measures an important working part of red blood cells.

➤ Restrict food and fluids except water for 12–14 hours prior to the test.

Perform Procedure

➤ Collect 3 mL of venous blood in a green-top tube.

Care After Test

➤ Assess the client for signs of infection including fever.

➤ Observe the client for signs and symptoms of anemia including pal-lor, dyspnea, chest pain, and fatigue.

➤ Encourage rest periods for client experiencing fatigue related to anemia.

➤ Evaluate client's ability to perform activities of daily living and refer to community health care services as needed.

➤ Review related tests such as hemoglobin, hematocrit, reticulocyte count, red blood cell indices, hemoglobin electrophoresis, ferritin level, total iron-binding capacity (TIBC), bone marrow and liver biopsies, urine porphyrins, and iron absorption and excretion studies.

Educate Your Client and Family

➤ If result is elevated, advise the client to avoid sun exposure, which may worsen symptoms.

➤ Advise the client diagnosed with porphyria and neurologic symptoms that attacks can be precipitated by infection, various phases of the menstrual cycle, not eating, and certain drugs.

Total Iron-Binding Capacity
toe tal • ie urn • bine ding • kah pas ih tee
(TIBC, Iron-Binding Capacity)

Normal Findings
ADULT, CHILD, ADOLESCENT, AND ELDERLY
240–450 µg/dL (SI units: 41–77 µmol/L)
PREGNANT
Values are slightly increased in the third trimester due to iron deficiency unless client is taking iron supplements.

NEWBORN
100–400 µg/dL (SI units: 17–68 µmol/L)

What This Test Will Tell You
This blood test evaluates the amount of iron, iron storage, and nutritional status in clients with anemia. The total iron-binding capacity (TIBC) measures the amount of free-floating

iron found in the plasma if all the transferrin protein were saturated with iron. Transferrin is a protein formed by the liver that has the primary function of transporting iron to the bone marrow for the synthesis of hemoglobin or to the body cells for use.

Abnormal Findings

▲INCREASED LEVELS may indicate hypochromic anemias, polycythemia vera, acute hepatitis with necrosis, late pregnancy, microcytic anemias, or iron salts therapy.

▼DECREASED LEVELS may indicate anemia (non–iron deficient), chronic infections, hemolytic anemia, sickle-cell anemia, rheumatoid arthritis, hemochromatosis, cirrhosis, neoplastic disease, renal disease, thalassemia, dysmenorrhea, hemorrhage, hypothyroidism, kwashiorkor, myocardial infarction, or pernicious anemia.

Interfering Factors

➤ Chloramphenicol fluorides and oral contraceptives can cause elevated test results.

➤ Adrenocorticotropic hormone can produce false negative results.

➤ Rough handling of the blood specimen can invalidate the results.

➤ Iron supplements will cause a false increase in the serum iron values, but will cause a false decrease in the total iron-binding capacity.

NURSING CONSIDERATIONS

Prepare Your Client

➤ Explain that the test will evaluate how much iron is in the body and available to make red blood cells.

Perform Procedure

➤ Collect 7–10 mL of venous blood in a red-top tube.

Care After Test

➤ Observe the client for signs and symptoms of anemia including pallor, dyspnea, palpitations, activity intolerance, and chest pain.

➤ Encourage rest periods for fatigue that occurs with anemia. Plan for consistent periods of light exercise but instruct the client to increase this slowly over time.

➤ Assist the client in gathering assistance with the usual activities of daily living including self-care and home maintenance activities.

➤ Instruct the client to maintain the usual patterns of sleep.

➤ Instruct the client to report any chest pain or palpitations to the primary health care provider.

➤ Obtain a dietary consult to assist the client in choosing a well-balanced diet, including foods high in vitamin C and iron.

➤ Investigate who plans and cooks the meals: is it the client or a caregiver? Instruct that person about foods high in iron and vitamin C.

➤ Review related tests such as serum iron, serum ferritin assay, transferrin, bone marrow biopsy, and liver biopsy.

Educate Your Client and the Family

➤ Instruct your client in the foods that are rich in iron such as liver, egg yolks, lean beef, and prune juice.

➤ Instruct your client in the foods that are rich in vitamin C, which is a promoter of iron absorption. Foods rich in vitamin C include oranges, grapefruit, cabbage, and potatoes.

> Teach your client to increase activity slowly after blood transfusion, as the blood does not become completely oxygenated for 12–36 hours after infusion. Excessive activity following the transfusion can result in undue fatigue and exhaustion for the client.

Toxoplasmosis Antibody Titer, Serum

tahk soe plaz moe sis • an ti bod ee • tie tur • see rum
(TPM Antibody Test, Indirect Fluorescent Antibody Tests, IFA)

Normal Findings

Titers < 1:16 indicate no previous infection.
Titers 1:16–1:256 are prevalent in the general population.
Titers > 1:256 suggest recent infection.

What This Test Will Tell You

This test diagnoses toxoplasmosis, a disease caused by the *Toxoplasma gondii* parasite. The disease may occur congenitally or following birth. Toxoplasmosis is transmitted to humans by ingesting undercooked meat of infected animals, from handling contaminated cat litter, and via the placenta of an infected mother to the fetus. Congenital toxoplasmosis is diagnosed either when the test levels are persistently elevated or with a rising titer in an infant for 2–3 months after birth. The Centers for Disease Control recommends that all pregnant clients be tested for this disease because one-quarter to one-half of adults are asymptomatically affected with toxoplasmosis.

Abnormal Findings

The test may reveal toxoplasmosis infection.

NURSING CONSIDERATIONS

Prepare Your Client

> Explain that this is a blood test to determine exposure to or the presence of toxoplasmosis, a disease that can occur from handling cat feces or raw meat.
> Ask if the client has handled cat feces during pregnancy.
> Ask if the client has eaten any raw or undercooked meat.

Perform Procedure

> Collect 5 mL of venous blood in a red-top tube.
> Write on the laboratory slip if the client has been exposed to cats or is pregnant.

Care After Test

> Assess infant for signs and symptoms of congenital toxoplasmosis including convulsions, hydrocephaly, microcephaly, developmental delays, cerebral calcification, and retinitis.
> Refer infant for developmental evaluation if congenital toxoplasmosis is diagnosed.

Educate Your Client and the Family

> Instruct the client regarding any repeat testing to detect a rising titer.

- ➤ Instruct a pregnant client who owns a cat to avoid handling cat litter.

- ➤ Instruct a pregnant client to thoroughly cook all meat.

Transferrin, Serum

trans fehr in • see rum

(Transferrin, Siderophilin, Tf Nelphelom, Transferrin Saturation)

Normal Findings

ALL AGES, TRANSFERRIN SATURATION

30%–40%

ADULT, SERUM TRANSFERRIN

200–400 μg/dL (SI units: 36–72 μmol/L)

PREGNANT, SERUM TRANSFERRIN

305 μg/dL (SI units: 55 μmol/L)

Elevations are seen in the third trimester.

NEWBORN, SERUM TRANSFERRIN

0–4 days: 130–275 μg/dL (SI units: 23–50 μmol/L)

3–9 months: 203–360 μg/dL (SI units: 36–65 μmol/L)

9 months and older: 305 μg/dL (SI units: 55 μmol/L)

CHILD AND ADOLESCENT, SERUM TRANSFERRIN

203–360 μg/dL (SI units: 36–65 μmol/L)

ELDERLY (OVER 60), SERUM TRANSFERRIN

180–380 μg/dL (SI units: 32–69 μmol/L)

What This Test Will Tell You

This blood test assists in determining the capacity of the red blood cells to carry iron. Transferrin, a protein found in the serum of the blood, is formed by the liver and is responsible for transporting iron obtained from dietary sources and from the breakdown of red blood cells. Most of the iron is taken to the bone marrow for use in the synthesis of hemoglobin. Low levels of transferrin will lead to inadequate amounts of hemoglobin and result in anemia. Transferrin is also believed to have important immune function in fighting bacterial infections.

Abnormal Findings

▲INCREASED LEVELS may indicate iron deficiency anemia, pregnancy, polycythemia vera, or estrogen or oral contraceptive therapy.

▼DECREASED LEVELS may indicate generalized malnutrition, chronic inflammation, tissue necrosis, nephrotic syndrome, hepatic damage, multiple myeloma, hemolytic anemia, or inherited atransferrinemia.

Interfering Factors

- ➤ Transferrin levels are increased with estrogen therapy and oral contraceptives.

- ➤ Transferrin levels are decreased with asparaginase, dextran, corticotropin, corticosteroids, and testosterone.

- ➤ Hemolysis due to rough handling of the sample may affect test results.

NURSING CONSIDERATIONS
Prepare Your Client
➤ Explain that this test will help to see how well the body is using iron to make red blood cells.

Perform Procedure
➤ Collect 7–10 mL of venous blood in a red-top tube.

Care After Test
➤ Observe the client for signs and symptoms of anemia including pallor, dyspnea, palpitations, activity intolerance, and chest pain.

➤ Encourage rest periods for fatigue that occurs with anemia. Plan for consistent periods of light exercise but instruct the client to increase this slowly over time.

➤ Assist the client in gathering assistance with the usual activities of daily living including self-care and home maintenance activities.

➤ Instruct the client to maintain the usual patterns of sleep.

➤ Instruct the client to report chest pain or palpitations to the primary health care provider.

➤ Obtain a dietary consult to assist the client in choosing a well-balanced diet including foods high in vitamin C and iron.

➤ Investigate who plans and cooks the meals: is it the client or a caregiver? Instruct that person in foods high in iron and vitamin C.

➤ Review related tests such as serum iron, serum ferritin assay, total iron-binding capacity, bone marrow biopsy, and liver biopsy.

Educate Your Client and the Family
➤ Instruct your client or caregiver in the foods that are rich in iron such as liver, egg yolks, lean beef, and prune juice.

➤ Instruct your client or caregiver in the foods that are rich in vitamin C, which is a promoter of iron absorption. Foods rich in vitamin C include oranges, grapefruit, cabbage, and potatoes.

Triglycerides, Serum
trie glis ur ides • see rum

Normal Findings
ADULT
Male: 40–160 mg/dL (SI units: 0.45–1.81 mmol/L)
Female: 35–135 mg/dL (SI units: 0.40–1.53 mmol/L)
PREGNANT
Levels may be increased during pregnancy.
NEWBORN
40–60 mg/dL (SI units: 0.45–0.68 mmol/L)

CHILD
30–138 mg/dL (SI units: 0.34–1.56 mmol/L)
ADOLESCENT, 10–19 YEARS OLD
Male: 36–163 mg/dL (SI units: 0.41–1.83 mmol/L)
Female: 41–128 mg/dL (SI units: 0.46–1.44 mmol/L)
ELDERLY
Up to 190 mg/dL may be acceptable (SI units: <2.14 mmol/L).

What This Test Will Tell You

This blood test helps evaluate the risk of coronary artery and peripheral vascular disease through identification of hyperlipidemia. The test measures the blood levels of triglycerides, an important form of stored fat. Triglycerides can be synthesized by the body or directly obtained from dietary intake of either vegetable or animal sources of fat and carbohydrates. Excess triglycerides are transported by very low density lipoproteins (VLDLs) and low-density lipoproteins (LDLs) to be stored in the body as adipose (fat) tissue. As they are needed, they can later be converted back to fatty acids to be used as an energy source. Serum triglyceride levels are an important component of a lipid profile to evaluate a client's risk of coronary artery and peripheral vascular disease.

Abnormal Findings

▲INCREASED LEVELS may indicate hyperlipidemia, pancreatitis, diabetes mellitus, pregnancy, hypothyroidism, obstruction of bile ducts, nephrotic syndrome, liver disease, glycogen storage disease, toxemia, myocardial infarction less than 1 year previously, or a metabolic disorder.

▼DECREASED LEVELS may indicate chronic obstructive pulmonary disease, hyperthyroidism, malnutrition, a malabsorption disorder, or cerebral infarct.

Interfering Factors

➤ Ingestion of a fatty meal can increase levels.
➤ Consumption of alcohol within 24 hours of blood sampling can increase levels.
➤ Pregnancy and oral contraceptives can increase levels.

➤ Many medications such as corticosteroids, estrogen, and furosemide may raise levels.
➤ Many medications such as heparin, ascorbic acid, asparaginase, and niacin may lower levels.

NURSING CONSIDERATIONS

Prepare Your Client

➤ Explain that this test is important in determining the risk of heart disease and heart attacks.
➤ Explain that you will need to draw blood from the vein for the test. Explain the venipuncture process clearly.
➤ Instruct the client not to consume alcohol for 24 hours before the test.
➤ Instruct the client not to eat for 12–14 hours before the test. Water is allowed.
➤ Advise the client not to make any drastic changes in normal diet for 2 weeks preceding the blood sampling.

Perform Procedure

➤ Perform a venipuncture to collect 7 mL of venous blood in a red-top tube (for neonate, draw blood from a heelstick if possible).
➤ Apply pressure or a pressure dressing to the venipuncture site.
➤ Label the sample and note any interfering factors or medications.
➤ Send the sample to the lab immediately.

Care After Test

➤ Evaluate the client's diet for the sources and amount of dietary fat. Refer to a registered dietician as indicated.
➤ Evaluate the client's history for coronary and vascular disease. Especially note pain in the legs with walking, chest pain, and family deaths from heart attacks.

> Evaluate other tests such as cholesterol and lipoproteins.

Educate Your Client and the Family

> Teach the client with elevated cholesterol the need to reduce fat intake from animal and vegetable sources. Total fat intake should not be more than 30% of the required daily calories.

> Emphasize foods that are part of a heart-healthy diet, rather than dwelling on foods that are not.

> Stress the importance of regularly scheduled exercise such as walking.

> Assist the client who weighs more than the ideal body weight to choose a reduced fat and calorie diet that incorporates personal food preferences. Be particularly attuned to including ethnic foods the client may value.

> Emphasize to the client that there are risk factors that can be controlled such as diet, exercise, weight, and smoking. Risk factors such as gender, family history, and diabetes cannot be eliminated, but can be minimized by addressing the risk factors they can control.

> Refer to counseling and support groups as indicated for client requiring a major lifestyle change.

Triiodothyronine

trie ie oe doe thie roe neen

(T_3, T_3 Radioimmunoassay, T_3 by RIA, T_3-RIA, Total Triiodothyronine, Total T_3)

Normal Findings

ADULT, ADOLESCENT, AND ELDERLY

80–230 ng/dL (SI units: 0.9–3.0 nmol/L)

PREGNANT

Values are increased during pregnancy.

NEWBORN

75–260 ng/dL (SI units: 0.8–2.8 nmol/L)

CHILD

90–250 ng/dL (SI units: 1.1–3.7 nmol/L)

What This Test Will Tell You

This blood test diagnoses various conditions of the thyroid gland and evaluates the effectiveness of therapy in the treatment of thyroid disorders. Triiodothyronine (T_3) is an important thyroid hormone that is five times more potent than thyroxine (T_4). T_3 is predominantly formed from a metabolic process that causes T_4 to lose an iodine atom, but a small amount is also produced by the thyroid gland itself. Even though triiodothyronine is present in the bloodstream for a shorter period of time than thyroxine, it is more powerful in its effects on the body. A T_3 level is the test of choice in diagnosing T_3 thyrotoxicosis. This test is of limited value in diagnosing hypothyroidism.

Abnormal Findings

▲ INCREASED LEVELS may indicate hyperthyroidism, T_3 thyrotoxicosis, toxic adenoma, or acute thyroiditis.

▼DECREASED LEVELS may indicate hypothyroidism (levels may be normal in some hypothyroid clients), chronic illness, or starvation.

Interfering Factors
➤ Estrogen, oral contraceptives, pregnancy, and methadone may increase levels.
➤ Levels are decreased with the use of anabolic steroids, androgens, beta blockers, high doses of salicylates, reserpine, and phenytoin.
➤ Testing with radioisotopes within 1 week of sampling may result in inaccurate findings.
➤ Hemolysis of blood sample.

NURSING CONSIDERATIONS

Prepare Your Client
➤ Explain that this is a blood test to see how well a gland in the neck called the thyroid gland is working.

Perform Procedure
➤ Collect 5–7 mL of venous blood in a red-top tube.
➤ If the client has been taking thyroid medication, note the medication and time of last dose carefully on the laboratory slip.

Care After Test
➤ Assess for signs of hypothyroidism including hypothermia, bradycardia, weight gain, thick and dry skin, thin hair, hypotension, cold extremities, masklike expression, fatigue, slowed mental processes, myalgia, weakness, and constipation.
➤ Assess for signs of hyperthyroidism including nervousness, apprehension, tachycardia, diaphoresis, flushed skin, tremor in hands, constipation, diarrhea, weight loss, weakness, amenorrhea, and cardiac dysrhythmias.
➤ Institute safety measures if weakness is noted.
➤ Review related tests such as levels of serum thyroxine, protein-bound iodine, thyrotropin-releasing hormone, thyroid-stimulating hormone, and triiodothyronine suppression test.

Educate Your Client and the Family
➤ Teach client that thyroid hormone replacement must be taken for life if hypofunction is found or if the thyroid is removed surgically.
➤ Teach client how to meet rest and nutritional needs required by a hyperfunctioning thyroid. This includes frequent rest periods and a high-calorie, high-protein diet.
➤ Instruct client on iodized salt sources for treatment of goiter.

T

Triiodothyronine Suppression Test
trie ie oe doe thie roe neen • suh **preh** shun • test
(Triiodothyronine Thyroid Suppression Test, T₃ Thyroid Suppression Test)

Normal Findings
Adult: Iodine uptake suppressed to at least 50% of baseline value.

What This Test Will Tell You
This nuclear scanning test helps determine if the cause of excessive iodine uptake in the thyroid gland is

related to a problem within the thyroid gland itself (autonomous) or is controlled by the pituitary gland. The test measures thyroid metabolic response to oral T_3 administration. Normally, administration of T_3 decreases the uptake of iodine by the thyroid. However, if there are autonomous hot spots in the thyroid gland, minimal if any suppression is achieved because the thyroid gland itself is responsible for increased iodine intake independently of other endocrine feedback or stimulation. If suppression to at least 50% of the client's baseline is achieved by the administration of T_3, then the thyroid gland is responding to the pituitary gland when iodine uptake is increased.

Abnormal Findings

▲ INCREASED LEVELS (failure to suppress uptake by 50%—autonomous thyroid hyperfunction) may indicate Graves' disease, toxic thyroid nodule, or thyroid cancer.

▼ DECREASED LEVELS (uptake suppressed to at least 50% of baseline—hot spot under pituitary control) may indicate iodine deficiency or thyroid cancer.

ACTION ALERT!

Assess clients carefully for allergic reaction to iodine, including dyspnea, itching, urticaria, flushing, hypotension, and shock. Life-threatening anaphylactic reactions can occur and need to be recognized and treated immediately.

Interfering Factors

➤ Dietary intake of iodine will interfere with the accuracy of test results.

Contraindications

➤ Pregnancy
➤ Lactation

➤ Infant/child
➤ Iodine allergy

Potential Complications

➤ Allergic reaction to iodine
➤ Radiation-induced tumor formation

NURSING CONSIDERATIONS

Prepare Your Client

➤ Explain that the test helps to evaluate how a gland in the neck called the thyroid gland is working by measuring how it responds to a certain hormone, called triiodothyronine or T_3.
➤ Assess for a history of allergy to iodine or shellfish.
➤ Instruct the client to avoid foods containing iodine, such as shellfish and iodized salt, prior to testing.
➤ Ensure triiodothyronine is administered as ordered prior to scheduled scans (usually 75–100 μg per day in divided doses by mouth for 5–10 days).

Perform Procedure

Nurses do not usually perform this procedure, but should understand the process to prepare the client and assist the physician. A baseline radioactive iodine uptake test is obtained. Radioactive iodine uptake tests are generally repeated during the last 2 days of T_3 administration to assess thyroid response.

Care After Test

➤ Client may resume a normal diet following test completion.
➤ Assess for signs of hyperthyroidism including nervousness, apprehension, tachycardia, diaphoresis, flushed skin, tremor in hands, constipation, diarrhea, weight loss, weakness, amenorrhea, and cardiac dysrhythmias.

➤ Institute safety measures if weakness is noted.

➤ Review related tests such as levels of serum thyroxine, protein-bound iodine, thyrotropin-releasing hormone, and thyroid-stimulating hormone.

Educate Your Client and the Family

➤ Provide information on normal thyroid function and on disease-specific interventions to normalize thyroid function following diagnosis.

➤ Teach client how to meet rest and nutritional needs required by a hyperfunctioning thyroid. This includes frequent rest periods and a high-calorie, high-protein diet.

➤ Instruct client on iodized salt sources for treatment of goiter.

T

Triiodothyronine Uptake Ratio

trie ie oe doe thie roe neen • up take • ray shoe

(T_3UR, T_3UP, T_3 Resin Uptake Test, Resin Triiodothyronine Uptake Test, RT_3U, T_3RU, Triiodothyronine Uptake Test, T_3 Uptake Test)

Normal Findings

ALL AGES

Normal uptake: 25%–35%

Normal ratio between client specimen and standard control: 0.8–1.30

T_3RU: 0.1–1.35

PREGNANT

Levels will be decreased during pregnancy.

What This Test Will Tell You

This resin exchange test helps diagnose hyperthyroidism or hypothyroidism, particularly when the thyroxine-binding globulin (TBG) level is abnormal. T_3 and T_4 levels may be artificially elevated or decreased in clients who have normal thyroids but have a condition that interferes with the T_3 and T_4 tests' accuracy (pregnancy, nephrotic syndrome, hormonal medications). This test is used to accurately assess thyroid function by quantifying TBG and thyroid-binding prealbumin (TBPA) levels.

Radioactive T_3 and a resin are added to serum, allowing the radioactive T_3 to bind to TBG sites that are vacant. Excess radioactive T_3 that was administered then combines with the resin and can be removed and measured. This excess amount is compared to the amount that bound to TBG sites and is reported as a percentage. The results of this test are an indirect reflection of free T_4.

Elevated results indicate decreased TBG and TBPA. Low results indicate increased TBG and TBPA.

Abnormal Findings

▲INCREASED LEVELS of T_3RU with high T_4 may indicate hyperthyroidism, T_3 toxicosis, or acute hepatitis.

▼DECREASED LEVELS of T_3RU with low T_4 may indicate hypothyroidism or renal failure.

▲INCREASED LEVELS of T_3RU with low T_4 may indicate hypoproteinemia or nephrosis.

▼ DECREASED LEVELS *of* T_3RU *with high* T_4 may indicate pregnancy or use of oral contraceptives or estrogens.

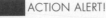 ACTION ALERT!

Assess clients carefully for allergic reaction to iodine, including dyspnea, itching, urticaria, flushing, hypotension, and shock. Life-threatening anaphylactic reactions can occur and need to be recognized and treated immediately.

Interfering Factors

➤ Levels may be decreased by estrogens, pregnancy, oral contraceptives, thiazides, clofibrate, and antithyroid medications.

➤ Levels may be increased by heparin, androgens, phenytoin, salicylates, thyroxine therapy, bishydroxycoumarin (Dicumarol), phenylbutazone, and steroids.

➤ Results may be altered or unreliable when the client has liver disease, renal disease, or cancer, or has recently been given radioactive material.

NURSING CONSIDERATIONS

Prepare Your Client

➤ Explain that the test helps to evaluate any problems in a gland in the neck called the thyroid gland.

Perform Procedure

➤ Collect 7 mL of venous blood in a red-top tube.

Care After Test

➤ Assess for signs of hypothyroidism including hypothermia, bradycardia, weight gain, thick and dry skin, thin hair, hypotension, cold extremities, masklike expression, fatigue, slowed mental processes, myalgia, weakness, and constipation.

➤ Assess for signs of hyperthyroidism including nervousness, apprehension, tachycardia, diaphoresis, flushed skin, tremor in hands, constipation, diarrhea, weight loss, weakness, amenorrhea, and cardiac dysrhythmias.

➤ Institute safety measures if weakness is noted.

➤ Review related tests such as levels of serum thyroxine, protein-bound iodine, thyrotropin-releasing hormone, and thyroid-stimulating hormone, and the triiodothyronine suppression test.

Educate Your Client and the Family

➤ Teach client that thyroid hormone replacement must be taken for life if hypofunction is found or if the thyroid is removed surgically.

➤ Teach client how to meet rest and nutritional needs required by a hyperfunctioning thyroid. This includes frequent rest periods and a high-calorie, high-protein diet.

➤ Instruct client on iodized salt sources for treatment of goiter.

➤ Monitor results of other endocrine testing.

Tryptophan Challenge Test

trip toe fan • chal enj • test

Normal Findings

ALL AGES

Excretion of xanthurenic acid <50 mg/24 hours (SI units: 250 μmol/24 hours)

PREGNANT

Generally not performed. Levels of xanthurenic acid will normally be elevated during pregnancy.

What This Test Will Tell You

This 24-hour urine test confirms deficiency of vitamin B_6 (pyridoxine). Adequate quantities of vitamin B_6 are essential for protein metabolism and for amino acid synthesis. Vitamin B_6 deficiency may result in serious metabolic problems or urinary calculi. Trytophan normally is converted to niacin, preventing the formation of xanthurenic acid. In vitamin B_6 deficiency, xanthurenic acid levels rise.

Abnormal Findings

▲INCREASED LEVELS (>100 mg/24 hours, SI units 500 μmol/24 hours) may indicate malnutrition, malignancy, or familial xanthurenic aciduria.

Interfering Factors

➤ Inaccurate test results will be obtained if all urine is not collected during the test period or if the urine specimen is stored improperly.

➤ Levels may be increased by pregnancy, estrogen therapy, oral contraceptives, hydralazine, isoniazid, and D-penicillamine.

NURSING CONSIDERATIONS

Prepare Your Client

➤ Explain that this test measures the amount of vitamin B_6 in the body.

➤ Review 24-hour urine collection procedure.

Perform Procedure

➤ Administer oral dose of L-tryptophan as ordered by the primary health care provider (50 mg/kg of body weight for children and up to 2 g/kg for adults).

➤ Collect 24-hour urine specimen.

➤ Ensure specimen contains the preservative thymol and refrigerate specimen or place it on ice during the collection period.

Care After Test

➤ Observe the client for signs and symptoms of anemia including pallor, dyspnea, chest pain, and fatigue.

➤ Encourage rest periods for client experiencing fatigue related to anemia.

➤ Evaluate client's ability to perform activities of daily living.

➤ Refer to community health care services as needed if client is unable to perform basic daily needs.

➤ Obtain a dietary consult to assist the client and family in choosing a well-balanced diet, including foods high in iron and vitamins B_{12} and B_6.

➤ Review related tests such as hemoglobin, hematocrit, reticulocyte count, red blood cell indices, hemoglobin electrophoresis, ferritin level, total iron binding capacity (TIBC), bone marrow and liver biopsies, and iron absorption and excretion studies.

Educate Your Client and the Family

➤ In confirmed cases of vitamin B$_6$ deficiency, review the role of vitamin B$_6$ in the body.

➤ Educate the client regarding dietary sources of vitamin B$_6$ including yeast, wheat, corn, and organ meats.

➤ Teach clients how to pace activities, taking frequent rest periods.

T-Tube Cholangiography

tee toob • kow lan jee og rah fee
(T-Tube Cholangiogram, Operative Cholangiogram)

Normal Findings

All ages: Patent biliary ducts. Normal filling of common bile duct, no dilatation or other filling abnormalities noted. Absence of cholelithiases. Normal progression of contrast material to the ampulla of Vater and duodenum.

What This Test Will Tell You

This radiographic test detects obstructions of the common bile duct caused by stones or strictures, or presence of a fistula. The T-tube cholangiography test is usually performed following cholecystectomy (5–10 days) to detect a residual stone that could potentially cause a blockage of the common bile duct. If no stones or restrictions are noted, the T-tube, which is a T-shaped tube that is placed into the common bile duct to drain bile, is usually removed.

A T-tube may be placed during a cholecystectomy to facilitate drainage of bile postoperatively. If there is a question of a residual stone, contrast material is instilled directly into the common bile duct during surgery. This is called an operative cholangiography.

Abnormal Findings

Abnormalities may indicate obstruction of common bile duct, congenital anomalies, tumor, cysts, cholelithiasis, or stricture of bile duct.

ACTION ALERT!

Assess clients carefully for allergic reaction to contrast material, including dyspnea, itching, urticaria, flushing, hypotension, and shock. Life-threatening anaphylactic reactions can occur and need to be recognized and treated immediately.

Interfering Factors

➤ Movement of client during required films may limit the clarity of images.
➤ Obesity, or presence of stool or barium in the intestine may decrease the clarity of x-ray films.

Contraindications

➤ Allergy to contrast media, unless the test is modified
➤ Pregnancy, due to radiation exposure to fetus

Potential Complications

➤ Allergic reaction/anaphylaxis
➤ Infection
➤ Cholangitis
➤ Sepsis

NURSING CONSIDERATIONS

Prepare Your Client

➤ Explain that this test is used to look inside the gallbladder to see if there are any problems with stones or the drainage of bile.

➤ Check to be sure the client has no allergy to contrast material.

➤ Ensure that an informed consent is obtained, because of the possible complications associated with this procedure.

➤ Check with your institution about restriction of food and fluids for 4–8 hours prior to the test.

➤ Consult with the primary health care provider about the need for bowel cleansing (laxatives or enemas) the night before and/or morning of the exam to prevent shadows on the x-rays.

➤ Confirm that adults and older children have voided before the procedure.

➤ Administer a sedative or tranquilizer prior to the procedure if ordered.

Perform Procedure

Nurses do not perform this procedure, but should understand the process to prepare the client. The client is positioned on an x-ray table. For a T-tube cholangiogram, the contrast agent is instilled into the T-tube, which was placed 4–10 days earlier during surgery. For an operative cholangiogram, a catheter is placed into the common bile duct during a cholecystectomy. In both methods, contrast material is injected into the common bile duct and x-rays are taken. Observe for reaction to contrast media such as nausea, rash, dyspnea, tachycardia, and hypotension. The T-tube may be removed at the end of either procedure, or left in place.

Care After Test

➤ Observe for signs of allergic reaction to the contrast material, which include urticaria, pruritus, fever, and dyspnea.

➤ The T-tube may be left in place after the procedure. Ensure a sterile, closed drainage system is used.

➤ Consult with a registered dietician to assist the family and client in meeting special dietary needs.

➤ Carefully monitor client for signs of infection or sepsis including fever, tachycardia, increased white cell count, and abdominal pain.

➤ Review related tests such as serum lipase levels, serum bilirubin, percutaneous transhepatic cholangiography, intravenous cholangiography, endoscopic retrograde cholangiopancreatography (ERCP), intravenous cholecystography, abdominal x-ray, and cholangiogram.

Educate Your Client and the Family

➤ Instruct overweight client on a low-calorie, low-fat, weight reduction diet with the assistance of a registered dietician.

Tuberculin Test

too bur kyu lin • test
(Tuberculin Skin Test, Mantoux's Test, PPD Test)

Normal Findings

All ages: Negative; zone of induration
< 5 mm in diameter at 48–72 hours.

What This Test Will Tell You

This skin test determines present or
past exposure to tuberculosis or previous vaccination with BCG (bacille
Calmette-Guérin). Purified protein
derivative tuberculin (PPD) is
injected intradermally. PPD is a protein fraction of tubercle bacilli, and
when it is introduced into the skin of
a person with active or dormant
tuberculosis infection it causes a
localized thickening of the skin
because of an accumulation of small,
sensitized lymphocytes. Sensitized T
cells react with the antigen at the
injection site, leading to edema and
fibrin deposits. The result is the
induration characteristic of a positive tuberculosis reaction.

Although the test is used to detect
tuberculosis infection, it is unable to
indicate whether the infection is
active or dormant. Additional studies, such as chest x-rays to detect
lesions in the lung and sputum testing for acid-fast bacilli, are performed to confirm the presence of
tuberculosis. The test may be done as
part of routine screening of high-risk
populations or as part of prenatal
evaluation of pregnant women and
routinely in health care workers.

Abnormal Findings

➤ *Positive reactions* may indicate
tuberculosis.
Suspicious: zone of induration > 5
mm but < 10 mm in diameter.

Positive: zone of induration > 10 mm
in diameter.
➤ *Negative reactions* may indicate
immunosuppression.

ACTION ALERT!

➤ The skin test should not be administered
to known tuberculin-positive reactors
because of the possibility of severe reactions including vesiculation, ulceration, and
necrosis. Epinephrine should be readily
available to use in the event of an anaphylactic reaction.
➤ Measures to prevent disease transmission should be implemented on all persons
with positive results until results from further testing are available.

Interfering Factors

➤ False negative results occur in
clients whose immune systems are
nonfunctioning.
➤ False negative reactions occur in
the following situations: bacterial
infections, immunosuppressive
agents, live virus vaccinations
(measles, mumps, polio, and
rubella), malnutrition, old age, newborns, overwhelming tuberculosis,
renal failure, and viral infections
(chicken pox, measles, and mumps).
➤ Previous vaccination with BCG
may produce a false positive result.
➤ False positive results occur with
nontuberculous *Mycobacteria* infections.
➤ Failure to store tuberculin as recommended by the manufacturer may
cause false negative results.
➤ Failure to administer PPD immediately after drawing it into the
syringe may produce false negative
results.

➤ Subcutaneous rather than intra-dermal injections may yield a false negative result.

➤ Serial testing may cause false positive results.

Contraindications

➤ Previous vaccination with BCG, because results will be positive without the client having tuberculosis

➤ Client with known active tuberculosis or history of previous positive PPD reaction, because severe local reactions including ulceration may occur

Potential Complications

➤ Severe local reactions in clients with active tuberculosis or previous history of positive PPD reaction.

➤ Anaphylaxis may occur in clients hypersensitive to PPD.

NURSING CONSIDERATIONS

Prepare Your Client

➤ Explain to the client that the test is to determine present or past exposure to tuberculosis.

➤ Assess for previous history of positive PPD reaction, history of tuberculosis or vaccination with BCG. Report a positive history to the physician.

➤ Assure client that they will not develop tuberculosis from this test. Answer any questions.

➤ Obtain a client history about hypersensitivity to skin tests.

Perform Procedure

➤ Cleanse the client's forearm with alcohol and allow to dry.

➤ Stretch the skin taut.

➤ Inject intradermally 0.1 ml of PPD into the lower, flexor surface of the forearm. A weal will appear.

➤ Remove the syringe.

➤ Mark the area with indelible ink so the site can be identified later.

Care After Test

➤ Mark the test area to locate for reading.

➤ Read the test 48–72 hours later by observing the forearm in good light for induration (hardening or thickening) and measuring the diameter of the induration (not erythema) zone in millimeters.

➤ Interpret the reaction based on the size of the zone of induration as follows:

Negative: zone <5 mm in diameter

Doubtful or probable: zone 5–10 mm in diameter

Positive: zone 10 mm or more in diameter

➤ Notify the primary health care provider if the test is positive or probable.

➤ If a positive skin reaction occurs, check the client's arm over the next 4–5 days to be certain that a severe skin reaction has not occurred.

➤ Evaluate related tests such as chest x-rays, sputum cultures, acid-fast bacilli, and sputum cytology. Follow-up chest x-rays should be performed with all positive reactions.

Educate Your Client and the Family

➤ Instruct client to return promptly on the instructed day and time. Inform the client that results of the skin test must be read during the stated time or they will be inaccurate.

➤ Tell the client that a positive reaction means that they have at some time been exposed to tuberculosis; it does not mean that they currently have tuberculosis.

> Explain that if results are positive, other tests such as chest x-ray and sputum cultures will be performed.

> Ask the client to report any severe skin reactions, difficulty breathing, itching, and hives.

Tubular Reabsorbed Phosphate, Serum and Urine

too byu lar • ree ab sorbd • fos fate • see rum • and • yur in
(Tubular Phosphate Reabsorption, TPR, Tubular Reabsorption of Phosphate, TRP)

Normal Findings
All ages: 80%–95%, or 0.80–0.95

What This Test Will Tell You
This urine and blood test evaluates the function of the parathyroid gland and examines the cause of hypercalcemia. Parathyroid hormone (PTH) is excreted by the parathyroid gland and is responsible for regulating the levels of ionized calcium as well as the excretion of both calcium and phosphorus by the kidneys. Measurement of urine and plasma levels of phosphate in the context of the serum creatinine and creatinine clearance values helps provide an indirect evaluation of parathyroid function. Increasing levels of PTH result in an increase of calcium reabsorption and a decrease of phosphorus absorption by the renal tubules. This test is most helpful in diagnosing hyperparathyroidism.

Abnormal Findings
▲ INCREASED LEVELS may indicate hyperparathyroidism, uremia, osteomalacia, malignancy, sarcoidosis, myeloma, renal disease, or autoimmune disorders.

▼ DECREASED LEVELS (<74%) may indicate hypoparathyroidism.

Interfering Factors
> Medications that may increase results include furosemide and gentamicin.
> Medications that may decrease results include chlorothiazide diuretics and amphotericin B.
> Uremia, renal tubular disease, and osteomalacia may cause false positive results.
> Hemolysis of sample.
> Failure to collect all urine during the timed period.
> Diet high in phosphate lowers tubular phosphate reabsorption (TPR) values. Diet low in phosphate raises TPR values.

NURSING CONSIDERATIONS

Prepare Your Client
> Explain that this test is performed to see how well a gland in the body called the parathyroid gland is working.
> Instruct client not to alter their usual intake of phosphorus-containing foods such as milk, eggs, meat, fish, poultry, nuts, beans, cheese, and cereal for at least 3 days before the test.
> Restrict food and fluids for 12 hours prior to the test.

➤ Consult with a registered dietician to assist the client in consuming a diet with 500–3000 mg of phosphate the day before testing.

Perform Procedure
➤ Collect a urine specimen for 1, 4, or 24 hours as ordered.
➤ Collect 10 mL of venous blood in a red-top tube 1 hour after 24-hour urine is started.
➤ Make sure a container with preservatives is used and that the urine is kept refrigerated or on ice during the collection period.

Care After Test
➤ Observe the client for signs of hypercalcemia including lethargy, bone pain, decreased muscle tone, nausea, vomiting, anorexia, constipation, flank pain, headache, thirst, and increased urinary output.
➤ Monitor intake and output carefully.
➤ Observe the client for signs of hypocalcemia including bone pain, lethargy, constipation, nausea, vomiting, cramps, shallow breathing, bronchospasm, dysrhythmias, decreased urinary output, increased abdominal girth, tetany, Chvostek's sign, and Trousseau's sign.
➤ Prepare to administer 10% calcium gluconate or calcium chloride by slow intravenous infusion in severe cases, or oral calcium supplements for less severe cases.
➤ Evaluate vitamin D and phosphorus balance as possible causes of calcium imbalance.
➤ Consult with a registered dietician to assist the family and client in meeting special dietary needs.
➤ Monitor electrocardiogram continuously, especially with hypocalcemia.
➤ Review related tests including serum phosphorus, serum albumin, urinalysis for calculi, chest x-rays, bone scans, clotting studies, parathyroid hormone levels, electrocardiogram, and serum digoxin level.

Educate Your Client and the Family
➤ If calcium is low, discuss increasing calcium-rich foods in diet. Provide a list of foods high in calcium content.
➤ If calcium is high, encourage fluids and anti-ash diet to prevent kidney stones.

Tubular Reabsorption of Phosphate
too byu lar • ree ab sorp shun • uv • foss fate
(TRP, Tubular Reabsorbed Phosphate, Tubular Phosphate Reabsorption, TPR)

Normal Findings
All ages: 82%–95%

What This Test Will Tell You
This blood and urine test helps establish the diagnosis of primary hyperparathyroidism and distinguish the etiology of hypercalcemia.

Values less than 80% are consistent with diminished renal tubular reabsorption of phosphate and primary hyperparathyroidism. The value is calculated by using the creatinine clearance, serum creatinine, and serum phosphate concentration.

Parathyroid hormone (parathormone) controls both calcium and phosphorus metabolism and excretion through a feedback mechanism leading to hypercalcemia and hypophosphatemia. Excessive amounts of parathyroid hormone are excreted in primary hyperparathyroidism, leading to a calcium-phosphate imbalance. Phosphate clearance and reabsorption are also controlled by serum calcium levels, potassium depletion, renal disorders, and calcitonin, estrogen, and adrenal steroids.

Abnormal Findings

▲ INCREASED LEVELS may indicate uremia, renal tubular disease, osteomalacia, sarcoidosis, myeloma, or prolonged heparin administration.

▼ DECREASED LEVELS may indicate primary hyperparathyroidism, parathyroid-hormone-secreting tumor, malignancy-induced hypercalcemia, or renal disorders.

■ ACTION ALERT!

Values less than 80% may indicate primary hyperparathyroidism and are associated with a high calcium level (>12 mg/dL). Monitor carefully for signs and symptoms of confusion, emotional lability, delirium, and stupor.

Interfering Factors

➤ Hemolysis.
➤ Failure to collect all urine or keep urine refrigerated or on ice during testing period.
➤ Low- or high-phosphate diet.
➤ Amphotericin B and chlorothiazide diuretics may decrease phosphate reabsorption.
➤ Furosemide and gentamicin may increase phosphate reabsorption.

NURSING CONSIDERATIONS

Prepare Your Client

➤ Explain that this is a test to evaluate the cause of an elevated body chemical, calcium.
➤ Instruct client to eat a normal calcium and normal phosphate diet (500–3000 mg/day) for 3 days prior to the testing. This diet would include moderate amounts of nuts, legumes, milk, egg yolks, poultry, fish, cheeses, and cereals. Consult with a registered dietician to assist the family and client in meeting special dietary needs if indicated.
➤ Restrict food and fluids for 8 hours prior to the test.

Perform Procedure

HOURLY TEST

➤ Have client drink 16 ounces of water.
➤ One hour later, have client void, emptying bladder, and discard specimen. Note time of voiding. Have client drink 8 ounces of water.
➤ One hour after first voiding, have client void again, emptying bladder. Save the urine specimen and label it with exact time and volume of voiding. Have the client drink 8 ounces of water. If urine specimen is less than 120 mL, restart the testing protocol.
➤ One hour after second voiding, have client void, emptying bladder. Save the urine specimen and label it with exact time and volume of voiding. Have the client drink 8 ounces of water. At this time, collect 10 mL of venous blood in a red-top tube for serum phosphorus and creatinine levels.
➤ One hour after third voiding, have client void, emptying bladder. Save the urine specimen and label it with

exact time and volume of voiding. At this time, collect 10 mL of venous blood in a red-top tube.

24-HOUR URINE TEST

➤ Use a 3-L, clean container with a preservative.

➤ Follow procedure for 24-hour urine collection.

➤ Also collect 10 mL of venous blood in a red-top tube.

➤ Keep the urine collection container on ice or refrigerated during the collection period.

Care After Test

➤ Assess for hypercalcemia including symptoms of polydipsia, polyuria, volume depletion, elevated blood pressure, dysrhythmias, electrocardiogram changes, anorexia, nausea, constipation, distention, back or joint pain, confusion, emotional lability, delirium, and stupor.

➤ With changes in mental status, provide for safety and protect for injury.

➤ Monitor for a history of fractures and assess history of renal calculi.

➤ Assess intake and output and monitor for signs and symptoms of renal calculi including hematuria and flank pain.

➤ Encourage client to drink at least 3000 mL of fluids per day unless contraindicated. Include juices such as cranberry juice and prune juice.

➤ Monitor vital signs every 4 hours for alterations in respiratory patterns, blood pressure, and heart rhythm.

➤ Monitor continuous electrocardiogram and assess for dysrhythmias.

➤ In primary hyperparathyroidism, limit intake of dietary calcium, particularly milk and milk products and calcium-containing medications such as Tums and Rolaids.

➤ Assess for pruritus, which is often associated with calcium and phosphorus imbalances, and provide comfort measures and antihistamines as ordered.

➤ Review related tests including blood urea nitrogen, serum potassium, creatinine, albumin, calcium, and parathyroid scan.

Educate Your Client and the Family

➤ Teach the client and family the importance of regular laboratory tests and regular follow-up care.

➤ Explain to client and family that when calcium is removed from the bones, there is an increased fragility and muscle weakness. Therefore, an effort should be made to avoid injury by using good body mechanics (keeping the back straight and using the arms and legs to lift) and by preventing falls.

➤ Encourage weight-bearing activity to reduce calcium loss.

➤ Explain to the client and family the importance of drinking 3 quarts (3000 mL) of fluids each day.

➤ Teach client and family the signs and symptoms of renal colic, such as cramping back pain.

Umbilical Blood Flow Studies

uhm **bil** ih kahl • **blud** • floe • **stud** eez

(Umbilical Velocimetry, Doppler Ultrasound Blood Flow Assessment)

Normal Findings

Fetus: Normal umbilical artery blood flow

What This Test Will Tell You

This ultrasound test is used most often to aid in diagnosing suspected intrauterine growth retardation (IUGR) related to decreased fetal-maternal blood exchange and increased vascular tone in the umbilical arteries. Doppler umbilical blood flow studies are also used in pregnancies with multiple gestation, prolonged pregnancy, diabetes, sickle-cell disease, and twin to twin transfusion. Umbilical blood flow studies measure the flow velocity in blood vessels (umbilical arteries). Red blood cells (RBCs) are moving objects that reflect sound. When the Doppler ultrasound wave is directed at blood moving through a blood vessel, echoes are created in response to systole and diastole. These echoes, or movement of blood through vessels, are displayed as wave forms.

Abnormal Findings

Abnormalities may indicate decreased umbilical arterial blood flow, intrauterine growth retardation (IUGR), or decreased fetal-maternal blood exchange.

ACTION ALERT!

Decreased umbilical arterial blood flow may indicate a serious health threat to the fetus resulting in the need to prepare for emergency delivery and immediate resuscitation of the infant.

Interfering Factors

➤ Nicotine and maternal smoking increase resistance in the placental vascular bed.

NURSING CONSIDERATIONS

Prepare Your Client

➤ Explain that this test measures blood flow going to the baby.

➤ Explain that the test is performed by a physician, ultrasound technician, or a nurse and takes about 20 minutes.

➤ Assure the client the test is noninvasive and will not be uncomfortable except for a full bladder. The test will not harm the fetus.

➤ If a vaginal probe is going to be used, the bladder is empty.

➤ Have the client drink 800–1000 mL of water or another liquid 1 hour prior to the exam to fill the bladder.

➤ Instruct the client not to void until the test is completed so that visualization is optimal.

Perform Procedure

➤ Assist the client into a supine position on the examining table. If she is short of breath, elevate the upper body.

➤ Apply a water-soluble conductive gel to the abdomen to enhance ultrasound transmission and reception.

➤ Move the transducer vertically and horizontally over the abdomen and pelvis.

➤ Pictures are then taken.

➤ Fetal structures may be pointed out to the mother during the exam.

Care After Test

➤ Ask the client if she is taking her prenatal vitamins as ordered by her primary health care provider. Stress the importance of supplemental vitamins in providing good nutrition and normal growth and development of her baby.

➤ Assess the client's knowledge of prenatal care including diet, activity, rest, signs and symptoms of labor, and danger signs in pregnancy. Provide instruction as indicated.

➤ Assess mother's readiness to meet parental role functions by reviewing infant care knowledge, methods of infant feeding, and ability to obtain needed supplies. Provide instruction and/or community health service referrals as indicated.

➤ Assess the client's ability to provide adequate nutrition for the fetus. Refer to social services and Women, Infants, and Children program (WIC) for assistance if needed.

➤ Assess the client for use of cigarettes, tobacco products, alcohol, over-the-counter medications, and street drugs. Instruct the client as necessary to avoid these substances as they may cause intrauterine growth retardation.

➤ If the client reports decreased fetal movements, assess recent maternal history for maternal activity and relationship to fetal movement. Assess also her recent consumption of food or fluids and its relationship to fetal movement. Consult with the primary health care provider about instructing the client to eat, drink, and then rest. During rest, tell her to concentrate on fetal movements for 1 hour. Three fetal movements in 1 hour are reassuring.

➤ Review related tests such as daily fetal movement count, nonstress testing, contraction stress test, and biophysical profile.

Educate Your Client and the Family

➤ Instruct the client about normal signs of labor such as a gush of fluid, bloody show, and contractions that increase in frequency, intensity, and duration.

➤ Instruct the client about danger signs in pregnancy such as a gush of fluid, vaginal bleeding, abdominal pain, temperature elevation, dizziness, blurred vision, persistent vomiting, severe headache, edema, muscular irritability, difficult urination, or decreased/absent fetal movements.

➤ Instruct client to notify the primary health care provider if they have less than three movements in 1 hour. A nonstress test or biophysical profile may be ordered.

➤ Teach the client the signs of preterm labor such as abdominal cramping with or without diarrhea, uterine contractions every 10 minutes or less, menstrual-like cramps in the lower abdomen, low backache, increase or change in vaginal discharge, or pelvic pressure.

➤ Advise the client to lie down on her left side and notify the primary health care provider if preterm labor is suspected.

➤ Teach daily fetal movement count.

Upper Gastrointestinal X-Ray Study

up ur • gas troe in tes ti nal • eks ray • stud ee

(UGI, Upper GI Series, Barium Swallow, Gastric Radiography, Gastrointestinal Motility Studies, Air Contrast Upper GI)

Normal Findings

All ages: Normal size, shape, patency, filling, and positioning of the structures of the esophagus, stomach, and upper duodenum. Normal peristalsis is observed. Mucosa is smooth, regular, and free of lesions or narrowing. Barium flows smoothly without leakage into the abdominal cavity. There is no reflux of the barium into the esophagus.

What This Test Will Tell You

This x-ray test visualizes the form and position, mucosal folds, peristaltic activity, and mobility of the esophagus, stomach, and upper duodenum to detect abnormalities of the gastrointestinal (GI) tract. An oral contrast substance such as barium sulfate is ingested. Barium sulfate is a chalky, thick substance that is visible on x-rays. If there is concern about a leakage into the abdominal cavity or possible perforation of the GI tract, a water-soluble contrast is used.

Abnormal Findings

The x-rays may reveal gastric ulcers, duodenal ulcers, hiatal hernias, gastritis, gastric inflammatory diseases, gastric cancer, esophageal cancer, stomach cancer, duodenal cancer, gastric polyps, esophageal varices, esophageal diverticulum, benign gastric tumors, extrinsic compression from pancreatic pseudocysts, cysts, pancreatic tumors, hepatomegaly, gastric perforation, duodenal diverticulum, foreign bodies, pyloric stenosis, volvulus of the stomach, duodenal web, or malrotation syndrome.

Interfering Factors

➤ Retained barium from previous gastrointestinal x-rays may obscure detail on the x-ray films.
➤ Failure to follow restrictions in diet, smoking, and/or medications may interfere with the test results.
➤ Failure to remove radiopaque objects in the x-ray field can obscure details on the x-ray films.
➤ Excessive air in the small bowel can obscure details on the x-ray films.
➤ Poor performance of the client or severe debilitation of the client may interfere as the client cannot assume the multiple positions required for the test.
➤ Smoking or anxiety may increase motility.
➤ Anticholinergics may decrease motility.

Contraindications

➤ Complete bowel obstruction, as the ingestion of contrast would further complicate the bowel obstruction
➤ Unstable vital signs
➤ Perforation of the GI tract, as the leakage of contrast into the abdominal cavity would lead to peritonitis
➤ Ileus, because the increased intake would complicate the ileus by increasing the abdominal distention and the client's discomfort

Potential Complications

➤ Aspiration of the contrast material
➤ Constipation or partial bowel obstruction as a result of unexpelled barium

NURSING CONSIDERATIONS

Prepare Your Client

➤ Explain that this test is used to look at the swallowing tube (esophagus), stomach, and upper gut (duodenum) to help find abnormalities in size, shape, or function of these organs.

➤ Ensure that an informed consent is obtained, because of the possible complications associated with this procedure.

➤ Instruct the client to maintain a low-residue diet for 2–3 days before the test (for example, decrease the amount of vegetables, nuts, grains, and fruit).

➤ Restrict food and fluids at least 8 hours before the test.

➤ Assure the client that the test is not painful, although they may experience fullness or nausea.

➤ Instruct the client to avoid smoking for 8 hours before the test as well as during the test because smoking may increase the GI motility.

➤ Collaborate with the primary health care provider regarding the need to withhold anticholinergics and narcotics for 24 hours before the test as these drugs could slow GI motility. Restrict the use of these drugs if ordered by the primary health care provider.

➤ If the client has a hyperactive bowel, atropine may be ordered to decrease the peristalsis of the bowel.

Perform Procedure

Nurses do not perform this procedure, but should understand the process to prepare the client. Assist the client to drink the 16 ounces of barium or contrast substance. In some studies, a carbonated powder is swallowed to create air in the bowel for an air contrast study. Following the ingestion of the barium, the client is placed on an x-ray table and assisted with moving through several position changes that promote filling of the upper GI tract. The client is instructed to lie still while x-rays are taken at a variety of times as the barium progresses through the upper GI tract. The flow of barium as it outlines various structures and passes through valves is noted and recorded.

Care After Test

➤ Inform the client that if water-soluble contrast was used, diarrhea may occur because this contrast material draws water into the gut (osmotic diuretic).

➤ As ordered, administer a cathartic such as milk of magnesia to prevent hardening of the barium, which could lead to a fecal impaction.

➤ Encourage the client to drink more fluids, unless contraindicated, to improve the passage of the barium through the GI tract.

➤ Encourage the client to rest for several hours following the procedure.

➤ Evaluate related tests such as abdominal ultrasounds, abdominal computed tomography (CT) scans, abdominal magnetic resonance imaging (MRI) scans, barium enema, and kidney, ureter, and bladder (KUB) x-rays.

Educate Your Client and the Family

➤ Educate the client on the prescribed treatments such as dietary restrictions, surgery, or medicines (if applicable) for the identified disease.

➤ Instruct the client or family to monitor the stool to ensure return to normal consistency within 3 days. Explain that it is normal for the stool to be clay-colored as the barium is being expelled for the first day or so after the x-ray.

➤ If a hiatal hernia was identified, instruct the client to remain in an upright position for several hours following a meal to decrease the risk of reflux of food into the esophagus.

➤ If a gastric ulcer was identified, instruct the client to avoid spicy or acidic food such as tomatoes, citrus fruits, pepper, and Mexican or Italian spices.

➤ Discourage the use of alcohol for the client with esophageal varices, hepatomegaly, or pancreatic disease.

Urea Clearance
yu ree ah • kleer ans

Normal Findings
ALL AGES
64–99 mL/minute (SI units: 1100–1700 µL/second
For flow rate < 2 mL/minute (33 µL/second): 41–68 mL/minute (SI units: 700–1130 µL/second)

What This Test Will Tell You
This urine and blood test measures overall renal function; however, this test is an indicator of both the excretory function of the kidney and metabolic function of the liver. Urea is the end product of protein and amino acid metabolism in the liver. The urea enters the blood and proceeds to the kidneys for excretion. Urea clearance measures both glomerular and tubular renal function. The reabsorption of urea by the renal tubules is affected by the amount of water reabsorbed and varies depending on the time of day and diet. For this reason, creatinine clearance is the preferred test to evaluate the glomerular filtration rate, whereas the urea clearance estimates overall renal function. Uremia is associated with urea clearances below 20 mL/minute. Urea clearance parallels renal parenchymal destruc-

tion after 50% of the tissue is nonfunctioning.

Abnormal Findings
Abnormal results may indicate dehydration, decreased renal blood flow, renal artery stenosis, renal artery thrombus, bilateral ureteral obstruction, congestive heart failure, acute or chronic glomerulonephritis, acute tubular necrosis, nephrosclerosis, polycystic kidney disease, renal tuberculosis, or malignancy of the kidneys.

Interfering Factors
➤ Failure to completely empty the bladder.
➤ Physical exercise during the testing period.
➤ Caffeine, milk, and small doses of epinephrine increase urea clearance.
➤ Corticosteroids, amphotericin, chloramphenicol, thiazide diuretics, and streptomycin affect levels.
➤ Hemolysis of blood sample.
➤ If urine flow rates are between 1 and 2 mL/minute, the results of this test may not be accurate.

Contraindications
➤ If urine flow rate is less than 1 mL/minute, this test should not be

performed because the flow rate is so low the results are inaccurate.

NURSING CONSIDERATIONS

Prepare Your Client

➤ Explain that this test mainly helps see how well the kidneys are working, but may also help identify if there is a problem in the liver.

➤ Instruct the client to refrain from physical exercise before and during the test.

➤ Instruct the client to limit tea, coffee, and meat for 24 hours before the test.

➤ Restrict food and fluids for 8 hours prior to the test.

Perform Procedure

➤ Prior to performing the procedure, assess urine output. In order for the test to be accurate, the rate of urine flow must be 2 mL/minute or higher.

➤ Have client void and discard specimen. This testing may be done as a 1-hour, 12-hour, or 24-hour collection.

➤ Encourage client to drink water during the collection period to ensure adequate urine output.

➤ Either collect two urine specimens 1 hour apart, or a 12-hour or 24-hour urine specimen. For the 1-hour testing, label each specimen for date and time. For the 24-hour or 12-hour urine specimen collections, follow timed collection procedure.

➤ Collect 7 mL of venous blood in a red-top tube at some point during the urine collection period.

Care After Test

➤ If blood urea nitrogen (BUN) levels are > 40 mg/dL without signs and symptoms of dehydration, monitor intake and output, complete dietary assessment, and check with primary health care provider regarding protein restriction.

➤ If client is dehydrated as manifested by poor skin turgor, increased pulse and respiration, dry mucous membrane, and decreased urine output, encourage an increased oral intake unless contraindicated.

➤ Monitor for lethargy, confusion, and change in mental status. Provide necessary safety precautions.

➤ Monitor for hyperkalemia including symptoms of weakness, paresthesia, irritability, nausea and vomiting, intestinal colic, and diarrhea.

➤ Monitor for signs and symptoms of uremia including nausea, vomiting, stupor, peripheral edema, decreased urine output, dyspnea, jugular vein distention, and weight gain.

➤ Compare BUN to serum creatinine. If both are elevated, suspect renal disease.

➤ Observe for signs and symptoms of anemia with an elevated BUN.

➤ Observe for signs and symptoms of gastrointestinal bleeding, which is associated with an elevated BUN.

➤ Review related tests including white blood cell count, blood urea nitrogen, creatinine, urine specific gravity, hemoglobin and hematocrit, serum electrolytes, total protein, urinalysis, and urine culture.

Educate Your Client and the Family

➤ Teach client and family regarding specific dietary prescription. In renal failure, the most common diet prescription is low protein, high calorie, low sodium, and low potassium.

➤ Teach client the importance of maintaining fluid restriction.

➤ Instruct the client to report evidence of any anemia including weakness, shortness of breath, palpitations, or bleeding.

➤ Instruct client to report signs and symptoms of worsening uremia including nausea, vomiting, stupor, peripheral edema, decreased urine output, dyspnea, jugular vein distention, and weight gain.

➤ Instruct the client to avoid exposure to infection.

➤ If the client is taking renal toxic drugs such as gold preparations, aminoglycosides, polymyxins, amphotericin B, or trimethadione, teach client and family the importance of regular and ongoing health care supervision.

Urea Nitrogen Blood Test

yu ree ah • nie troe jen • blud • test
(Blood Urea Nitrogen, BUN, Serum Urea Nitrogen, SUN)

Normal Findings

ADULT, PREGNANT, AND ADOLESCENT
7–20 mg/dL (SI units: 2.5–7.2 mmol/L)
NEWBORN
4–15 mg/dL (SI units: 1.4–5.4 mmol/L)
CHILD
5–18 mg/dL (SI units: 1.8–6.4 mmol/L)
ELDERLY
8–21 mg/dL (SI units: 2.9–7.5 mmol/L) This level is slightly higher due to decreasing ability of the kidneys to concentrate urine.

What This Test Will Tell You

Blood urea nitrogen measures renal function and hydration. Urea, the end product of protein and amino acid metabolism in the liver, enters the blood and passes to the kidneys for excretion. The blood urea nitrogen (BUN) is, therefore, an indicator of both the metabolic function of the liver and the excretory function of the kidney. A damaged liver is unable to synthesize urea, and diseased kidneys have a limited ability to excrete urea.

The test is performed on plasma or serum. Levels depend on protein intake, hydration, and rate of urea production and excretion by the kidneys. Azotemia is the term used to describe an elevated urea nitrogen.

The BUN cannot be used as a single measure for renal function; however, it is frequently used as a screening test for renal function. The creatinine is a much more specific test of kidney function, and it is often used in conjunction with the BUN. The BUN/creatinine ratio is used to determine whether renal failure is prerenal, renal, or postrenal azotemia.

Abnormal Findings

▲INCREASED LEVELS may indicate renal failure, glomerulonephritis, pyelonephritis, acute tubular necrosis, hypovolemia, shock, congestive heart failure, urinary tract obstruction, excessive protein catabolism, gastrointestinal bleeding, burns, myocardial infarction, high-protein diet, dehydration, malnutrition, or starvation.

▼ DECREASED LEVELS may indicate liver failure, hypervolemia, malnutrition, acromegaly, alcohol abuse, celiac disease, cirrhosis, hepatitis, or liver destruction.

 ACTION ALERT!

Value over 100 mg/dL indicates severe renal impairment. Carefully observe for dyspnea related to fluid overload and dysrhythmias related to electrolyte imbalances. With elevated levels, alterations in cognitive function are common, requiring careful attention to safety.

Interfering Factors

➤ Protein intake.

➤ Hydration status.

➤ Drugs that can decrease levels include chloramphenicol and streptomycin.

➤ Drugs that increase levels include corticosteroids, tetracyclines, rifampin, furosemide, triamterene, aminoglycosides, antineoplastic drugs, phenacetin, cephalosporins, methyldopa, amphotericin B, vancomycin, probenecid, neomycin, polymyxin B, methicillin, bacitracin, carbamazepine, allopurinol, chloral hydrate, diuretics, indomethacin, propranolol, salicylates, and non-steroidal anti-inflammatory drugs.

➤ Pregnancy.

➤ Acromegaly.

➤ Severe liver damage.

➤ Celiac disease.

➤ Hemolysis.

NURSING CONSIDERATIONS

Prepare Your Client

➤ Explain that this test is helpful in discovering any problems in the kidney.

➤ The most accurate BUN testing occurs when food, fluids, or medications have been restricted for 8 hours.

Perform Procedure

➤ Collect 5 mL of venous blood in a red-top tube.

Care After Test

➤ If BUN levels are >40 mg/dL without signs and symptoms of dehydration, monitor intake and output, complete a dietary assessment, and check with health care provider regarding protein restriction.

➤ Assess for dehydration by noting poor skin turgor, increased pulse and respiration, dry mucous membrane, and decreased urine output. Encourage an increased oral intake unless contraindicated.

➤ Monitor for lethargy, confusion, and change in mental status. Provide necessary safety precautions.

➤ Monitor for hyperkalemia including weakness, paralysis, irritability, nausea and vomiting, intestinal colic, and diarrhea. Administer ion exchange resins, calcium, or insulin and glucose as ordered to treat hyperkalemia.

➤ Monitor for signs and symptoms of uremia including nausea, vomiting, stupor, peripheral edema, decreased urine output, dyspnea, jugular vein distention, and weight gain.

➤ Compare BUN to serum creatinine. Elevations in both strongly suggest renal disease.

➤ Observe for signs and symptoms of anemia, as an elevated BUN is associated with decreased red blood cells.

➤ Observe for signs and symptoms of gastrointestinal bleeding, which is associated with an elevated BUN.

➤ Review related tests including white blood count, creatinine, urine specific gravity, hemoglobin and hematocrit, serum electrolytes, total protein, urinalysis, and urine culture.

U

Educate Your Client and the Family

➤ Teach client and family regarding specific dietary prescription. In renal failure, the most common diet prescription is low protein, high calorie, low sodium and low potassium.

➤ Teach client the importance of maintaining fluid restriction where indicated.

➤ Instruct the client to report evidence of any anemia (weakness, shortness of breath, palpitations) or bleeding.

➤ Teach client the purpose, action, and side effects of any prescribed medications.

➤ Instruct client to report signs and symptoms of worsening uremia including nausea, vomiting, stupor, peripheral edema, decreased urine output, dyspnea, jugular vein distention, and weight gain.

➤ Teach client and family regarding importance of ongoing follow-up health care.

➤ Encourage the client to avoid exposure to infection.

➤ If the client is taking renal toxic drugs, teach client and family the importance of regular and ongoing health care supervision.

Urethral Pressure Profile

yu ree thrahl • presh ur • proe file
(UPP, Urethral Pressure Measurements, Urethral Pressure Profile Procedure, UPPP, Urodynamic Study)

Normal Findings
See data at top of next page.

What This Test Will Tell You

This measured pressure study evaluates stress incontinence, prostatic obstruction, and other conditions that affect urine flow from the bladder through the urethra. By measuring variations from normal pressure, alterations in normal voiding patterns can be quantified and specific information obtained to guide therapy.

Abnormal Findings

Abnormalities may indicate prostatic hypertrophy, stress incontinence, adverse effects of medications, neuromuscular abnormalities, or inadequate implanted artificial urethral sphincter.

ACTION ALERT!

Clients with cervical cord lesions may sustain an autonomic reflex, known as autonomic dysreflexia, that produces an elevated blood pressure, severe headache, lower pulse rate, flushing, and diaphoresis. This can lead to a cerebrovascular accident or death if not recognized and treated promptly with catheter removal and administration of propantheline bromide.

Interfering Factors

➤ Client movement during the procedure may interfere with results.

Contraindications

➤ Urinary tract infections

Potential Complications

➤ Autonomic dysreflexia
➤ Urinary tract infection

Normal Findings

Age	Female	Male
<25	55–105 cm H_2O	37–125 cm H_2O
25–44	31–115 cm H_2O	31–115 cm H_2O
45–64	40–100 cm H_2O	40–125 cm H_2O
>64	35–75 cm H_2O	35–105 cm H_2O

All ages: Normal urethral closing mechanism revealed.

U

NURSING CONSIDERATIONS

Prepare Your Client

➤ Explain that the test is performed to see how well the pathway from the bladder (urethra) is able to let urine leave the body when they urinate.

➤ Ensure that an informed consent is obtained, because of the possible complications associated with this procedure.

➤ Inform the client that they will experience some discomfort and may feel the urge to void during the procedure, slightly more than during routine urethral catheterization.

➤ Assure the client that drapes will be used to ensure privacy although the perineum must be exposed during the procedure.

Perform Procedure

Nurses do not perform this procedure, but should understand the process to prepare the client and assist the physician. The test is usually performed by a urologist in about 20 minutes. Place the client in the lithotomy position and drape the client with the perineum exposed.

The procedure may be performed in three different ways. One way is to insert a catheter, fill the bladder with fluid or gas, and measure pressure within the urethra as the catheter is withdrawn. A second method involves inserting small, inflated intraluminal balloons that provide pressure on the urethral walls, which can be measured. Finally, catheter tip transducers can be used to directly measure pressure resistance. The factors measured include the pressure along the length of the urethra, intraluminal closing forces, and effective urethral length. In all three methods, the catheter is withdrawn slowly while pressures along the urethra are recorded, then removed.

Care After Test

➤ Evaluate patterns of urinary elimination for difficulty initiating urination, weak stream, leakage of urine with increased intra-abdominal pressure, dribbling, and any other abnormalities.

➤ Evaluate related tests such as uroflowmetry, cystometry, excretory urography, and electromyography. Note results of the urinalysis to determine if abnormalities are present.

Educate Your Client and the Family

➤ Encourage the client to drink more fluids to dilute the urine and to minimize bladder sensitivity.

➤ Explain that some minor discomfort or burning may be noted soon after the procedure is completed, especially if carbon dioxide is used.

➤ Describe signs and symptoms of lower urinary tract infection, such as burning or discomfort on urination, urgency, frequency, chills, and malaise. Tell the client to contact the primary care provider if this occurs.

➤ Teach Kegel exercises to client with apparent stress incontinence.

Uric Acid, Serum
yur ik • ass id • see rum
(Uric Acid, Blood)

Normal Findings
ADULT
Male: 2.1–8.5 mg/dL (SI units: 0.15–0.48 mmol/L)
Female: 2.0–6.8 mg/dL (SI units: 0.09–0.36 mmol/L)
PREGNANT
Levels fall by about one-third in early pregnancy but rise to normal ranges by term.
INFANT
2.0–6.2 mg/dL (SI units: 0.11–0.34 mmol/L)
CHILD
2.5–5.5 mg/dL (SI units: 0.12–0.32 mmol/L)
ADOLESCENT
3.6–5.5 mg/dL (SI units: 0.19–0.30 mmol/L)
ELDERLY
3.5–8.5 mg/dL (SI units: 0.19–0.47 mmol/L)
Values tend to increase slightly in the elderly.

What This Test Will Tell You
This blood test evaluates a variety of conditions where there is excessive production and destruction of cells, identifies clients at risk for renal calculi, and evaluates the severity of toxemia of pregnancy. Uric acid is formed during the breakdown of nucleic acids and is an end product of purine metabolism in the liver. Most uric acid produced daily is excreted by the kidneys, with a small amount excreted in the stool. Abnormally high levels of uric acid may indicate excessive cell breakdown and catabolism of nucleic acids as in gout, or excessive production and destruction of cells as in leukemia. Elevated levels may also occur with ketoacidosis since the ketoacids compete with uric acid for tubular excretion and result in decreased uric acid excretion. Decreased uric acid levels may indicate defective tubular absorption or acute hepatic atrophy.

Abnormal Findings
▲INCREASED LEVELS may indicate renal failure, gout, leukemia, severe eclampsia, mononucleosis, multiple myeloma, alcoholism, metastatic cancer, excessive dietary purines, metabolic acidosis, multiple myeloma, arthritis, starvation, shock, strenuous exercise, stress, lead poisoning, or cancer chemotherapy.
▼DECREASED LEVELS may indicate treatment with uricosuric drugs, Fanconi's syndrome, neoplastic disease, Wilson's disease, or liver disease.

ACTION ALERT!
Values greater than 12 mg/dL uric acid in blood may indicate serious renal impairment and place the client at high risk for formation of uric acid renal stones. Strain all urine to assess for passage of calculi.

Interfering Factors

➤ Stress may increase uric acid levels.

➤ Starvation, fasting, dieting, a high-purine diet, caffeine, and alcohol abuse may raise levels.

➤ Drugs that increase levels include ascorbic acid, low-dose aspirin, bishydroxycoumarin, corticosteroids, cytotoxic agents, diuretics, probenecid, levodopa, methyldopa, nicotinic acid, epinephrine, phenothiazines, and theophylline.

➤ Glucose infusions may decrease levels.

➤ Drugs that may decrease levels include allopurinol, acetazolamide, clofibrate, corticosteroids, high-dose aspirin, estrogens, guaifenesin, probenecid, warfarin, azathioprine, and mannitol.

➤ Recent use of x-ray contrast agents may cause decreased levels.

➤ Febrile illnesses may affect results.

NURSING CONSIDERATIONS

Prepare Your Client

➤ Explain that this test is performed to look for gout, kidney problems, or other conditions where tissues may be damaged. Explain that it is valuable in assessing eclampsia if it is being performed for this purpose.

➤ Instruct the client to fast for 8 hours before the test, if appropriate. (Check with the laboratory as this requirement varies.)

➤ Instruct the client to avoid foods high in purines for 24 hours prior to the test if this has been ordered. Foods high in purines include organ meats, scallops, sardines, caffeine-containing beverages, legumes, mushrooms, spinach, and yeast.

Perform Procedure

➤ Collect 5–7 mL of venous blood in a red-top tube.

Care After Test

➤ Assess client with suspected hyperuricemia for signs and symptoms of gout, such as tophi of the ear lobe and joints, joint pain, and edema in the great toe.

➤ Increase fluid intake, unless contraindicated, to prevent formation of renal stones if hyperuricemia is suspected.

➤ If hyperuricemia is present, check the urine pH.

➤ Evaluate related tests such as the blood urea nitrogen and creatinine to evaluate kidney function. Monitor the pH of the urine since an acid urine is conducive to the formation of uric acid stones. Check urine uric acid levels to determine if the hyperuricemia is related to kidney dysfunction or overproduction.

Educate Your Client and the Family

➤ Instruct client with high uric acid levels to avoid foods high in purines such as organ meats, sardines, scallops, anchovies, broth, mincemeat, shellfish, legumes, mushrooms, and spinach. Request dietary consultation if indicated.

➤ Advise the client to decrease or eliminate alcoholic intake, since ethanol causes renal retention of urate.

➤ Teach the client, if appropriate, about drugs that are used to treat an acute attack of gout such as colchicine and indomethacin and maintenance drugs such as probenecid, sulfinpyrazone, or allopurinol.

➤ Advise the client with hyperuricemia to maintain a liberal fluid intake to decrease the risk of renal stone formation.

U

Uric Acid, Urine
yur ik • ass id • yur in

Normal Findings
ALL AGES

For normal or low-purine diet: 250–750 mg/24 hours (SI units: 1.48–4.43 mmol/24 hours)
For purine-free diet: 120 mg/24 hours (SI units: 2.48 mmol/24 hours)
For high-purine diet: 1000 mg/24 hours (SI units: 5.90 mmol/24 hours)
Sometimes high- and low-purine diets are ordered during the test.

What This Test Will Tell You
This 24-hour urine collection test is used as a supplement to the serum uric acid test for identifying disorders that alter production or excretion of uric acid such as gout, renal dysfunction, or leukemia. Uric acid is formed from the breakdown of nucleic acids and is an end product of purine metabolism. Most uric acid produced daily is excreted by the kidneys, with a small amount excreted in the stool. Abnormally high levels of uric acid in a 24-hour urine specimen may indicate excessive cell breakdown and catabolism of nucleic acids as in gout, or excessive production and destruction of cells as in leukemia. Decreased levels are found in kidney disease because impaired renal function depresses uric acid excretion. Elevated amounts of urinary uric acid precipitate into urate stones in the kidneys, so this test helps to identify people at risk for stone formation.

Abnormal Findings
▲INCREASED LEVELS may indicate gout (with excessive uric acid production), chronic myelogenous leukemia, ulcerative colitis, poly- cythemia vera, liver disease, multiple myeloma, febrile illness, toxemia of pregnancy, high-purine diet, lymphosarcoma, pernicious anemia, sickle-cell anemia, Fanconi's syndrome, or Wilson's disease.

▼DECREASED LEVELS may indicate gout (with poor uric acid excretion), renal failure, eclampsia, lead poisoning, or chronic alcoholism.

Interfering Factors
➤ Allopurinol increases urine uric acid content.
➤ Medications that can increase *or* decrease urine uric acid content include diuretics, low doses of aspirin, phenylbutazone, and probenecid.
➤ Radiographic contrast media can increase urine uric acid levels.
➤ Urine uric acid concentrations rise with a high-purine diet and fall with a low-purine diet.

NURSING CONSIDERATIONS

Prepare Your Client
➤ Explain to the client that this test measures how well the body and kidneys in particular are able to get rid of a waste product called uric acid.
➤ Instruct the client on how to collect a 24-hour urine sample.
➤ If a special diet is ordered during the testing period, instruct the client on the diet for high or low purine content.

Perform Procedure
➤ Obtain a 3L container from the laboratory, and follow requirements for a 24-hour urine collection.
➤ Place the collection container on ice or in the refrigerator according to

laboratory policy.

➤ Keep urine refrigerated or on ice throughout the collection period.

Care After Test

➤ Assess client with suspected elevated uric acid levels for signs and symptoms of gout, such as tophi of the ear lobe and joints, joint pain, and edema in the great toe.

➤ Increase fluid intake, unless contraindicated, to prevent formation of renal stones if high uric acid levels are suspected.

➤ Evaluate related tests such as the blood urea nitrogen (BUN) and creatinine to evaluate kidney function. Monitor the pH of the urine since acidic urine is conducive to the formation of uric acid stones. Check scrum uric acid levels to determine if the elevated level is related to renal dysfunction or overproduction of uric acid.

Educate Your Client and the Family

➤ Instruct client with high urine uric acid levels to avoid foods high in purines such as organ meats, sardines, scallops, anchovies, broth, mincemeat, shellfish, legumes, mushrooms, and spinach.

➤ Instruct the client to decrease or eliminate alcoholic intake, since ethanol causes renal retention of urate.

➤ Teach the client, if appropriate, about drugs that are used to treat an acute attack of gout such as colchicine and indomethacin and maintenance drugs such as probenecid, sulfinpyrazone, or allopurinol.

➤ Advise the client with elevated urine uric acid levels to maintain a liberal fluid intake to decrease the risk of renal stone formation, unless contraindicated.

Urinalysis
yur in al ah sis

What This Test Will Tell You

Urinalysis screens for abnormalities within the urinary system as well as for systemic problems that may manifest symptoms through the urinary tract. Visual examination, microscopic examination, reagent strip testing, and refractometry are various methods used in performing a complete urinalysis. Abnormalities in any finding warrant further related testing and investigation.

Interfering Factors

APPEARANCE

➤ Urine normally becomes hazy or

cloudy on standing, but this can be reversed in the laboratory by adding a few drops of acid.

➤ Vaginal contamination from female clients is a common cause of cloudy urine.

➤ After ingestion of food, urates or phosphates may produce cloudiness in normal urine.

➤ Greasy-appearing cloudiness may be caused by large amounts of fat in the urine.

➤ Contamination of the specimen with feces may produce cloudy urine.

COLOR

➤ The normal color of urine darkens

on standing for longer than 30 minutes, due to the oxidation of urobilinogen to urobilin.

➤ Some foods affect urine color. Beets can cause a red-colored urine. Rhubarb can cause the color to be brown. Carrots can cause a dark yellow color.

➤ Many drugs cause the urine to change color:

Red or red-brown–Cascara and senna laxatives, sulfisoxazole with phenazopyridine, phenytoin, chlorpromazine, and Ex-Lax.

Red–Aminopyrine, phenazopyridine, aniline dyes, PSP and BSP dyes in alkaline urine, phenolphthalein and phenazopyridine in acid urine, or deferoxamine.

Orange to orange red–Phenazopyridine, aminopyrine, oral anticoagulants, furazolidone, nitrofurantoin, and sulfonamides.

Orange to purple red–Chlorzoxazone.

Orange yellow–In alkaline urine: salicylazosulfapyridine, rifampin, sulfasalazine.

Bright yellow–Riboflavin.

Pale–Diuretics or diuresis due to alcohol ingestion.

Green or blue–Some diuretics, methylene blue, amitriptyline, methocarbamol, vitamin B complex, and yeast concentrate.

Brown–Phenolic drugs, phenylhydrazine, cascara, furazolidone, levodopa, metronidazole, nitrofurantoin, some sulfonamides.

Black–Cascara, ferrous sulfate, phenols, Lysol poisoning, porphyrin, and chloroquine.

➤ Contamination of the specimen with vaginal discharge, blood, or feces will discolor the urine.

GLUCOSE

➤ Stress and emotional excitement may cause false positives. Usually it is a trace reaction.

➤ Testing after a heavy meal may reveal a transient glycosuria.

➤ Intravenous administration of dextrose-containing fluids, especially hyperalimentation, usually produces glycosuria because the pancreas cannot produce insulin fast enough.

➤ Pregnancy and lactation may cause a false positive on some reagent strips due to lactose or galactose. About 70% of pregnant women show a temporary glycosuria that appears to be of no clinical significance.

➤ Drugs that produce false positive results for glucose in the urine include ascorbic acid, cephalosporins, chloral hydrate, nalidixic acid, oxytetracycline, paraldehyde, penicillins, salicylates, streptomycin, morphine, levodopa, and radiographic contrast media.

➤ False negatives may be obtained if deteriorated reagent strips have been used, or if directions are not followed exactly.

➤ Large amounts of ketones may yield a false negative.

➤ False positive test results with Clinitest® may occur when the client is taking vitamin C, aspirin, aminosalicylic acid, cephalothin, nitrofurantoin, streptomycin, sulfonamides, or chloral hydrate.

➤ False negative results may occur with Clinistix® and Tes-Tape® when the client is taking vitamin C or phenazopyridine.

➤ Levodopa may cause false negative results with Clinistix®.

LEUKOCYTE ESTERASE TEST

➤ False positive results may occur if the sample is contaminated with vaginal secretions, trichomonas, parasites, or heavy mucus.

➤ False negative results may occur if

high levels of protein and ascorbic acid are present in the urine.

pH

➤ Urine that is allowed to stand unrefrigerated or urine in which urea-splitting bacteria are present becomes more alkaline.

➤ Uncovered urine specimens tend to become alkaline because carbon dioxide will vaporize from the urine into the air.

➤ Alkaline urine after meals is a normal response to the secretion of hydrochloric acid in gastric juices.

➤ Dietary factors that produce an alkaline urine include large quantities of citrus fruits, dairy products, and vegetables.

➤ Drugs that may cause an alkaline urine include certain antibiotics, such as kanamycin, neomycin, and streptomycin, sulfonamides, excess salicylates, sodium bicarbonate, acetazolamide, and potassium citrate.

➤ Highly concentrated urine is strongly acidic.

➤ Dietary factors that produce an acidic urine include large quantities of meat protein and/or cranberries.

➤ Drugs that may cause an acidic urine include ammonium chloride, methenamine mandelate (mandelic acid), ascorbic acid, and diazoxide.

SPECIFIC GRAVITY

➤ Specific gravity is highest in the morning specimen since the kidneys normally concentrate the urine during the night.

➤ Refrigerated urine has a falsely high specific gravity.

➤ Recent use of radiographic dyes in the urinary tract increases the specific gravity.

➤ Drugs or intravenous fluid that may cause increased levels include dextran, sucrose, and albumin.

➤ Moderate amounts of glucose or protein in the urine may raise values.

PROTEIN

➤ Severe emotional stress, strenuous exercise, and exposure to cold may cause proteinuria because of renal vasoconstriction.

➤ Transient proteinuria may occur after eating large amounts of protein, immediately following delivery, or in newborn infants.

➤ Urinary tract infections or urine contaminated with vaginal secretions or menstrual flow may cause proteinuria because of pus or red blood cells in the urine.

➤ Radiopaque dye received within the last 3 days and alkaline urine may cause false positive results.

➤ Incorrect use and assessment of the color strip test can lead to inaccurate findings.

➤ Drugs that may cause increased protein levels include acetazolamide, aminoglycosides, amphotericin B, cephalosporins, colistin, griseofulvin, lithium, methicillin, nafcillin, nephrotoxic drugs, gold salts, oxacillin, penicillamine, penicillin G, phenazopyridine, polymyxin B, salicylates, sulfonamides, tolbutamide, and viomycin.

ODOR

➤ Urine which stands for a long time has a strong ammonia-like smell due to the formation of ammonia caused by bacterial activity decomposing the urea in the specimen.

➤ Some foods, such as asparagus, produce characteristic odors.

➤ Antibiotics and vitamins may affect urine odor.

KETONES

➤ High-protein, carbohydrate-free, and high-fat diets may result in ketonuria.

➤ Medications that cause false positive results include phenazopyridine,

U

ascorbic acid, ether, insulin, isopropyl alcohol, metformin, isoniazid, isopropanol, paraldehyde, valproic acid, levodopa, and bromosulfophthalein.

WHITE BLOOD CELLS
➤ Contamination with vaginal discharge or vaginal infections.
➤ Heavy mucus.
➤ Dilute, alkaline urine or urine that has been standing at room temperature for more than 2 hours causes disintegration of WBCs.

RED BLOOD CELLS
➤ Vigorous exercise.
➤ Traumatic catheterization to collect sample.
➤ Contamination with menstrual blood flow.
➤ Failure to test the sample quickly may yield false negative results.
➤ Alkaline urine hemolyzes red cells and dissolves casts.
➤ Heavy smoking causes red blood cells to appear in the urine.
➤ Medications including salicylates, anticoagulants, sulfonamides, and cyclophosphamide may increase the number of RBCs in urine.
➤ Reagent strip method of detection may yield false positive results if the client is receiving tetracycline, oxytetracycline, or copper therapy.
➤ High specific gravity or elevated protein content may make the reagent strip method less sensitive.

CRYSTALS
➤ Contrast dye.
➤ Ampicillin and sulfonamides may increase the levels of crystals.
➤ Prolonged standing at room temperature or refrigeration may increase the numbers of crystals.

BACTERIA
➤ Contamination with skin or vaginal bacteria.

➤ Contamination with stool.
➤ The number of bacteria will increase if the specimen is not analyzed promptly.

CASTS
➤ Expelling urine through a needle may destroy casts.
➤ Alkaline urine may dissolve casts.
➤ Strenuous physical exercise or contact sports may cause red cell casts to appear.

NURSING CONSIDERATIONS

Prepare Your Client

➤ Explain that this test is to look for problems with the urine and the organs that help form it.
➤ Advise the client to wash the perineal area prior to collecting the specimen to avoid contamination with vaginal secretions or stool.
➤ Inform the client that a specimen from the first morning urination is preferred since it is usually concentrated and more likely to reveal abnormalities and formed substances.
➤ Describe the procedure for collecting a clean-catch or midstream specimen if indicated.

Perform Procedure

➤ Collect approximately 50 mL of urine, freshly voided into a clean, dry container. A fresh specimen may be taken from a urinary catheter according to agency policy.
➤ Collect a clean-catch or midstream specimen if the specimen is likely to be contaminated by vaginal discharge, bleeding, or feces.
➤ Follow manufacturer's directions when using reagent or dipstick methods to test urine for glucose, ketones, erythrocytes, or leukocytes (leukocyte esterase test).

Care After Test

➤ Note the appearance of the specimen and document this according to policy.

➤ Review the specimen collection process with the client to rule out contamination with other substances.

➤ Assess the client for signs and symptoms of urinary tract infection such as dysuria, urgency, and frequency.

➤ Evaluate contraceptive method for female client. The use of a diaphragm and spermicidal jellies and creams are often associated with increased urinary tract infections.

➤ Because this test is done for a large variety of different conditions and illnesses, review indications for the test carefully and plan nursing care according to the suspected problem.

➤ Evaluate related tests such as the microscopic urinalysis, renal ultrasound, serum glucose, renal arteriogram, cystogram, cystourethrogram, and urine culture and sensitivity.

Educate Your Client and the Family

➤ Teach the client about signs and symptoms of urinary tract infection and appropriate treatment such as increasing fluid intake, dietary modifications, and drug therapy if indicated.

➤ Review with female clients and children proper toileting habits, including wiping from front to back and not holding urine in the bladder for prolonged periods, to help avoid urinary tract infections.

➤ Teach women the importance of emptying the bladder at least every 4–6 hours to prevent stasis of urine. Also, advise them to void immediately after intercourse. Pregnant women should empty their bladders every 2 hours.

➤ Advise women to shower rather than tub bathe, especially with bubble bath, due to the irritation to the urethra.

➤ Inform women that cotton underpants provide better absorbency and protection.

➤ If antibiotics are prescribed, stress the importance of taking all the medication, even after symptoms have disappeared.

Normal Macroscopic Findings in Routine Urinalysis

Characteristic	Normal finding	Abnormal finding
Appearance	Clear to slightly hazy	**Hazy or cloudy urine** may indicate the presence of white blood cells, red blood cells, bacteria, pus, phosphates, urates, uric acid, prostatic fluid, or spermatozoa. **Milky urine** may indicate the presence of fat or pyuria.
Color	Pale, straw-colored to amber-colored	**Pale or straw-colored urine** may indicate a large fluid intake, diuretic therapy, untreated diabetes mellitus, alcohol ingestion, or chronic interstitial nephritis.

➤

Color, *continued*

Orange-colored urine may indicate restricted fluid intake, dehydration, excess sweating, fever, or bile pigment related to hepatobiliary dysfunction. **Brownish-yellow to greenish-yellow urine** may indicate bilirubin in the urine or jaundice related to hepatobiliary dysfunction. **Green-colored urine** may indicate *Pseudomonas* infection.

Red or reddish dark-brown urine may indicate blood in the urine (dark red from bleeding from the kidneys; red to bright red from bleeding from the lower urinary tract), hemoglobin, myoglobin, or porphyrins in the urine.

Dark brown urine may indicate porphyrins, melanin, melanotic tumor, or Addison's disease.

Brown-black urine may indicate excessive hemoglobin in the urine, Lysol poisoning, or melanin.

Black urine may indicate alkaptonuria.

Smoky-colored urine may indicate the presence of red blood cells.

Glucose

Adult, child, adolescent, elderly: Negative; <0.5g/24 hours (SI units: <2.78 mmol/24 hours) **Pregnant:** Negative to small amounts of glucose in the urine. **Newborn:** Negative. However, may be positive in 25% of normal premature infants and infants up to the third day.

Increased levels with hyperglycemia may indicate diabetes mellitus, gestational diabetes, severe stress (e.g., trauma, surgery), infection, metabolic derangements (shock, severe burns, liver disease), medication-induced hyperglycemia (adrenal corticosteroids, adrenocorticotropic hormone, thiazides, oral contraceptives, excessive intravenous glucose, dextrothyroxine), Cushing's syndrome, carcinoma of the pancreas, severe chronic pancreatitis, cerebrovascular accident, brain tumor, hypothalamic dysfunction, pheochromocytoma, or

Glucose, *continued*

advanced cystic fibrosis. **Increased levels without hyperglycemia** may indicate pregnancy, or renal tubular dysfunction (Fanconi's syndrome, galactosemia, lead poisoning, multiple myeloma).

pH

Adult, pregnant, adolescent, and elderly: 4.5–8.0
Newborn: 5.0–7.0
Child: 4.8–7.8

Increased levels (alkaline urine) may indicate a urinary tract infection, metabolic alkalosis, respiratory alkalosis, renal tubular acidosis, renal failure, contamination with urea-splitting bacteria, diuretic therapy, or vegetarian diet.
Decreased levels (acidic urine) may indicate metabolic acidosis, respiratory acidosis, diarrhea, dehydration, starvation, uncontrolled diabetes mellitus, or high-protein diet.

Specific gravity

Adult, pregnant, child, or adolescent: 1.003–1.035
Infant: 1.001–1.020—lower values are usually seen until 3 months of age when concentration ability of the kidneys reaches normal level.
Elderly: Lower limits of normal due to decreased concentration ability.

Increased levels may indicate dehydration, syndrome of inappropriate antidiuretic hormone, glycosuria, proteinuria, fever, diaphoresis, or vomitting and diarrhea.
Decreased levels may indicate overhydration, diuretic therapy, diabetes insipidus, renal failure, glomerulonephritis, or pyelonephritis.

Protein

Adult, pregnant, child, adolescent, elderly: 2–8 mg/dL or negative by reagent strip test.
Infant: Negative to trace amounts in urine. May be positive in up to 25% of premature infants and newborns up to the third day.

Nephrotic syndrome, pre-eclampsia or toxemia of pregnancy, glomerulonephritis, urinary tract infection, fever, trauma, diabetes mellitus, congestive heart failure, acute infections, hypertension, postural proteinuria, systemic lupus erythematosus, polycystic kidney disease, liver disease, heavy metal poisoning, nephrotoxic drug therapy, or bladder tumors. ▶

U

Odor	**All ages:** Aromatic or faintly ammonia-like.	Diabetes mellitus, starvation, malnutrition, dehydration, urinary tract infection, maple syrup urine disease, or phenylketonuria.
Leukocyte esterase	**All ages:** Negative	Urinary tract infection.
Ketones	**All ages:** Negative	Diabetes mellitus, starvation, fasting, high-protein diets, weight reduction diets, anorexia, fever, alcoholism, post-anesthesia, diarrhea, or vomiting.

Normal Microscopic Findings in Routine Urinalysis

Characteristic	Normal finding	Abnormal finding
Red blood cells (RBCs)	0–3 with a high-power field 1 or 2 with a low-power field	Bleeding in the urinary tract, infection, trauma, tumors, glomerulonephritis, renal hypertension, lupus erythematosus, transfusion reaction, hemolytic anemia, hydronephrosis, cystitis, prostatitis, acute tubular necrosis, bacterial endo-carditis, hemorrhagic disorders, pyelonephritis, tuberculosis, cancer, renal calculi, or trauma from catheterization of the bladder.
White blood cells (WBCs)	0–5 with a high-power field 0 in a low-power field	Bacterial urinary tract infections, prostatitis, bladder tumors, strenuous exercise, tuberculosis, cystitis, or pyelonephritis.
Epithelial cells	Few	Renal tubular destruction.
Crystals	Absent	Renal calculi, inborn error of metabolism, gout, leukemia, lymphoma, severe chronic renal disease, hypercalcemia, high cholesterol, hepatic disease, cystinuria, and urinary tract infection.
Epithelial casts	Absent or scant	Glomerulonephritis, rejection of transplanted kidney, toxemia of pregnancy, ethylene glycol ingestion, heavy metal poisoning, and amyloidosis. ▶

Fatty casts	Absent	Diabetic nephropathy, glomerulonephritis, chronic renal disease, renal transplant rejection, malignant hypertension, localized nephron obstruction, or nephrotic syndrome.
Hyaline casts	Absent or 1–2 hyaline casts in a low-powered field	Inflammatory diseases, trauma, renal parenchymal disease, congestive heart failure, chronic renal failure, diabetic nephropathy, malignant hypertension, fever, strenuous exercise, or stress.
Red blood cell casts	Absent	Glomerulonephritis, bacterial endocarditis, sickle-cell anemia, hypertension, lupus erythematosus, kidney infarction, vascular diseases, collagen diseases, acute inflammatory diseases, or Goodpasture's syndrome.
Waxy casts	Absent	Chronic renal disease, diabetes mellitus, malignant hypertension, renal transplant rejection, glomerulonephritis, localized nephron obstruction, and nephrotic syndrome.
Granular casts	Absent or scant	Urinary tract infection, acute tubular necrosis, stress, renal transplant rejection, glomerulonephritis, chronic renal failure, pyelonephritis, lead poisoning, or nephrosclerosis.
White blood cell casts	Absent	Pyelonephritis, interstitial inflammation of the kidney, glomerulonephritis, lupus nephritis, nephrotic syndrome, or renal infection.
Bacteria	Less than 3 in a high-powered field Less than 1000/mL	Urinary tract infection, prostatitis, cystitis, urethritis, or pyelonephritis.
Parasites	Absent	Genitourinary tract infection with *Trichomonas vaginalis* or other parasites.
Yeast cells	Absent	Genitourinary tract infection.

U

Urinary Calculi Analysis

yur ih **nair** ee • **kal** kyu lie • ah **nal** ah sis
(Urolithiasis, Urinary Stones, Renal Calculi)

Normal Findings

All ages: Negative, no calculi present in urine

What This Test Will Tell You

This urinalysis detects the presence of gross or microscopic calculi and determines their mineral content. Urinary calculi are stones within the urinary system, which may be formed in the kidney or bladder. Urinary calculi are insoluble substances formed from calcium, phosphate, oxalate, uric acid, struvite, and cystine crystals. The vast majority of stones contain calcium as one component. Certain factors contribute to the ease of stone formation (urolithiasis). These factors include the pH of the urine, the amount of solute in the urine, and the amount of urine. Problems with purine metabolism predispose one to the formation of uric acid stones. Prolonged immobility leads to urinary stasis and, because of calcium mobilization from the bones, an increase in serum and urine calcium. If fluid intake is also inadequate, then the calcium saturating the urine is more likely to precipitate out and form stones. Because different types of stones are treated differently, both in terms of dietary modifications and drug therapy, it is essential that the components of the stone are identified.

Abnormal Findings

Stones may be calcium oxalate calculi, calcium phosphate calculi, cystine calculi, urate calculi, or magnesium ammonium phosphate calculi and may indicate gout, idiopathic hypercalciuria, primary hyperparathyroidism, primary cystinuria, dehydration, hepatic dysfunction, or *Proteus* infection of the urinary tract.

Interfering Factors

➤ Failure to properly collect and strain *all* urine may allow the stone to pass and go undetected.

NURSING CONSIDERATIONS

Prepare Your Client

➤ Explain to the client that this test detects urinary or kidney stones, and that if stones are found, the laboratory will analyze them to find out what medications or changes in the diet will help avoid forming more.

➤ Tell the client that all urine must be collected and strained.

➤ Keep the urinal or bedpan within easy reach of the client who has received analgesics, as drowsiness may make it unsafe for the client to get out of bed to void.

➤ Reassure the client that symptoms will subside immediately after excretion of any stones.

➤ Encourage the client to drink 3000–4000 mL of fluid per day, unless contraindicated, to help wash out the stones and to hinder their formation by diluting the urine.

➤ Provide a urinal or bedpan for collection of urine.

➤ Encourage the client to call for assistance with urination if needed.

➤ Administer medication to control pain as ordered.

Perform Procedure

➤ Collect all urine quickly after the client voids.

➤ Pour the entire specimen carefully through a urine strainer (a fine-mesh sieve) or an unfolded 4" × 4" gauze dressing.

➤ Inspect the filter or gauze dressing carefully for stones. Calculi may be minute, and may look like gravel or sand.

Care After Test

➤ Observe for symptoms of urolithiasis, such as flank pain, dysuria, and urinary retention, frequency, or urgency. Note hematuria.

➤ Document the appearance of the calculi and the number, if possible.

➤ Place the calculi in a properly labeled container, and send the container to the laboratory immediately for prompt analysis.

➤ Continue to collect and strain all urine until the primary health care provider deems it no longer necessary.

➤ Consult with a registered dietician to assist the family and client in meeting special dietary needs to reduce formation of calculi.

➤ Evaluate related test findings from the urinalysis such as the presence of red blood cells, white blood cells, bacteria, or crystals. Note the white blood cell count if infection is suspected. Evaluate radiographic findings such as the x-ray of the kidneys, ureters, and bladder (KUB); intravenous pyelogram (IVP); computed tomography (CT) scans; or other tests such as renal ultrasonography that may demonstrate calculi. If renal calculi are present, the urinalysis report may include findings of red blood cells (due to direct trauma caused by the calculi on the endothelial lining of the ureter, bladder, or urethra), or white blood cells or bacteria (both resulting from urinary stasis). Microscopic examination of the urine may allow identification of crystals from which stones could form. Increases in the serum calcium, serum phosphate, or serum uric acid levels suggest that excess minerals are present and contributory to the stone formation. Review urine pH level; uric acid and cystine stones tend to form in acidic urine while struvite and calcium phosphate stones tend to form in alkaline urine.

Educate Your Client and the Family

➤ Teach the client the primary prevention of stone formation: avoiding immobility and fluid-depleted states.

➤ Educate the client about measures taken to prevent recurrences of stone formation including medications to combat infection and alter the pH of the urine, testing the pH of the urine with reagent strips daily, dietary modification based on the type of stone-forming process (avoiding calcium-containing or other foods that are known to promote calculus formation), eating a well-balanced diet, and maintaining a liberal fluid intake.

➤ Instruct the client about the importance of recognizing any signs of recurrence.

U

Urinary Tract Brush Biopsy

yur in air ee • trakt • brush • bie op see
(Retrograde Renal and Ureteral Brush Biopsy)

Normal Findings

All ages: No abnormal cells or tissue present

What This Test Will Tell You

This endoscopic technique collects tissue specimens from the renal pelvis or ureters for microscopic examination to differentiate between benign and malignant lesions, or monitors recurrent lesions for malignant changes. This test is useful in evaluating lesions involving the bladder, ureter, renal pelvis, or calyx, especially if there is evidence of a bladder tumor on radiological examination or if hydroureter is present without stones.

Abnormal Findings

Positive findings may include benign or malignant lesions.

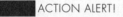 ACTION ALERT!

Brush biopsy may cause such complications as perforation, hemorrhage, sepsis, or contrast medium extravasation. Monitor for signs and symptoms of hemorrhage or shock including apprehension, anxiety, tachycardia, tachypnea, pain, hypotension, pallor, diaphoresis, and mental status changes.

Interfering Factors

➤ Improper specimen collection

Contraindications

➤ Known hypersensitivity to contrast media or iodine-containing foods, such as shellfish
➤ Urinary tract infection
➤ Obstruction at or below the biopsy site
➤ Bleeding disorders

Potential Complications

➤ Hemorrhage
➤ Perforation of the bladder, ureter, or urethra
➤ Sepsis
➤ Shock
➤ Contrast medium extravasation
➤ Complications related to general, spinal, or local anesthesia
➤ Hypersensitivity reaction to the contrast medium

NURSING CONSIDERATIONS

Prepare Your Client

➤ Explain that this test is performed to get a sample of tissue from inside the system that makes urine to see if there are any problems or changes in the tissues.
➤ Ensure that an informed consent is obtained, because of the possible complications associated with this procedure.
➤ Assess and record baseline vital signs.
➤ Consult with the primary health care provider regarding the need for sedation prior to the procedure.
➤ Withhold food and fluids for 8 hours prior to the procedure if general anesthesia is used. If local anesthesia is to be used, only clear liquids may be taken for 8 hours prior to the test.
➤ Inform the client that the procedure will take only 30–60 minutes, and that they will be monitored closely during and immediately after the test.
➤ Review the client's history for hypersensitivity to anesthetics, con-

trast media, or iodine-containing foods, such as shellfish. Alert the urologist if these findings are positive.

Perform Procedure

Nurses do not perform this procedure, but should understand the process to prepare the client and assist the physician. Position the client on the examination table with the legs placed in stirrups and draped. If general or local anesthesia is to be used, it is administered prior to positioning the client on the table. Cleanse the external genitalia with antiseptic solution. Local anesthesia may be instilled into the urethra. Encourage the client to retain it for 5–10 minutes.

The cystoscope is inserted into the bladder and a guide wire passed up the ureter, followed by a urethral catheter over the guide wire. Contrast medium is instilled through the catheter, which is positioned next to the lesion under fluoroscopic guidance. The contrast medium is washed out with normal saline. A biopsy brush is passed through the catheter to brush the lesion. This procedure is repeated several times, using a new brush each time. Each brush is removed from the catheter, and a smear made on a slide for Papanicolaou staining. Each brush tip is cut off and placed in a formalin solution.

The catheter is irrigated with normal saline as the last brush is removed and the saline is collected for laboratory analysis. The cystoscope is withdrawn, and the client's legs removed from the stirrups.

Label specimen containers indicating the site and method utilized in obtaining the specimen, and transport to the laboratory immediately. If client has received local anesthesia, allow them to rest in the supine position for several minutes before being assisted from the table. If client has received general or spinal anesthesia, transport them to the recovery room following hospital procedure.

Care After Test

➤ Monitor vital signs closely until stable; usually every 15 minutes for the first hour, every 30 minutes for the next hour, and then every 4 hours for 24 hours.

➤ Record the time, color, and amount of the first and subsequent voidings, being alert for hematuria and abdominal or flank pain. Urine should be clear by the third voiding.

➤ Assess the client for bladder distention, incomplete emptying of the bladder, suprapubic or flank pain, chills, and fever.

➤ Monitor for signs of hypersensitivity reaction such as hives, itching, difficulty breathing, or changes in vital signs. Report any abnormal findings to the primary health care provider immediately.

➤ Administer analgesics or warm sitz baths if bladder spasms occur.

➤ Administer antibiotics if ordered.

➤ Resume food and fluids unless contraindicated. A fluid intake of 3000 mL within 24 hours after the test is desirable.

➤ Evaluate related tests such as an x-ray of the kidneys, ureters, and bladder (KUB), intravenous pyelography, retrograde pyelography, cysto-urethrography, and excretory urogram. Note results of kidney function tests such as the blood urea nitrogen and serum creatinine to be alert for possible coexisting kidney problems.

Educate Your Client and the Family

➤ Instruct the client to report immediately any severe abdominal or flank pain, bright blood in the urine, or signs of hypersensitivity such as hives, itching, and dizziness.

➤ Teach outpatient client how to monitor urinary output and the necessity of reporting symptoms such as pain, chills, and fever immediately.

Urine Concentration and Dilution

yur in • kon sen tray shun • and • die loo shun

(Water Loading, Water Deprivation Tests, Fishberg Test, Addis Test, Mosenthal Test, Volhard's Test)

Normal Findings

CONCENTRATION TESTS

Fishberg test:

Specific gravity greater than or equal to 1.025 and 300 mL of urine

Osmolality > 500 mOsm/L water

Mosenthal's test:

>1.020 and at least a 7-point difference between the highest and lowest specific gravities measured

Volhard's test:

Greater than or equal to 1.025

Osmolality > 800 mOsm/L water

DILUTION TEST

Specific gravity < 1.003

Osmolality < 100 mOsm/kg water

PREGNANT

The test is unreliable in pregnant women because the tubules may be unable to concentrate urine.

NEWBORN

The test should not be performed on newborns because of the risk imposed from fluid deprivation or overload. Also, infants do not gain the ability to concentrate urine until about 3 months of age. While the infant's capacity to dilute urine is comparable to that of an adult, the infant kidney is not as well equipped to process a sudden large quantity of fluid.

ELDERLY

In the elderly, depressed values can be associated with normal renal function.

What This Test Will Tell You

This urine test measures specific gravity and osmolality to evaluate the kidney's ability to concentrate urine in response to fluid deprivation, or to dilute urine in response to fluid overload. The loss of the kidney's ability to concentrate and dilute urine indicates significant renal tubular damage. Normally as the body becomes fluid depleted, larger volumes of water are reabsorbed, resulting in more concentrated urine with a specific gravity over 1.020 and urine osmolality three to four times that of plasma (normal plasma osmolality is 275–300 mOsm/kg). Conversely, with increased fluid intake, more water is excreted, causing more dilute urine with a specific gravity often as low as 1.005 and a urine osmolality less than 100 mOsm/kg. One of the first kidney functions to be lost is the ability to concentrate and dilute urine. In severe renal damage, the specific gravity may become fixed at a level of 1.008 to 1.012, regardless of the fluid intake.

This test is frequently done in conjunction with the administration of vasopressin to diagnose diabetes insipidus (water deprivation antidiuretic hormone stimulation test).

Abnormal Findings

Abnormal results may indicate renal tubular damage, decreased renal blood flow, excessive or prolonged overhydration, diabetes insipidus, hypokalemia sarcoidosis, bone disease, or hyperparathyroidism.

ACTION ALERT!

Some clients may have decreased cardiac function and poorly tolerate the increased fluid load. Assess closely for dyspnea, neck vein distention, a galloping heart rhythm, and crackles in the lungs, which may indicate fluid overload. Notify the primary health care provider promptly if these symptoms occur.

Interfering Factors

➤ Failure to adhere to dietary and fluid restrictions will interfere with accurate determination of results.
➤ Presence of disorders that alter serum protein or sodium levels.
➤ Pregnancy, fluid and electrolyte imbalances, and low salt may affect results.
➤ Low-protein diets may invalidate results.
➤ Liver disease and congestive heart failure may invalidate the results.
➤ Diuretics cause increased urine volume and dilution.
➤ Nephrotoxic drugs may decrease renal concentrating ability.
➤ Acute or chronic water or electrolyte imbalance before the test may produce inaccurate results.
➤ Administration of radiographic dyes within 7 days prior to the test may cause increased urine osmolality.

➤ Glucosuria invalidates the results.
➤ Edema, sweating, diarrhea, and fever interfere with the dilution test.

Contraindications

➤ Advanced renal, liver, or cardiac disease, because fluid overload can precipitate water intoxication, sodium diuresis, or congestive heart failure

Potential Complications

➤ Dilution tests may precipitate congestive heart failure in clients with impaired cardiac function.
➤ Withholding diuretics may cause a fluid overload in clients with congestive heart failure or renal dysfunction.

NURSING CONSIDERATIONS

Prepare Your Client

➤ Explain to the client that this test is performed to see how well the kidneys are able to make urine or hold onto water in the body as needed.
➤ Advise the client that a normal protein diet with adequate fluids should be followed for 3 days before the test.
➤ Withhold diuretics for 48–72 hours prior to the test and during the test.
FOR THE CONCENTRATION TEST
➤ Explain to the client that a high-protein meal with only a small amount of fluids will be provided the evening before the test.
➤ Instruct the client to withhold food and fluids after the evening meal (at least 14 hours).
➤ Emphasize to the client that cooperation is necessary to obtain accurate results.
➤ Instruct the client to completely empty the bladder before retiring for the night, and to save any urine voided during the night. This urine

should be sent to the lab in a separate container and labeled for time of collection.

➤ Inform the client that several urine specimens will be collected at specified times the next morning.

FOR THE DILUTION TEST

➤ Explain to the client that this test usually follows the concentration test and necessitates no additional preparation.

➤ Explain to the client that after voiding, they will be instructed to drink approximately 3 pints (1500 mL) of water within 30 minutes and that after this, urine specimens will be collected at timed intervals for 4 hours.

Perform Procedure

CONCENTRATION TEST

➤ Withhold diuretics, as ordered.

➤ Provide a high-protein meal and only 200 mL of fluid the evening before the test.

➤ Restrict food and fluids for at least 14 hours after the evening meal.

➤ Provide clean 500-mL specimen containers.

➤ Collect urine specimens the next morning at the specified times, such as 6 A.M., 8 A.M., 10 A.M.

➤ Obtain specimens from a urinary catheter, if the client is catheterized, and clamp the catheter between collections.

➤ Keep specimens separate.

DILUTION TEST

➤ Perform this test upon completion of the concentration test.

➤ Give the client 1500 mL of water to drink within 30 minutes.

➤ Administer intravenous solutions, as ordered by the primary health care provider, if this approach is to be utilized rather than using oral intake.

➤ Collect urine specimens every half hour or hour, as ordered, for 4 hours after ingestion or administration of the fluid.

➤ Obtain specimens from an indwelling catheter, if the client is catheterized, and clamp the catheter between collections. Keep specimens separate.

Care After Test

➤ Measure and record the volume of each specimen and the total volume of all specimens.

➤ Label and time the specimens appropriately and send immediately to the laboratory.

➤ Assess the client for symptoms of fluid overload, such as tachypnea, dyspnea, rales, tachycardia, or cardiac arrhythmias.

➤ Provide a balanced meal or snack and resume normal fluid intake.

➤ Evaluate related tests such as the blood urea nitrogen, serum creatinine, urinalysis, urinary electrolytes, creatinine clearance, water deprivation antidiuretic hormone stimulation test, and radiographic examinations of the kidneys.

Educate Your Client and the Family

➤ Advise the client to report any symptoms of fluid overload, such as palpitations or shortness of breath, immediately.

➤ Instruct client who is unable to concentrate urine to monitor for signs of dehydration such as dry mucous membranes, thirst, and dizziness upon standing.

➤ Teach safety precautions to persons who have diabetes insipidus. Caution them to move slowly when changing positions or standing up, and to wear medical alert identification.

➤ Stress the importance of taking medication throughout their lives.

Urine Culture and Sensitivity

yur in • kul chur • and • sen sih tiv ih tee

(Urine C & S)

Normal Findings

All ages: Less than 10,000 organisms per mL. Urine in the bladder normally contains no organisms, but upon collection it becomes contaminated with organisms present in the perineal area. Less than 10,000 organisms per mL is probably contamination rather than an abnormal finding.

What This Test Will Tell You

This microscopic urinalysis determines the presence of pathogenic organisms in the urinary tract and tests for antimicrobial sensitivity by determining the effects of various antibiotics on a particular microorganism. This test involves the direct microscopic inspection of a sample of urine for Gram-stain, culture, and sensitivity studies. Once the urine is collected and sent to the laboratory, it is initially Gram-stained to identify the organism as gram-positive or gram-negative. This test can be performed quickly (less than 10 minutes), and provides guidelines to begin appropriate antimicrobial therapy. The urine is then incubated for 24 and then 48 hours on the appropriate culture medium and studied by a microbiologist. The culture allows further identification of the infecting organism. Once the organism is identified, its sensitivity or resistance to various antimicrobial agents is tested and appropriate antibiotic therapy may then be prescribed.

Merely finding organisms in the urine sample does not signify clinical urinary tract infection. The distal portion of the urethra is typically colonized by organisms from the perineal area. Levels below 10,000 organisms per mL usually represent contamination of the specimen rather than infection. Concentrations of 100,000 organisms per mL generally constitute significant infection. If the client is symptomatic, however, a culture of a single organism at a level of 10,000 organisms per mL may be significant and require treatment.

Abnormal Findings

➤ *Bacterial counts less than 10,000/mL* may indicate contamination of the specimen, or urinary tract infection in clients who are symptomatic.

➤ *Bacterial counts greater than 100,000/mL* may indicate urinary tract infection.

➤ *Bacterial counts from 10,000 to 100,000/mL* indicate probable urinary tract infection.

ACTION ALERT!

If urinary tract infection is strongly suspected, initiation of antimicrobial therapy may be instituted after obtaining cultures but before confirmation by culture results.

Interfering Factors

➤ Improper specimen collection may result in bacterial contamination from sources such as the perineal area, vaginal secretions, stool, hands, skin, or clothing.

➤ Antibiotic therapy initiated before specimen collection may yield false negative results.

> The number of bacteria will increase if the specimen is allowed to stand at room temperature for several hours. Urine is an excellent culture medium. Collection of specimens should be as aseptic as possible, and samples should be sent to the laboratory immediately for prompt analysis.

> Falsely low colony counts may be observed in the urine of clients who are receiving forced fluids or diuretic therapy, since the urine will be dilute.

NURSING CONSIDERATIONS

Prepare Your Client

> Explain to the client that this test is performed to detect possible infections of the urinary system and to determine the best medication.

> Advise the client that an early morning specimen should be obtained, if possible, because bacterial counts are highest at that time.

> Describe the procedure for collecting a clean-catch (midstream) urine sample. This method of specimen collection is preferred over catheterization to obtain a specimen because catheterization increases the risk of introducing an infection.

Perform Procedure
CLEAN-CATCH TECHNIQUE

> Obtain a urine culture using a clean-catch technique. For infants and children who are not yet toilet trained, a sterile urine collection bag may be attached to the perineal area for collection.

INDWELLING CATHETER

> Clamp the catheter tubing for 15 minutes to allow urine to accumulate in the upper portion of the tubing.

> Cleanse the needle port of the rubber catheter with an alcohol wipe and allow to dry.

> Insert a sterile needle through the port and withdraw 10 mL of urine.

> Remove the syringe. Expel the urine into a sterile specimen cup and cap tightly.

> Remove the clamp from the tubing.

Care After Test

> Label the specimen container with the specific collection site and method of collection, client's name, date, and time. Note any antibiotic therapy the client is receiving.

> Institute antibiotic therapy if ordered.

> Assess the client for signs and symptoms of urinary tract infection such as dysuria, urgency, frequency, fever, chills, and malaise.

> Identify risk factors for urinary tract infections such as the use of diaphragms and contraceptive jellies, foam, and suppositories.

> Review related test results such as a urinalysis for the presence of bacteria, white blood cells, red blood cells, and casts. Note if findings for nitrates or leukocyte esterase are positive. Check the serum white blood cell count and differential for evidence of systemic infection.

Educate Your Client and the Family

> Inform the client that results will not be available for 1–2 days and that antibiotic therapy may be initiated prior to laboratory confirmation of infection.

> Instruct client on the importance of compliance with antibiotic therapy, especially completing the prescribed course of treatment.

> Encourage the client to increase fluid intake, unless contraindicated, if urinary tract infection is suspected.

> Teach the client about signs and

symptoms of urinary tract infection and appropriate treatment, including dietary modifications and drug therapy, if appropriate.

➤ Teach female client to wipe from the front to the back after voiding or a bowel movement.

➤ Teach client to shower rather than bathe, and to avoid any bubble bath products, which can increase risk of infection.

Urine Cytology

yur in • sie tol oe jee
(Cytologic Study of Urine)

Normal Findings

All ages: Negative for abnormal cells. Epithelial and squamous cells are normally present in the urine.

What This Test Will Tell You

This microscopic urinalysis examines cells shed (exfoliated) from the urinary tract to detect cell changes due to malignancies or inflammatory conditions of the bladder, the renal pelvis, the ureters, and the urethra. Cytology is the microscopic study of cells to determine their origin, structure, function, and pathology. Because cells from the epithelial lining of the urinary tract exfoliate readily into the urine, a simple cytologic examination of these cells can aid in the diagnosis of urinary tract disease. Urine cytology is not done routinely. However, it is especially useful for detecting cellular changes in persons at high risk for bladder cancer, such as smokers, people who work with aniline dyes, and persons previously treated for bladder cancer. This test can also detect cytomegalovirus infection and other viral disease. In these disorders, abnormal cells are shed into the urine and can be detected upon examination of the sample. Cytologic studies will commonly be reported as inflammatory, benign, atypical, suspicious for malignancy, or positive for malignancy.

Abnormal Findings

➤ *Inflammatory conditions* may indicate benign prostatic hypertrophy, kidney stones, diverticula of bladder, strictures, or malformations.

➤ *Infectious conditions* may indicate bacterial, viral, or fungal infection of the urinary tract; cytomegalovirus infection; or measles.

➤ *Malignant conditions* may indicate cancer of the bladder, renal pelvis, ureters, kidney, or urethra; or metastatic cancer.

Interfering Factors

➤ An early morning specimen is not suitable since cell death occurs overnight in the bladder.

➤ An improper specimen collection may be contaminated with extraneous cells.

➤ Delay in sending the sample to the laboratory allows cells to begin to disintegrate.

➤ False positive findings may result if instruments have recently been used in the urinary tract and may have produced cellular injury or changes.

➤ Chemotherapeutic drugs may alter the results.

NURSING CONSIDERATIONS

Prepare Your Client

➤ Explain that this test is performed to detect abnormal cells that may be present in the urinary tract.

➤ Advise the client that a random urine specimen, not an early morning specimen, is needed, and to collect at least 6 ounces (180 mL) of urine.

➤ Provide supplies and privacy for proper specimen collection. A sterile specimen cup and antiseptic sponges should be available. Depending on the laboratory, a special container and/or preservative may be needed.

➤ Describe the procedure for collecting a clean-catch (midstream) urine sample.

➤ Tell the client if additional specimens will be needed and when they should be obtained. Usually three random specimens are collected for cytologic evaluation and compared before concluding that abnormal cells are present or absent.

Perform Procedure

➤ Instruct client to perform a clean-catch technique to obtain urine sample.

➤ Obtain a catheterized specimen if it is difficult to obtain the specimen, or if a high urinary tract lesion is suspected.

➤ Label the specimen container and transport to the laboratory immediately before cell degeneration begins.

➤ Note on the laboratory requisition if the specimen was obtained by catheterization, because epithelial cells from the urethra or bladder may have been added to the urine by the catheter.

Care After Test

➤ Review related tests such as the urinalysis for abnormal cells and cellular debris, results of x-ray studies of the urinary tract, and cystoscopy and biopsy findings.

Educate Your Client and the Family

➤ Inform the client if additional urine specimens will be needed.

➤ Explain to the client that results will be interpreted by the pathologist, who will relay results to their primary health care provider. Cytologic studies may take 2 or more days for final interpretation.

➤ Encourage the client to increase fluid intake, unless contraindicated, if infection or inflammation is suspected.

Urine Flow Studies

yur in • floe • stud ees

(Uroflowmetry, Urodynamic Studies)

Normal Findings

Normal urine flow curve for age and sex.

ADULT

Total flow of >200 mL is needed for flow study.

Male: 12–21 mL/second
Female: 12–18 mL/second
PREGNANT
Flow rate may normally be decreased in advanced stages of pregnancy due to pressure on the bladder.
CHILD
>100 mL
Male: 10–12 mL/sec
Female: 10–15 mL/sec
ADOLESCENT
>200 mL
Male: 12–20 mL/second
Female: 12–18 mL/second
ELDERLY
>200 mL
Male: 9 mL/second
Female: 10 mL/second

What This Test Will Tell You

This urodynamic test diagnoses voiding problems or loss of bladder control, and evaluates the effectiveness of reconstructive bladder surgery. Uroflowmetry is a simple, noninvasive procedure that measures the volume of urine expelled from the bladder per second. It involves measuring the voiding duration, amount, and rate of urine voided by having the client void into a special commode chair equipped with a funnel and a load cell mechanism that measures weight over time. The uroflowmeter measures flow rate, continuous flow, and intermittent flow. The volume of urine voided is recorded and plotted on graph paper as a curve over the time of voiding, and is interpreted taking the client's age and sex into consideration.

Abnormal Findings

▲INCREASED FLOW RATE may indicate reduced urethral resistance associated with external sphincter dysfunction or decreased outflow resistance due to stress incontinence, especially high peak flow over short voiding time.

▼DECREASED FLOW RATE may indicate outflow obstruction caused by urethral stricture, prostatic hypertrophy or cancer, or hypotonia of the detrusor muscle.

More than one distinct peak in a normal curve may indicate abdominal straining and detrusor muscle weakness.

Interfering Factors

➤ Optimal amounts of urine in the bladder for evaluation are between 200 and 400 mL. Too little urine impedes accurate measurement. Quantities over 400 mL interfere with bladder extrusor muscle function.

➤ Client movement while seated on the commode chair may result in an inaccurate flow recording.

➤ Client hesitancy due to nervousness may cause inaccurate results.

➤ Toilet tissue in the funnel or commode will invalidate results.

➤ Inaccurate leveling of the transducer or centering of the beaker beneath the funnel will invalidate results.

➤ Overflow of urine, if the beaker is not large enough, will invalidate results.

➤ Drugs that affect bladder and sphincter tone, such as anticholinergics and urinary spasmolytics, will alter test results.

➤ Recent use of instruments in the urethra may cause decreased flow rates.

➤ Failure to gain client understanding or cooperation will make the test unreliable.

NURSING CONSIDERATIONS

Prepare Your Client

➤ Explain to the client that this test

is performed to evaluate patterns of urination.

➤ Tell the client not to void for several hours prior to the test.

➤ Instruct the client how to void into the urine flowmeter, including assuming a normal voiding position, performing a normal void, and completely emptying the bladder into the funnel.

➤ Emphasize the need to remain still while voiding to help ensure accurate results.

➤ Tell the client not to let stool or toilet tissue enter the funnel.

➤ Assure the client that they will have complete privacy during voiding.

Perform Procedure

➤ Follow manufacturer's instructions and institutional protocol for the exact procedure, which will vary according to the type of urine flowmeter.

➤ Assure that the client's bladder is adequately full and that the client has a normal urge to void.

➤ Check cable connections to the flowmeter.

➤ Leave the client alone to ensure that embarrassment does not interfere with normal voiding.

➤ Activate the flowmeter, according to manufacturer's directions, just prior to the void.

➤ Ask the client to assume a normal voiding position and void, completely emptying the bladder without straining.

➤ Perform serial recordings over 2 to 3 days, if necessary, to provide the most accurate evaluation of urine flow patterns.

Care After Test

➤ Perform nursing assessments related to the client's voiding patterns, paying close attention to voiding patterns, amounts in normal voiding, and episodes of incontinence.

➤ Assist the client, if necessary, to assume a comfortable position.

➤ Record the position of the client and the amount and route of fluid intake or method of filling the bladder.

➤ Analyze the uroflow curve, noting the volume voided and the rate, pattern, and duration of voiding.

➤ Evaluate related tests, such as the routine urinalysis and other urodynamic studies such as cystometry, voiding cystourethrography, measurement of residual urine, and urethral pressure profiles.

Educate Your Client and the Family

➤ Inform the client if and when successive urine flow tests will be performed.

➤ Teach the client about symptoms related to urinary retention or urinary tract infection, if indicated.

➤ Inform client of support groups for incontinence, if indicated.

➤ Offer suggestions to prevent incontinence, if appropriate, such as voiding schedule, and pelvic floor muscle (Kegel) exercises.

Urobilinogen, Urine and Fecal

yur oh bie lin oe jen • yur in • and • fee kuhl

Normal Findings

URINE

Females: 0.1–1.1 Ehrlich units/2-hour sample

Males: 0.3–2.1 Ehrlich units/2-hour sample

0.5–4.0 mg/24-hour sample

0.1–1.0 Ehrlich unit/mL

FECAL

40–300 mg/24 hours

What This Test Will Tell You

This urine and fecal test helps diagnose extrahepatic obstruction and differentiates between hepatic and hematologic disorders. This test measures urine levels of urobilinogen, which is formed in the duodenum where intestinal bacteria change bilirubin to urobilinogen. Most urobilinogen is eliminated in the feces, but approximately 1% is reabsorbed into the bloodstream to be excreted by the kidneys in urine. In the presence of normal serum bilirubin levels, elevated urobilinogen levels may indicate early hepatitis or mild hepatotoxic injury.

Abnormal Findings

▲INCREASED LEVELS may indicate hepatocellular damage (early hepatitis, portal cirrhosis), intravascular hemolysis, hemorrhage into tissues, hemolytic diseases, biliary obstruction with infection of biliary tract, congestive heart failure with hepatic dysfunction, infectious mononucleosis, or malaria.

▼DECREASED LEVELS may indicate cholelithiasis, biliary obstruction without infection of biliary tract, massive hepatocellular damage, renal insufficiency, cancer of the head of the pancreas, and severe diarrhea.

Interfering Factors

➤ Para-aminosalicylic acid, cascara, formaldehyde, phenothiazines, procaine, acetazolamide, sodium bicarbonate, and sulfonamides may cause increased levels.

➤ Extremely alkaline urine may cause elevated urobilinogen levels.

➤ Extremely acidic urine may depress urobilinogen levels.

➤ Bananas and high-carbohydrate meals eaten within 48 hours of test may cause elevated levels.

➤ Chloramphenicol, neomycin, ammonium chloride, and ascorbic acid may decrease urobilinogen levels.

➤ Failure to use a preservative for a 24-hour collection.

➤ Consumption of wine containing nitrates may result in false negative findings.

NURSING CONSIDERATIONS

Prepare Your Client

➤ Inform client and family that this test is to help diagnose a problem with red blood cells or the liver.

➤ Tell client not to eat bananas for 48 hours prior to testing. Instruct them also to avoid meals high in carbohydrates for 24 hours before venous sampling.

➤ For the urine test, explain that you will need either a random urine, a 2-hour specimen, or a 24-hour specimen. For more accurate testing, the 2-hour specimen is obtained between noon and 4 P.M. when urine levels will be the highest.

Perform Procedure

➤ Collect as required a random or a 2-hour specimen in a clean, dry container. For a 2-hour specimen have client void and discard this urine, then collect all urine, protecting it from light, during the following 2-hour period. Have the client void at the end of the time period and include this urine in the collection.

➤ Collect urine for 24 hours if ordered, protecting it from light.

➤ Send specimen to laboratory immediately. Test must be performed within 30 minutes. Urobilinogen is very unstable at room temperature and when exposed to fluorescent lighting. Protect container from light.

➤ Urobilinogen levels may also be quantified with commercial reagent strips. Follow directions carefully when using these products.

➤ For fecal study, collect a random stool sample. Keep specimen protected from light to prevent the breakdown of urobilinogen to urobilin.

➤ Send specimen to lab immediately. If testing cannot be performed within 30 minutes, specimen should be refrigerated.

Care After Test

➤ Assess client for unusual bruising or prolonged bleeding from venipuncture site. Delayed clotting is a complication of severely impaired liver function.

➤ Assess skin, sclera of eyes for jaundice and note findings.

➤ Consult with a registered dietician to design a high-calorie, well-balanced diet. People with advanced liver disease have poor absorption of nutrients due to decreased bile flow into the intestines. As appropriate, reduce sodium or protein in the diet if edema and ascites, or increased ammonia levels are present.

➤ Evaluate other liver function tests such as aspartate aminotransferase (AST), alanine aminotransferase (ALT), direct and indirect bilirubin levels, alkaline phosphatase, serum ammonia, and prothrombin time. Also evaluate hemopoietic tests including the red blood cell (RBC) count, RBC indices, hematocrit, and hemoglobin.

Educate Your Client and the Family

➤ Instruct the client and family to report any jaundice—yellow discoloration of skin or whites of eyes.

➤ As appropriate, instruct client and family on a high-calorie, well-balanced diet. If sodium restrictions or protein restrictions are indicated, assist client and family to choose dietary selections with these limitations.

➤ People with impaired liver function have prolonged bleeding times. Instruct the client and family on safety measures such as electric razors, non-skid shoes, and soft toothbrushes.

➤ Instruct the client and family to report prolonged or unusual bleeding or bruising. Also report very dark-colored or tarry stools, because esophageal varices are a complication of liver disease.

Urogenital Secretions, Examination for Trichomonads

yur oe jen ih tahl • se kree shuns • eg zam ih nay shun • for • tri ko moe nads (*Trichomonas*)

Normal Findings
Negative, no *Trichomonas* identified

What This Test Will Tell You
This microscopic analysis of urine or secretions detects trichomoniasis, a sexually transmitted infection of the genitourinary tract. It is transmitted by direct contact with vaginal and urethral fluids of infected individuals. *Trichomonas* infection causes foamy yellow drainage, petechiae, vaginal burning, and itching in females. It causes a white urethral discharge or no symptoms in males.

Abnormal Findings
Positive results for *Trichomonas* may reveal trichomoniasis.

Interfering Factors
➤ Improper collection technique may interfere with the detection of *Trichomonas*.
➤ Collection of the specimen after therapy begins decreases the parasites in the specimen.
➤ Failure to send the specimen to the laboratory immediately causes decreased motility of trichomonads.

NURSING CONSIDERATIONS

Prepare Your Client
➤ Explain that this test is to determine the cause of a urogenital infection.
➤ Explain that the test will be performed by a physician or advanced practice nurse.
➤ Tell the female client that the test requires a specimen of vaginal secretions, urethral discharge, or urine. The only discomfort for the female will be the speculum insertion.
➤ Instruct the female client not to douche before the test.
➤ Instruct the male client that the test requires a specimen of urethral or prostatic secretions or urine. Some discomfort may be experienced as the swab touches the urethral opening.

Perform Procedure
Nurses do not usually perform this procedure, but should understand it to prepare the client and assist with the process.

Vaginal: Assist the female into lithotomy position. An unlubricated vaginal speculum is inserted and the specimen is collected with a cotton-tipped applicator. Place the applicator in the tube with normal saline.

Urethral: Insert the end of a cotton-tipped sterile applicator into the male or female urethral meatus. Rotate the swab and hold in place for 10 seconds to collect secretions. Transfer applicator to the tube of saline.

Male prostatic specimen: Instruct the male client to produce ejaculation via masturbation, and give him a clean container to collect semen. If unable to do this, the client may collect ejaculate at home in a condom. Instruct the client to bring the specimen to the laboratory in a clean covered container within 1 hour.

U

Urine specimen: Instruct the male or female to cleanse the urethral opening with soap and water and then rinse and dry the area. Give them a clean container with cover and indicate how full it must be to contain at least 20 mL of urine. Tell them to urinate into the container and then cover the container.

Send all specimens to the laboratory immediately.

Care After Test

➤ Assess client for presence of frothy discharge, painful urination, itching, and odor.

Educate Your Client and the Family

➤ Instruct the client with positive results to notify their sexual partner(s) to be tested.

➤ Educate client on the use of condoms.

➤ Teach client that finishing all perscribed medications is essential to resolving the infection.

➤ Teach the client that infected sexual partners need to be treated in order to prevent the client from becoming reinfected.

➤ Provide guidelines on retesting or finishing medication before having intercourse again.

Vanillylmandelic Acid

vah **nil** il man **del** ik • **ass** id

(VMA, Urine Catecholamines, Epinephrine, Norepinephrine, Metanephrine, Normetanephrine, Dopamine)

Normal Findings

VMA

Adult, pregnant, and elderly: 2–7 mg/24 hours (SI units: 10–35 µmol/24 hours)

Newborn: <1.0 mg/24 hours (SI units: <5 µmol/24 hours)

Infant: <2.0 mg/24 hours (SI units: <10 µmol/24 hours)

Child: <4.0 mg/24 hours (SI units: <20 µmol/24 hours)

Adolescent: 1–5 mg/24 hours (SI units: 5–25 µmol/24 hours)

CATECHOLAMINES

Epinephrine 0–20 µg/24 hours (SI units: 0–81.9 µmol/24 hours)

Norepinephrine 0–100 µg/24 hours (SI units: 0–591 µmol/24 hours)

Metanephrine 25–96 µg/24 hours (SI units: 1.3–4.1 µmol/24 hours)

Dopamine 65–400 µg/24 hours (SI units: 424–2612 µmol/24 hours)

What This Test Will Tell You

This 24-hour urine test diagnoses and monitors hypertension secondary to catecholamine-secreting tumors such as pheochromocytoma. Urine VMA levels measure the amount of vanillylmandelic acid (VMA), a metabolite of epinephrine and norepinephrine, in a 24-hour urine specimen. VMA levels reflect endogenous production of epinephrine and norepinephrine, major catecholamines in the body. This test helps detect catecholamine-secreting tumors and helps evaluate the function of the adrenal medulla, the primary site of catecholamine production.

An analysis of more than one catecholamine metabolite is usually performed, because not every client with a catecholamine-producing tumor will have elevated levels of VMA. Total catecholamine levels in a 24-hour urine collection may be measured, as may individual catecholamines such as epinephrine, norepinephrine, and dopamine and catecholamine metabolites such as metanephrine, normetanephrine, and homovanillic acid (HVA), a metabolite of dopamine. The laboratory test for VMA is easier to do than the other urine tests for catecholamines. However, because many foods and drugs cause false positive VMA results, other tests are often performed as the screening procedure. Serum tests for catecholamines may also be performed to aid in the diagnosis.

Abnormal Findings

▲INCREASED LEVELS may indicate pheochromocytoma, neuroblastoma, ganglioneuroma, ganglioblastoma, multiple endocrine neoplasia, severe stress or anxiety, or strenuous exercise.

ACTION ALERT!

Excessively high levels of VMA may indicate pheochromocytoma, a catecholamine-secreting tumor that causes dangerously high blood pressure. Carefully monitor systemic blood pressure and report elevations promptly to the primary health care provider.

Interfering Factors

➤ Increased levels of VMA may be caused by certain foods containing phenolic acid ingested up to 3 days prior to the test, including coffee, tea, anything containing vanilla, chocolate, fruits (especially bananas), avocados, cheese, cider vinegar, gelatin foods, salad dressing, carbonated drinks except ginger ale, jelly and jam, candy and mints, cough drops, chewing gum, and foods containing artificial flavoring, coloring, or licorice. However, newer laboratory methods are not affected by food intake.

➤ Drugs that may alter catecholamine levels are ampicillin, chloral hydrate, epinephrine, hydralazine, methyldopa, nicotine, tetracycline, and vitamin B complex.

➤ Prolonged fasting can alter both VMA and catecholamine levels.

➤ Stress, fever, and anxiety can elevate both VMA and catecholamine levels.

➤ Fasting or starvation increases VMA levels.

➤ Many drugs will cause increased VMA levels, including caffeine, insulin, epinephrine, levodopa, lithium, nitroglycerin, salicylates, sulfonamides, aminophylline, penicillin, chlorpromazine, isoproterenol, clyteryl guaiacolate, methenamine, quinidine, and methocarbamol.

➤ Drugs that may cause decreased VMA levels include antihypertensives, reserpine, chlorpromazine, monoamine oxidase (MAO) inhibitors, clonidine, salicylic acid, disulfiram (Antabuse), guanethidine, reserpine, levodopa, salicylates, and imipramine.

➤ Failure to adhere to dietary or drug restrictions may interfere with test results.

➤ Vigorous exercise or stress can cause increased VMA levels.

➤ Falsely decreased levels may be associated with alkaline urine, uremia, or radiographic contrast agents.

➤ Improper specimen collection and storage may alter test results.

Potential Complications

➤ Withholding medications prior to the test in order to obtain accurate results may result in loss of symptom control achieved with that drug, especially hypertension.

NURSING CONSIDERATIONS

Prepare Your Client

➤ Explain that this test is to measure the amount of certain hormones present in the urine that can be related to high blood pressure.

➤ Instruct the client to restrict foods and beverages containing phenolic acid. Provide a complete list of these foods and inform the client the restrictions must take place for 48 hours prior to the test and during the collection period. Check with the individual laboratory to determine specific restrictions.

➤ Tell the client to avoid vigorous physical exercise and stressful situations during the collection period. Encourage rest and adequate food and fluids.

➤ Explain the 24-hour urine collection procedure to the client.

Perform Procedure

➤ Obtain a clean, 3-L container with hydrochloric acid (HCl) or acetic acid preservative.

➤ Follow the procedure for collecting a 24-hour urine sample.

➤ Keep the specimen refrigerated or on ice during the collection period.

➤ Empty a Foley catheter bag hourly

into the collection container, if the client has an indwelling catheter.

➤ Encourage the client to drink fluids during the 24 hours, unless contraindicated.

➤ Encourage rest and decrease stress and anxiety during the test to minimize increased secretion of epinephrine and norepinephrine, which may interfere with obtaining accurate results.

➤ Maintain food and fluid restrictions and withhold drugs as ordered during the collection period.

➤ Observe the client closely for symptoms related to withdrawal of prescribed medications.

➤ Transport the urine specimen promptly to the laboratory after the 24-hour period.

Care After Test

➤ Resume administration of medications withheld before the test.

➤ Allow the client to resume their normal diet and activity.

➤ Observe the client for symptoms of excess catecholamines by closely monitoring for hypertension, tachycardia, palpitations, headache, and feelings of anxiety or nervousness.

➤ Evaluate related tests such as other catecholamines and their metabolites in the urine or serum, and x-ray, computed tomography scans, or ultrasound studies.

Educate Your Client and the Family

➤ Teach the client with suspected or confirmed pheochromocytoma about drug therapy, specifically alpha-blocking agents, and the need for surgery as definitive treatment for the tumor.

➤ Inform family members of client with confirmed pheochromocytoma that they need to be evaluated as well.

Venography of the Legs

vee nah grah fee • uv • the • legs
(Venogram)

Normal Findings

All ages: Normal anatomical structure, and normal and patent veins

What This Test Will Tell You

This radiographic test diagnoses venous occlusive disease as well as anatomical abnormalities of veins, most commonly in the legs. The study is performed by inserting a venous catheter into a vein in the foot under fluoroscopy. Once the catheter is placed, contrast material is injected and motion films are taken to record the flow of contrast (dye) through the venous system. The structure of the venous system can be visualized and occlusive areas identified.

Abnormal Findings

Abnormalities may indicate venous thrombosis or partial or complete venous occlusion.

Interfering Factors

➤ Lack of client cooperation

Contraindications

➤ Allergy to contrast material, unless test is modified

➤ Renal insufficiency or renal failure, because contrast material is excreted through the kidneys
➤ Pregnancy, due to radiation exposure of the fetus

Potential Complications
➤ Allergic reactions including anaphylaxis
➤ Hemorrhage
➤ Vasospasm
➤ Thrombus or embolus resulting in vascular occlusion in the extremity
➤ Embolus of blood clot or atherosclerotic plaque to other body areas
➤ Infection
➤ Renal failure

NURSING CONSIDERATIONS
Prepare Your Client
➤ Explain to the client and family that this test is used primarily to detect blood clots in the veins, those blood vessels that return blood to the heart.
➤ Ensure that an informed consent is obtained, because of the possible complications associated with this procedure.
➤ Explain that once the needles are inserted, the procedure itself is painless, but there may be some feelings of warmth from the contrast medium.
➤ Check the chart to be sure the client has no allergy to contrast material, shellfish, or iodine.
➤ Explain the procedure to the client and family.
➤ Record baseline vital signs.
➤ Restrict food and fluids (NPO) for at least 4–8 hours preceding the venography.
➤ Check with the primary health care provider to determine if medications should be administered while the client is NPO.

➤ Administer sedatives or tranquilizers as ordered before the procedure, especially for client who is anticipated to have difficulty lying still.
➤ Confirm that adults and older children have voided before the procedure.
➤ Do not remove glasses, dentures, or hearing aids unless dictated by your hospital policy. The client may need these in order to communicate and cooperate during the procedure.

Perform Procedure
Nurses do not perform this procedure, but should understand the process to prepare the client and assist the physician. Monitor vital signs throughout the procedure. Access to a superficial vein in the foot is accomplished by percutaneous or cutdown access. Before contrast material is injected into the vein, alert the client that a warm, flushed feeling may be experienced. X-ray pictures are taken of the flow of contrast material during injection. Observe the client immediately for any signs or symptoms of allergic reaction. If the intravenous line is removed in the laboratory, apply pressure and dress the wound.

Care After Test
➤ Monitor vital signs closely.
➤ Assess the venous puncture site(s) carefully for bleeding and hematoma.
➤ Assess for a positive Homan's sign, as well as other signs of venous occlusion such as edema and discoloration of the affected extremity.
➤ Observe for signs of allergic reaction to the contrast material, which include urticaria, pruritus, conjunctivitis, dyspnea, and apprehension.
➤ Evaluate for signs of systemic infection including elevated temper-

ature and chills, as well as local infection at the venipuncture site.

➤ Encourage fluids, due to the diuretic effect of the contrast material.

➤ Evaluate very young and older clients for signs of renal dysfunction related to the contrast material.

➤ If venous circulation is compromised by thrombus formation, consult with the primary health care provider about the level of activity and need for bed rest.

➤ Evaluate related tests such as Doppler studies and clotting studies.

Educate Your Client and the Family

➤ Explain to the client and family that the only pain that should be felt is when the needle is placed into a vein in the foot.

➤ Teach the client to inspect the feet daily, to wear comfortable shoes, and to elevate legs whenever possible.

Ventriculography
ven **trik** yu **log** rah fee
(Ventriculogram)

Normal Findings
Normal structure of ventricular system

What This Test Will Tell You
This radiographic test diagnoses tumors and abnormal structure of the brain ventricles. The ventricles are four interconnected chambers within the brain that have a specialized structure, the choroid plexus, that secretes cerebrospinal fluid (CSF). This is a very invasive test that must be performed by injecting air or contrast media through burr holes drilled into the skull. Computed tomography (CT) scan and magnetic resonance imaging (MRI) have largely replaced this test, which should only be performed when no other testing options exist. Ventriculography is still used for detecting small tumors in the ventricles or suprasellar region.

Abnormal Findings
Abnormalities may indicate ventric-

ular tumors, suprasellar tumors, or hydrocephalus.

ACTION ALERT!

Assess client carefully for allergic reaction to contrast material including dyspnea, itching, urticaria, flushing, hypotension, and shock. Life threatening anaphylactic reactions can occur and need to be recognized and treated immediately.

Interfering Factors

➤ Movement of the client during radiography will result in shadowed or unclear images.

➤ The client needs to remove metal objects such as hairpins, dental bridges, or glasses that will obstruct visualization of ventricles of the brain.

Contraindications

➤ X-rays are discouraged during the first trimester of pregnancy. If x-rays are necessary, the woman should wear a lead apron.

➤ Allergy to contrast media, unless

modifications in the testing procedure are made. Antihistamines or steroids may be given several days before the procedure and/or during the procedure.

➤ Infection at or near the insertion site.

➤ Increased intracranial pressure.

Potential Complications

➤ Allergic reaction to the contrast media

➤ Meningitis

➤ Brain herniation

➤ Headache

NURSING CONSIDERATIONS

Prepare Your Client

➤ Explain that this test is performed to diagnose abnormalities of the brain that can't be found by x-ray and other imaging tests.

➤ Restrict food and fluid for at least 6–8 hours before the test is performed.

➤ Tell the client there is no need to restrict medications before the exam.

➤ Ensure that an informed consent is obtained, because of the possible complications associated with this procedure.

Perform Procedure

Nurses do not perform the procedure, but should understand the process to explain it to the client. Either general or local anesthetic may be used. The scalp area where the needle will be inserted needs to be shaved.

The client is positioned in a chair. Small burr holes are made through the skull to allow the physician to place a needle into the ventricles of the brain. Air or contrast material is injected into the ventricles after cerebrospinal fluid is removed, in order to visualize structures by x-ray. The radiographic pictures are taken from several directions in order to visualize all the ventricles. The wounds are sutured closed as needed and covered with a sterile dressing.

Care After Test

➤ Assess the client for delayed allergic reaction to the contrast media such as skin rash, itching, headache, and vomiting. An oral antihistamine may be given for mild reactions.

➤ Observe dressings for bleeding or leakage of CSF.

➤ Assess for signs and symptoms of increased intracranial pressure such as seizures, headache, changes in vital signs, and decreased level of consciousness.

➤ Implement headache relief measures including ice packs, dim and quiet environment, and analgesics as ordered.

➤ Assess for nuchal rigidity.

➤ Encourage drinking fluids to prevent dehydration resulting from the diuretic effect of the contrast media.

➤ Elevate the head of the bed less than 20 degrees for the first 24 hours.

➤ Review related tests such as CSF analysis, computed tomography, magnetic resonance imaging, brain scan, cerebral angiography, and electroencephalography.

Educate Your Client and the Family

➤ Assist the parents of children with hydrocephalus to locate community resources.

➤ Provide psychosocial, spiritual, and emotional support to the client and family with a diagnosis of brain tumor.

➤ Teach client and family ways to compensate for any motor or sensory losses.

Von Willebrand Antigen, Plasma

von • wil eh **brand** • an ti jen • plaz mah

(Von Willebrand Factor, VIIIR:Ag, vW Antigen, vWF ag, Factor VIII R:Ag, Factor VIII Related Antigen)

Normal Findings

ALL AGES
45%–185% of control sample
PREGNANT
Values tend to increase with pregnancy.

What This Test Will Tell You

This blood test differentiates between classic hemophilia (hemophilia A) and von Willebrand's disease when bleeding times are inconclusive. Von Willebrand's disease is a genetically transmitted disease that results in both a deficiency in Factor VIII and a decrease in adhesiveness of platelets. These put the client at risk for bleeding, with prolonged coagulation and bleeding times. Von Willebrand factor functions in hemostasis and acts as a carrier for the portion of the Factor VIII compound that is responsible for coagulation.

Abnormal Findings

▲INCREASED LEVELS may indicate neoplastic disorders, hepatic damage, renal disease, thrombosis, myocardial infarction, oral contraceptive use, exercise, or stress.
▼DECREASED LEVELS may indicate hereditary or acquired von Willebrand's hemophilia.

Interfering Factors

➤ Hemolysis of the blood sample will invalidate the results.
➤ Contamination with tissue thromboplastin will invalidate the results.
➤ Use of oral contraceptives, exercise, or stress may increase levels.

Potential Complications

➤ Prolonged bleeding at the venipuncture site

NURSING CONSIDERATIONS

Prepare Your Client

➤ Explain that this test is used to assess the blood's ability to clot.

Perform Procedure

➤ Perform a venipuncture and withdraw 2 mL of venous blood and discard if your laboratory requires. Without removing the needle, withdraw 7 mL of venous blood and fill a blue-top tube. Gently rotate and invert the tube several times to thoroughly mix the blood with the anticoagulant.
➤ Apply pressure or a pressure dressing to the venipuncture site.

Care After Test

➤ Hold pressure at the venipuncture site for 5 minutes to prevent hematoma formation. Assess client for unusual bruising or prolonged bleeding from venipuncture site. Delayed clotting is a complication of severely impaired clotting.
➤ Test all body secretions including stool, gastrointestinal aspirate, and tracheal aspirate for occult blood. Closely inspect mucous membranes for bleeding.
➤ Review related tests such as complete blood count, bone marrow biopsy, direct Coombs' (antiglobulin) test, serum protein electrophoresis, clot retraction, bleeding time,

prothrombin consumption test, platelet aggregation, platelet survival, hemoglobin and hematocrit, and platelet count.

Educate Your Client and the Family

➤ Teach the client and family members about bleeding precautions including using a soft-bristled toothbrush, using electric razors rather than straight razors, avoiding constipation, avoiding picking their nose, and avoiding constricting clothing. If menses is experienced, the client should maintain a pad count and note the saturation of each pad.

➤ Teach the client and family members the signs and symptoms of bleeding including petechiae (small purplish spots on the skin), bruising, blood in urine and stool, vaginal bleeding, and bleeding from invasive lines.

➤ Teach the client to avoid over-the-counter aspirin and aspirin-containing drugs, phenothiazines, codeine, non-steroidal anti-inflammatory drugs, and alcohol.

White Blood Cell with Differential Count
white · blud · sel · with · dif ur en shul · kownt
(WBC with Diff, CBC with Diff, Differential Leukocyte Count)

Normal Findings

ADULT

Total WBC: 4,000–10,000/mm³

Neutrophils 50%–70%: 2,000–8,400/mm³

Eosinophils 1%–4%: 200/mm³

Lymphocytes 20%–40%: 2,500/mm³

Monocytes 2%–8%: 300/mm³

Basophils 0.3%–1%: 10/mm³

Bands (stabs) 8%: 620/mm³

PREGNANT

Total WBC: Slight increases seen during pregnancy

Neutrophils: Slight increases seen during the third trimester of pregnancy

Eosinophils 1%–4%: 200/mm³

Lymphocytes 20%–40%: 2,500/mm³

Monocytes 2%–8%: 300/mm³

Basophils: Slight decreases seen during pregnancy

Bands (stabs) 8%: 620/mm³

NEWBORN

Total WBC: 9,000–30,000/mm³

Neutrophils 47%: 8,870/mm³

Eosinophils 2.4%: 450/mm³

Lymphocytes 31%: 5,800/mm³

Monocytes 5.8%: 1,100/mm³

Basophils 0.5%: 100/mm³

Bands (stabs) 14.2%: 2,680/mm³

CHILD (UNDER 3)

Total WBC: 6,000–17,000/mm³

Neutrophils 25%–45%: 2,650/mm³

Eosinophils 2.6%: 200–250/mm³

Lymphocytes 40%–60%: 6,300/mm³

Monocytes 4.2%–5%: 350–650/mm³

Basophils 0.6%: 50/mm³

Bands (stabs) 8%: 850–1,150/mm³

ADOLESCENT

Total WBC: 4,000–10,000/mm³

Neutrophils 38%–77%: 3,800/mm³

Eosinophils 0.8%–8.5%: 200/mm³

Lymphocytes 16%–52%: 2,700/mm³

Monocytes 0.9%–11.6%: 350–400/mm³

Basophils 0.25%–1.4%: 40/mm³

Bands (stabs) 8%: 620–640/mm³

ELDERLY

Values are within same range as for a normal adult but may trend toward lower normal limits. This is secondary to physiologic slowing of bone marrow activity in the elderly.

What This Test Will Tell You

This blood test evaluates a number of conditions and differentiates causes of alterations in the total white blood cell (WBC) count including inflammation, infection, tissue necrosis, and or leukemic neoplasia. The differential white cell count identifies the five specific types of white blood cells present in the blood. The presence of these cells is expressed most accurately in percentages (based upon a 100-cell sample) but may also be expressed in numbers of cells per cubic millimeter of blood. These five cell types reflect the integrity of the client's immune system.

Abnormal Findings

▲INCREASED *total white blood cell count (leukocytosis)* may indicate infection, inflammation, trauma, tissue necrosis, stress, leukemia neoplasia, hemorrhage, trauma, malignancies (particularly gastrointestinal, liver, bone, and metastasis), toxins, or serum sickness.

▼DECREASED *total white blood cell count (leukopenia)* may indicate autoimmune disease, bone marrow failure or depression, overwhelming infection, dietary deficiency, or drug toxicity.

▲ INCREASED *neutrophil count* may indicate bacterial infection including osteomyelitis, septicemia, otitis media, gonorrhea, salpingitis, endocarditis, or pneumonia; parasitic infection; tissue necrosis including burns, myocardial infarction, or carcinoma; metabolic disorder including eclampsia, thyrotoxicosis, uremia, or diabetic acidosis; or inflammatory disorder including rheumatic fever, rheumatoid arthritis, trauma, Cushing's disease, myositis, vasculitis, or acute gout.

▲ INCREASED *numbers of bands (stabs)*, which are immature neutrophils, is associated with disorders of cell production and bone marrow depression and response to infection.

▼ DECREASED *neutrophil count* may indicate infection including typhoid, brucellosis, hepatitis, influenza, measles, rubella, mononucleosis, or tularemia; bone marrow depression secondary to radiation or myelotoxic medications; deficiency of folic acid; systemic lupus erythematosus; lymphoblastic leukemia; aplastic anemia; or pernicious anemia.

▲ INCREASED *eosinophil count* may indicate allergic response including asthma, hay fever, food allergy, medication allergy, or serum sickness; parasitic infection including hookworm, roundworm, amebiasis, or trichinosis; skin disorder including eczema, pemphigus, psoriasis, or shingles; neoplastic disorder including Hodgkin's disease, chronic myelocytic leukemia, necrosis of solid tumors, lung cancer, or bone cancer; ulcerative colitis; polyarteritis nodosa; pernicious anemia; scarlet fever; strenuous/excessive exercise; autoimmune disease; or a splenectomy.

▼ DECREASED *eosinophil count* may indicate Cushing's syndrome; stress response associated with trauma, burns, shock, surgery; congestive heart failure; aplastic anemia; or pernicious anemia.

▲ INCREASED *basophil count* may indicate chronic myelocytic leukemia, polycythemia vera, Hodgkin's disease, myxedema, ulcerative colitis, nephrosis, or a chronic hemolytic anemia.

▼ DECREASED *basophil count* may indicate hyperthyroidism, pregnancy, stress response, ovulation, anaphylactic reactions, or steroid therapy.

▲ INCREASED *lymphocyte count* may indicate viral infection including tuberculosis, hepatitis, mumps, pertussis, syphilis, rubella, mononucleosis, cytomegalovirus, or other viral illnesses; lymphocytic leukemia; ulcerative colitis; hypoadrenalism; thyrotoxicosis; chronic bacterial infection; or an immune disease.

▼ DECREASED *lymphocyte count* may indicate defective lymphatic circulation; immunodeficiency secondary to immunosuppressive therapy; high levels of adrenal corticosteroids; chronic debilitating conditions such as congestive heart failure, renal failure, or advanced tuberculosis; lupus erythematosus; leukemia; human immunodeficiency virus (HIV); radiation treatment; Hodgkin's disease; or burns.

▲ INCREASED *monocyte count* may indicate infection such as tuberculosis, hepatitis, malaria, Rocky Mountain spotted fever, or subacute bacterial endocarditis; systemic lupus erythematosus; rheumatoid arthritis; polyarteritis nodosa; monocytic leukemia; lymphomas; chronic ulcerative colitis; or other carcinoma.

▼DECREASED *monocyte count* does not have clinical significance related to disease; it may indicate positive response to prednisone treatment.

███████ ACTION ALERT!

Total WBC < 2,500 or > 30,000/mm³. Leukopenia of <2,500/mm³ indicates bone marrow depression and may reflect results of viral infection, cancer chemotherapies, exposure to toxins, mononucleosis, measles, rubella, typhoid fever, and hepatitis A. Interventions depend on the cause of the alteration of white cells, and the specific white cells affected. Take immediate steps to prevent infection (reverse isolation, no fresh fruits, no fresh flowers, etc.).

Interfering Factors

➤ Hemolysis of the sample due to rough handling during collection and transport will affect test results.

➤ Failure to use the correct anticoagulant in the collection tube or to mix the sample with the anticoagulant adequately will adversely affect the test results.

➤ Pregnancy, particularly during the last trimester, will cause an increase in neutrophils and total WBCs. A reduction in basophils is also noted during pregnancy.

➤ Methysergide and desipramine may produce either increases or decreases in the eosinophil count.

➤ Individuals who have had a splenectomy will demonstrate a mild elevation of WBC counts.

➤ Indomethacin and procainamide may produce a lowered eosinophil level.

➤ Cigarette smoking.

➤ Adrenocorticotropic hormone (ACTH) therapy may cause elevated counts in the absence of infection, but mask leukocytosis with infections.

➤ Any medication or substance that stimulates an allergic response will produce an increase in eosinophil.

➤ Medications that may increase total WBC counts include heparin, steroids, chloroform, epinephrine, allopurinol, adrenaline, and triamterene.

➤ Lowered total WBC levels may occur with administration of anticonvulsants, antihistamines, antimetabolites, antithyroid drugs, barbiturates, steroids, diuretics, sulfonamides, and antibiotics.

NURSING CONSIDERATIONS

Prepare Your Client

➤ Explain to your client that this test helps to assess the body's ability to fight infection, to tell the difference between an infection and an allergy, or to find problems with the way bone marrow makes blood cells.

➤ Instruct your client to avoid strenuous physical activity for 24 hours prior to testing, if possible.

Perform Procedure

➤ Collect 7 mL of venous blood in a lavender-top tube.

➤ Gently invert the collection tube several times immediately after collection to mix the sample with the anticoagulant in the tube.

Care After Test

➤ If WBC differential indicates an infection, assess client responses to antimicrobials. Interventions will include assessment of vital signs, focused physical assessment of body systems affected, administration and maintenance of fluids, monitoring intake and output, and assistance with activities of daily living as required.

➤ If WBC differential indicates an allergic or inflammatory response, monitor the client's response to therapies. Inflammatory responses may worsen or involve more than one body system. Monitor the client for worsening of the inflammatory condition, particularly respiratory compromise.

➤ If WBC differential indicates the presence of tissue necrosis, identify the body system involved (such as myocardial infarction). Plan nursing care to provide for limitations in activity tolerance, alterations in comfort, and increased nutritional requirements. Monitor your client's progress during the recovery phase.

➤ If the WBC differential indicates depressed bone marrow function, monitor your client for evidence of infection. Protect your client from exposure to potential sources of transmission of infection. Plan care to compensate for limitations in energy resulting from a possible anemia.

➤ Review related tests, such as hemoglobin, hematocrit, red blood cell count, red cell indices, and platelets.

Educate Your Client and the Family

➤ When decreased bone marrow activity is demonstrated on the WBC differential, instruct your client about the importance of obtaining immunizations that may provide some level of protection (pneumococcal vaccine, flu vaccine, hepatitis B vaccine). Also instruct the client and family about the importance of avoiding individuals with acute illnesses and upper respiratory infections. If the client lives with young children, it is important to maintain the immunization schedule of these children to prevent unnecessary exposure of the client to infections.

➤ Instruct the client and family in the plan of care when infection is identified. This may include the antimicrobials or other medications prescribed and how they are to be administered, requirements for fluid intake, comfort measures, management of temperature elevations, and nutritional needs.

➤ When an allergic or inflammatory condition is identified, explore possible interventions for prevention of recurrences with the client and family. If the substance to which the client is allergic can be identified, discuss methods of avoiding that substance. If a medication allergy is identified, instruct the client and family in communication tools such as a medical alert bracelet or necklace. Discuss management steps for allergic responses that can be taken at home prior to access to the health care system.

➤ Explain the similarities and differences in treatment and management of parasitic, viral, and bacterial illnesses to the client and family. Discuss routes of transmission to help the client and family identify means of limiting exposure of others.

WHITE BLOOD CELL DIFFERENTIAL

Neutrophils	Increased in:	Neutrophil count must always
	parasitic or bacterial infections, inflammatory diseases, ischemia processes.	be evaluated in relation to total WBC count. If neutrophil count is

Neutrophils, *continued*	Decreased in: bone marrow depression, pernicious anemia, acute lymphoblastic leukemia, and aplastic anemia.	significantly greater than overall WBCs, immune function may be poor or an overwhelming infection is present. A shift to the left means that there is a significant increase in numbers of bands.
Monocytes	Increased in: bacterial, viral and parasitic infections, collagen diseases, blood dyscrasias. Decreased: No significance.	Monocytes function as phagocytic scavengers to remove foreign material.
Lymphocytes	Increased in: bacterial and viral infections, immune diseases, lymphocytic leukemia, ulcerative colitis. Decreased in: immunodeficiency from immunosuppressive therapy, systemic lupus erythematosus, burns, elevated adrenal corticosteroid, poor lymphatic circulation, chronic debilitating conditions.	Primary cause for increase in lymphocytes is viral infection. Bacterial and parasitic infection may also cause increases.
Eosinophils	Increased in: allergic responses, such as asthma, hay fever, or food or drug reactions; parasitic infections; skin disorders; neoplastic disorders; and after a splenectomy. Decreased in: Cushing's syndrome, congestive heart failure, aplastic and pernicious anemia, stress response to severe illness.	Primarily influenced by antigen-antibody responses. Eosinophils demonstrate a diurnal rhythm: in most people, eosinophils are highest in the late evening and lowest in the early morning. This pattern is reversed in individuals who work nights or who are asthmatic.
Basophils	Increased in: chronic myelocytic leukemia, polycythemia vera, chronic hemolytic anemia, Hodgkin's disease, ulcerative colitis, myxedema. Decreased in: pregnancy, ovulation, anaphylactic reactions, hyperthyroidism, stress response, steroid therapy.	Basophil function not understood as well as other white cell types; basophils believed to be related to allergic and anaphylactic responses (basophil count decreases).

W

THERAPEUTIC DRUG MONITORING

DRUG	FREQUENCY FOR DRAWING LEVELS	THERAPEUTIC LEVEL	TOXIC LEVEL	TUBE[1]
ANTIDYSRHYTHMICS CLASS I				
disopyramide	trough level	2.0–5.0 µg/mL	≥8.0 µg/mL	red top
flecainide	peak collection after steady state has been reached	0.2–1 µg/mL	≥1.0 µg/mL	red top
lidocaine	collect 45 min after a bolus	1.5–5 µg/mL	>6.0 µg/mL (after MI) 2.0–6.0 µg/mL (non-MI)	red top
mexiletine	trough level	0.5–2.0 µg/mL	>2.0 µg/mL	red top
moricizine	—	0.1 µg/mL	—	—
phenytoin	trough level	10–20 µg/mL	>20 µg/mL	red top
procainamide	trough level	4–10 µg/mL	>10 µg/mL	red or green top
procainamide + NAPA	trough level	10–30 µg/mL	>30 µg/mL	red or green top

DRUG	FREQUENCY FOR DRAWING LEVELS	THERAPEUTIC LEVEL	TOXIC LEVEL	TUBE[1]
propafenone	—	0.2–3.0 µg/mL	—	—
quinidine	random	2.0–5.0 µg/mL	>7.0 µg/mL	red top
tocainide	—	6–12 µg/mL	>15 µg/mL	red top
ANTIDYSRHYTHMICS CLASS II				
acebutolol	serum concentration assays have not been useful in monitoring antiarrhythmic or toxic effects	—	—	—
esmolol	serum concentration assays have not been useful in monitoring antiarrhythmic or toxic effects	—	—	—
propranolol	trough level	0.01–0.34 µg/mL	>2 µg/mL	red top

1 Always check with the laboratory at your facility regarding current tube for blood collection.

THERAPEUTIC DRUG MONITORING (continued)

DRUG	FREQUENCY FOR DRAWING LEVELS	THERAPEUTIC LEVEL	TOXIC LEVEL	TUBE[1]
ANTIDYSRHYTHMICS CLASS III				
amiodarone	—	0.5–2.5 µg/mL SI: 0.8–3.9 µmol/L	>2.5 µg/mL >3.9 µmol/L	—
bretylium	—	0.04–0.9 µg/mL	not defined	—
ANTIDYSRHYTHMICS CLASS IV				
diltiazem	—	40–200 ng/mL	>200 ng/mL	—
nicardipine	—	30–50 ng/mL	—	—
nifedipine	—	25–100 ng/mL	>100 ng/mL	—
verapamil	—	0.125–0.40 µg/mL	90 µg/mL	red top

DRUG	FREQUENCY FOR DRAWING LEVELS	THERAPEUTIC LEVEL	TOXIC LEVEL	TUBE[1]
CARDIAC GLYCOSIDES				
digitoxin	draw 6–12 hours after administration of drug	10–30 ng/mL SI: 26–45 nmol/L	>30 ng/mL >59 nmol/L	red top
digoxin	collect 12 hours after dose	0.5–2.0 ng/mL SI: 1.0–2.6 nmol/L	>2.5 ng/mL >3.2 nmol/L	green top
TRICYCLICS		Steady state plasma levels are usually achieved in 1 to 4 weeks.		
amitriptyline	sample blood 10–15 hours after last drug intake			
	trough level	125–250 ng/mL SI: 430–900 nmol/L	>500 ng/mL >1800 nmol/L	royal blue or red top
nortriptyline	collect at steady state trough; collect >12 hours after dose	50–150 ng/mL	>500 ng/mL	royal blue or red top
amoxapine (transport specimen frozen)	sample blood 10–15 hours after last drug intake	200–500 ng/mL	>500 ng/mL	red top

THERAPEUTIC DRUG MONITORING (continued)

DRUG	FREQUENCY FOR DRAWING LEVELS	THERAPEUTIC LEVEL	TOXIC LEVEL	TUBE[1]
desipramine	for daily dosing: 10–14 hours after dose; for divided doses: 4–6 hours after last dose	75–300 ng/mL SI: 281–1125 nmol/L	>400 ng/mL >1500 nmol/L	orange-green top
doxepin	trough level: collect 12 hours after dose	30–250 ng/mL SI: 107–537 nmol/L	>500 ng/mL >1790 nmol/L	red top
imipramine	trough level: collect 12 hours after dose	100–300 ng/mL	>500 ng/mL	royal blue top (no heparin)
maprotiline	sample blood 10–15 hours after last drug intake	200–300 ng/mL	>500 ng/mL	—
protriptyline	trough level: collect 12 hours after dose	160–250 ng/mL SI: 266–950 nmol/L	>500 ng/mL >1900 nmol/L	—

DRUG	FREQUENCY FOR DRAWING LEVELS	THERAPEUTIC LEVEL	TOXIC LEVEL	TUBE[1]
ANTIBIOTICS				
amikacin	IV: draw peak 30 minutes after dose IM: draw peak 1–2 hours after dose	trough: 0–5 µg/mL	peak: >35 µg/mL	red top
chloramphenicol	trough level	10–20 µg/mL	>25 ng/mL	red top
gentamicin	peak and trough levels	peak: 5–10 µg/mL trough: <2–4 µg/mL	peak: >12 µg/mL trough: >2–4 µg/mL	red or green top
kanamycin (transport specimen on ice)	peak and trough levels	peak: 25–35 µg/L trough: 1–8 µg/L	peak: >35 µg/L trough: >10 µg/L	red top
netilmicin	peak and trough levels	peak: 5–10 µg/mL trough: <2–4 µg/mL	peak: >12 µg/mL trough: >2–4 µg/mL	—
streptomycin (transport specimen on ice)	—	peak: 4–8 µg/mL trough: <5 µg/mL	peak: 40 µg/mL trough: 40 µg/mL	red top

THERAPEUTIC DRUG MONITORING (continued)

DRUG	FREQUENCY FOR DRAWING LEVELS	THERAPEUTIC LEVEL	TOXIC LEVEL	TUBE[1]
tobramycin	peak and trough levels	peak: 5–10 µg/mL trough: <2–4 µg/mL	peak: >12 µg/mL trough: >2–4 µg/mL	red or green top
NON-STEROIDAL ANTIINFLAMMATORY				
acetaminophen	4 hours or 12 hours after drug ingestion	10–30 µg/mL	>200 µg/mL	red, green, or royal blue top
salicylic acid	trough level	<100 µg/mL	>150–300 µg/mL	red top
BRONCHODILATORS				
aminophylline	collect at steady state for continuous infusion; intermittent IV dose: peak level	10–20 µg/mL	>20 µg/mL	red or green top
theophylline	peak and trough level	10–20 µg/mL	>20 µg/mL	red or green top

DRUG	FREQUENCY FOR DRAWING LEVELS	THERAPEUTIC LEVEL	TOXIC LEVEL	TUBE[1]
ANTICONVULSANTS				
carbamazepine	trough level	multiple anticonvulsant therapy: 4–8 μg/mL; single agent therapy: 8–12 μg/mL	multiple anticonvulsant therapy: >8.0 μg/mL; single agent therapy: >12.0 μg/mL	red top
clonazepam	trough level	30–60 ng/mL	>70 ng/mL	red top
diazepam	trough level	0.2–2.0 μg/mL	>5–20 μg/mL	red or royal blue top
ethosuximide	trough level	25–100 μg/mL	>150 μg/mL	red top
magnesium sulfate	random	1.8–2.2 mg/dL	level increased or decreased from normal	green top
mephenytoin	—	15–30 μg/mL	>50 μg/mL	—
methsuximide	trough level	10–40 μg/mL	>40 μg/mL	—

▶

THERAPEUTIC DRUG MONITORING (continued)

DRUG	FREQUENCY FOR DRAWING LEVELS	THERAPEUTIC LEVEL	TOXIC LEVEL	TUBE[1]
paraldehyde	—	10–100 µg/mL for sedation; >200 µg/mL for anesthesia	200–400 µg/mL for sedation; >500 µg/mL for anesthesia	—
phensuximide	—	4–14 µg/mL	80–150 µg/mL	—
phenytoin	trough level	10–20 µg/mL	>20 µg/mL	red top
primidone	trough level	5–12 µg/mL	>15 µg/mL	red top
valproic acid	trough level	50–100 µg/mL	>100 µg/mL	red top
BARBITURATES				
amobarbital	—	1–5 µg/mL	10–30 µg/mL	red or lavender top (no heparin)

DRUG	FREQUENCY FOR DRAWING LEVELS	THERAPEUTIC LEVEL	TOXIC LEVEL	TUBE[1]
aprobarbital	—	—	—	red top
butabarbital	—	1–5 μg/mL	10–30 μg/mL	red top
pentobarbital	trough level	hypnotic: 1–5 μg/mL; therapeutic coma: 20–50 μg/mL	>10 μg/mL	red top
phenobarbital	trough level	15–40 μg/mL	>40 μg/mL	red top
secobarbital	—	3–5 μg/mL	>5 μg/mL	red top
talbutal	—	—	—	red top
thiopental	trough level	hypnotic: 1–5 μg/mL; therapeutic coma: 30–100 μg/mL; anesthesia: 7–130 μg/mL	>10 μg/mL	red top

➤

THERAPEUTIC DRUG MONITORING (continued)

DRUG	FREQUENCY FOR DRAWING LEVELS	THERAPEUTIC LEVEL	TOXIC LEVEL	TUBE[1]
IMMUNOSUPPRESSANT				
cyclosporine	random	kidney transplant: 75–300 ng/mL; heart, liver, or lung transplant: 150–300 µg/mL	—	lavender or green top
FK-506	weekly	unknown method at this time; new method is being designed	—	green top
ALCOHOL	random	none	>100 mg/dL (intoxication per National Safety Council)	red or green top
BENZODIAZEPINE				
chlordiazepoxide	trough level	1–3 µg/mL	>5 µg/mL	red top

DRUG	FREQUENCY FOR DRAWING LEVELS	THERAPEUTIC LEVEL	TOXIC LEVEL	TUBE[1]
clonazepam	trough level	0.005–0.012 ng/mL	—	red top
diazepam	trough level	0.1–1.0 µg/mL	>2 µg/mL	red or royal blue top
flurazepam[2]	—	none detected	>2000 ng/mL	red, black, or gray top
haloperidol	—	3–20 ng/mL	>50 ng/mL	green top
lorazepam	—	50–240 ng/mL	not defined	—
oxazepam	—	10–100 ng/mL	>200 ng/mL	—
prazepam	—	not defined	not defined	—
temazepam	—	not defined	not defined	—
triazolam	—	not defined	not defined	—

➤

THERAPEUTIC DRUG MONITORING (continued)

DRUG	FREQUENCY FOR DRAWING LEVELS	THERAPEUTIC LEVEL	TOXIC LEVEL	TUBE[1]
ANTIMANIC				
lithium	collect 30 minutes after bolus	0.5–1.3 mEq/L	>1.5 mEq/L	red top
ANTINEOPLASTIC				
fluorouracil[3]	plasma assays are available but are not routinely used in clinical practice	—	—	—
methotrexate (protect specimen from light)	collect 0.5–2 hours after low dose therapy; collect at 24 hours, 48 hours, and 72 hours after high-dose therapy	$>2 \times 10^{-7}$ M/L 48 hours postinfusion	—	red top

1 Always check with the laboratory at your facility regarding current tube for blood collection.
2 Desalkylflurazepam metabolite: 0–140 ng/mL; hydroxyethylflurazepam metabolite: 4–7 ng/mL.
3 Use of this drug may precipitate angina.

COMMON ADULT LABORATORY VALUES

Laboratory value	Conventional units	SI units
Albumin	3.2–5.0 g/dL	32–50 g/L
Bilirubin		
Total	0.1–1.0 mg/dL	5.1–17.0 μmol/L
Direct (conjugated)	0.1–0.3 mg/dL	1.7–5.1 μmol/L
Indirect (unconjugated)	0.2–0.8 mg/dL	3.4–12.0 μmol/L
Blood urea nitrogen	7–20 mg/dL	2.5–7.2 mmol/L
Calcium		
Total	8.5–10.5 mg/dL	1.98–2.44 mmol/L
Ionized	4.5–5.6 mg/dL	1.05–1.30 mmol/L
Chloride	95–110 mEq/L	95–110 mmol/L
CO_2 content	22–30 mEq/L	22–30 mmol/L
Creatinine		
Male	0.6–1.5 mg/dL	53–132 μmol/L
Female	0.5–1.1 mg/dL	44–97 μmol/L
Erythrocyte (RBC) count		
Female	4.2–5.4 million/mm^3	$4.2–5.4 \times 10^{12}$/L
Male	4.5–6.2 million/mm^3	$4.5–6.2 \times 10^{12}$/L
Glucose (fasting)	80–140 mg/dL	4.4–7.7 mmol/L
Hematocrit		
Male	39%–49%	0.39–0.49
Female	33%–43%	0.33–0.43
Hemoglobin		
Male	10–17 g/dL	6.2–10.5 mmol/L
Female	11.5–15.5 g/dL	7.1–9.6 mmol/L
Leukocyte (WBC) count	3100–9000/mm^3	$3.1–9.0 \times 10^9$/L
Magnesium	1.2–1.9 mEq/L	0.50–0.78 mmol/L
Partial thromboplastin time	60–70 seconds	
Phosphorus	2.7–4.5 mg/dL	0.87–1.45 mmol/L
Platelet count	130,000–450,000/mm^3	$130–450 \times 10^9$/L
Potassium	3.5–5.1 mEq/L	3.5–5.1 mmol/L
Prothrombin time	11–14 seconds	85%–100%
Sodium	138–145 mEq/L	138–145 mmol/L

COMMON PEDIATRIC LABORATORY VALUES

Laboratory Value	Conventional Units	SI units
Albumin	4.0–5.9 g/dL	40–59 g/L
Bilirubin		
Total	0.1–1.0 mg/dL	5.1–17.0 μmol/L
Direct (conjugated)	0.1–0.3 mg/dL	1.7–5.1 μmol/L
Indirect		
(unconjugated)	0.2–0.8 mg/dL	3.4–12.0 μmol/L
Blood urea nitrogen	5–18 mg/dL	1.8–6.4 mmol/L
Calcium		
Total	8.8–10.8 mg/dL	2.2–2.7 mmol/L
Ionized	4.8–5.9 mg/dL	1.12–1.37 mmol/L
Chloride	98–105 mEq/L	98–105 mmol/L
CO_2 content	20–28 mEq/L	20–28 mmol/L
Creatinine	0.3–0.7 mg/dL	26–61 μmol/L
Erythrocyte (RBC) count	4.6–5.5 million/mm³(μL)	$4.4–7.1 \times 10^{12}$/L
Glucose (fasting)		
<24 months of age	60–100 mg/dL	3.3–5.5 mmol/L
24 months		
to adolescence	70–105 mg/dL	3.8–5.8 mmol/L
Hematocrit	31%–43%	0.31–0.43
Hemoglobin	11–16 g/dL	6.8–9.9 mmol/L
Leukocyte (WBC) count	6,000–17,000/mm³	$6.0–17.0 \times 10^9$/L
Magnesium		
5 months–6 years	1.4–1.9 mEq/L	0.58–0.78 mmol/L
6–12 years	1.4–1.7 mEq/L	0.58–0.70 mmol/L
12–20 years	1.4–1.8 mEq/L	0.58–0.74 mmol/L
Partial thromboplastin time	60–70 seconds	
Phosphorus	4.5–5.5 mg/dL	1.45–1.78 mmol/L
Platelet count	150,000–450,000/mm³	$150–450 \times 10^9$/L
Potassium	3.4–4.7 mEq/L	3.4–4.7 mmol/L
Prothrombin time	11–14 seconds	85%–100%
Sodium	138–145 mEq/L	138–145 mmol/L

COMMON GERIATRIC LABORATORY VALUES

Laboratory value	Conventional units	SI units
Albumin	3.2–5.0 g/dL	32–50 g/L
Bilirubin		
Total	0.1–1.0 mg/dL	5.1–17.0 μmol/L
Direct (conjugated)	0.1–0.3 mg/dL	1.7–5.1 μmol/L
Indirect (unconjugated)	0.2–0.8 mg/dL	3.4–12.0 μmol/L
Blood urea nitrogen	8–21 mg/dL	2.9–7.5 mmol/L
Calcium		
Total	8.5–10.5 mg/dL	1.98–2.44 mmol/L
Ionized	4.5–5.6 mg/dL	1.05–1.30 mmol/L
Chloride	95–110 mEq/L	95–110 mmol/L
CO_2 content	22–30 mEq/L	22–30 mmol/L
Creatinine	0.4–1.9 mg/dL	35–167 μmol/L
Erythrocyte (RBC) count		
Female	4.2–5.4 million/mm^3	4.2–5.4 × 10^{12}/L
Male	4.5–6.2 million/mm^3	4.5–6.2 × 10^{12}/L
Glucose (fasting)	52–135 mg/dL	2.9–7.4 mmol/L
Hematocrit		
Male	38%–54%	0.38–0.54
Female	35%–49%	0.35–0.49
Hemoglobin		
Male	10–17 g/dL	100–170 g/L
Female	11.5–15.5 g/dL	115–155 g/L
Leukocyte (WBC) count	3100–9000/mm^3	3.1–9.0 × 10^9/L
Magnesium	1.2–1.9 mEq/L	0.50–0.78 mmol/L
Partial thromboplastin time	60–70 seconds	
Phosphorus	2.7–4.5 mg/dL	0.87–1.45 mmol/L
Platelet count	130,000–450,000/mm^3	130–450 × 10^9/L
Potassium	3.5–5.1 mEq/L	3.5–5.1 mmol/L
Prothrombin time	11–14 seconds	85%–100%
Sodium	138–145 mEq/L	138–145 mmol/L

SELECTED REFERENCES

Balows, A. (1991) *Manual of Clinical Microbiology*. Washington, D.C.: American Society for Microbiology.

Baum, G. L. and Wolinsky, E. (1989) *Textbook of Pulmonary Diseases*. Boston: Little, Brown & Co.

Beischer, N. A. and MacKay, E. V. (1986) *Obstetrics and the Newborn*. Philadelphia: W. B. Saunders Co.

Black, J. M., and Matassarin-Jacobs, E. (1993) *Luckmann's and Sorensen's Medical-Surgical Nursing: A Psychophysiologic Approach*. Philadelphia: W. B. Saunders Co.

Elta, G. H. (1991) Approach to the patient with gross gastrointestinal bleeding. In J. B. Lippincott Co., Philadelphia: *Textbook of Gastroenterology*, Vol. 1, edited by Tadataka Yamada.

Emanuelson, K. L. and Densmore, M. J. (1981) *Acute Respiratory Care*. New York: John Wiley & Sons.

Farley, D. R., and Donohue, J. H. (1992) Early gastric cancer. *Surgical Clinics of North America*, 72 (2): 401–421.

Finegold, S. M., and Baron, E. J. (1986) *Bailey and Scott's Diagnostic Microbiology*. St. Louis: C. V. Mosby Co.

Foster, R. R., Hunsberger, M. H. and Anderson, J. T. (1989) *Family-Centered Nursing Care of Children*. Philadelphia: W. B. Saunders Co.

GI Bleeding: The choices in endoscopic therapy. (1988) *Emergency Medicine* 20 (1): 88–107.

Harmon, R. G., Bagby, J. R., Donnell, H. D., and Malone, B. R. (1986) *Tuberculosis Control Manual*. Jefferson City MO: Missouri Department of Health.

Ignatavicius, D. D. and Bayne, M.V. (1991) *Medical-Surgical Nursing: A Nursing Process Approach*. Philadelphia: W. B. Saunders Co.

Kozier, B., Erb, G., Blaiser, K., and Wilkinson, J. M. (1995) *Fundamentals of Nursing*, 5th ed. Redwood City, CA: Addison-Wesley Nursing.

Ladewig, P. W., London, M. L., and Olds, S. B. (1990) *Essentials of Maternal-Newborn Nursing*. Redwood City, CA: Addison-Wesley Nursing.

Myers, J. O., Ragland, J. J., and Candelaria, L. A. (1990) Fiberoptic endoscopy of the gastrointestinal tract in surgical training. *Surgery, Gynecology and Obstetrics*, 170 (4): 283–286.

Olds, S. B., London, M. L., and Ladewig, P. W. (1992) *Maternal-Newborn Nursing—A Family-Centered Approach*. Redwood City, CA: Addison-Wesley Nursing.

Rosen, S. D., and Rogers, A. I. (1991) Clinical recognition and evaluation of peptic ulcer disease. *Postgraduate Medicine* 88 (5): 42–55.

Schroeder, Krupp, Tierney, and McPhee, eds. (1991). *Current Medical Diagnosis and Treatment*, 30th ed. Norwalk, CT: Appleton-Lange.

Sims, D'Amico, Steismeyer, and Webster (1995) *Health Assessment in Nursing*. Redwood City, CA: Addison-Wesley Nursing.

Society of Gastroenterology Nurses and Associates. (1993) Gastroenterology nursing: A core curriculum. *St. Louis: Mosby-Year Book.*

Tabibian, N. (1991) Endoscopy versus X-ray studies of the gastrointestinal tract: Future health care implications. *Southern Medical Journal*, 84 (2): 219–221.

Thomas, C., ed. (1989) *Taber's Cyclopedic Medical Dictionary*, 16th ed. Philadelphia: F. A. Davis.

Wallach, J. (1992) *Interpretation of Diagnostic Tests: A Synopsis of Laboratory Medicine.* Boston: Little, Brown & Co.

Wilson, S. F., and Thompson, J. M. (1990) *Respiratory Disorders.* St. Louis: C. V. Mosby Co.

NOTE: A *t* following a page number indicates tabular material and an *f* following a page number indicates an illustration.

Microcytes, 107
Microsomal antibody, 62–63
Mielke bleeding time, 99–102
Milk/milk products, digestion of, lactose tolerance test in evaluation of, 432–433
Minute volume/minute ventilation, 589
MIP, 590
Mitogen assay, 469–470
Mixed lymphocyte culture, 469–470
MLC, 469–470
Mono-spot test (mononucleosis spot test), 283–285, 481–482
Mono-test, 283–285, 392–393, 481–482
Monocytes
    in bone marrow, 115t
    decreased numbers of, 107, 751
    differential count of, 753
    increased numbers of, 106, 750
    normal values for, 749
Monocytopenia, 107, 751
Monocytosis, 106, 750
Mononucleosis, infectious, tests for, 283–285, 392–393, 481–482
Monospot test (mononucleosis spot test), 283–285, 481–482
Monotest, 283–285, 392–393, 481–482
Monostican, 283–285
Mosenthal test, 728–730
Motility, esophageal, tests of, 294–297
MR blood flow scanning, 473–475
MRA (MR angiography), 473–475
MRF, 473–475
MRI (MR imaging), 473–475
MRS, 473–475
MS screening panel (MS panel), 483–484
MSAFP, 26–27
Multiple myeloma, Bence-Jones protein in, 93
Multiple sclerosis screening panel (multiple sclerosis panel/expanded evaluation), 483–484
Multitest (delayed hypersensitivity skin tests), 627–629
Muramidase, urine and serum, 484–486
Muscular diseases
    electroencephalography in evaluation of, 269–271
    serum aldolase levels in, 19–20
    serum myoglobin levels in, 492–493
    urine myoglobin levels in, 493–494

MV, 589
Myasthenia gravis, acetylcholine receptor antibody test for (myasthenia gravis test panel), 1–2, 486–487
Mycobacterium tuberculosis, acid-fast bacilli test in identification of, 2–4
Mycoses, serologic tests for, 331–332
Myelin basic protein, 487–489
Myeloblasts, in bone marrow, 115t
Myelocytes, in bone marrow, 115t
    increased/decreased levels of, 114–115
Myelography/myelogram, 489–482
Myeloid/erythroid ratio, in bone marrow
    increased/decreased, 116
    normal, 115t
Myeloma, Bence-Jones protein in, 93
Myelomeningocele, alpha-fetoprotein in screening for, 26–27
Myocardial function, exercise stress test in evaluation of, 308–310
Myocardial infarction
    CPK-MB levels in, 225, 226t
    lactic dehydrogenase levels in, 430–431
    serum myoglobin levels in, 492–493
    urine myoglobin levels in, 493–494
Myocardial scan, 148–150
Myoglobin
    serum, 492–493
    urine, 493–494
Myopathies, electromyography in evaluation of, 271–273

N

Na+, 635–638
Nasoenteric intubation, for duodenal contents culture, 260, 261
Nasogastric intubation, for gastric cytology and culture, 344–345
    care after, 345
    client preparation for, 344
Nasopharyngeal cancer, Epstein-Barr virus antibody in, 283–284
Nasopharyngeal (nasopharynx) culture, 495–496
Natriuretic hormone (atrial natriuretic factor/hormone), 84–85
Nausea/vomiting, caloric study causing, 128, 275
Needle biopsy
    bone, 113

Right ventricular pressure, normal, during cardiac catheterization, 145t

Ristocetin cofactor, disorders involving, platelet aggregation in evaluation of, 544–545

RNP, 52

Rocky Mountain spotted fever, febrile and cold agglutinin test for, 312t

Rotavirus antigen, fecal, 615–616

RPR test, 655–656

RSV antigen, 604–606

RT$_3$U, 691–692

Rubella
antibody to, 617
TORCH test in identification of, 680–681

Rumpel-Leed positive pressure (capillary fragility), 131–133

RV, 588–589

S

SACE, 42–43

Salivary ducts, x-ray studies of (sialography), 623–624

Sarcoidosis, angiotensin-converting enzyme in evaluation of, 42–43

SBFT (SBF), 633–635

Scalp electrodes, 269, 270

Schiller's iodine test, 161

Schilling test, 618–620

Scintigraphy. See also Radionuclide imaging
abdominal, 351–352
gastrointestinal, 351–352
hepatobiliary, 334–335

Scintiphotography, pulmonary, 462–464

Scout film (abdominal plain film), 426–427, 504–505

Secretin, for gastrin stimulation test, 348, 349

Sed rate (erythrocyte sedimentation rate), 291–292

Seizure disorders, electroencephalography in evaluation of, 269–271

Sella turcica x-ray, 620–621

Semen analysis/examination, 621–623

Semen collection
for antispermatozoal antibody test, 56–57, 642
for semen analysis, 622–623

Seminal cytology, 621–623

Septicemia, blood culture and sensitivity in, 102–104

Serology
acquired immune deficiency, 8–10
fungal, 331–332
for syphilis, 655–656

Serotonin, metabolites of (5-hydroxyindoleacetic acid), 404–407

Serum hepatitis, 387–389

Serum levels. See specific compound measured

Serum osmolality, 507–508

Serum thrombin time, 541–542

72-hour stool collection, for fecal lipid analysis, 445, 446

Sex (gender), fetal
amniocentesis in determination of, 31–33
amniotic fluid analysis in determination of, 35–37

Sex chromatin mass/body/test (Barr body analysis), 92–93

SGOT (serum glutamic oxaloacetic transaminase), 80–82

SGPT (serum glutamic-pyruvic transaminase), 17–19

Shake test, 538–539

Shell vial assay, for cytomegalovirus, 252–253

Shoulder
abnormal arthrographic findings in, 73
normal arthrographic findings in, 72

Sialography, 623–624

Sickle-cell disease/trait, abnormal hemoglobin in, 378

Sickle-cell test/preparation (Sickledex), 380–381

Sickle prep, 380–381

Siderocyte stain (hemosiderin stain), 386–387

Siderophilin (transferrin), serum, 685–686

Sigmoidoscopy, 624–626

Silverman-needle-aspirated breast biopsy, 124

Sims-Huhner test, 560–561

Single-photon emission computed tomography, cardiac, 148

Skeletal diseases. See also Bone
serum phosphorus in evaluation of, 540–541

814

Ventricular pressure, normal, 145t
Ventriculography/ventriculogram,
    745–746
Vertebrae, myelography in evaluation of,
    489–482
Very low-density lipoproteins (lipids),
    447–449
  normal values for, 179, 447
Vestibular function
  caloric study in evaluation of,
    128–130
  electronystagmography in evaluation
    of, 274–276
Vestibulo-ocular reflex response
  caloric study of, 128–130
  in electronystagmography, 274–276
Vibroacoustic stimulation test, 6–7
Viral hepatitis, serum studies for,
    387–389
Visual evoked potential studies, 306–308
Vital capacity, 589
  forced, 589
Vitamin A (retinol), serum, 608–609
Vitamin B_1 (thiamine), serum and urine,
    660–662
Vitamin B_2 (riboflavin), urine, 614–615
Vitamin B_6 (pyridoxine), tryptophan
    challenge test in identification of
    deficiency of, 693–694
Vitamin B_{12} (cyanocobalamin), 240–242
  absorption of (Schilling test),
    618–620
Vitamin C (ascorbic acid), urine and
    plasma levels of, 79–80
Vitamin D_3 (cholecalciferol), 175–177
VLDL. See Very low-density lipoproteins
    (lipids)
VMA, 741–743
Voiding, urine flow studies in evaluation
    of, 734–736
Voiding cystography/cystogram (voiding
    cystourethrography/ cystourethro-
    gram), 245–247
Voiding electromyography, 521–523
Volhard's test, 728–730
Volumes, lung, 588
Vomiting, 128, 275
von Willebrand antigen/factor, plasma,
    747–748
von Willebrand's disease
  abnormal findings in, 195

platelet aggregation in evaluation of,
    544–545
VPS (ventilation/perfusion scan),
    462–464
VST, 6–7
vW antigen (vWF ag), 747–748

W

Waldenström's macroglobulinemia,
    Bence-Jones protein in, 93
Water balance
  serum chloride in evaluation of,
    170–172
  serum osmolality in evaluation of,
    507–508
  urine osmolality in evaluation of,
    508–510
Water caloric test, 128–130, 275
Water loading/water deprivation tests,
    728–730
Waxy casts, in urine, 723
WBCs, 749–753
Weils-Felix reaction test, for febrile and
    cold agglutinins, 311–313
Westergren method for erythrocyte sedi-
    mentation test, normal findings in,
    291
Western Blot test, for HIV, 8–10
White blood cell (WBC) count, 749–753
  decreased, 107
  with differential, 749–753
  elevated, 106
White blood cell (WBC) smear, 106–109
White blood cells (leukocytes)
  alkaline phosphatase in, 441–443
  antibodies to, 440–441
  casts of, in urine, 723
  in cerebrospinal fluid, 155–156
  in pericardial fluid, 529
  in peritoneal fluid, 531, 532
  in pleural fluid, 662, 663
  precursors of, increased/decreased
    levels of in bone marrow,
    114–115
  in urine, 718, 722
Widal's test, 311–313
Willebrand antigen/factor, plasma,
    747–748
Willebrand's disease
  abnormal findings in, 195

BODY SYSTEM INDEX

Cardiovascular

Arterial Blood Gases, 63
Arteriography of the Arms and Legs, 68
Atrial Natriuretic Factor, 84
Carboxyhemoglobin, Serum, 135
Cardiac Catheterization and Angiography, 144
Cardiac Isotope Imaging, 148
Carotid Duplex Scanning, 150
Chest X-ray, 162
Cholesterol, Serum, 179
Chromium, Serum, 186
Digital Subtraction Angiography, 256
Doppler Studies, 258
Echocardiogram, 265
Electrocardiogram, 267
Exercise Stress Test, 308
Lactic Acid, Serum, 428
Lactic Dehydrogenase, 430
Lipoproteins, 447
Lung Scan, 462
Magnetic Resonance Imaging, 473
Mediastinoscopy, 478
Oximetry, 514
Pericardiocentesis, 529
Plethysmography, Arterial, 549
Plethysmography, Venous, 55
Pulmonary Angiography, 583
Triglycerides, Serum, 686
Venography of the Legs, 743

Digestive

Alkaline Phosphatase, Serum, 23

Endocrine

Adrenal Angiography, 10
Adrenal Venograph, 12
Adrenocorticotropic Hormone Stimulation, 16
Adrenocorticotropic Hormone, 14
Aldosterone, Serum and Urine, 21
Androstenedione, 41
Anti-Insulin Antibody, 49
Antidiuretic Hormone, 48

Antithyroglobulin Antibody, 61
Antithyroid Microsomal Antibody, 62
Blood Glucose, Random, 104
Catecholamines, Serum, 151
Chloride, Serum, 170
Computed Tomography of the Adrenals, 207
Cortisol, Serum, 220
Cortisol, Urine Free, 222
Cyclic Adenosine Monophosphate, 242
Estriol Excretion, 300
Follicle-Stimulating Hormone, Serum, 326
Free Fatty Acids, 329
Free Thyroxine T_4, 330
Galactose-1-phosphate Uridyl Transferase, 333
Glucagon, Serum, 356
Glucose Tolerance, 363
Glucose, Fasting, 357
Glucose, Postprandial, 359
Glucose-6-Phosphate Dehydrogenase, 361
Glycosylated Hemoglobin, 365
Hexosaminidase A and B, 394
17 Hydroxycorticosteroids, 403
Insulin, serum, 414
17-Ketosteroids, 423
Lactose Tolerance, 432
Luteinizing Hormone Assay, 465
Metyrapone, 479
Oxalate, Urine, 512
Parathyroid Hormone, 517
Phenylalanine Screening, 537
Prolactin, Serum, 567
Radioactive Iodine Uptake, 593
Radioallergosorbent Test, 594
Renin Assay, 603
Sella Turcica X- Ray, 620
Somatotropin Suppression Test, 640
Somatotropin, 639
Testosterone, Serum, Plasma, 659
Thorn Test, 665
Thyroid Biopsy, 668
Thyroid Scan, 669

819

Genitourinary

Hematologic